Fertility Control

Fertility Control

EDITORS

Stephen L. Corson, M.D.

Assistant Clinical Professor, Department of Obstetrics and Gynecology, The University of Pennsylvania School of Medicine; Attending Physician, Pennsylvania Hospital; Director, Philadelphia Fertility Institute, Philadelphia

Richard J. Derman, M.D., M.P.H.

Clinical Assistant Professor of Obstetrics and Gynecology, Cornell University Medical College; Attending Physician, The New York Hospital, New York

Louise B. Tyrer, M.D.

Vice President for Medical Affairs, Planned Parenthood Federation of America, Inc., New York, New York

Little, Brown and Company
Boston/Toronto

Library of Congress Catalog Card No. 84-81161

ISBN 0-316-15748-1

Printed in the United States of America

DON

DEDICATED TO THE MEMORY OF
CHRISTOPHER TIETZE
(1909–1984)

Christopher Tietze was probably the world's leading
authority in statistical analysis of data in the field of
birth control and social and biomedical research related to fertility regulation. He was the first to ana-
lyze and compare the mortality rates of the various
methods of fertility control and compare them with
the rates when no method was used—a graphic por-
trayal of the benefits of fertility control. His analysis
and presentation of the data showing the safety of
legal abortion will always remain a classic and likely
had more impact on changing the laws around the
world to permit safe and legal abortion than any
other activity. Additionally, the availability of safe
and legal abortion has saved the lives and reproductive capabilities of millions of women. He distinguished, ennobled, and humanized the field and was
a zealous and effective advocate for reproductive
freedom. His work will always remain a source of inspiration to all of us in the field of fertility regulation.

Contents

Contributing Authors

Fredrick R. Abrams, M.D.
Assistant Clinical Professor of Obstetrics and Gynecology, University of Colorado Health Sciences Center; Director, Center for Biomedical Ethics, Rose Medical Center, Denver
Chapter 1

Nancy J. Alexander, Ph.D.
Professor, Departments of Anatomy, Obstetrics/Gynecology, and Urology, University of Oregon Health Sciences Center School of Medicine, Portland; Scientist, Reproductive Physiology, Oregon Regional Primate Research Center, Beaverton
Chapter 27

Deborah J. Anderson, Ph.D.
Assistant Professor in Pathology, Harvard Medical School and Dana-Farber Cancer Institute, Boston, Massachusetts
Chapter 27

William C. Andrews, M.D.
Professor of Obstetrics and Gynecology, Eastern Virginia Medical School; Attending Obstetrician and Gynecologist, Norfolk General Hospital, Norfolk
Chapter 12

Frances R. Batzer, M.D.
Assistant Clinical Professor, Department of Obstetrics and Gynecology, The University of Pennsylvania School of Medicine; Attending Physician, Pennsylvania Hospital; Assistant Director, Philadelphia Fertility Institute, Philadelphia
Chapter 4

Gary S. Berger, M.D., M.S.P.H.
Adjunct Associate Professor of Maternal and Child Health, University of North Carolina School of Public Health, Chapel Hill; Director, Chapel Hill Fertility Services, Chapel Hill
Chapter 21

Michael S. Burnhill, M.D., D.M.Sc.
Professor of Clinical Obstetrics and Gynecology, University of Medicine and Dentistry of New Jersey-Rutgers Medical School; Attending Physician and Director, Ambulatory Care Department, Middlesex General Hospital, New Brunswick
Chapter 23

Jill A. Cobrin, J.D.
Director of Insurance and Claims Administration, Planned Parenthood Federation of America, Inc., New York, New York
Chapter 3

Elizabeth B. Connell, M.D.
Professor of Gynecology and Obstetrics, Emory University School of Medicine; Attending Physician, Grady Memorial Hospital, Atlanta, Georgia
Chapter 26

Jay M. Cooper, M.D.
Chairman, Department of Obstetrics and Gynecology, Phoenix Baptist Hospital, Phoenix, Arizona
Chapter 9

Stephen L. Corson, M.D.
Assistant Clinical Professor, Department of Obstetrics and Gynecology, The University of Pennsylvania School of Medicine; Attending Physician, Pennsylvania Hospital; Director, Philadelphia Fertility Institute, Philadelphia
Chapter 8

Joseph E. Davis, M.D., F.A.C.S.
Clinical Professor, Department of Urology, New York Medical College, Valhalla
Chapter 10

Richard J. Derman, M.D., M.P.H.
Clinical Assistant Professor of Obstetrics and Gynecology, Cornell University Medical College; Attending Physician, The New York Hospital, New York
Chapter 19

Michael J. Free, Ph.D.
Director of Research and Development, Program for Introduction and Adaptation of Contraceptive Technology, Seattle, Washington
Chapter 22

Myron Gordon, M.D.
Professor and Chairman, Department of Obstetrics and Gynecology, Albany Medical College of Union University; Obstetrician and Gynecologist in Chief, Albany Medical Center Hospital, Albany, New York
Chapter 1

Stanley H. Greenberg, M.D.
Clinical Assistant and Professor of Surgery (Urology), Medical University of South Carolina School of Medicine, Charleston
Chapter 11

David A. Grimes, M.D.
Clinical Associate Professor, Department of Gynecology and Obstetrics, Emory University School of Medicine; Clinical Research Investigator, Division of Sexually Transmitted Disease, Center for Disease Control, Atlanta, Georgia
Chapter 5

Marianne A. Jackson, M.D.
Resident Physician, Department of Obstetrics and Gynecology, University of Washington School of Medicine, Seattle
Chapter 21

Andrew M. Kaunitz, M.D.
Assistant Professor, Department of Obstetrics and Gynecology, University of Florida, Gainesville; Director, Division of Ambulatory Care, Department of Obstetrics and Gynecology, University Hospital, Jacksonville, Florida; formerly Epidemic Intelligence Officer, Division of Reproductive Health, Center for Disease Control, Atlanta, Georgia
Chapter 5

Louis G. Keith, M.D.
Professor of Obstetrics and Gynecology, Northwestern University Medical School; Attending Physician, Department of Obstetrics and Gynecology, Prentice Women's Hospital and Maternity Center of Northwestern Memorial Hospital, Chicago, Illinois
Chapter 21

Janet E. Kornblatt, M.P.H.
Consultant, Medical Division, Planned Parenthood Federation of America, Inc., New York, New York
Chapter 3

Carl J. Levinson, M.D.
Clinical Professor, Department of Obstetrics and Gynecology, University of California, San Francisco, School of Medicine; Chairman, Department of Obstetrics and Gynecology, Children's Hospital of San Francisco, San Francisco
Chapter 7

Daniel R. Mishell, Jr., M.D.
Professor and Chairman, Department of Obstetrics and Gynecology, University of Southern California School of Medicine; Chief Physician of Obstetrics and Gynecology, Los Angeles County-University of Southern California Medical Center, Los Angeles
Chapter 16

Herbert B. Peterson, M.D.
Department of Obstetrics and Gynecology, University of North Carolina at Chapel Hill School of Medicine, Chapel Hill
Chapter 7

Diana B. Petitti, M.D.
Assistant Professor, Division of Family and Community Medicine, University of California, San Francisco, School of Medicine, San Francisco
Chapter 2

Malcolm Potts, M.B., B.Chir., Ph.D.
President, Family Health International, Research Triangle Park, North Carolina
Chapter 25

Allan Rosenfield, M.D.
Acting Chairman of Obstetrics and Gynecology and Professor of Obstetrics/Gynecology and Public Health, Columbia University College of Physicians and Surgeons; Director, Center for Population and Family Health, Columbia University College of Physicians and Surgeons, New York, New York
Chapter 14

Subir Roy, M.D.
Associate Professor of Obstetrics and Gynecology, University of Southern California School of Medicine; Physician Specialist, Obstetrics and Gynecology, Los Angeles County-University of Southern California Medical Center, Los Angeles
Chapter 16

Sheldon Schlaff, M.D.
Assistant Professor of Obstetrics and Gynecology and of Medicine, The University of Pennsylvania School of Medicine; Attending Physician, Pennsylvania Hospital; Director, Pennsylvania Endocrine Laboratory, Philadelphia
Chapter 17

Richard M. Soderstrom, M.D.
Clinical Professor of Obstetrics and Gynecology, University of Washington School of Medicine; Chief of Obstetrics and Gynecology, Reproductive Health Specialists, Seattle
Chapters 15, 20

Phillip G. Stubblefield, M.D.
Associate Professor of Obstetrics and Gynecology, Harvard Medical School, Boston; Chairman, Department of Obstetrics and Gynecology, Mount Auburn Hospital, Cambridge, Massachusetts
Chapter 6

Louise B. Tyrer, M.D.
Vice President for Medical Affairs, Planned Parenthood Federation of America, Inc., New York, New York
Chapters 3, 13

Andrew T. Wiley, M.D., M.P.H.
Public Health Physician, Information and Training Division, Office of Population, Agency for International Development, Department of State, Washington, D.C.
Chapter 18

Stephen S. York, J.D.
Attorney, Law Firm of Bower and Gardner, New York, New York
Chapter 3

A. Albert Yuzpe, M.D., M.Sc., F.R.C.S.(C)
Professor, Department of Obstetrics and Gynecology, The University of Western Ontario Faculty of Medicine; Chief, Department of Gynaecology, University Hospital, London, Ontario, Canada
Chapter 24

Preface

More and more individuals voluntarily seek to control their fertility so that they may have only the number of children they want at an appropriate time in their lives. According to statistical calculations by Christopher Tietze, if a woman did not practice contraception at least once during her fertile life—from menarche to menopause—she could expect to have at least 14 births or 31 abortions (or any combination of the two) before age 45. Based on increased demand for medical services to assist individuals in regulating their fertility, this aspect of medical practice now occupies new prominence, as well as a considerable amount of the time of the busy practitioner. In fact, new health care practitioners who have a special commitment to the provision of family planning services, such as the Family Planning Nurse Practitioners, have emerged.

In addition to increased demand for services in fertility control, the medicolegal climate in the United States continues to become more litigious, particularly for the discipline of obstetrics and gynecology within which most of the aspects of fertility regulation services fall. To ensure quality care, it is especially important that a practitioner of fertility-related services keep continually updated on the ever-changing medical practices in this field. Additionally, it is essential to understand and adhere to the concepts of voluntarism, patient education, informed consent, and quality assurance so as to better serve the interests of the patient, while at the same time assuming maximum protection from medical malpractice actions.

Independently, and then collectively, the editors of this volume perceived a need for a text devoted exclusively to the various aspects of fertility regulation. From the outset we wanted to achieve two major goals. The first was to assemble a work that contained information useful to the clinician in everyday practice. Our second goal was to provide a text with sufficient documentation so as to qualify as an authoritative reference source of value to students, resident physicians, and academicians. Although these goals may at first glance appear dissimilar, we did not consider them to be mutually exclusive.

To meet these goals the editors chose the authors of each chapter with care. The contributing authors are recognized experts in their particular topic. But equally important, they are practical clinicians as well as skillful communicators.

The editors wanted to incorporate new concepts in the book. Therefore, we chose to lead off with a section entitled Special Issues in Fertility Control. The initial chapter, Ethical Issues in Fertility Control, by Myron Gordon, M.D., and Fredrick R. Abrams, M.D., sets the tone and framework of the book. Dr. Gordon was the first chairperson of the Committee on Bioethics of the American College of Obstetricians and Gynecologists. This chapter focuses on the importance of patient voluntarism in all matters related to fertility control, emphasizing that although fertility-related decisions appropriately are a matter of deliberations between the patient and the doctor, the locus of control is and always must be with the patient. We have faithfully adhered to this concept throughout the text.

The chapter by Diana B. Petitti, M.D., entitled Statistical Aspects of the Evaluation of the Safety and Effectiveness of Fertility Control Methods, is replete with illustrations of interesting situations in fertility regulation practice that guide the reader through the maze of statistical jargon leading to a clear understanding of how to evaluate data presented in studies on fertility control in the medical literature.

The chapter on Medicolegal Issues and Risk Reduction in Family Planning Practice written by Jill A. Cobrin, J.D., Stephen S. York, J.D., et al. contains important information on how the clinician can assure the quality of the services provided and at the same time reduce the risk of lawsuits—a matter of great concern to all physicians.

The major categories of surgical fertility regulation techniques are covered by chapters on abortion, sterilization, and sterilization reversal by the following outstanding authors: Andrew M. Kaunitz, M.D., David A. Grimes, M.D., Phillip G. Stubblefield, M.D., Carl J. Levinson, M.D., Herbert B. Peterson, M.D., Stephen L. Corson, M.D., Jay M. Cooper, M.D., Joseph E. Davis, M.D., and Stanley H. Greenberg, M.D. Surgical methods of fertility regulation are utilized by more individuals of the world to control unwanted fertility than are the temporary methods of contraception. Additionally, as the reader will see, surgical methods are the most highly effective means of birth control and further offer an exceptional degree of safety. Since sterilization is now being requested by younger individuals, and since some people may later change their minds and wish to reestablish their fertility following sterilization, we considered it essential to cover the topic of sterilization reversal as well.

The section on Hormonal Methods of fertility regulation leads off with a classic discussion of the Principles of Oral Contraception by William C. Andrews, M.D. As past president of the American Fertility Society and long recognized as an expert in hormonal contraception, Andrews brings a well-balanced perspective to the discussion of oral contraception. In this chapter he weighs the values of the numerous studies on oral contraceptives and emerges with a convincing summation of the benefits and risks associated with their use. To make the discussion of the pill practical for the clinician, Louise B. Tyrer, M.D., details, with comprehensive referencing, the latest concepts in Oral Contraceptive Practice. The various hormonal methods currently being studied that may have a considerable impact on the future practice of fertility control are detailed by such leading researchers in the field as Daniel R. Mishell, Jr., M.D., and Sheldon Schlaff, M.D. An additional horizon chapter by Nancy J. Alexander, Ph.D., on contraceptive vaccines is fascinating.

All other methods of contraception are discussed by authors of note with equal attention to detail, including implications for clinical practice, to ensure that the text *Fertility Control* provides a comprehensive coverage of the field of fertility regulation.

S. L. C.
R. J. D.
L. B. T.

Acknowledgments

First and foremost, the editors of the book *Fertility Control* wish to acknowledge the superb contributions of each of the authors. No one (or even three) author could have possibly achieved the medical credibility which is now found on the pages of this multiple-authored text.

Second, we wish to express our gratitude to Curtis Vouwie, Medical Editor, and Jane MacNeil, Senior Book Editor, of Little, Brown and Company, Publishers, who encouraged, advised, and prodded all of us to ensure the publication of a superbly accurate and readable product of which we all are proud.

Additionally, our sincere thanks go to those often unsung collaborators who prepared the excellent illustrations, spent hundreds of hours juggling phrases on word processors, and proofed the manuscripts.

Also, our gratitude goes to the meaningful others in our lives who assisted and supported us through the completion of this monumental task: here's to Judy, Kate, and Chuck, with our love and thanks.

I. Special Issues in Fertility Control

1. Ethical Issues in Fertility Control

Myron Gordon
Fredrick R. Abrams

Within this volume the reader will find expert commentary on a spectrum of techniques designed to alter the consequences of the expression of sexual drives. Contained herein are valuable data for rational decisions regarding the control of reproduction; however, such decisions, concerned as they are with procreation, sexual function, sexual identity, and the social fabric of society, are rarely made devoid of emotional and subjective factors. Therefore, an examination of ethics in general and the historic evolution of the current ethics of reproduction is necessary.

BASIS FOR ETHICS

Being human is a social enterprise. Regulation of interaction is necessary, and guidance for decisions is essential. At some happy time, the idea surfaced that to convince rather than coerce was a worthy goal. Men and women of good will have wished to live ethically with their fellows. Such a relationship required that the rational pursuit of self-interest be tempered by justice, abstention from behavior injurious to others, and the promotion of the welfare of others as well as one's own. Dubious dogmas were intermingled with these principles, which, in the light of history, served only as expedient temporary adaptations to circumstances and always maintained the status quo of those in power. These masqueraders—for example, the "divine right" of kings—have tended to be revealed by time and public scrutiny as false models of what was actually needed and desired.

Some basic principles have stood the test of time, but within the confines of those principles, changing circumstances cry for different rules. However, inertia works on minds as well as masses, and the loss of security that comes with change has always resulted in a lag between social behavior and the reaction of the establishment—acknowledgment, tolerance, and finally acceptance. This lag also serves to buffer society against faddists and truly disruptive behavior by withholding approval until new ideas are time-tested.

TOLERANCE OF VALUES—PRIVATE AND PUBLIC

What does one learn from a review of the influence of ethics on current thought regarding the sex act and its consequences? First, regardless of the justification, whether political, economic, or religious, the interests of society as contemporaneously structured were and are served by ethical considerations. Second, it is apparent that no segment of our society has had a monopoly on the truth. Every time science, politics, or

3

religion speaks without regard for human fallibility (or the inability to interpret divine infallibility correctly), they stub their toes on the facts: When papal authority made Galileo recant, the earth nevertheless continued to revolve around the sun; if a majority of the geographers of the world maintained that the earth were flat, still no one would fall off the edge. Third, the expansion of knowledge has both created and solved ethical problems. For an example close to this special sphere of interest, take that of the severely deformed child. Whether dealing with Stone Age Africa, the Australian aborigine, the Spartan law for deformed children, the Justinian Code bidding the father of deformed children to destroy them, or the Platonic recommendations for parentage of inferior stock, the birth of defective children has been a problem of panhistoric social concern. The state of technology for centuries gave little practical alternative to infanticide until, with the advent of amniocentesis, prenatal diagnosis for some abnormalities became possible, and selective abortion could solve some of the social problems. Further technical advance involving preconceptional genetic analysis permitted the detection of carriers, thus obviating the problem if the partners agree to abstain from conception. If the partners desire children, the option of selective abortion remains, permitting those fetuses without the defect to survive. Technology again may rescue us from this less-than-optimal choice, because the next almost-certain event will be the ability to exchange undesired genetic material from the gametes or the zygote for normal DNA: In this way, the dilemma confronted in dealing with many seriously deficient or deformed children may be solved technologically. Then a new problem is created, the risks and benefits of altering genetic heritage. We will struggle with this as well, having learned that in science what *can* be done *will* be done. It is clear that some of our dilemmas have been and will be solved by knowledge, but that guideposts are needed for direction at the crossroads.

It is with these observations in mind that tolerance is sought for the different ranking of values. Those activities that society feels are of great importance to daily civil orderly function have been codified as law. They are society's "musts." Thus, a person's minimum requirements in dealing with another are regulated by law. On a larger scale are varieties of behavior that are of greater daily importance to individuals. These do not threaten social order but without guidance could lead to chaos in individual transactions. The guides for these are ethics and morals, society's "oughts" as compared to "musts." Obligations and rules defined by role (e.g., child-parent, lovers, teacher-student, patient-doctor) are more extensively regulated by ethics than by law. Ethics often calls for more self-restraint than does the

law, and its application is usually recognized as commendable, even by those who fail to practice it.

There is inevitably a spectrum of private behavior that at one extreme has public consequences. It is here that society as represented by law must tread carefully to avoid trespass upon the individual's right to self-determination with which the state has no legitimate interest. It is not unreasonable to adopt differing private and public morality. In weighing values, one can find behavior in which one would not participate but which one would not feel justified preventing for others. The behavior, while not personally condoned, may be less odious than the limitation of another's right to make decisions for himself or herself—even disagreeable decisions, even unethical decisions, even tragic decisions. This is the fulcrum about which sexual ethics in a pluralistic society revolves. It can be the rationale that enables persons with conflicting values to coexist, until knowledge eliminates the basis for conflict. Rules can be agreed upon by society that may never be proved to be based on eternal truths but nevertheless serve society well as rational guides in the pursuit of individual goals without hindrance from, or harm to, society.

POLITICAL AND RELIGIOUS FACTORS INFLUENCING BIRTH CONTROL

Political Influences

By becoming familiar with the history of birth control, one can see that it is inextricably entangled with politics and religion. A contentious political factor that never fails to arouse an initial emotional response must be carefully and objectively considered: the politics of male subjugation of the female. A significant argument has been advanced that the central issue of contraception and abortion is fear of the return of the control of reproduction to the female, something the male has resisted, using all the power of the institutions of politics and religion. In a society where property rights were invested in males, a man had to be certain that his own genetic line was continued. Suspicion of female infidelity could not be tolerated. In times when technology to prevent pregnancy was uncertain at best, separation of procreation and the sex act was too dangerous, and female extramarital sex threatened one's very birthright. Dr. William Lafferty [1] propounded this viewpoint as follows:

If you have always thought the proscription against abortion is based on widespread belief that abortion involves the destruction of human life rather than on the sexist oppression of women, consider what the abortion laws would be like, if, overnight, men got pregnant instead of women. It is unthinkable that men would be much solaced by womanly assurances that the joys of "motherhood" would compensate for interrupting their work and other activities, keeping them at home and giving them the primary responsibility for child care during the next eighteen years. Naturally, in this hypothetical world where men rather than women bear children, some men would want to carry their pregnancies to term, but certainly others would insist on their right to abort pregnancies on the grounds that they have the right to control their bodies and their lives. Men have always enjoyed personal control over their lives and it seems unlikely that many would be put off by religious rhetoric or want to jeopardize their careers, risking professional supplantation by women. Since men make the laws, there would probably be a sudden lifting of the ban on abortion, the emergence of laws forbidding doctors to refuse to perform abortions on request, and the establishment of abortion clinics at every local shopping center. Law probably would not require pregnant men to get the consent of their wives before having abortions and men in general probably would not talk so much about the advisability of those who want abortions first consulting with clergymen or submitting to examination by a psychiatrist to make sure that they were doing the right thing.

The evolution from women-as-property to an oppressed minority and on to citizens of equal stature is not completed yet.

Another political factor was the need for population control to meet the contemporaneous need of the society. Warlike societies such as ancient Rome encouraged fertility because of military needs, with Justinian's imperial laws regulating contraceptives and abortifacients [14]. Modern Nazi Germany established houses for young women of good racial stock to be impregnated by suitable Aryan soldiers to provide eugenically sound citizens for the Thousand-Year Reich [15].

The politics of the Australian aborigines where survival was difficult punished women for having too many children, and infanticide was an accepted solution, as it was in other communities across the world. A modern-day parallel is the enactment of laws permitting abortion in the Soviet Union in 1920, Japan in 1948, Great Britain in 1968, and many other Eastern and Western countries in response to perceived overpopulation.

The Influences of Religion

A substantial segment of our society believes that certain rules relating to procreation have divine origins and therefore are universal and immutable. Interdiction of contraception is based on Old Testament statements in Genesis and Deuteronomy. The rules of the theocratic society provided for inheritance through male offspring. Should a man die before he produced an heir, it was incumbent upon his brother to fertilize the widow; the child would be recognized as that of the deceased.

Onan, when directed to perform this duty, failed to honor the commitment, instead practicing coitus interruptus: "And the thing which he did was evil in the sight of the Lord and he slew him also" (Gen. 38:8–10). Later, when the duty was explained in the Mosaic era, the punishment for failure to honor the commitment was not so severe, although it carried social stigma (Deut. 25).

The second basis is the command given to Adam and Eve (Gen. 1) to be fertile and multiply. Those who argue that the Bible was interpreted very selectively for the contemporaneous needs of society suggest that the statement was a blessing, not a command, given much the same way to Noah and to Jacob. They also point out that there are other clear instructions—for example, to forgive debts every 7 years and not to charge interest to a countryman on loans—but these less acceptable commandments have been expediently overlooked. Nevertheless, in this way an authoritative basis was formed for an interdiction of nonprocreative sexual activity, which has lingered throughout the ages. Like other dogma, the rule often supersedes the reason. For example, masturbation for semen analysis or husband insemination to promote pregnancy remains interdicted for the orthodox, a result at cross-purposes with the original command to be fertile and multiply.

JUDAIC

From the same roots barring coitus interruptus, the Judaic tradition has evolved into the twentieth century without any strong prohibition against contraception. Rabbinic interpretations have determined an obligation for two children; more is meritorious, but not obligatory. Talmudic writings have pointed out that the messianic age cannot arise until all souls are born. Abortion is prohibited by the Orthodox except to save the life of the mother; the exception is derived from the acknowledgment that killing in self-defense is permissible, and the fetus can sometimes be considered an aggressor. Jews, who are loosely divided into Reform, Conservative, and Orthodox groups, have no single voice that speaks with authority for all.

CATHOLIC

From an early position of total rigidity in which it was maintained that coitus had no purpose except procreation (Clement of Alexandria, Augustine), a reinterpretation of its role in Catholic doctrine has emerged. Medieval recognition that marital coitus might be for pleasure without sin was further reinforced by the nineteenth century Jesuit Jean Gury, who wrote that it might reinforce conjugal affection. When the Second Vatican Council reaffirmed that love was a moral end in conjugal relations and that oral contraceptives seemed defensible, Pope John XXIII appointed a commission to evaluate ovulation suppressants in the 1960s. Despite the positive recommendation of the majority of the commission, including the leading moral theologian Josef Fuchs, Pope Paul VI repeated the established position in the (fallible) encyclical *Humanae Vitae* in 1968 [14]. In some Western countries outside the United States, such as Belgium, Canada, France, Germany, and the Netherlands, this encyclical was not accepted without some reservations.

PROTESTANT

Luther and Calvin were passionately anticontraception, and once again the fact that political control of the Low Countries lay in numbers helped to promote that position, which produced more people of the sect that wished to remain in power. Nevertheless, Calvin did emphasize the companionship between marriage partners (and their relation in turn together with God). Later, in keeping with the emphasis on individual relationships to God and the dominion over earth as ordained by God, the rationale of controlling nature for God's purpose began to clear the way for contraceptive control over procreation. Affirmational value in addition to procreational value for marital relations became more acceptable. In 1930 the Lambeth Conference of the Anglican church officially recognized the use of birth control as acceptable within the marital relationship.

ISLAM

The position of Islam is that all is preordained, so that any contraceptive practice is permissible if it has the possibility of failure or success (for example, coitus interruptus). Birth control is permissible but not recommended. The feeling is that procreation itself is meritorious, and in using contraception a person is abstaining from a meritorious act. The act of contraception was accepted because birth control often had good reasoning. The liberal attitude noted that contraception impinged upon a woman's right to fulfillment and to progeny; therefore, her consent was needed for the male to practice contraception (primarily in reference to coitus interruptus). The position on abortion varies among the sects. The Hanafy permit abortion before the end of the fourth month, when ensoulment occurs, and the Maliki found it permissible up to 40 days. In general, abortion was tolerated even when it was not recommended. Medieval secular literature discussed contraception widely and in detail. The current modern interpretation is that Moslems have the right to limit their own reproduction but that governments cannot, although they may inform and encourage.

HINDU

At the basis of the Hindu position is the ethical ideal of dharma or righteousness for the betterment of life, both secular and spiritual. Marriage is felt to serve numerous purposes, among which are pleasure, parenthood, companionship, sacrificial service, and spiritual bliss. Generally, reproduction was discouraged by custom, such as prohibiting a widow from remarrying, and by taboo, which prevented sexual relations during lactation. Currently, there are no moral or religious objections to birth control, but abortion is considered sinful because of killing a sentient being. However, even under the religious precepts, a case can be made on the Hindu concept of sympathy, permitting abortion out of compassion for an afflicted woman. Sterilization is voluntary, but one or two children are necessary to satisfy religious requirements.

INTUITION OR NATURAL LAW

Intuition at first glance may not seem a religious factor; however, it derives from a revelation (from within oneself) and depends on faith in its truth, so it is not far afield. Some people do not base their anti–birth control stance on formal religious grounds but rather on an intuitive position of what is normal or natural or "meant to be." Few of them would opt for a natural extraction of a decaying tooth or refuse an antibiotic in order to let pneumonia run its natural course. Some short-sighted teenagers, in their urge for the natural, have forgotten the natural consequences of urge. This argument, natural versus unnatural, lost its basis when the first hominid threw a stone when hunting. There appears to be nothing more human than the pattern of altering the environment because of basic biologic needs. For shelter we have abandoned the cave, for clothing we have improved upon fur and fiber, for food we have eliminated the undependability of hunting and gathering. Prestressed concrete, nylon, and refrigeration are not unnatural. They are triumphantly human, and humans have only the natural with which to fabricate, regardless of origin or inspiration. "Ironically, to believe that 'playing God' is even possible would itself be hubris according to some religious thought, which maintains that only God can interfere with the descriptive laws of nature (that is, perform miracles)"[17].

HISTORIC PERSPECTIVE

One certainty exists: Across the entire scroll of history there are references to methods designed to alter the consequence of coitus. The Petri papyrus (1850 B.C.), the Ebers papyrus (1550 B.C.), Aristotle (fourth century B.C.), and Soranus (second century B.C.) referred to potions, fumigants, and mechanical barriers to conception. The Upanishads in the seventh century B.C. offered birth control incantations. Avicenna in the eleventh century described in detail in the "Canon of Medicine" many contraceptives that worked both as barrier techniques and as spermicides. Chaucer in the fourteenth century mentioned contraception in his writings [7].

Infanticide has been practiced in many cultures for various reasons—excess population, birth defects, incestuous parentage, uncertain parentage, as a religious offering, etc. In nineteenth century China, where population problems were felt earlier than in the Western world (population of about 430 million in 1850), infanticide of female children was the widest mode of population control, whereas the people remained generally ignorant of contraceptive modalities. In most Western cultures the current law distinguishes infanticide from "ordinary" homicide, and probation or mental treatment is ordered for the former [8].

The modern history of public advocacy of contraceptive techniques begins in London in 1822, when Francis Place published a treatise and thereafter distributed handbills addressed "To the Married of Both Sexes of the Working People," describing birth control techniques. Ten years later in America, a young physician, Charles Knowlton, was fined and jailed for publishing a detailed book on birth control technique [8]. Over 40 years after Knowlton's death in 1850, an English reformer, Annie Besant, forced a trial in England by publishing a book on birth control; as a consequence, her children were taken from her as an unfit mother, but ultimately she won the right to distribute the book. In America the Comstock Law was passed in 1873, which classified birth control literature as obscene. In 1912 Margaret Sanger published her first birth control articles and later a pamphlet. After charges were dropped for the latter, she opened her first clinic in 1916 and spent 30 days in jail for "maintaining a public nuisance." Later court decisions and changes in public and government policy reversed the suppression of birth control programs and in fact began their support nationally and internationally through foreign aid programs and United Nations agencies. Yet it was not until 1965 that the Supreme Court of the United States finally struck down the last state law that in Connecticut prohibited the use of contraception [7].

ETHICAL CONSIDERATIONS FOR PHYSICIANS AND OTHER HEALTH WORKERS

If there is a presumption of the right to noninterference with self-affecting actions, upon what ethical grounds might a physician decline a request for contraception? Even religious constraints permit "natural" techniques. Should a request for a religiously objectionable technique be made, what then? Certainly, religious view should not be confused with medical opinion. A woman has the right to expect medical advice from her physician and theological guidance from her clergy, and any overlap must clearly be identified. If a physician feels so strongly about a position that he cannot with clear conscience refer the patient to another source of help, most patients are sophisticated enough to seek help elsewhere, if the refusal is properly identified as a religious position, not medical. Such values should not be disguised as medical issues. An example of how such skewed reasoning influenced medical advice in the past appears in an 1888 treatise on masturbation by Lawson Tait: "The best remedy was not to tell the poor children that they were damning their souls, but to tell them that they might seriously hurt their bodies"[7]. In much the same way the recent outbreak of herpes has been invoked not as a viral infection but as divine retribution for swinging singles (without any explanation for those who contracted herpes in a sanctioned monogamous relationship from a partner with latent disease). So, too, has pregnancy been miscast as the punishment for unsanctioned intercourse by those too short-sighted to measure the consequences of and to an unwanted child.

The morality of out-of-wedlock sexual relations is controversial. Social disapproval of extramarital coitus originated with the need for protection of the offspring as the primary social value. In some Polynesian cultures where coitus was haphazard, children belonged to the community and their welfare was ensured by all. But in most societies, perhaps because food and shelter were less easily obtained, such protection could not be assured without a responsible male. With the technological separation of procreation from sexual activity this reason is invalid, since pregnancy need not result.

Philosophers pondering the ethics of behavior have always distinguished actions affecting others from actions affecting only oneself. Hence, for the physician who believes that his task is to promote and restore the patient's autonomy [8], a request for contraception from an adult patient offers little problem. A physician would be correct to introduce the subject of the health aspects of extramarital coitus, aside from the potential pregnancy that the patient is seeking to avoid. Sexually transmitted diseases ought to be discussed in a balanced and realistic manner. The principle of informed consent is applicable, and a review of the medical risks and benefits of the various methods of contraception, comparing them with each other and with the omission of contraception, is an expected function of the physician.

Since truly individual sexual activity is a paradoxical term (except for masturbation, which is certainly no longer a medical concern), what other ethical concerns might be raised? A segment of society sees contraception as the means by which family-oriented social organization might break down. Eleanor Garst [11] wrote in 1966:

Almost every individual now living would have lived quite differently if reproduction had been subject to free mutual choice . . . . Will life be the same when every girl at the onset of puberty takes The Pill as routinely as she sees her dentist?— When the psychological separation of intercourse and reproduction has become as complete as the physical separation now can be? . . . . Will women choose to marry? (Sex) will not necessarily (be) confined to one partner for life (how often is it now?) . . . . What social pattern will emerge? Will children be bred selectively? Will bonuses be paid for not having children? What of the time when the fertilized ovum can be implanted into the womb of a mercenary and one's progeny be selected from a sperm bank? Will (the children) become the responsibility of the total community? Will communal love develop the human qualities that we assume emerge from the present rearing of children?
I don't raise the question in advocacy. What disturbs me is the real possibility of the disappearance of our humane, life-giving qualities with the speed of development in the life sciences, and the fact that nobody seems to be discussing the alternative possibilities for good and evil in these developments.

Subsequently, there has been a vast increase in discussion of these issues with the resurgence of interest in normative ethics. One of the most comprehensive approaches is by Leon R. Kass [13]. His article includes a thought-provoking examination of the need to evaluate carefully the use of all available new technology:

The de-humanizing consequences of programmed reproduction extend beyond the mere acts and processes of life-giving. Transfer of procreation to the laboratory will no doubt weaken what is presently for most people the best remaining justification for the existence of marriage and the family. Sex is now comfortably at home outside of marriage; child rearing is progressively being given over to the state, the schools, the mass media, and the child-care centers. Some have argued that the family, long the nursery of humanity, has outlived its usefulness.
Some of its virtues are too often overlooked. The family is rapidly becoming the only institution in an increasingly impersonal world where each person is loved not only for what he does or what he makes, but simply because he is. The family is also the institution where most of us . . . . acquire a sense of continuity to the past and a sense of commitment to the future. Without the family we would have little incentive to take interest after our own deaths . . . . Elimination of the family would throw us to the mercy of an impersonal lonely present.

Since sex and contraception are here to stay, it behooves us to consider whether the values we regard highly might be threatened by contraception. An argu-

ment even more cogent can be made that contraception, by eliminating the risk of inadvertent childbearing outside the traditional family structure, serves to preserve that model best. We might examine a little more skeptically those reproductive techniques that might disrupt bonding or other psychological functions, serving those ends we call *humane*, or techniques such as donor artificial insemination, which could be used outside the traditional family structure.

Where else might the ethical use of contraception be called into question? The minor or adolescent patient poses a dilemma. The argument is that the availability of contraception promotes sexual activity. There appears to be no basis for the position that there is something *intrinsically* bad about sexual activity in the young female except the risk of undesired reproduction. Psychological problems, not intrinsic but culturally imposed, are discussed below.

Teenage pregnancy is a problem because sexual activity is undertaken without regard for contraception, not because contraception is available [19]. Teenage sexual activity cannot be separated from significant psychosocial factors, but placing obstacles in the path of those teenagers who would avoid compounding the problem with a pregnancy is not productive. The objective of promoting parental instruction for appropriate sexual behavior is laudable. The idea that the time for parents to become involved is after the child seeks contraception, as some government interventions promote, is fallacious. Such an invasion of privacy, even if ever warranted, is too late to be helpful.

In a study of 193 teenagers in New York City seeking birth control, abortion, or prenatal care, Cobliner [5] learned that of the 143 (unintentionally) pregnant, 71 percent believed they wouldn't get pregnant or simply "took a chance," 13 percent were misinformed about the time pregnancy could occur, 10 percent were poor users of contraception, and 6 percent had device failures. All of them had been sexually active for more than 6 months.

Interviews showed that those at high risk of pregnancy had few long-range goals, conformed greatly to peer pressures, had very conflictive relationships with their mothers and their sexual partners, obtained contraceptive information by hearsay, and did not seek authoritative help. These characteristics were essentially opposite from those of the teenagers who had avoided pregnancy.

Domeena C. Renshaw [16], in a plea for physician-centered sexual education for adolescents, pointed out that in 1979 there were a million teenage pregnancies (12,642 under age 15), one-third of which were aborted; 70 percent of these young women failed to finish high school. She noted that the causes of pregnancy were complex, but certainly some could have been avoided with proper education. The ethical obligation of the physician to the teenage patient is to deal with sexuality with no less care than with other organ symptoms. Renshaw points out that sex education should emphasize that sexual expression is a choice with an important role in character development and the ability to sustain deep personal relationships, in family ties, and in religious beliefs. Further, she points out, the physician, more than the parent, might be able to caution the teenager about peer pressures that are manipulative and exploitative. Finally, nonsexual affection and caring must be emphasized in a world where primarily erotic phenomena abound in the daily environment.

Although contraception has been the means to dissociate procreation from the sexual act, it cannot be blamed for sexual activities under socially disapproved conditions. Such extramarital and premarital behavior certainly is not unique to contemporary society. The value of contraception for planning, in order to make children the result of a jointly considered familial undertaking, is undeniable. The opportunity for contraception for the couple, who recognize, for whatever reason, their inability to assume a parental role, is certainly better than imposing such a role on them or their unwanted child. Since the sexual drive is clearly a compelling one, contraception avoids the unwanted extramarital pregnancy as well. Unwanted pregnancy is not the only reason to be wary of extramarital sexual expression. It is appropriate to discuss this with the patient, since there is a second echelon of psychological complexities arising from taboos. A patient should also be aware of the potential for exploitation if the sexual expression has a different meaning for the partners (e.g., if one believes it is affirming a commitment, while the other believes it is purely recreational). It is part of the complete role of the physician to explore these positions on behalf of the patient. An experienced counselor may feel duty-bound to discuss his or her own values, but they should be identified as values, not disguised as medical information, and be presented with empathy and without threat. Further discussion of the health aspects are part of the informed consent owed to a patient when any medication is prescribed.

For the teenager whose sophistication is presumably less than that of the adult, even more information may be needed. Rarely will a teenager who is engaged in sexual activity (as the vast majority of them are by the time they reach the physician's office) be immediately dissuaded (if that were desired) from continuing sexual activity. One would be remiss to send such patients away unprotected or at least unreferred to a source for contraception. It would be helpful if the patient had sufficient rapport with her parents to discuss this issue, but as Zelnick [19], Cobliner [5], and others have shown, it is precisely those teenagers who do not relate well to parents who, left unprotected, are more likely to have unwanted pregnancies. Encouraging the patient to try to establish sufficient rapport to discuss these needs might be the beginning of a better overall relationship with parents, but violating her privacy will only confirm her isolation and mistrust of the adult world.

STERILIZATION—SPECIAL ETHICAL ISSUES

Sterilization, as a form of contraception, raises additional ethical questions because it requires an operative procedure and is frequently irreversible. Ethically, the major issues surrounding sterilization have been those that relate to informed consent. Thus, in addition to the general characteristics of such consents for medical procedures, the requirements for informed consent for sterilization usually include added precautions against coercion, full discussion of alternatives, and a period of time for reflection and reconsideration. After reconsideration in general, the request for sterilization should proceed from the patient to the physician and should not originate from institutional or governmental administration. Additional precautions against coercion may include an age floor (21 years), assurances of mental competence, and prohibition against initiation of the request for sterilization during hospital admission for delivery or abortion [6]. In dealing with the issue of mental incompetence, the major ethical issues are (1) assurance of maximal autonomy for the patient in the decision-making, (2) determination of who can speak for the best interests of the patient, and (3) exclusion of institutions and the state from initiating or participating coercively in the decision-making process.

Other issues that deserve special emphasis were noted by the American College of Obstetricians and Gynecologists in the statement "Ethical Considerations in Sterilization" [2]. The statement emphasizes that the patient should be encouraged to include other appropriate persons in the decision, that linkage of sterilization to the denial of other medical care is "unethically coercive," and that central to free and informed consent is that it be volitional, that is, freely given in the presence of recognized alternatives. Thus, access to other forms of contraceptive care must be available, and the risks and benefits should be clearly explained, including the risks of failure.

Lastly, in providing sterilization service the health care professional should guard against playing a purely technical role, in particular, as the "instrument" of other individuals, groups, or the state. As in other health care, the professional should evaluate the indications and contraindications for any particular patient and should assist the patient in selecting the best procedure for the clinical situation.

ABORTION—ETHICAL CONSIDERATIONS IN A PLURALISTIC SOCIETY

If one holds that life itself is *the* ultimate value, then abortion can never be justified (except under some rare circumstance where fetal and maternal life are being balanced). If this value is derived from religious revelation, there is no rationale for questioning further (unless one wishes to doubt the infallibility of those interpreting the revelation). But we should dispose of the premise that this is only a religious issue. The fact that political activity is spearheaded by the Catholic church and fundamentalist Protestant groups has been a source of confusion. The church's position on nuclear war does not make nuclear war solely a religious issue. (Some physicians, for example, feel that nuclear war is a cogent medical issue, holding that there is no adequate local medical response to a nuclear explosion.) Searching for a value on which to base a logical progression leading to rules by which to live, one need not be theistic to find great worth in respect for life. If such a value is to be translated into law, however, the issue is not the identity of the supporters, but whether that law is unjustly discriminatory. I have heard of no one who is in favor of abortion; those who accept it find it better than an unwanted pregnancy. It would be far preferable for the pregnancy to have been avoided, when undesired. Confronted with the fact of pregnancy, many acknowledge that they may no longer be dealing with a problem in which the solution is readily identified as right or wrong. Absolutists on either pole appear to have the least difficulty with the problem. Others, realizing that there may be no right answer, fall back on solutions that are, for those involved, the least undesirable. The tension arises not because life is not valued but rather because the prevention of suffering is valued more highly. For some, personhood is not either present or absent but rather a spectrum distinguishable by degree of development, from potential (as a zygote) to actual (as a self-conscious being aware of the future). Persons holding this position may be able to opt for early abortion because they value highly the here-and-now avoidance of conscious suffering, and they feel that it outweighs the destruction of a life that is potential but neither sentient nor conscious early in development. Were the decision one of justice versus injustice, freedom versus slavery, beneficence versus maleficence, no ethical problems would appear; such values standing unopposed would readily be acknowledged as decisive. A dilemma is created when something of value must be sacrificed, when there are worthy values on each side of the scale. In the debate over abortion, the ultimate value of right to life conflicts with the value of relief or avoidance of suffering. Physical pain is abhorrent, but emotional distress is also suffering, of which not all living things are capable. As in most human endeavors, equities and individual circumstances must be measured, because the two opposing weighty and worthy principles simply will not tip the scale either way [18].

The problem of abortion is unique. There simply is no analogous situation. One of many possible pairs of living human cells combine in only one available environment. One should note that an infinite number of other unique pairs are gone forever, having failed to combine. If the combined cells survive an early 20 to 50 percent natural mortality, they will grow and develop, usually as a single entity, the majority without significant physical abnormality. Electrical brain activity, the significance of which is unknown, does not appear until 8 weeks of intrauterine life. Pain as we know it could not be perceived without brain activity; hence, this is the earliest possible time fetal destruction could be painful to the fetus (although it is unlikely to be perceived until much more integrated activity occurs [12]. If this entity passes the hurdle of prematurity (with intrinsic morbidity and mortality), it will come to delivery. Then, if no anomaly incompatible with extrauterine life exists, it will continue growth and development. At this time *and only in retrospect* can one say that a human life began at conception. At some later point, long after birth, it will become aware of itself, and only much later will it be physically self-sufficient. The unique aspect is its absolute physical dependence for a substantial number of months in utero on only one person in the universe. If that person is unwilling to support it, does the state have a compelling interest sufficient to force her to subjugate her decision to promote the survival of the conceptus? So far, courts have assumed a compelling fetal interest in a maternal-fetal conflict only as term approaches, but is compulsion appropriate? Bowes and Selgestad [3] have reviewed the literature, in reporting a court-ordered cesarean section for fetal distress at term in a recalcitrant mother. The legal literature cited asserted the state's interest primarily at what promises to become a progressively more difficult point to determine, given the nature of neonatal intensive care technology: viability. Additionally, concerns about the issue of prematernal responsibility to the fetus in areas where fetal diagnosis and therapy may be indicated or where the pregnant woman is involved in practices harmful to the fetus (e.g., substance abuse) are now being raised.

The practicalities of the situation were acknowledged by the authors as follows:

The directive of the court was clear that necessary medical treatment could be administered against the will of the patient. Fortunately, the court's decision had a salutary effect on the patient, and her attitude became one of reluctant acceptance and compliance. Had the patient steadfastly refused, it might not have been either safe or possible to administer anesthesia to a struggling, resisting woman who weighed in excess of 157.5 kilograms.

Society can prove its humanity by collectively providing for the disabled of any age whose parents (or children) are unwilling or unable to care for them. Society can agree to take damaged infants at birth and relieve the agony of the parents and the necessity for devoting family resources, emotional and material, competitive with and disproportionate to those needed by the family's intact children. Serving as a "catastrophic insurance" arm, society can eliminate many of the utilitarian reasons for abortion based on genetic abnormalities predicted in advance of birth. In such a society, where a damaged or unwanted child may be relinquished to good social care without stigma, some people confronting this dilemma may be more inclined to sacrifice self-interest at least for the duration of the pregnancy, opting not to abort. For some people, in this way, the issue of not wanting any pregnancy can be separated from that of not wanting a defective child. For those who do not wish to carry a pregnancy, some fetal rights will probably continue to be conferred pragmatically by courts in late pregnancy. There will be maternal-fetal conflict until contraception is technically perfected, psychological blocks are avoided, and social lag is overcome, virtually eliminating the problem that so preoccupies us now.

Privately, we may condone or condemn abortion. Once again, the duality of a private and public morality is needed to enable those committed to the "peaceable" community [10] to govern themselves without violent confrontation. Imposing a law (by playing constitutional word games) on a substantial number of people who conscientiously oppose it effectively imposes on an individual involuntary use of her body. If tragic choices must be made, the burden of proof falls on an impersonal and distant society to demonstrate a clearly superior basis for contravening the choice of those fully-formed, sentient, and self-aware individuals who must live with the consequences of that choice.

The control of reproduction, as a part of health care, receives special ethical emphasis because it is linked to procreation, sexual identity, and sexual function. Thus, although the individual patient's rights and autonomy are of central concern in providing the related health services, society takes specific interest in such services. As such, society will seek to exercise this interest through its various agencies in the form of standards, regulations, and controls. Health care professionals, through understanding the historic and current perspectives of the ethical issues, can help to maintain and enhance their patients' autonomy and access to appropriate care.

REFERENCES

1. Adams, E., and Briscoe, M. L. *Up Against the Wall, Mother.* Macmillan, Calif.: Glencoe Press, p. 362, 1971.
2. American College of Obstetricians and Gynecologists. Ethical Considerations in Sterilization. Approved June 6, 1979.
3. Bowes, W., and Selgestad, B. Fetal versus maternal rights: Medical and legal perspectives. *Obstet. Gynecol.* 58:209, 1981.
4. Cassell, H., The function of medicine. *Hastings Cent. Rep.* 7:16, 1977.
5. Cobliner, W. G. Teen age pregnancy: Who is most at risk? *The Female Patient* 6:63, 1981.
6. Department of Health, Education, and Welfare. Sterilizations and Abortions. *Federal Register,* November 8, 1978. Part V, pp. 52146–52175.
7. Encyclopaedia Britannica (14th ed.). Birth control. Vol. 3, pp. 706 B–708, 1969.
8. Encyclopaedia Britannica (14th ed.). Infanticide. Vol. 12, p. 217, 1969.
9. Engelhardt, H. T. The disease of masturbation: Values and the concept of disease. *Bull. Hist. Med.* 48:234–248, 1974.
10. Engelhardt, H. T., Jr. Bioethics in pluralistic societies. *Perspect. Biol. Med.* 26: 64, 1982.
11. Garst, E. The Asexual Society. In *Annals of America.* Chicago: Encyclopaedia Britannica, Inc., Vol. 18, p. 348. 1968.
12. Goldblatt, D. *Nervous System and Sensory Organs, Intrauterine Development.* Philadelphia: A. C. Barnes, 1968.
13. Kass, L. A. The new biology: What price relieving man's estate? *Science* 174:779, 1971.
14. Noonan, J. T. Contraception. In W. T. Reich (ed.), *Encyclopedia of Bioethics.* New York: Macmillan, The Free Press, p. 206, 213, 1978.
15. Petersen, W. History of Population Theories. In W. T. Reich (ed.), *Encyclopedia of Bioethics.* New York: Macmillan, The Free Press, p. 1230, 1978.
16. Renshaw, D. C. Sex education: Why the physician must help. *The Female Patient* 7:33, 1982.

17. Splicing Life: A Report on the Social and Ethical Issues of Genetic Engineering with Human Beings. President's Commission for the Study of Ethical Problems in Medicine and Biomedical and Behavioral Research, p. 55. Washington, D.C.: Superintendent of Documents, November 1983.
18. Toulmin, S. The tyranny of principles, *Hastings Cent. Rep.* December, 1981.
19. Zelnick, M., and Kanter, J. F. Sexual activity, contraceptive use, and pregnancy among metropolitan teenagers. *Fam. Plann. Perspect.* 12: p. 230, 1980.

BIBLIOGRAPHY

Brody, H. *Ethical Decisions in Medicine* (2nd ed.). Boston: Little, Brown 1981.

Childress, J. F., King, P., Dworkin, G., and Pelligrino, E. D. (eds.) *Bioethics Reporter.* University Publishing of America, Maryland, 1983.

Levine, C. (ed.) *Hastings Cent. rep.* Vol. 10–13, 1981–1983.

Reich, W. T. (ed.) *Encyclopedia of Bioethics.* New York: Macmillan, The Free Press, 1978.

2. Statistical Aspects of the Evaluation of the Safety and Effectiveness of Fertility Control Methods

Diana B. Petitti

Because millions of otherwise healthy people use fertility control methods, their safety is a particularly important issue. With several possible fertility control methods available to most people, the relative effectiveness of the methods becomes a crucial factor in decision making. In response to the need for information on the safety and effectiveness of fertility control methods a large body of research literature has evolved; statistical aspects of study design and data analysis play an important role in the interpretation of this literature. This chapter is aimed at making understandable the most important statistical aspects of research on the safety and effectiveness of fertility control methods so that practicing clinicians may themselves judge information on these subjects.

EFFECTIVENESS

The effectiveness of a drug, device, or procedure to control fertility is its ability to prevent conception or birth. Quantifying effectiveness is less easy than defining it. To begin with, effectiveness can refer either to the ability to prevent birth in ideal circumstances when the method functions perfectly and the patient uses it perfectly, termed *theoretic-effectiveness* or *method-effectiveness;* or to the ability to prevent birth in circumstances of actual use, termed *use-effectiveness* (Table 2-1). Second, there are several statistical methods for calculating effectiveness, and the choice of method influences those values and subsequent conclusions based upon them.

Theoretic- Versus Use-Effectiveness

Each method of fertility control has biologic or mechanical characteristics that determine its effectiveness. For example, an oral contraceptive with a very low dose of steroid hormones might inhibit ovulation in some but not all menstrual cycles. Its theoretic-effectiveness is determined by the number of cycles in which ovulation is inhibited. The low-dose contraceptive would have lower theoretic-effectiveness than a contraceptive that inhibited all ovulations, because even when the low-dose contraceptive did all it could do, some pregnancies would occur. In addition to the biologic and mechanical properties of the method that determine its theoretic-effectiveness, a method's convenience of use, ease of use, and immediate side effects influence whether or not the method is actually used, one determinant of use-effectiveness. For example, an oral contraceptive that caused immediate vomiting in 50 percent of those who tried to use it is likely to be abandoned by those who were nauseated, and its use-effectiveness would consequently be low.

Table 2-1. Theoretic- versus use-effectiveness

Type	What it measures	Comments
Theoretic-effectiveness	Ability to prevent pregnancy in ideal situation where method works perfectly and is used properly	Represents the upper limit of effectiveness of the method
Use-effectiveness	Ability to prevent pregnancy in real-life situations	May be affected by characteristics of users such as age, social class, education, and culture

Table 2-2. Use-effectiveness of the diaphragm in two studies

Study	Characteristics of study group	Use-effectiveness[a]
Vessey et al. [43]	White, married, 25 or more years, high social class	0.98[b]
Vaughan et al. [39]	Married, 18–44 years, middle-high class	0.89[c]
	Married, 18–44 years, high class	0.96[c]

[a]Number of pregnancies per woman-year of use.
[b]By the Pearl method.
[c]By the life-table method.

Whenever presented, measures of effectiveness should be appropriately identified as being either of theoretic-effectiveness or of use-effectiveness. Both quantities are important, theoretic-effectiveness representing the upper limit of effectiveness of a method and use-effectiveness representing the likely performance of the method in a real-life group of users. For some methods, theoretic-effectiveness and use-effectiveness are identical, whereas for other methods they are greatly disparate. For example, oral contraceptives have both high theoretic- and high use-effectiveness because the mechanism of control of fertility, ovulation inhibition, is reliable and because, at least in Western cultures, taking a pill every day is a task that can be performed regularly by most women. The diaphragm, in contrast, is a method with high theoretic- but low use-effectiveness. If it is inserted correctly at the proper time with every act of intercourse and if it is left in place for 6 to 8 hours, few pregnancies will occur. In real life some women may neglect to use the device on some days and some may fail to leave it in place for an adequate length of time. The actual number of pregnancies may then be high, and the method will have low use-effectiveness.

Theoretic-effectiveness is fixed by the biologic or mechanical mechanism by which the method prevents birth. Use-effectiveness may vary according to the characteristics of users. To illustrate, Table 2-2 shows the results of two studies of the use-effectiveness of the diaphragm in three groups [39, 43]. The diaphragm had a use-effectiveness of 0.96 in women of high social class and a use-effectiveness of 0.89 in women of middle-high social class. In cultures where pill-taking is an unusual event, oral contraceptives may have low use-effectiveness. Counseling of patients about the

use-effectiveness of a fertility control method should ideally take into account differences in use-effectiveness according to characteristics such as age, education, and social class. Cultural differences also alter use-effectiveness rates. This should be taken into consideration during counseling. Unfortunately, studies that measure the use-effectiveness of methods in relation to these characteristics are rare.

Calculating Effectiveness

Until the mid-1960s the effectiveness of fertility control methods was almost always calculated using the Pearl pregnancy rate, named after Raymond Pearl [20], the statistician who first suggested it. To calculate the Pearl pregnancy rate, the number of accidental pregnancies is divided by the total months of contraceptive use, and this result is then multiplied by 12. This calculation gives the number of accidental pregnancies per woman-year of contraceptive use; subtraction from 1 yields use-effectiveness by the Pearl method.

The inadequacies of the Pearl method were delineated almost simultaneously by several authors [23, 24, 32]. To understand these inadequacies, imagine a study of 100 women all of whom begin use of a hypothetical fertility control method. Imagine that 50 become pregnant in the first month of use. The other 50 women are observed to use the method for 10 years, and none of them become pregnant. The use-effectiveness of the method calculated by the Pearl method is 0.90 (Table 2-3). This quantity does not reflect one's intuitive notion about the effectiveness of the method—that the method is very poor. The longer a group of users is observed, the higher the use-effectiveness will be when calculated by the Pearl method [23, 32]. This happens because women who do not conceive early in the study are less accident prone and also may be less fertile [36]. That length of use

Table 2-3. The Pearl method for calculating use-effectiveness: Hypothetical example showing inadequacies

Women in the study	100
Women pregnant in month 1	50
Months of use in them	50
Women never pregnant	50
Months of use in them	6,000

$$\text{Pearl pregnancy rate} = \frac{50}{50 + 6,000} \times 12 = .10 \text{ per woman-year}$$

$$\text{Use-effectiveness by Pearl method} = 1 - .10 = .90 \text{ per woman-year}$$

among subjects influences the estimate of use-effectiveness when calculated by the Pearl method is its major deficiency.

A refinement of the Pearl method is to use only the first 12 months of observation to calculate use-effectiveness. Using the refinement, an intuitively better measure of use-effectiveness is obtained. For the hypothetical data shown in Table 2-3, the refinement yields a use-effectiveness for the hypothetical method of 0.08. This figure more accurately reflects the obvious lack of effectiveness of the method. Yet even this refinement is deficient since the estimated use-effectiveness still depends on the length of time that subjects remain in the study. Returning to the hypothetical example, imagine that five of the 50 women who did not conceive in the first month of use discontinued using the method after 9 months in order to conceive. The other 45 women continue to use the method for 12 full months without conceiving. In this case, use-effectiveness by the Pearl method, refined by using only the first 12 months of observation, is 0.06. In all of the three cases described, the same 50 women of the original 100 users became pregnant in the first month of use, and none of them became accidentally pregnant after the first month. Yet the estimates of use-effectiveness using the Pearl method, even with its refinement, are 0.90, 0.08, and 0.06. Although a situation as extreme as this one probably occurs rarely in real life, the dependence of the Pearl method on the length of observation of subjects is a serious flaw.

In recognition of the inadequacy of the Pearl method, beginning in the mid-1960s life-table techniques have been used increasingly to estimate the use-effectiveness of fertility control methods [25, 35]. Life-table techniques take into account varying lengths of observation of subjects in a study. Extensions of life-table techniques are used to estimate not only use-effectiveness but the probabilities of other events of interest in evaluating the overall performance of a method of fer-

tility control, particularly the intrauterine device (IUD) [4, 16, 26, 38].

In its simplest form a life-table is used to estimate the cumulative probability of having an accidental pregnancy in some period of time after initiation of use, usually 1 year. Use-effectiveness is calculated by subtracting this estimate from 1. Table 2-4 shows the calculation by a life-table of use-effectiveness for the hypothetical situation described previously. Using this technique, the use-effectiveness of the hypothetical method is estimated to be 0.50, which is the intuitively correct figure. The life-table estimate of use-effectiveness will not change if more women stop using the method to become pregnant; nor will it change if some women use the method for a very long period of time whereas others become pregnant immediately.

The example in Table 2-4 is the simplest possible life-table, a single decrement life-table. Even using the simplest technique, issues arise in deciding how to count observation of women who drop out and how to deal with subjects who stop using the method and restart it. Several papers discuss solutions to the complex questions that arise in using life-table techniques to calculate use-effectiveness [4, 16, 37], which are beyond the scope of this presentation. With the simple single-decrement life-table only a single quantity can be estimated—here, the pregnancy rate. There are situations where estimating the rates of several events while removing, by statistical methods, the influence of others is also important. In the hypothetical example, it might be the case that all the pregnancies in the first month were a result of the expulsion of IUDs. In women who did not expel the device in the first month the method performs perfectly. An estimate of what the pregnancy rate would have been in the absence of expulsions is important information, and the simple life-table estimate does not yield it.

Formally, the problem of estimating the probability of one event while removing, by statistical methods, the influence of others is a problem of competing risks [26]. Particularly in the evaluation of IUD performance, it is of considerable interest to estimate what the rate of pregnancy would have been in the absence of, say, expulsions. Life-table techniques that allow estimation of the rate of one event and removal of the effects of others by a statistical method have been developed. They are called multiple-decrement life-tables, and they are discussed in detail by Tietze [37, 38] and others [26].

For the practicing clinician, however, an understanding of the meaning of the final rate estimates is necessary in order to interpret information from studies that use the techniques. Table 2-5 shows the final results of an experimental study that compared the performance of two different copper IUDs [34]. The rates calculated by the simple life-table technique (a single-decrement

Table 2-4. Life-table calculation of cumulative probability of an accidental pregnancy: Hypothetical data

Month of use	Number of women using method (a)	Number of accidental pregnancies (b)	Number who stopped use or terminated for reasons other than pregnancy (c)	Accidental pregnancy rate [(b) ÷ (a)] (d)	Use-effectiveness [1 − (d)] (e)	Cumulative use-effectiveness (f)
1	100	50	0	0.50	.50	.50
2	50	0	0	0.00	1.00	.50
3	50	0	0	0.00	1.00	.50
4	50	0	0	0.00	1.00	.50
5	50	0	0	0.00	1.00	.50
6	50	0	0	0.00	1.00	.50
7	50	0	0	0.00	1.00	.50
8	50	0	0	0.00	1.00	.50
9	50	0	5	0.00	1.00	.50
10	45	0	0	0.00	1.00	.50
11	45	0	0	0.00	1.00	.50
12	45	0	0	0.00	1.00	.50

Table 2-5. Two-year net and gross cumulative rates of selected events for the CU 380A and CU 200 intrauterine contraceptive devices

Event	Net rate[a]		Gross rate[a]	
	380A	200	380A	200
Pregnancy	0.8	5.0	1.0	6.6
Expulsion	7.5	9.9	8.8	11.3
Removal for bleeding/pain	21.8	15.0	25.2	22.9
Total discontinuation for above	36.8	34.6	n.a.[b]	n.a.[b]

[a]Per 100 woman-years.
[b]The individual rates cannot be added to obtain the discontinuation rate.
Source: From I. Sivin and J. Stern. Long-acting, more effective TCU IUDS: A summary of U.S. experience 1970–1975. *Stud. Fam. Plann.* 10:263, 1979.

life-table) are called *gross rates*; the rates calculated by the life-table technique that allows for competing risks (a multiple-decrement life-table) are called *net rates*. The gross rate measures the overall occurrence of the event; the net rate estimates what the rate of the event would have been if the effects of the other events were removed. In the study in Table 2-5, the estimated gross pregnancy rate for the 380A IUD is 1.0. This estimate of the pregnancy rate includes pregnancies that result from expulsions as well as those from pregnancy with the IUD in place. The estimated net pregnancy rate for the 380A IUD is 0.8. This estimate of the pregnancy rate is interpreted as what the pregnancy rate would have been had there been no expulsions and no removals for bleeding and pain. The gross rates cannot be added to obtain a total discontinuation rate; net rates can. Gross rates are used to compare the overall performance of two or more different IUDs for a specific event; net rates are used to examine the performance of a single IUD with respect to different events and to compare discontinuation rates between IUDs. Thus, in the study shown in Table 2-5, the 380A, with a gross pregnancy rate of 1.0, is obviously superior to the 200, which has a pregnancy rate of 6.6. The 380A has a net discontinuation rate for pregnancy, expulsion, and removal for bleeding and pain of 36.8; for the 200, it is 34.6. From the point of view of device discontinuation, the IUDs perform similarly.

SAFETY

Safety refers to a fertility control method's short-term and long-term risks and to its benefits other than the prevention of birth. Most of the statistical aspects of research on safety apply equally to studies of short-term and long-term safety, although the terminology used in the following sections more often has been applied to studies of long-term safety, which are epidemiologic studies. Here, both types of studies are called *analytic studies*. The critical evaluation of the literature on the safety of fertility control methods requires knowledge of study design, measures of "risk," significance testing and confidence intervals, and bias.

Study Design

Analytic studies can be experimental or nonexperimental. In experimental studies subjects are assigned randomly to treatments or exposures and followed forward in time to determine the occurrence of disease or of a condition other than disease. In nonexperimental studies three designs are commonly used: cross-sectional, cohort, and case-control. In a cross-sectional study the existence of the disease and of the exposure is determined in a group of individuals at a point in time and compared. In a cohort study groups of exposed and unexposed subjects are identified, and the occurrence of the disease after exposure is determined and compared. In a case-control study people with and without the disease are identified, and their exposure at that time or a time in the past is determined and compared.

The terms *prospective* and *retrospective* are often used as synonyms for cohort and case-control studies, respectively. These terms properly refer to temporal relationships between the conduct of the investigation and either ascertainment of exposure or the occurrence of disease. *Prospective* means "forward"; describing studies, the term denotes those in which data collection proceeds forward in time from the initiation of the study. *Retrospective* means "looking back"; describing studies, the term is used whenever some aspect of the study involves looking back.

A cohort study may be either prospective, involving data collection that proceeds forward from definition of exposure; or it may be retrospective, involving a "look back" by the investigator to determine exposure and disease occurrence. Retrospective cohort studies are also called *historic cohort studies*. The Royal College of General Practitioners oral contraceptive study [29] is a prospective cohort study because in 1968 Dr. Kay and colleagues identified women using oral contraceptives and other methods of contraception (the cohort) and followed them forward in time to determine disease occurrence (the prospective component). Recently, Walker et al. [44] published results from a study of rates of hospitalization in relation to vasectomy. In this study the investigators looked back at pathology files and membership records from the Puget Sound Health Cooperative (the retrospective component) to identify men with and without vasectomy (the cohort) and studied hospitalization rates after vasectomy. The

study was, therefore, a retrospective cohort study. Bhiwandiwala, Mumford, and Feldblum [5] have studied the short-term safety of several different methods of laparoscopic tubal sterilization using a prospective cohort design.

Case-control studies are always retrospective because exposure is determined by looking back, either by reviewing records or by asking subjects to recall exposure. Burkman et al. [7] used a case-control design to study IUD use and pelvic inflammatory disease (PID). The retrospective component of this study was an interview in which subjects were asked to recall their past general, contraceptive, and gynecologic histories.

The validity of the results of a study of contraceptive safety is not dependent on whether the study was cross-sectional, cohort, or case-control; retrospective or prospective; experimental or nonexperimental. That is, there are no magic properties attached to results of studies of one or another design. Rather, a study's results must be considered in relation to whether the study was conducted well; whether there were biases that account for the results; whether the investigators considered alternative explanations for their findings; and whether the data support the conclusions. Some advantages and disadvantages of the different types of studies are inherent in their design, however, and some designs have important limitations (Table 2-6).

The major advantage of an experimental study is that it is assumed that the random assignment of subjects to treatment or exposure assures that the groups are comparable for factors except the exposures that are known to influence or might influence development of the disease. Thus, when an investigator assigns women randomly to IUD and oral contraceptive use, it is assumed that the mean number of prior sexual partners, age, parity, and age at first intercourse are comparable in both groups. A difference in the rate at which women using the two methods of contraception develop cervical cancer could thus be attributed solely to use of the contraceptive method. A second advantage of experimental studies is the assignment of exposure before the onset of disease. The importance of this will become apparent in the discussion of case-control studies.

A major disadvantage of experimental studies is that they are expensive and time consuming. A very large number of subjects need to be studied to yield valid information on rare diseases. Rarely is it possible to assign methods randomly in experimental studies of the safety of fertility control methods. Even when methods are assigned randomly, the necessity for use of the methods for an amount of time sufficient to study late events limits the practical usefulness of this design for the study of safety.

The advantages of a cohort study are that exposure is determined before disease occurs; that many different

Table 2-6. Advantages, disadvantages, and limitations of different study designs

| | Nonexperimental | | | |
	Cohort	Case-control	Cross-sectional	Experimental
Advantages	Exposure defined before onset of disease Many different outcomes can be studied in the same group Relative safety of several methods can be compared	Relatively inexpensive Can be finished in a short time Rare diseases can be studied	Inexpensive Easy to conduct Can make use of existing data	Random assignment assures comparability on factors that affect disease outcome Exposure defined before onset of disease
Disadvantages and limitations	Expensive Time consuming Ability to detect associations is limited by number of subjects and frequency of the disease	Control selection subject to many biases Relative safety of different methods cannot be compared Ascertainment of exposure may be affected by knowledge of the presence of the disease No feeling about the frequency of the disease obtained directly	Time relationships uncertain Ascertainment of exposure may be affected by knowledge of presence of disease	Impossible to assign most fertility control methods randomly Expensive Time consuming Ability to detect associations limited by number of subjects and frequency of the disease

diseases can be studied in one effort; and that the relative safety of one or more methods of fertility control can be compared. In the Oxford Family Planning study [40], a cohort study, the relation of oral contraceptive use to a large number of diseases was determined. In addition, because approximately equal numbers of users of the IUD, the diaphragm, and oral contraceptives entered the study, the overall risk of morbidity and mortality according to use of the different methods was determined.

The principal disadvantage of cohort studies is their tendency to be expensive and time consuming. An exception is the conduct of retrospective cohort studies such as that of Walker et al. [44]. Here, the ability to identify easily a large group of men vasectomized in the past and to link this information by computer with information on hospitalizations allowed a cohort study to be carried out quickly and at low cost.

The most serious limitation of cohort studies is that practical constraints on the number of subjects who can be included make it impossible for the study to yield

definitive results on the relation between the exposure and the risk of rare diseases. For example, because vasectomy increases levels of circulating antisperm antibodies [2, 22], it would be interesting to know whether vasectomy increases the risk of systemic lupus erythematosus, which is an autoimmune disease. The incidence of the disease in men is probably less than 1 in 5000. A cohort study with equal numbers in vasectomized and nonvasectomized men would need almost 250,000 subjects to rule out with 90 percent confidence a twofold increase in the risk of the disease in vasectomized men. Recruiting this number of subjects would be extremely difficult and costly.

The major advantage of case-control studies is their ability to study rare diseases. In general, they are less expensive than cohort or experimental studies, and they usually can be completed in a shorter period of time.

The most obvious problem with case-control studies is that exposure is determined after the occurrence of disease, and this procedure may result in recall bias.

Recall bias is the tendency of subjects to recall or doctors to report the existence of an exposure because a diagnosis has been made. If a woman is diagnosed as having PID, for example, the attending physician may be more likely to ask about IUD use and to record its use in the medical chart. A case-control study that relied on medical records to determine IUD use and enrolled, for example, women with fractured legs as controls might well find a higher proportion of IUD users in PID cases. The difference could be because of the greater likelihood of women with PID to have been asked about IUD use. When the subjects in a case-control study are themselves asked about their exposure, cases, because they are ill, may be more likely to remember or to report their exposure. For example, in case-control studies of complications of pregnancy in relation to previous induced abortion, women with complications may be more likely to report their prior abortion to "explain" the complication.

Another disadvantage of case-control studies is the difficulty in designing them. For the results of a case-control study to be valid, the chances of being selected as a case or control must not be related to probability of exposure. It is not always easy to ensure this. To illustrate, take a study of cervical dysplasia and oral contraceptive use. Cervical dysplasia is generally diagnosed on the basis of a cytologic smear. For this reason, women with known cervical dysplasia are, by definition, users of medical care services. Users of medical care services may be more likely not only to get smears but also to use methods of fertility control such as oral contraceptives that require a visit to a physician. A control group that comprised women who were not as frequent users of medical services would not be appropriate for a case-control study of cervical dysplasia and oral contraceptive use: Fewer are likely to use oral contraceptives.

A limitation of case-control studies is the ability to study only one disease at a time. Another limitation is that estimates of risk derived from case-control studies make comparison of the relative safety of different methods of fertility control virtually impossible. For example, in a case-control study the Centers for Disease Control found that the risk of ovarian cancer was reduced by a factor of 2 in pill users [9]; several case-control studies have found that the risk of venous thromboembolism is elevated in oral contraceptive users by a factor of 8 to 10 [31, 42]. These case-control studies taken together do not yield information on whether, overall, oral contraceptives cause more disease than they prevent.

The advantages of a cross-sectional study are that they are inexpensive; they are easy to carry out; and they can often make use of existing data. Duguid, Parratt, and Traynor [11] did a cross-sectional study of the prevalence of *Actinomyces*-like organisms in users of IUDs and oral contraceptives. They determined rapidly and easily that the presence of this finding on Pap smear is confined to IUD users and, in them, the finding is strongly associated with increasing duration of IUD use.

Cross-sectional studies have two major disadvantages. First, the relationship between the exposure and the condition being studied is uncertain. Thus, it is possible, although improbable, that women with *Actinomyces*-like organisms on Pap smear had the IUD inserted because they had this finding. More realistic concerns related to temporal relationships arise in other settings. The second disadvantage is that, as in a case-control study, reporting of a given symptom or disease may be affected by having the exposure. For example, oral contraceptive users may be more likely to report weight gain in a cross-sectional survey because they "know" there is a relationship of weight gain to oral contraceptive use.

Risk

In analytic studies the term *risk* is used for measures of the magnitude of the association of an exposure or treatment with a disease or condition. It is important to know whether a difference in disease rate between users and nonusers of a fertility control method is large or small. The size of the probability value (*p*) associated with a statistical test of significance does not measure the size of an association. That is, a study with a statistically more significant *p* value, say $p = .0001$, has not found a larger association than a study with a statistically less significant *p* value, say $p = .05$. This point is illustrated in Table 2-7 using hypothetical data.

In the hypothetical example, two separate studies were done, each comparing the rate of uterine perforation for two different methods of laparoscopic sterilization, called methods A and B. In study 1 the perforation rates for methods A and B are statisically significantly different; *p* is equal to .04. In study 2 the perforation rates for methods A and B are also statistically significantly different; *p* is equal to .00001. Yet the perforation rates for methods A and B are identical in the two studies. The "risk" of method B is higher by the same amount, even though the value is more statistically significant in study 2. This example illustrates the need for measures of risk that are not dependent on the results of a statistical test.

A number of methods with this property have been proposed and are in general use. Fleiss [14] discusses many of them critically. Fortunately, in analytic studies of the safety of fertility control methods, attributable risk, relative risk, and the odds ratio are used almost exclusively to measure the size of associations.

Table 2-7. Hypothetical studies of uterine perforation rates for two methods of laparoscopic sterilization

| | Study 1 | | Study 2 | |
	Method A	Method B	Method A	Method B
Number of procedures	1,000	1,000	5,000	5,000
Number of perforations	2	10	10	50
Rate of perforation*	2.0	10.0	2.0	10.0
Probability value for statistical test *(p)*		.04		.00001

*Per 1,000 procedures.

Table 2-8. Calculation of the odds ratio

	With disease (case)	Without disease (control)
Exposed	a	b
Not exposed	c	d
	Odds ratio = (a × d) ÷ (b × c)	

Attributable risk is the difference in incidence or mortality between the exposed and the unexposed or an estimate of this difference. Attributable risk is calculated directly using data from a cohort study; methods to estimate it using data from a case-control study are also available [45, 46]. Relative risk is the ratio of incidence or mortality in the exposed or unexposed; it is calculated using data from a cohort study. The odds ratio is calculated as shown in Table 2-8; it is used to estimate relative risk using data from a case-control or a cross-sectional study.

Attributable risk has an easy intuitive interpretation: It is the amount of the disease among the exposed that can be attributed uniquely to the exposure. For example, in 1974 the incidence of cerebrovascular disease in oral contraceptive users enrolled in the Oxford Family Planning study was 43 per 100,000 woman-years; in users of the diaphragm, it was 6 per 100,000 woman-years [40]. The attributable risk of cerebrovascular disease in oral contraceptive users is calculated by subtracting the incidence in diaphragm users from that in oral contraceptive users: It is 37 per 100,000. This quantity is interpreted to mean that 37 of 43 cases of cerebrovascular disease in a group of 100,000 oral contraceptive users can be attributed directly to oral contraceptive use.

Relative risk and the odds ratio do not have as easy an intuitive interpretation as attributable risk. In the preceding example, the relative risk of cerebrovascular disease in oral contraceptive users is calculated by dividing the incidence in oral contraceptive users by the incidence in diaphragm users: It is 7.2. This quantity is interpreted to mean that the chances of developing cerebrovascular disease are 7.2 times higher in oral contraceptive users than in diaphragm users. An odds ratio of this magnitude would have the same interpretation.

Putting relative risk and odds ratio estimates in proper perspective in the absence of information on the rate of the disease in the population can be difficult. For example, Rooks et al. [28] did a case-control study of hepatocellular adenoma and oral contraceptive use. From their data an odds ratio of 12.5 for oral contraceptive use of more than 1 year can be calculated, implying that the chances of developing hepatocellular adenoma are 12.5 times higher in oral contraceptive users than in nonusers. Sartwell et al. [31] did a case-control study of venous thromboembolism and oral contraceptive use. In their study an odds ratio of 4.4 for current oral contraceptive use can be calculated, implying that the chances of developing venous thromboembolism are 4.4 times higher in oral contraceptive users than in nonusers. The incidence of hepatocellular adenoma and venous thromboembolism in oral contraceptive nonusers is probably different by at least a factor of 10, however, and comparison of the odds ratios can be misleading for this reason. To illustrate why, assume an incidence of hepatocellular adenoma in nonusers of oral contraceptives of .00001 and an incidence of venous thromboembolism of .0001. In this case there would be 11 "extra" cases of hepatocellular adenoma and 102 "extra" cases of venous thromboembolism in 1 million oral contraceptive users based on the odds ratios. Yet the largeness of the odds ratio for hepatocellular adenoma makes this disease seem the greater "risk" of oral contraceptive use. If a disease is very rare, even with a high relative risk or odds ratio, few of those who are exposed will develop the disease. If a disease is common, even a small relative risk or odds ratio may translate to many more cases of the disease in those who are exposed.

Significance Tests and Confidence Intervals

The purpose of a test of statistical significance is to decide whether what is observed could have occurred by chance. Statistical significance testing is based on the theory of probability, whose fundamentals can be grasped intuitively. Imagine, for example, that one observes a coin being tossed 20 times and that all the tosses are heads. The intuitive suspicion is that this coin is not a fair coin. A formal statistical test of this suspicion could be performed, basing the test on probability theory. In this example the chances of observing 20 heads in 20 tosses of a fair coin—that is, a coin with an equal chance of heads and tails—are less than 1 in 1 million (0.5^{20}). Thus, the observed event—20 heads in 20 tosses—is unlikely to be due to chance.

The question asked by the observer in the coin tossing example is analogous to the question asked by an investigator who, in a study of glucose tolerance, observes a 1-hour glucose concentration of 139.5 mg per deciliter in oral contraceptive users and one of 132.1 mg per deciliter in nonusers of oral contraceptives [47]. That is, could the observed difference in 1-hour glucose concentration between oral contraceptive users and nonusers be due to chance? If, based on a statistical test, the difference is not likely to be due to chance, the investigator may then offer another explanation for the observation.

A large number of statistical tests exist. Commonly used statistics can be divided broadly into those that are parametric and those that are nonparametric. Tests based on parametric statistics require that assumptions about the distribution of the factor being studied be met. Tests based on nonparametric statistics make no assumptions about the distribution of the factor being studied. The most commonly used parametric and nonparametric statistics and some of their uses are shown in Table 2-9. The details for calculating these statistics in order to perform a test of significance can be obtained in statistical texts [3, 35].

Understanding the mechanics of the calculation of a statistic and the procedure for performing the test is less important to the critical interpretation of information from analytic studies than is an appreciation for the limitations of significance testing. Most important, a statistically significant result does not establish the truth of the investigator's hypothesis. Conversely, the absence of a statistically significant result does not prove that the hypothesis is false. Last, statistical significance does not necessarily mean biologic importance.

To illustrate the first point, that a statistically significant result does not prove the investigator's hypothesis, return to the coin tossing example. The observer's hypothesis is that the coin is not fair. Based on the formal statistical test, the observer concludes that 20 heads in 20 tosses is not likely to be due to chance. The performance of the statistical test and the unlikeliness of chance as an explanation of the observation do not, however, prove that the coin is not fair.

Similarly, in the study of serum glucose concentration, Wingerd and Duffy [47] found that the difference in 1-hour glucose concentrations between oral contraceptive users and nonusers was statistically significant. Based on the results of the statistical test, the investigators can properly conclude that the difference in glucose concentration is not likely to be due to chance. It would be incorrect to conclude on the basis of the statistical test that oral contraceptive use raises 1-hour serum glucose concentration, however.

To illustrate the second point, that the absence of statistical significance does not prove that the hypothesis is false, imagine a second coin tossing experiment. In this experiment, the same coin is tossed only three times, and all three tosses are heads. Could the observation of three heads in three tosses of a fair coin be due to chance? A formal statistical test would yield a probability of three heads in three tosses of a fair coin of 0.13; thus, three heads in three tosses could be due to chance. However, one cannot conclude on the basis of the statistical test that the coin *is* fair. Similarly, if in the previously mentioned study of 1-hour glucose concentration and oral contraceptive use, the difference in concentration had not been statistically significant, it would be an error to conclude on the basis of the statistical test that oral contraceptive use is unrelated to 1-hour glucose concentration. Rather, one can conclude that chance cannot be ruled out as an explanation for the difference.

To illustrate the third point, that statistical significance does not necessarily mean biologic importance, take as an example a study of selected physiologic measures in men with and without vasectomy [21]. In the study the mean serum potassium concentration in 4,385 men with a prior vasectomy was 4.6 mEq per liter; in 13,155 men without vasectomy the mean potassium concentration was 4.5 mEq per liter. The difference in

Table 2-9. Commonly used statistical tests

Statistics test	Use
Parametric	
t	To compare the difference in two means
F	To compare the difference in variances of two or more groups
Nonparametric	
X^2	To compare the difference in proportions or to test for association in tables
McNemar	To compare the difference in two proportions when groups are related or when there are "before" and "after" measures
Fisher's Exact	To compare the difference in two proportions when the numbers are very small

potassium concentration was highly statistically significant ($p < .0001$). Hence the difference is unlikely to be due to chance, although, in keeping with the first point, the statistical test does not establish that vasectomy causes an increase in serum potassium. More important, even if vasectomy did cause an increase in serum potassium of 0.1 mEq per liter, this increase probably is not of biologic importance.

Interpretation of the results of analytic studies requires not only recognition of the limitations of statistical tests of significance but also an appreciation of the concept of the confidence interval. A confidence interval is a formal expression of the uncertainty attached to an estimate of a mean, a relative risk, an odds ratio, or a proportion [3]. A confidence interval is specified as two numbers, the lower and the upper bound of the interval, and a probability value, which by convention is usually 90 or 95 percent.

The formal statistical interpretation of the 95 percent confidence interval is that, if a study were repeated many times, over the long run 95 percent of the confidence intervals would include the true value of the mean, relative risk, odds ratio, or proportion. The more common but formally less correct interpretation of a confidence interval is that the true mean, relative risk, odds ratio, or proportion has a 95 percent chance of being within the interval. The common interpretation is a useful way of thinking about confidence intervals, despite its being formally less correct.

Table 2-10 shows the results of three studies of the long-term safety of two methods of fertility control [7, 8, 27]. In the first study the odds ratio estimate is more than 1, suggesting an increase in the chances of developing the disease in users of the method. In the other two studies the odds ratio estimates are near 1, implying no increase in the chances of developing the disease in users. Inspection and understanding of the meaning of the 95 percent confidence intervals for the odds ratio estimates yield a more accurate interpretation of the studies. Thus, in the study by Burkman et al. [7] of pelvic inflammatory disease and IUD use the 95 percent interval for the odds ratio has a lower bound of 1.8 and an upper bound of 2.5. Based on the narrowness of this interval, one can be fairly certain that the true risk of PID in IUD users is close to 2.

In contrast, in the study by Ramcharan et al. [27] of acute myocardial infarction and oral contraceptive use the 95 percent confidence interval has a lower bound of 0.4 and an upper bound of 11.5. The wideness of this interval indicates the large uncertainty associated with this study's estimate of the chances of developing an acute myocardial infarction in oral contraceptive users compared with nonusers. On the basis of this study alone, because of the wide confidence interval, it cannot be concluded that the risk of myocardial infarction is not increased in oral contraceptive users. In contrast, in the Centers for Disease Control study [8] of breast cancer and oral contraceptive use the confidence interval has a lower bound of 0.9 and an upper bound of 1.3. Based on this study and the narrowness of the confidence interval, it can be concluded with considerable certainty that the risk of breast cancer is not increased in oral contraceptive users overall.

Problem of Bias

Bias means distortion; bias in research produces a distortion of the truth. An appreciation of how bias may arise is essential to the critical evaluation of all medical literature, but it is particularly important in weighing the validity of studies of contraceptive safety. Sackett [30] has catalogued 35 biases that arise in analytic studies. Table 2-11 lists the biases that are most common in studies of the safety of fertility control methods.

The first common bias in studies of the safety of fertility control methods is negative results bias. This refers to the tendency of authors to report and journals to publish positive results more frequently than negative results. Negative results may not even be of interest until positive results have been published. Thus, a study that shows that tubal sterilization is not associated with atherosclerosis in humans is less likely to be published than a study that shows vasectomy is not associated with atherosclerosis, because positive results in animals have been reported for vasectomy [1] but not for tubal sterilization. It is also probably the case that a

Table 2-10. Risk estimates and confidence intervals in three studies of long-term contraceptive safety

Study	Subject of study	Estimated risk	95% confidence interval for estimated risk
Burkman et al. [7]	PID and IUD use	2.1	1.8, 2.5
Ramcharan et al. [27]	Acute myocardial infarction and oral contraceptive use	1.1	0.4, 11.5
Centers for Disease Control [8]	Breast cancer and oral contraceptive use	1.1	0.9, 1.3

IUD = intrauterine device; PID = pelvic inflammatory disease.

Table 2-11. Biases most commonly encountered in studies of the safety of fertility control methods

Positive results bias

No or improper control group bias

Noncontemporaneous control group bias

Misclassification bias

Small sample size bias

Diagnostic suspicion bias

Source: After D. L. Sackett. Bias in analytic research. *J. Chronic Dis.* 32:51, 1979.

negative result following a positive result tends to be published in a journal of lesser stature, causing the negative result to carry less scientific weight. The overall effect of negative results bias is for the medical literature to be weighted with positive results, often in prestigious medical journals. This gives a false impression of the overall safety of fertility control methods.

The second common bias arises from the absence of a control group or from the use of an inappropriate control group. Some early studies of IUD safety concluded that the rate of PID was not elevated in IUD users based largely on anecdotal observations that the rate of PID appeared to be the same in IUD users as in the clinical practices of the investigators or in hospitals. On the basis of the observation that 71 percent of women with amenorrhea and hyperprolactinemia who were treated for a pituitary adenoma had used oral contraceptives, Sherman et al. [33] concluded that oral contraceptives were a likely causal agent. In both these instances proper control groups were not used. In the first case, the "control" was a vague notion of PID rates in a not necessarily comparable population. In the second case the proportion of users of oral contraceptives among women without a pituitary adenoma was not determined. Subsequent research with proper control groups has shown an increased risk of PID in IUD users [7, 12, 13, 15, 17, 19, 40] and no relationship of oral contraceptive use to pituitary adenomas [10, 48]. Choice of a proper control group for an analytic study is one of the most difficult areas for researchers in the field.

A related bias is noncontemporaneous control group bias. This bias arises when changes over time in definitions, diseases, or treatments occur, rendering a historic comparison invalid. This bias is particularly problematic in studies that attempt to correlate trends in exposures over time with trends in disease rates over time, as the presumption of such studies is that everything else has remained the same. Wiseman and Macrae [49] analyzed data on mortality from all circulatory disease in women aged 15 to 44 in England and Wales

from 1957 through 1976 and found a decline from 36.8 per 100,000 to 21.7 per 100,000. They concluded that, because oral contraceptive use had increased over this time whereas mortality had declined, oral contraceptive use did not increase mortality from circulatory disease. This conclusion ignores the possibility that changes in mortality from cardiovascular diseases unassociated with oral contraceptive use may have occurred; or that treatment may have altered the probability of mortality, given the existence of the disease. The possibility of bias from use of a noncontemporaneous control group should always be considered as an explanation of results of trend studies.

Misclassification bias occurs when the investigator's classification of exposure or disease is erroneous. Of course, an investigator does not purposely misclassify subjects. Misclassification may arise because the test used to define disease is flawed or because the method for determining exposure has error. The Pap smear, for example, is known to have a high error rate [18]. In a study of cervical neoplasia that is based on the results of a single Pap smear, some women with neoplasia will be misclassified as having no disease because their Pap smears are falsely negative. Other disease-free women will be classified as having the disease because their Pap smears are falsely positive. Similarly, exposure may be misclassified in a study of prior induced abortion that relies on patient reports because some subjects may deny having had a prior abortion. In general, misclassification of either disease or exposure tends to compromise the ability of a study to reveal a true association [6].

Small sample size bias arises when the number of subjects is too small to demonstrate an association even if one, in truth, exists. The problem was discussed earlier with regard to the disadvantages of cohort studies. Erroneous conclusions based on too small a sample can be avoided by more reliance for conclusions on inspection of the confidence interval.

Membership bias arises when membership in one group may imply a degree of health that differs systematically from that in the general population. For example, users of barrier methods of contraception may be more health conscious than users of other contraceptive methods. They may, therefore, have a set of habits and behaviors that put them at less risk for many diseases. When a disease rate in users of other contraceptive methods is compared with the disease rate in them, it may be higher not because of the use of the contraceptive method but because of the difference in habits and behaviors.

Diagnostic suspicion bias arises when knowledge of a person's exposure affects the interpretation or outcome of the diagnosis process. If knowledge that a woman is an oral contraceptive user leads a physician to do a lung scan in the presence of chest pain, then cases of pulmonary embolism based on the presence of a positive lung scan may be biased, oral contraceptive users being overrepresented. Diagnostic suspicion bias may even become diagnostic certainty bias when a diagnosis is made because of a particular exposure. Further studies of PID and IUD use in the 1980s may be particularly prone to this bias because some physicians would consider pelvic pain, IUD use, and fever to determine PID. The question of pituitary adenomas in relation to oral contraceptive use is yet another example of a subject for which care must be taken to consider diagnostic suspicion bias. A woman with postpill amenorrhea may be more likely to have an extensive workup for an adenoma than a woman with amenorrhea who does not use an oral contraceptive.

In this chapter examples have been used to help the reader become more discerning when reading the literature on contraceptive efficacy and safety rates. Proper patient counseling has as its first prerequisite a well-informed health provider capable of accurate interpretation of the literature.

REFERENCES

1. Alexander, N. J., and Clarkson, T. B. Vasectomy increases the severity of diet-induced atherosclerosis in *Macaca fascicularis. Science* 201:538, 1978.
2. Ansbacher, R. Sperm agglutinating and sperm immobilizing antibodies in vasectomized men. *Fertil. Steril.* 22:629, 1971.
3. Armitage, P. *Statistical Methods in Medical Research.* Oxford: Blackwell, 1980.
4. Azen, S. P., et al. Some suggested improvements to current statistical methods of analyzing contraceptive efficacy. *J. Chronic Dis.* 29:649, 1976.
5. Bhiwandiwala, P. P., Mumford, S. D., and Feldblum, P. J. A comparison of different laparoscopic sterilization occlusion techniques in 24,439 procedures. *Am. J. Obstet. Gynecol.* 144:319, 1982.
6. Bross, I. Misclassification in 2 × 2 tables. *Biometrics* 10:478, 1954.
7. Burkman, R. T., and The Women's Health Study. Association between intrauterine device and pelvic inflammatory disease. *Obstet. Gynecol.* 57:269, 1981.
8. The Centers for Disease Control Cancer and Steroid Hormone Study. Long-term oral contraceptive use and the risk of breast cancer. *J.A.M.A.* 249:1591, 1983.
9. The Centers for Disease Control Cancer and Steroid Hormone Study. Oral contraceptive use and the risk of ovarian cancer. *J.A.M.A.* 249:1596, 1983.
10. Coulam, C. B., et al. Pituitary adenoma and oral contraceptives: A case-control study. *Fertil. Steril.* 31:25, 1979.

11. Duguid, H. L. D., Parratt, D., and Traynor, R. *Actinomyces*-like organisms in cervical smears from women using intrauterine contraceptive devices. *Br. Med. J.* 281:534, 1980.
12. Eschenbach, D. A., Harnisch, J. P., and Holmes, K. K. Pathogenesis of acute pelvic inflammatory disease: Role of contraception and other risk factors. *Am. J. Obstet. Gynecol.* 128:838, 1977.
13. Faulkner, W. L., and Ory, H. W. Intrauterine devices and acute pelvic inflammatory disease. *J.A.M.A.* 235:1851, 1976.
14. Fleiss, J. L. *Statistical Methods for Rates and Proportions* (2nd ed.). New York: Wiley, 1981.
15. Flesh, G., et al. The intrauterine contraceptive device and acute salpingitis: A multifactor analysis. *Am. J. Obstet. Gynecol.* 135:402, 1979.
16. Jain, A. K., and Sivin, I. Life-table anaylsis of IUDs: Problems and recommendations. *Stud. Fam. Plann.* 8:26, 1977.
17. Kaufman, D. W., et al. Intrauterine contraceptive device use and pelvic inflammatory disease. *Am. J. Obstet. Gynecol.* 136:159, 1980.
18. Maisel, F. J., et al. Papanicolaou smear, biopsy, and conization of the cervix: An evaluation of their reliability in the diagnosis of cervical cancer. *Am. J. Obstet. Gynecol.* 86:931, 1963.
19. Osser, S., Liedholm, P., and Sjoberg, N.-O. Risk of pelvic inflammatory disease among users of intrauterine devices, irrespective of previous pregnancy. *Am. J. Obstet. Gynecol.* 138:864, 1980.
20. Pearl, R. Factors in human fertility and their statistical evaluation. *Lancet* 225:607, 1933.
21. Petitti, D. B., et al. Physiologic measures in men with and without vasectomies. *Fertil. Steril.* 37:438, 1982.
22. Phadke, A. M., and Padukone, K. Presence and significance of autoantibodies against spermatozoa in the blood of men with obstructed vas deferens. *J. Reprod. Fertil.* 7:163, 1964.
23. Potter, R. G. Length of observation as a factor affecting the contraceptive failure rate. *Milbank Mem. Fund Q.* 38:140, 1960.
24. Potter, R. G. Additional measures of use-effectiveness of contraception. *Milbank Mem. Fund Q.* 41:400, 1963.
25. Potter, R. G. Application of life table techniques to measurement of contraceptive effectiveness. *Demography* 3:297, 1966.
26. Potter, R. G. Use-effectiveness of Intrauterine Contraception as a Problem in Competing Risks. In R. Freedman and J. Y. Takeshita (eds.), *Family Planning in Taiwan.* Princeton: Princeton University Press, 1969.
27. Ramcharan, S., et al. *The Walnut Creek Contraceptive Drug Study* (Vol. III). NIH Publication No. 81-564, Jan., 1981.
28. Rooks, J. B., et al. The association between oral contraception and hepatocellular adenoma: A preliminary report. *Int. J. Gynaecol. Obstet.* 15:143, 1977.

29. Royal College of General Practitioners. *Oral Contraceptives and Health*. London: Pitman Medical, 1974.
30. Sackett, D. L. Bias in analytic research. *J. Chronic. Dis.* 32:51, 1979.
31. Sartwell, P. E., et al. Thromboembolism and oral contraceptives: An epidemiologic case-control study. *Am. J. Epidemiol.* 90:365, 1969.
32. Sheps, M. C. On the person years concept in epidemiology and demography. *Milbank Mem. Fund Q.* 44:69, 1966.
33. Sherman, B. M., et al. Pathogenesis of prolactin-secreting pituitary adenomas. *Lancet* 2:1019, 1978.
34. Sivin, I., and Stern, J. Long-acting, more effective TCu IUDs. A summary of U.S. experience 1970–1975. *Stud. Fam. Plann.* 10:263, 1979.
35. Swinscow, T. D. V. *Statistics at Square One* (4th ed.). London: The Mendip Press, 1978.
36. Tietze, C. Differential fecundity and effectiveness of contraception. *Eugenics Review* 50:231, 1959.
37. Tietze, C. Intrauterine contraception: Recommended procedures for analysis. *Stud. Fam. Plann.* (Suppl. 18):1, 1967.
38. Tietze, C., and Lewitt, S. Recommended procedures for the statistical evaluation of intrauterine contraception. *Stud. Fam. Plann.* 4:35, 1973.
39. Vaughan, B., et al. Contraceptive failure among married women in the United States, 1970–1973. *Fam. Plann. Perspect.* 9:251, 1977.
40. Vessey, M., et al. A long-term follow-up study of women using different methods of contraception: An interim report. *J. Biosoc. Sci.* 8:373, 1976.
41. Vessey, M. P., et al. Pelvic inflammatory disease and the intrauterine device: Findings in a large cohort study. *Br. Med. J.* 282:855, 1981.
42. Vessey, M. P., and Doll, R. Investigation of relation between use of oral contraceptives and thromboembolic disease. *Br. Med. J.* 1:199, 1968.
43. Vessey, M. P., Lawless, M., and Yeates, D. Efficacy of different contraceptive methods. *Lancet* 1:841, 1982.
44. Walker, A. M., et al. Hospitalization rates in vasectomized men. *J.A.M.A.* 245:2315, 1981.
45. Walter, S. D. The estimation and interpretation of attributable risk in health research. *Biometrics* 32:829, 1976.
46. Whittemore, A. S. Estimating attributable risk from case-control studies. *Am. J. Epidemiol.* 117:76, 1983.
47. Wingerd, J., and Duffy, T. J. Oral contraceptive use and other factors in the standard glucose tolerance test. *Diabetes* 26:1024, 1977.
48. Wingrave, S. J., Kay, C. R., and Vessey, M. P. Oral contraceptives and pituitary adenomas. *Br. Med. J.* 280:685, 1980.
49. Wiseman, R. A., and Macrae, K. D. Oral contraceptives and the decline in mortality from circulatory disease. *Fertil. Steril.* 35:277, 1981.

BIBLIOGRAPHY

Armitage, P. *Statistical Methods in Medical Research*. Oxford: Blackwell, 1980.

Fleiss, J. L. *Statistical Methods for Rates and Proportions* (2nd ed.). New York: Wiley, 1981.

Fletcher, R. H., Fletcher, S. W., and Wagner, E. H. *Clinical Epidemiology—The Essentials*. Baltimore: Williams & Wilkins, 1982.

Friedman, G. D. *Primer of Epidemiology* (2nd ed.). New York: McGraw-Hill, 1980.

Glantz, S. A. *Primer of Biostatistics*. New York: McGraw-Hill, 1981.

Lillienfeld, A. M., and Lillienfeld, D. E. *Foundations of Epidemiology* (2nd ed.). New York: Oxford University Press, 1980.

Schlesselman, J. J. *Case-Control Studies: Design, Conduct, Analysis*. New York: Oxford University Press, 1982.

Swinscow, T. D. V. *Statistics at Square One* (4th ed.). London: The Mendip Press, 1978.

3. Medicolegal Issues and Risk Reduction in Family Planning Practice

Jill A. Cobrin
Janet E. Kornblatt
Louise B. Tyrer
Stephen S. York

THE SPECTER OF MEDICAL MALPRACTICE IN THE SPECIALTY OF OBSTETRICS AND GYNECOLOGY: AN OVERVIEW

The current trend in medical malpractice litigation represents nothing less than a full-blown assault on the specialty of obstetrics and gynecology. More than the practitioner of almost any other medical specialty, it is the obstetrician/gynecologist who is at risk of being sued for medical malpractice. As of this writing, there are 24 recognized medical specialties in the United States represented by separate specialty boards. If the medicolegal risk in the practice of medicine were evenly distributed among the various specialties, each specialty should account for 4.16 percent of the total risk. The unfortunate truth for the obstetrician/gynecologist is that this is simply not the case.

In September of 1980 the National Association of Insurance Commissioners (NAIC) published the results of a study of 71,782 medical malpractice claims closed by insurance companies in the United States between July 1975 and December 1978. This resulted in a finding that 12.6 percent of all the claims included in the study were attributable to the specialty of obstetrics and gynecology. Further, it was found that these claims accounted for 14.3 percent of the total indemnity paid for all claims [13].

More recently, one of the largest commercial insurance companies in the United States which insures medical professional liability reviewed 3,574 medical malpractice claims opened between May 1982 and March 1983. This study [8] found that 19.9 percent of the claims involved the specialty of obstetrics and gynecology and that these claims were responsible for 23.4 percent of the total claims cost (indemnity paid on closed claims and indemnity reserves for open claims).

The question remains as to why the obstetrician/gynecologist is invariably the favorite target of plaintiffs' attorneys. The answer to this appears to lie in the fact that treatment rendered by the practitioners of this particular specialty is known to result in injuries that involve very significant monetary potential. For example, it is this specialty that is responsible for birth-related injuries, including the potentially devastating case of the brain-damaged infant. The NAIC study found that the average indemnity payment for claims involving birth-related injuries was $219,752 in 1978. Today, litigated cases involving these injuries frequently result in both settlements and verdicts well in excess of $1 million.

THE MEDICOLEGAL RISKS OF FAMILY PLANNING PRACTICE

While the specific practice of family planning medicine is not usually implicated in the causation of birth-

27

related and other injuries that generally involve the practice of obstetrics, it is known to produce other types of injuries that also involve very significant monetary potential. For example, hysterectomy is a frequently litigated injury in this area of practice, and the case of a young woman in the prime of her childbearing years who has sustained the permanent loss of her reproductive capacity is a highly significant case indeed. Another example is the increasing incidence of litigation involving the rather significant claims known as wrongful life, wrongful birth, and wrongful conception. Thus, the practitioner of family planning medicine should not assume that this area of practice is low risk in terms of the possibility of being sued for medical malpractice.

As a general rule, medical malpractice claims in family planning medicine can be separated into two broad categories, those involving surgical treatment and those involving nonsurgical treatment. For the purposes of the following discussion, the first category will include abortion procedures and male and female sterilization procedures. Of course, the practice of family planning medicine does involve the performance of other types of surgical procedures, including diagnostic laparoscopy and diagnostic colposcopy to name but two. However, it is the experience of the authors that claims in the category of surgical treatment are largely limited to abortion and sterilization procedures.

The category of nonsurgical treatment will include contraceptive treatment and errors of diagnosis. Again, however, this category is fairly self-limiting insofar as claims involving contraceptive treatment are concerned. Of all the available methods of birth control, it is the authors' experience that only oral contraceptives and intrauterine devices (IUDs) result in any significant number of medical malpractice claims. Such claims involving the so-called barrier methods are few and far between and in the opinion of the authors statistically insignificant.

CLAIMS INVOLVING SURGICAL TREATMENT

Abortion Procedures

When considering the medicolegal risks inherent in the performance of abortion procedures, it is important to distinguish the typical first-trimester suction curettage procedure from the more technically difficult second-trimester procedures such as dilatation and evacuation (D&E) and the various amnioinfusion techniques. Claims that result from second-trimester procedures generally involve injuries that are more significant from a medicolegal standpoint. This is not to say that claims that relate to first-trimester procedures do not involve

significant injuries. However, the percentage of significant claims appears to be higher with second-trimester procedures.

With respect to first-trimester procedures, based on the experience of the authors the most frequent claim is that of incomplete abortion. Fortunately, such claims are relatively insignificant from the standpoint of monetary potential as they usually involve only a minimal amount of subsequent treatment with no claim of permanent injury. Data from the NAIC study show that the average indemnity payment for all claims in that study involving suction curettage abortion procedures was $26,927. However, this was only $7,791 when the claimed injury was an incomplete abortion.

Claims for postabortion hemorrhage are much less frequent than those for incomplete abortion, and they are also relatively insignificant in terms of severity. The average indemnity payment for such claims in the NAIC study was $10,179.

The most serious claims in the context of first-trimester abortion procedures are also the most infrequent; these are the claims involving operative trauma to the uterus and other abdominal organs, usually the small bowel. Of course, the typical case of a minor uterine perforation, which involves a 24-hour hospital admission for observation and results in spontaneous closure of the defect without surgical repair, is not a serious claim. However, when the perforation is of major proportions such that a hysterectomy is necessary, the resulting claim must be considered as having significant severity. In the NAIC study claims for hysterectomy following operative trauma had an average indemnity payment of $84,063. When the trauma also involves the small bowel such that a bowel resection is necessary, the severity of the claim is, of course, even greater. These types of claims involve significant monetary potential because of the permanent disability that follows the underlying injury. In the case of a hysterectomy the patient's reproductive capacity is obviously compromised on a permanent basis. If a bowel resection has been necessary, then the result can be a claim of permanent lower gastrointestinal problems, and this is particularly true if the resection has resulted in the removal of a significant portion of terminal ileum.

Claims involving second-trimester abortion procedures are much more infrequent than those involving first-trimester procedures, and this is undoubtedly a function of relative performance frequency. However, these claims generally involve greater severity than those from first-trimester procedures because the injuries are usually more significant. In the case of D&E procedures, the most frequently claimed injury is abdominal trauma with subsequent surgical repair. Amnioinfusion procedures have never accounted for a very significant percentage of abortion-related claims;

however, it is these procedures that have been responsible for most of the very few abortion-related wrongful death claims.

Female Sterilization Procedures

In the experience of the authors, claims involving tubal ligation procedures are less frequent than those involving first-trimester abortion procedures. As a general rule, they also seem to be less severe, and this appears to be confirmed by the NAIC study, which found that the average indemnity payment for a tubal ligation claim was $14,495.

There are, of course, a myriad of medically accepted procedures for the performance of a bilateral tubal ligation. However, the two techniques that appear to account for the vast majority of claims are the laparoscopic technique and the minilaparotomy. Accordingly, the following discussion will focus on the medicolegal risks inherent in the these two techniques.

According to the current medical literature, laparoscopic tubal ligation has become the most popular method of interval female sterilization in the United States. As such, it is not surprising that it has also become the most popular subject of sterilization malpractice litigation among plaintiffs' attorneys. Whether the procedure is performed by coagulation of the fallopian tubes by electrical current or the application of occlusive clips or rings, it is known to have a recognized failure rate. A small percentage of the claims involving the laparoscopic technique are based on a failure of the procedure; however, the majority involve traumatic and electrical injuries to abdominal viscera.

Traumatic injury to abdominal viscera can occur with any of the techniques that are currently in use for the performance of laparoscopic sterilization. However, claims experience indicates that these types of injuries occur more frequently in closed laparoscopy rather than with open laparoscopy, and this would seem to be a result of the fact that closed laparoscopy involves blind entry into the abdomen. The traumatic intraabdominal injuries that are known to occur during closed laparoscopy are almost always caused by one of the two instruments that are used in this procedure, namely, the pneumoperitoneum needle or the sharp pyramidal trocar. Given the claims that have resulted from the performance of this procedure, it can fairly be said that almost every structure in the abdomen is subject to injury by the needle or trocar. Most claims involve injury to the uterus, small bowel, and urinary bladder. However, a smaller number of claims have also involved injury to the colon, bowel mesentery, stomach, and both major and minor blood vessels. Subsequent surgical repair of such injuries is essential.

With respect to electrical injuries to abdominal vis-

cera, claims experience indicates that this situation almost always involves inadvertent radio-frequency burns of the small bowel. There have been some claims in which electrical current was directly applied to an anatomic structure other than the fallopian tube. However, the vast majority of claims of electrical injury represent inadvertent bowel burns, and almost all of these appear to be caused by the electrosurgical equipment itself rather than operator error.

The incidence of claims for bowel burns seems to have decreased since bipolar laparoscopic equipment began to replace the unipolar equipment that was originally developed. However, the bipolar equipment seems to have a higher failure rate due to decreased voltage and lower frequency current, and the authors are aware that many physicians now prefer to use the more advanced unipolar equipment that utilizes a low-voltage, high-frequency current and a floating or isolated ground system. Unfortunately, regardless of the technological improvements that have been made in laparoscopic equipment inadvertent bowel burns still occur, and they still result in malpractice claims.

Claims with respect to bilateral tubal ligation by means of minilaparotomy rarely involve an intraabdominal injury, and this is to be expected, given the fact that generally the fallopian tube is delivered through the surgical incision such that there is only a minimum of instrumentation within the peritoneal cavity itself. Rather, most claims that result from minilaparotomy sterilization involve a failure of the procedure resulting in a subsequent pregnancy. Claims experience indicates that these failures are occasionally caused by the ligation of an anatomic structure other than the fallopian tube, such as the round ligament. More frequently, such failures are the result of a recanalization of the tube, and it is not infrequent that this situation may be attributable to poor technique on the part of the surgeon.

Male Sterilization Procedures

The number of claims that result from vasectomy procedures is quite minimal, and it is fair to say that the male sterilization procedure represents the lowest medicolegal risk in the practice of family planning medicine. It is the authors' experience that almost all vasectomy claims involve the two primary complications of the procedure, namely, postoperative hematoma and postoperative infection. Such claims are clearly insignificant in terms of their monetary potential when they are compared to the mainstream of medical malpractice litigation. In fact, the NAIC study found that the average indemnity payment for vasectomy claims was $7,624, a figure that is even less than the average indemnity payment for an incomplete abortion.

There are, however, a small number of vasectomy claims that involve more than minimal monetary potential. These are the claims in which one or both of the patient's testicles are damaged by either disruption of the vascular supply to the testicle or damage to the spermatic plexus nerve. The resulting damage to the testicle generally varies from testicular atrophy to surgical removal of the injured organ. In either case, the claim carries more significant monetary potential. Adherence to postoperative semen testing protocols avoids most cases of litigation for failure to sterilize.

The Medicolegal Implications of a Failed Family Planning Surgical Procedure

With increasing incidence the failure of a family planning surgical procedure is known to result in the initiation of a medical malpractice claim. When an abortion procedure is ineffective such that the pregnancy continues or when a sterilization procedure fails resulting in a subsequent conception, the patient has the option of either terminating the pregnancy or continuing with it. If the pregnancy is terminated and a claim results, the situation is one of rather limited monetary potential. If, however, the pregnancy continues and results in the birth of a living infant, the practitioner faces the possibility of a claim for wrongful life, wrongful birth, or wrongful conception. As such, any discussion of the medicolegal risks in the practice of family planning medicine would be inadequate without consideration of these relatively new legal issues.

Wrongful life and wrongful birth claims involve an infant who has been born in a deformed or defective condition. Until recently, the two claims were not distinguished semantically, and the term *wrongful life* was used to denominate any claim in this regard whether it was brought by the infant or the parents. Recent case law has drawn a distinction, and a claim for wrongful life is now said to be the infant's claim for being born in the first instance. The parents' claim is denominated as *wrongful birth*, and the basis for this claim is the parents' allegation that, had they known of the possibility of the deformity or defect, they would have terminated the pregnancy so that the infant would not have been born at all. In either case, the claim is not that the deformity or defect could have been prevented but rather that the birth itself would have been prevented but for the alleged medical malpractice of the defendant. The malpractice is usually claimed to be a failure on the part of the defendant to be aware of the possibility of the deformity or defect through either genetic counseling or the performance of diagnostic tests such as amniocentesis and ultrasonography and a further failure to advise the parents accordingly.

In terms of damages, the infant in a wrongful life claim seeks to recover monetary compensation for being born in the first instance. In their contemporaneous wrongful birth claim, the parents seek a variety of monetary damages as follows: the medical expenses associated with the pregnancy and the birth; the mother's loss of earnings occasioned by the pregnancy and the birth; the mother's physical pain and suffering associated with the pregnancy and birth; loss of the infant's services, society, companionship, and comfort as occasioned by the deformity or defect; the extraordinary expenses for specialized care and training of the infant as occasioned by the deformity or defect; and the mental anguish and emotional distress of the parents occasioned by the deformity or defect.

The courts in a number of jurisdictions in the United States have considered the legal sufficiency of claims for wrongful life and wrongful birth. As of this writing, all states that have considered the issue have rejected the claim for wrongful life and have held that the infant has no legally cognizable claim. A few commentators have suggested that both California [21] and Washington [10] permit a claim for wrongful life: However, the cases in those two states merely permit the infant to recover damages in his or her own right in connection with the extraordinary expenses to be incurred for specialized care and treatment occasioned by the deformity or defect after the child attains the age of majority.

Neither California nor Washington nor any other state permits the infant to recover damages on the theory that he or she should not have been born. The other 15 states that have considered the issue specifically prohibit the infant from maintaining any claim [2]. The general rationale of the courts is that the judicial system is not equipped to make a determination as to whether or not the value of nonlife exceeds the value of impaired life.

With respect to the claim for wrongful birth, the courts in eight states have held that any monetary recovery made by the parents must be limited to the extraordinary expenses for specialized care and treatment occasioned by the infant's deformity or defect [5]. However, four states permit recovery by the parents beyond these extraordinary expenses, and while there are minor variations as to exactly what is recoverable in these jurisdictions, they all hold that the parents may recover for the one item of damage that involves the most significant monetary potential, namely, their mental anguish and emotional distress [3].

The specific practice of family planning medicine is directly involved in wrongful life and wrongful birth claims on a fairly infrequent basis. However, the same cannot be said for wrongful conception claims, as family planning medicine is the only practice involved in such claims. A wrongful conception claim occurs when a completely normal and healthy, albeit unplanned, infant is born following an unsuccessful family planning surgical procedure. The claim is made by the parents rather than the infant, and the usual theory is that the procedure in question was performed in a negligent manner, thereby resulting in the unplanned birth of an unwanted child.

With respect to damages, the parents in a wrongful conception claim seek to recover monetary compensation for the expenses in connection with the failed surgical procedure, the expenses and the physical pain and suffering in connection with the pregnancy and the birth, and, most important, the expenses they will incur in raising the allegedly unwanted child to the age of support, which, in almost every state, is 21 years.

As of this writing, the courts in 25 states have considered the legal sufficiency of claims for wrongful conception. All these states permit the parents to recover monetary damages for the failed procedure as well as for the expenses and the physical pain and suffering in connection with the subsequent pregnancy and birth. However, 18 states reject the remainder of the claimed damages and hold that a claim to recover the expenses of raising a normal and healthy infant is not legally cognizable [1]. Only seven states permit the recovery of such damages [4].

CLAIMS INVOLVING NONSURGICAL TREATMENT

Nonsurgical Contraception

As previously indicated, consideration of the medicolegal risks involved in nonsurgical methods of contraception will be limited to oral contraceptives and intrauterine devices. It should be noted that, in terms of overall severity, claims involving contraception appear to be on a par with those involving first-trimester abortion procedures. According to the NAIC study, the average indemnity payment for contraception claims was $24,364.

ORAL CONTRACEPTIVES

Without question, oral contraceptives represent the greatest medicolegal risk in the practice of family planning medicine, and this is a function of the rare but severe injuries that are known to result from the increased risk of cardiovascular disorders that has been attributed to birth control pills. Of course, the minor risks and side effects of oral contraceptive use occur far more frequently than the serious complications. However, the minor problems seldom result in claims; it is the serious cardiovascular complications that account for the vast majority of claims for injuries allegedly caused by oral contraceptives.

The injuries that are claimed most frequently are thrombophlebitis (occasionally resulting in an above-the-knee amputation), pulmonary embolism, occlusive stroke, and myocardial infarction. These are, of course, serious injuries, and they involve significant monetary potential. Other serious injuries that are claimed less frequently include retinal thrombosis, mesenteric artery thrombosis, and thrombosis causing renal failure. A review of the data from the NAIC study reveals the relative severity of these injuries in terms of average indemnity paid as follows: cerebral and spinal paralysis—$235,262; cardiac arrest and brain damage—$184,753; above-knee amputation—$140,979; blindness—$99,518; renal failure—$96,352; respiratory arrest and lung complications—$66,679; myocardial infarction—$51,678; pulmonary embolism—$47,157; and circulatory problems—$43,945.

The relative monetary potential of these severe and debilitating injuries clearly represents a significant medicolegal risk for the practitioner who prescribes oral contraceptives, and this risk appears to be greater today than ever before. In the authors' experience, until recently it was the general rule that oral contraceptive claims were usually products liability claims directed against the pharmaceutical company that manufactured and marketed the birth control pill in question rather than medical malpractice claims against the physician who prescribed the pill. Under a legal doctrine known as strict tort liability, the plaintiff's attorney is only required to prove that there was some inherent defect in the product (usually claimed to be a labeling defect with respect to the package insert) as well as causal connection between the alleged defect and the claimed injury. Under this doctrine it is not necessary for the plaintiff's attorney to prove that the defect was the result of any negligence on the part of the pharmaceutical company. Proof of the defect and causal connection is enough to support a recovery of monetary damages against the manufacturer.

Oral contraceptive claims are still directed at the various pharmaceutical companies as products liability claims. However, in the past several years such claims have been directed at the prescribing physician on a more frequent basis, and sometimes exclusively, as medical malpractice claims. Consequently, if the patient who uses birth control pills is at increased risk of developing a serious cardiovascular complication the physician who prescribes oral contraceptives is clearly at increased risk of developing a serious medicolegal complication.

INTRAUTERINE DEVICES

The historic development of IUD claims is similar to that of oral contraceptive claims. In the past it was usually the pharmaceutical company that manufactured and marketed the IUD that was on the receiving end of a claim, although it was not unheard of for the physician who inserted the IUD to also be involved in the claim. Today, however, the physician is involved on a much more frequent basis.

This procedural similarity between IUD claims and oral contraceptive claims does not extend to the issue of severity. In the experience of the authors, IUD claims involve an overall monetary potential significantly less than that associated with oral contraceptive claims. This experience seems to be confirmed by data from the NAIC study that show the average indemnity payment for IUD claims to be $21,644, a figure that is even less than the average indemnity payment for first-trimester abortion claims.

Some IUD claims have alleged that the device has perforated through the uterine fundus or that it has become embedded in the uterine wall. However, the most common IUD claim is that the device has caused pelvic inflammatory disease, and the more serious claims in this regard allege that this disease process has caused permanent sterility as a result of either adhesions in and around the fallopian tubes or hysterectomy. In either case the monetary potential of such a claim is about the same as claims involving hysterectomies following first-trimester abortion procedures. In the case of hysterectomy it is not uncommon for the surgical procedure to include a bilateral salpingo-oophorectomy due to the presence of tubo-ovarian abscesses. Such a claim generally involves increased monetary potential because the patient will experience early symptoms of menopause.

It must be emphasized that the current climate regarding IUDs does not enhance the defense of claims for injuries allegedly caused by one of the devices. In large part this situation seems to be the result of an unsubstantiated public perception that IUDs are simply not safe, a perception undoubtedly caused by the well-publicized problems reported in connection with the Dalkon Shield. In any event, the practitioner should be aware of the experience of many defense attorneys that, as a result of this situation, IUD claims are difficult to defend regardless of the facts of the individual case.

Failures of Diagnosis

It is not unusual for a medical malpractice claim to allege a failure to diagnose and treat a particular condition, and this is true of claims directed at every medical specialty. In fact, the NAIC study found that 27 percent of all claims included in the study were based on alleged diagnostic errors. As such, it should come as no surprise that the medicolegal risk inherent in the practice of family planning medicine includes claims for failures of diagnosis.

Such claims are often made in the context of specific surgical or nonsurgical treatment. For instance, a fairly frequent allegation in an incomplete abortion claim is that the physician failed to accurately diagnose the gestational age before performing the procedure. Another example is the allegation that the practitioner failed to diagnose and treat pelvic inflammatory disease when the patient wearing an IUD complained of lower abdominal pain and a vaginal discharge. However, there have been a variety of incidents in which the condition that allegedly should have been diagnosed was not directly related to the treatment that was rendered.

The most frequent claim in this regard is failure to diagnose an ectopic pregnancy. The patient claims that the alleged failure caused her to lose a fallopian tube, and defense attorneys generally view such a claim as one of rather limited monetary potential, as the patient would have lost the fallopian tube whether or not the diagnosis was made before the ectopic pregnancy ruptured. The other typical diagnosis claim is a failure to diagnose breast, cervical, or endocervical carcinoma; these claims usually involve an allegation of failure to repeat or properly evaluate the results of a Pap smear or colposcopic examination. Juries tend to be disturbed by cases in which cancer is the claimed injury, and such claims must be considered as having very significant monetary potential.

In any event, the lesson of the diagnosis claims is that, while family planning practice is fairly limited in terms of the conditions for which treatment is sought, the practitioner must be observant for any unusual signs and symptoms and must be prepared to refer the patient for appropriate treatment when indicated.

MEDICOLEGAL RISK REDUCTION

Given the level of medicolegal risk inherent in the practice of family planning medicine, it is certainly in the interest of the practitioner to reduce that risk as much as possible. High quality medical care is the best protection against the existing risk. However, such a level of care is often not enough, an unfortunate truth that is demonstrated by the fact that a significant percentage of claims are medically defensible. While the technical skills of the medical practitioner may be excellent, they do not necessarily protect the practitioner from exposure to a medicolegal claim.

The fact that high quality medical care does not provide complete protection from claim exposure illustrates the crucial need for the implementation of an effective risk reduction program. In addition to decreasing medicolegal risk, such a program also facilitates the provision of high quality services and enhances patient satisfaction, both of which are important components of health care delivery. The essential elements of risk reduction in practice are administration; patient education; record keeping; follow-up; quality assurance; insurance; and handling of claims and lawsuits. The role played by each element in risk management will be explored.

Administration

WRITTEN PROTOCOLS

The importance of a well-organized and comprehensive administrative system cannot be overstated. Before the first patient is seen, office policies and procedures must be clearly established. The best way to accomplish this is to develop written protocols. Protocols should describe what will happen from the moment the patient arrives at the office or clinic until the time that the patient is discharged.

The protocols should provide complete details on the following aspects of patient care:

Personnel
Equipment lists (hardware and consumables)
Criteria for patient selection
Intake procedure(s)
Patient flow patterns
Patient history
Physical examination
Documentation
Description of procedures provided
Referral procedures
Preoperative and postoperative management and procedures, where applicable
Recovery procedures
Discharge procedures
Emergency procedures
Management of complications
Triage and recording of telephone inquiries and emergencies
Follow-up
Financial practices
Data collection

Ancillary activities should also be described:

Pharmacy services—information on medications available, where and how they are stored, who has responsibility for inventory and dispensing
Laboratory services—range of tests provided on-site; logging and follow-up of tests sent to laboratories
Credentials of referral laboratories, especially cytology

Sample forms should be included:

Medical history
Medical record
Fact sheets
Consents
Record release
Referral

Protocols should include descriptions of the functions of both medical and nonmedical staff. Explicit protocols will be valuable tools for the orientation and training of staff. All staff members must read and understand these documents; this will facilitate patient management and should serve to make clear the lines of communication and responsibility. Staff input should be sought in order to ensure adherence as well as accuracy. Protocols should be written in such a way that they can be easily amended and updated, and a system for routine review and revision in accord with changing medical, legal, and administrative standards should be implemented. Protocols should be frequently referred to and should reflect the actual operations of the practice. Such protocols may then represent a key element of a quality assurance and audit mechanism.

STAFFING

Appointment of Quality Staff. The recruitment and selection of quality staff is crucial to the effective functioning of a medical care office or agency. Care must be taken to retain only qualified, competent, and committed individuals. Interpersonal skills and the ability to cooperate with others are nonquantifiable skills that are nevertheless of critical importance [12]. While there are no formulas for success in this very subjective area, a few basic guidelines should prevail.

The licensing, degree, and professional credentialing requirements of all personnel (medical as well as nonmedical) must be specified and adhered to [9]. To determine these requirements, appropriate state licensure and regulatory agencies should be consulted. Additionally, detailed functional job descriptions must be developed for every position. These should be revised and updated on a regular basis.

An important personnel policy to adopt is a routine check of both previous employers and character references. Careful assessment of the value of these references is as important as obtaining them. An explanation for any gaps in employment history should be sought. An attempt should be made to secure a work sample or observe a demonstration procedure before hiring, wherever possible.

Once staff have been selected, there should be a predetermined probationary period. It is important that the work load be shared and that no one staff member becomes overburdened or overwhelmed, as this may force that person to take shortcuts or to become careless and perhaps overlook important details. Such mistakes can be not only costly but dangerous.

Staff Training and Continuing Education. A general orientation program for new employees should be developed and offered to all new staff either before their appointment date or immediately thereafter. Position-oriented training must also be available; this should be intense and concentrated on new employees and those assuming new positions. This training should then be supplemented by formal and informal in-service training and continuing educational opportunities.

Patient Education

PATIENT COMMUNICATION

Treatment for any type of reproductive health care requires that the patient be given a comprehensive explanation of the treatment rendered and the reasons it is required. Consumers of health care services are becoming increasingly sophisticated and are expressing an active interest in what is happening to them. They have begun questioning the risks and benefits of prescribed therapies and requesting clarification of technical information. This is a positive trend that should be encouraged. An understanding patient is more likely to be cooperative.

Patients should receive instructions regarding general reproductive functions. Explanations can be provided individually or in groups but must be given simply and in a manner comprehensible to the lay person. Equally important, an effort must be made to determine if the patient understands the content of the material being presented. If the target community is largely non-English-speaking, translations must be made available. If a pharmaceutical or other company sends brochures or pamphlets in a language other than English, these should be proofread for tone and accuracy before distribution. It may be useful to employ such teaching aids as instructional films, plastic models, diagrams, charts, and other audiovisual aids. It should be remembered that these are a supplement to interaction with the patient and not a replacement for a detailed question-and-answer period, extensive direct communication, and a written fact sheet.

When a patient first requests a means of fertility control, it is important to explain all available methods, even if the patient has requested a specified method of contraception. It must be assumed that the patient does not possess adequate knowledge of all the risks and benefits of other methods. The method chosen may not be appropriate or may have been chosen on the basis of misinformation or inapplicable information. As patient education usually takes place before the physical examination, it should be explained to the patient that the findings of the examination, considered in conjunction with the individual's medical history and laboratory tests and coupled with the patient's preference, will

have an effect upon the method of contraception selected.

Patient education should concern itself mainly with the method being selected. However, questions relating to reproduction in general should be covered. Each office visit represents an opportunity to educate patients in all aspects of health care. This can be accomplished by means of a structured educational program or simply by training patients to use waiting time constructively by offering audiovisual services (e.g., films on various aspects of fertility control) or having written materials available in the waiting room for patient information and education.

FACT SHEETS

Simply written, clear and concise fact sheets on each method of contraception or procedure offered should be available. Use of simple, accurate diagrams is a good technique for clarification. Fact sheets should be written in a language in which the patient is fluent. Additionally, the information provided must be objective and verifiable. It is important to be certain that fact sheets are not open to interpretation as endorsements of any particular method or product.

Fact sheets should contain, at a minimum, the following information: a description of the method or procedure; a detailed explanation of the benefits and risks, using numbers such as 1 per 1,000, as percentages are not as easily interpreted (care must be taken to make certain that this listing of known risks is not presented as all-inclusive); potential and known side effects; and instructions in the event of any questions or emergency. This information must be routinely reviewed and updated as new data become available and dispensed to patients as soon as practicable.

Fact sheets must be coordinated with consent forms, which must be signed by patients and witnessed before any treatment or procedure, as they are part of the informed consent process.

INFORMED CONSENT

The most difficult question facing physicians today is how much information they should give to a patient regarding the proposed course of treatment to enable the patient to make an informed decision relating to his or her medical care. Informed consent is the duty of a physician to explain to a patient the nature of the problem or illness and the proposed treatment as well as to warn of any material risks or dangers in or related to the therapy so that the patient can make an intelligent and informed choice about whether to undergo such treatment [6]. This should be done before any course of treatment is undertaken.

This means that the physician must explain the nature of the treatment, known risks of the treatment, alternatives to the treatment, the right to refuse treatment, and the risks involved if the treatment is not taken. This must be done in an objective manner so as not to influence or induce a patient to act in a certain manner. One must not make any guarantees or warranties.

Two standards are used in defining the scope of a physician's obligation to disclose. Historically, courts used a "standard of practice" approach, which measured the obligation to disclose against what a reasonable physician in the same or a similar community would disclose under the same or similar circumstances. Considerations by the physician would include the individual patient's health, his or her mental condition, and whether or not the risks are usual possibilities versus remote ones [16]. In recent years another approach has developed, which emphasizes a patient's right to self-determination; it measures the scope of the informed consent against a "reasonable man" standard. In these instances the information that a reasonable patient would need in order to make an informed decision would be considered the key determining factor. This does not mean that the physician must discuss all risks; the standard is that the practitioner must disclose those risks that are *material* to the patient's decision. A risk is material when a "reasonable person, in what the physician knows or should know to be the patient's position, would be likely to attach significance to the risk or cluster of risks in deciding whether or not to forego the proposed therapy" [6].

There are no set rules or definitions. As one court noted, "The disclosure doctrine, like other marking lines between permissible and impermissible behavior in medical practice, is in essence a requirement of conduct prudent under the circumstances" [6].

It is important to note that there may be statutory exceptions to the requirements of informed consent. In fact, while this legal doctrine is one that has generally evolved through case law, 23 states have enacted statutes regarding the elements of informed consent as well as exceptions to the traditional common law rules [7]. The following exceptions have been codified in some jurisdictions:

1. When the patient waives the informed consent. There are some patients who do not want to know the risks involved in a procedure. In such instances this waiver must be documented, witnessed, and recorded in the patient's chart.
2. In an emergency situation. If a patient is unconscious and a situation of urgency arises requiring treatment immediately, the risk of harm from the failure to treat far outweighs the risk of treatment. If it is possible to obtain the consent of a relative, the physician should do so.

3. When the physician is unaware of the risks of a particular treatment. A physician cannot be held liable if he or she did not know of the risks involved in a procedure as long as a reasonable physician under like circumstances in the same or a similar community would not have known of these risks.
4. When disclosure would harm the patient. The question facing the physician is whether disclosing information pertaining to the risks of a treatment would be a threat to the patient's health.
5. When the risk involved is obvious to the patient or known to the average person.
6. When the risk involved is so remote so as not to be considered material.

It is impossible to say when these exceptions will be deemed applicable by the courts. The practitioner must always act with caution.

Consent Forms. A patient's consent to any course of treatment is essential. Failure to obtain consent may lead to a claim of battery. Accordingly, a signed consent form certifying that the risks and benefits of the proposed treatment have been explained should be obtained. The form should detail the nature of the procedure, the inherent risks, the benefits, and possible complications. As with fact sheets, it is important that consent forms be written in a language in which the patient is fluent. If the consent form is being used in conjunction with a fact sheet, these two documents must be consistent. The consent form should contain an indication that the patient has read and understood the fact sheet.

Although consent forms are evidence that the necessary steps have been taken to thoroughly inform the patient so that he or she can make an appropriate decision regarding treatment, this can be disputed if the circumstances under which the consent was obtained indicate that the patient actually had no understanding of the situation, was in some way coerced, or was given false information about the procedure.

Informed Consent for Minors. Historically, minors could not consent for medical treatment. However, there have always been exceptions to the rule. Minors could consent in an emergency or if they were "emancipated." Although the definition of *emancipated* varies by state, in general it means being free of parental control and being self-supporting. Because of public health concerns, minors can, in all states, consent to treatment for sexually transmitted diseases.

Recently, a "mature minor" doctrine has been adopted by courts and state legislatures, which permits minors to consent to certain types of treatment. A mature minor is one who understands the nature and consequences of the treatment and can, therefore, make an informed decision [18]. This doctrine is clearly demonstrated in cases involving a minor's ability to obtain reproductive health care. The Supreme Court has established that minors have a right of access to sex-related health care, including contraceptive services and abortion [17].

The issue of parental involvement in the case of minors is important and should be thoroughly explored with the minor patient. In fact, one study [20] demonstrates that most teenagers advise their parents when they decide to seek contraception. However, a number of teens are unwilling to involve their parents and have stated that a parental notification requirement would deter them from a visit for family planning; the result would be the use of less reliable but more easily accessible methods or nonuse of contraception. Both of these options would likely result in increased incidence of teenage pregnancy. Therefore, the authors believe that a parental notification requirement is inappropriate.

A number of states have either by statute or case law grappled with these issues. Several have affirmed a minor's right to consent for contraception services and pregnancy-related health care, but others specifically limit the minor's right. Such laws are often challenged and found to be unconstitutional [22]. Review with an attorney of the applicable laws in a given jurisdiction is essential.

Mentally Disabled Patients. Mentally handicapped people have a right to treatment; the problem is whether they can consent to such treatment. A determination must be made as to their competency in understanding the nature of the treatment and the benefits and risks involved. If the individual is found to be unable to give such consent, a third party who is legally responsible for the patient (parent, spouse, or legal guardian) may give the consent. When necessary, the court will appoint a guardian. These patients must not be treated without the appropriate consent for such treatment.

Record Keeping

The medical record provides permanent and continuous documentation of patient care. Included in a medical record are a medical history of the patient; a family history; physician notes; laboratory reports; x-ray reports; consent forms; and fact sheets.

The medical record is the means by which a provider knows what has occurred and what is intended to occur in the course of treatment for a particular patient. Although used primarily by the physician and office staff, it is also the only means any other provider who renders services has of ascertaining a patient's past medical treatment.

The medical record itself should be a well-organized, easy-to-read document that limits the need for narrative. Compliance is a major problem in maintaining adequate accounts of medical procedures and occurrences; therefore, the need for the practitioner to write extensive explanations should be minimized. There are a variety of ways in which this can be accomplished—for example, using questions worded so that they require yes or no answers, providing check lists with space for commentary should it be necessary, and utilizing anatomic diagrams that can be marked to indicate findings.

The keeping of accurate records is a great responsibility for any practitioner. The records will be referred to time and time again and may be seen by other medical professionals, insurance companies, attorneys, and the patient. A medical record should, therefore, be accurate, legible, and neat.

Language is the key to record keeping. Accurate, appropriate, and precise language is essential. Words should not be used out of context. Vague or ambiguous language should be avoided; direct statements should be used. A record should not be cluttered with comments not germane to the treatment in question. Entries made in the record should be objective. Statements and opinions should be supported by factual observations, not conjecture on the part of the clinician.

Only standard abbreviations commonly used in the medical profession are acceptable for use in a medical record. Unofficial abbreviations or personal shorthand not immediately recognizable by other practitioners should be avoided.

The record needs to be completely filled in and must list in a conspicuous manner any allergic history, detailing the types of medication involved and the manifestations of apparent sensitivity. Maintenance of a separate medication sheet facilitates the identification of past and current medications.

A record should be completed promptly. It is much easier to record such things as the patient's condition at the time treatment is given rather than trying to recall the details at a later date.

Note on all charts every test or procedure performed, even if they are routine. Many clinicians document only positive findings; it is equally important to document negative findings.

The fact that the risks and benefits of a treatment were explained and that a patient has given an informed consent must be noted on the chart. Note also if the patient indicates that he or she does not want to know the risks and benefits but wishes to go ahead with a proposed treatment. Likewise, if a patient refuses treatment, state that it was the patient's decision to decline treatment after being given an explanation of the risks and benefits, including the possible effects of failure to get treatment. Noncompliance by a patient should also be charted (e.g., if a patient is referred for further treatment and fails to go or if the patient refuses to follow instructions).

A cardinal rule in charting is that never under any circumstances should a record be altered. In a court-room situation alterations could easily appear as though someone attempted to camouflage errors. If a mistake is actually made when writing in the chart, one line should be drawn through the mistake so that the original wording can still be determined, and the word "error," the date, and the practitioner's initials should appear next to it. Obliteration with pen or eradicating liquid is inappropriate. Corrections should be noted in the margin or if necessary on a separate sheet of paper attached to the record.

Historically, patients' accessibility to their records has been limited, in the belief that disclosure to a patient of the record might cause emotional trauma or injury. In recent years courts and legislatures have tended to make the information contained in these records available to patients and their authorized representatives [11]. Patient confidentiality should be ensured by re-leasing records only when a signed authorization is obtained from the patient. The signatures on the au-thorization should be compared with any signatures in the record. Information should not be provided over the telephone except in an emergency situation to a known provider with consent documented on the record.

Under most circumstances it is good medical practice to permit the patient to review his or her record. The authors believe that making the record accessible to patients may discourage malpractice suits. We suggest that either the physician or other qualified staff member review the record together with the patient. In this way abbreviations and terminology can be explained. This will also serve to ensure that no alterations are made by the patient and that nothing is removed from the record. Remember that the original record should not leave the office. Original records should be released only to a judge or pursuant to court order.

The length of time one needs to keep patient records varies by state, and several have statutes that deal with this issue. In those states that do not have specific stat-utes on the subject, consider the statute of limitations—the time period in which a lawsuit may be filed—for medical malpractice claims. In general, the statute be-gins to run from the time the treatment is given. A number of jurisdictions, however, have a "discovery rule" in which the statute does not begin to run until the patient knows, or should have known, that an in-jury has taken place.

In the case of minors the statute of limitations does not begin to run until the minor reaches the age of majority or an age specified by state statute. Therefore, it is a good policy to keep the records of minors until the statute has expired for these patients.

Records should be easily accessible to authorized personnel and kept in locked files. Limited access should be maintained. Care should be taken to protect patient confidentiality, which can easily be jeopardized if the record is not handled and stored appropriately. Records should be used only by authorized persons and returned to the file immediately once they are no longer required. A good medical record system is one in which it becomes immediately apparent when a chart is removed for any reason.

A logical, easy-to-follow record-keeping system should be established. Records should be retrievable by patient name. They should have a unique patient identification number in order to maintain confiden-tiality. A system for retrieval by method or treatment modality is also useful in the event of a manufacturer's recall and in carrying out medical audits of specific top-ics [19]. Color coding the exterior folder as well as the forms or tables within the record is one way of organiz-ing records. Computer coding of diagnoses, laboratory results, procedures, medications, and allergies is in-creasingly utilized by clinics and private offices. There should be a clear distinction between active and inac-tive patients, and inactive charts should be purged on a regular basis.

A system for chart notation should be agreed upon and used consistently. Everyone working with the charts should be familiar and comfortable with the sys-tem and adhere to it. Staff training sessions should be devoted to this subject.

Follow-Up

Protocols and tickler systems should be developed for follow-up. The computer is invaluable in this area. There should also be a written protocol for handling problem cases. This should include telephone follow-up procedures and instructions on acceptable docu-mentation of a (predetermined) minimum number of telephone attempts to reach the patient. In the event this fails, a certified return-receipt-requested letter should be sent and the receipt kept in the record.

The system for contacting the patient should facilitate maintaining confidentiality. This is especially true in the case of minors.

If a patient is referred for services, notes in the chart should reflect not only the referral but the date of the referral visit, treatment regimens given and prescribed, outcome, and discharge data.

Additionally, if the patient refuses a referral, this should also be recorded.

Quality Assurance

Good patient care requires that a quality assurance program be implemented [15]. The preceding sections have attempted to outline the elements of practice necessary to ensure quality care and to facilitate review and evaluation of the patterns of practice.

A formal quality assurance program should be designed in light of both medical and legal considerations. There are several quality assurance mechanisms that can be easily adapted to accommodate different practice needs.

A key component of a quality assurance program is patient care audit. This can be accomplished by having the person responsible for medical records routinely review charts before they are returned to the files. This person should look for such inaccuracies as incomplete or illegible notes, loose pages, and incomplete or missing forms. The reviewer should also assess if the protocol has been followed. If the persons to whom this task is designated are capable of doing a more detailed review and identifying complications associated with method/procedure or operator, they should do so.

Random chart review should take place at regularly scheduled intervals. This review may be either prospective or retrospective. In the former case, for example, a certain number of charts of patients in a given age group being placed on a particular treatment regimen may be reviewed periodically to ascertain if they are being followed up in accord with the protocol. A retrospective review may involve review of charts of patients who previously experienced a particular therapy or diagnosis. The information gained from this process should be shared immediately when necessary or on a regular basis, not only with those directly concerned but with the entire staff as an object lesson.

Consensual agreement is another valuable technique that can be employed for purposes of quality assurance. While chart review focuses on the process involved in rendering care, consensual agreement examines both the process of delivering care and the outcome. Representatives from all areas—administrative, nursing, physician, and secretarial personnel—are included for a comprehensive assessment and an exchange of ideas and experiences. The group selects a procedure, treatment modality, disease entity complication, or problem and reviews relevant cases from all possible angles. This multidimensional review can yield interesting and important findings that might not have emerged by consideration of process alone. There have been situations in which an applicable protocol has been scrupulously adhered to and yet an unexpected outcome resulted. Consensual agreement, by examining all the variables, might be a useful tool in identifying exactly what factors contributed to unexpected results.

Periodic staff meetings should be held to discuss problem cases, charting problems, and consumer feedback. This will elicit staff input as to areas of concern and suggestions for improvement.

Consumer feedback forms are a valuable mechanism for assessing quality of care and patient satisfaction. These forms should be made available to all patients, including those who are referred for service.

Insurance

Insurance is a means of transferring risk. By purchasing an insurance policy to cover a specific risk, you are transferring the risk of loss to an insurance company. The private practitioner needs various kinds of insurance to protect his or her practice, including fire, property, and general liability coverage. Your insurance needs should be fully explored with your insurance broker after a detailed review of your physical space and practical needs.

One essential kind of coverage is medical professional liability insurance. This insures you against claims or suits by patients alleging that the medical treatment you provided harmed them. In recent years the cost of this coverage has increased dramatically. Some physicians, especially those who have never experienced a loss, have decided to "go bare" and not be insured. The authors strongly recommend that any physician contemplating such an action reevaluate the situation. Although you may never have been sued, there is always a first time, and it can happen to you. In a litigious society such as ours, with the high jury verdicts, we believe that it would be terribly unwise to practice without adequate professional liability insurance.

Adequacy of coverage (limits of liability) cannot easily be defined; it will depend on what procedures and types of treatment you perform as well as your geographic location and should be discussed with brokers or insurance representatives. They will also be able to describe the kinds of policies available, claims made or occurrence, and help you in deciding what to purchase [14].

Most people agree that insurance policies are boring and difficult to read. We cannot stress enough, however, the need for you to review your policies with an insurance expert.

Claims and Lawsuits

Often dissatisfied patients will call to complain about the treatment they received. It is important to hear them out and to explain what you did and why. If the problem stems from something your staff did, this incident should be fully explored with them. If the problem is applicable to other staff persons' duties, discuss it in general terms with all staff. There will always be incidents and complaints; the important thing is to learn from them.

The patient may ask you to pay for additional medical expenses incurred. Although many believe that this will deter someone from taking further action, we suggest that you consult with your professional liability carrier. Some policies expressly forbid making such payments.

If you are served with a summons, do not panic, unless you are uninsured! Call your insurance company immediately. The company will assign a qualified attorney to represent you. You should cooperate fully with this attorney, and he or she should be the only person with whom you discuss the case. Do not contact the patient in an attempt to rectify the situation yourself. If the patient's attorney contacts you directly, refer him or her to your counsel. Do not provide copies of the records to anyone, unless instructed to do so by your attorney.

Medical malpractice lawsuits are often a time-consuming and demanding process. You must be available for pretrial discovery as well as the actual trial. Most medical malpractice cases are settled before trial. If your case goes to trial, stay calm. Before the trial date your attorney will explain what will take place and prepare you for what to expect. He or she will advise you as to dress, demeanor, and the kinds of questions to expect. Listen carefully and ask questions. Once in the courtroom, be calm, objective, and completely professional. Most importantly, listen to your attorney.

Delivering quality health care and minimizing the medicolegal risk are compatible, indeed complementary, goals. They can, in fact, largely be achieved by the same process. The elements of this process have been outlined in this chapter. Open lines of communication between the patient and the physician with maintenance of good patient relationships are one of the most significant elements in medicolegal risk reduction. But such will not suffice unless the provision of quality services is assured. It is important to remember that a formal risk reduction program must be instituted from the inception of services or as soon thereafter as possible, that resources must be allocated for this purpose, and that it must be clearly designated as a priority. The specific vehicles chosen for use are not so crucial to the success of a risk reduction program. One medical record form may not be clearly superior or appropriate in all circumstances. No method of quality assurance is without its deficits; in fact, a combination of review procedures or the use of multiple approaches may prove most effective. What is important is careful review of all the aspects of a health care delivery setting with a view toward integration of the basic elements of risk reduction.

REFERENCES

1. Alabama—*Boone v. Mullendore*, 416 So. 2d 718 (1982); Arkansas—*Wilbur v. Kerr*, 628 S.W.2d 568 (1982); Delaware—*Coleman v. Garrison*, 349 A.2d 8 (1975); District of Columbia—*Hartke v. McKelway*, 707 F.2d 1544 (1983); Florida—*Public Health Trust v. Brown*, 388 So.2d 1084 (1980); Georgia—*White v. U.S.*, 510 F. Supp. 146 (1981); Illinois—*Cockrum v. Baumgartner*, 477 N.E.2d 385 (1983); Kentucky—*Shork v. Huber*, 648 S.W.2d 861 (1983); Missouri—*Miller V. Duhart*, 637 S.W.2d 183 (1982); New Hampshire—*Kingsbury v. Smith*, 442 A.2d 1003 (1982); New Jersey—*P. v. Portadin*, 432 A.2d 556 (1981); New York—*Weintraub v. Brown*, 470 N.Y.S.2d 634 (1983); Pennsylvania—*Mason v. Western Pennsylvania Hospital*, 453 A.2d 974 (1982); Tennessee—*Montgomery v. Henry* (unreported, Tennessee Court of Appeals, 1980); Texas—*Sutkin v. Beck*, 629 S.W.2d 131 (1982); Virginia—*McNeal v. U.S.*, 689 F.2d 1200 (1982); Wisconsin—*Reick v. Medical Protective Co.*, 219 N.W.2d 242 (1974); and Wyoming—*Beardsley v. Wierdsma*, 650 P.2d 288 (1982).

2. Alabama—*Elliot v. Brown*, 361 So.2d 546 (1978); Delaware—*Coleman v. Garrison*, supra (1); Florida—*DiNatale v. Lieberman*, 409 So.2d 512 (1982); Georgia—*White v. U.S.*, supra (1); Kentucky—*Shork v. Huber*, supra (1); Massachusetts—*Payton v. Abbott Laboratories*, 437 N.E.2d 171 (1982); Michigan—*Eisbrenner v. Stanley*, 208 N.W.2d 209 (1981); Missouri—*Miller v. Duhart*, supra (1); New Jersey—*Berman v. Allen*, 404 A.2d 8 (1979); New York—*Becker v. Schwartz*, 413 N.Y.S.2d 895 (1978); Pennsylvania—*Speck v. Feingold*, 439 A.2d 110 (1981); South Carolina—*Phillips v. U.S.*, 508 F. Supp. 537 (1980); Texas—*Nelson v. Krusen*, 635 S.W.2d 582 (1982); Wisconsin—*Dumer v. St. Michael's Hospital*, 233 N.W.2d 372 (1975); and Wyoming—*Beardsley v. Wierdsma*, supra (1).

3. Alabama—*Robak v. United States*, 658 F.2d 471 (1981); Pennsylvania—*Speck v. Feingold*, supra (2); Virginia—*Naccash v. Burger*, 290 S.E.2d 825 (1982); and Washington—*Harbeson v. Parke-Davis*, 656 P.2d 483 (1983).

4. Arizona—*University of Arizona Health Sciences Center v. Superior Court of the State of Arizona, Maricopa County*, 667 P.2d 1294 (1983); California—*Morris v. Frudenfeld*, 185 Cal. Rptr. 76 (1982); Connecticut—*Ochs v. Borrelli*, 445 A.2d 883 (1982); Michigan—*Troppi v. Scarf*, 187 N.W.2d 511 (1971); Minnesota—*Sherlock v. Stillwater Clinic*, 260 N.W.2d 169 (1977); North Carolina—*Pierce v. Piver*, 262 S.E.2d 320 (1980); and Ohio—*Bowman v. Davis*, 356 N.E.2d 496 (1976).

5. California—*Turpin v. Sortini*, 182 Cal. Rptr. 337 (1982); Florida—*DiNatale v. Lieberman*, supra (2); Michigan—*Eisbrenner v. Stanley*, supra (2); New Jersey—*Schroeder v. Perkel*, 432 A.2d 834 (1981); New York—*Becker v. Schwartz*, supra (2); Tennessee—*Montgomery v. Henry*, supra (1); Texas—*Jacobs v. Theimer*, 519 S.W.2d 846 (1976; and Wisconsin—*Dumer v. St. Michael's Hospital*, supra (2).

6. *Canterbury v. Spence,* 464 F.2d 772 (1972).

7. Danzon, P. M. The Frequency and Severity of Medical Malpractice Claims. The Rand Corporation, Institute for Civil Justice, Santa Monica, Calif., February, 1983. (The 23 states are Alaska, California, Delaware, Florida, Hawaii, Idaho, Iowa, Kentucky, Louisiana, Maine, Nevada, New Hampshire, Nebraska, New York, North Carolina, Ohio, Pennsylvania, Rhode Island, Tennessee, Texas, Utah, Vermont, and Washington.)

8. Department of Professional Liability of The American College of Obstetricians and Gynecolgists (resource).

9. Gorosh, M., and Martin, E. Improving management through evaluation: Techniques and strategies for family planning programs. *Stud. Fam. Plann.* 9:163, 1978.

10. *Harbeson v. Parke-Davis,* supra (3).

11. Hirsch, H., and Bromberg, J. Physician responsibilities in keeping medical records. *Malpractice Dig.* November–December, 1979.

12. Johnson, J. M. Reproductive health care: Delivery of services and organizational structure. *Family and Community Health,* May, 1982.

13. *Malpractice Claims.* National Association of Insurance Commissioners, Vol. 2, No. 2, September, 1980.

14. Mehr, R., and Cammack, E. *Principles of Insurance* (6th ed.). Homewood, Ill.: Richard D. Irwin, 1976. (C.f. Williams and Heins, *Risk Management and Insurance* [3rd ed.]. New York: McGraw-Hill, 1976.)

15. Michnich, et al. *Ambulatory Care Evaluation: A Primer for Quality Review.* Ambulatory Care Evaluation Project, School of Public Health, University of California at Los Angeles, 1976.

16. Mills, D. Whither informed consent? *J.A.M.A.* 229:305, 1974.

17. Paul, E., and Pilpel, H. Teenagers and pregnancy: The law in 1979. *Fam. Plann. Perspect.* 11:297, 1979.

18. Paul, E., and Scofield, G. Informed consent for fertility control services. *Fam. Plann. Perspect.* 11:159, 1979.

19. Planned Parenthood Federation of America. *Patient Care Audit Manual,* 1980.

20. Torres, A. Does your mother know. . .? *Fam. Plann. Perspect.* 10:280, 1978.

21. *Turpin v. Sortini,* supra (5).

22. The Federal Court of Appeals in Washington, D.C. ruled in July 1983 that the federal regulations requiring parental notification of the provision of prescription contraceptives by federally funded family planning clinics violated Title X of the Public Health Service Act. Title X is the major source of federal funds for family planning. *Planned Parenthood Federation of America, Inc. v. Heckler,* No. 712 S.2d 650 (D.C. Cir. 1983).

4. Early Pregnancy Detection: Past, Present, Future

Frances R. Batzer

Early pregnancy detection is based on the recognition of both the maternal hormonal response to fertilization and the anatomic presence of a gestational sac. While hormonal detection of pregnancy has been an accepted technique since 1927 when Ascheim and Zondek demonstrated gonadotropic activity in the urine of pregnant women [72], anatomic parameters as defined by ultrasound are only now beginning to be relatively precise [31, 55]. Their combined use in the diagnosis of pregnancy pathology such as ectopic pregnancy and trophoblastic disease is indicative of the current understanding of normal and abnormal gestational development. The specificity, sensitivity, and accuracy of the various techniques and tests available for pregnancy detection will be discussed.

HORMONAL PREGNANCY EVALUATION

The ideal molecule for pregnancy testing should have as its properties

1. Unique to pregnancy
2. Short half-life to accurately reflect current pregnancy status
3. Integral to pregnancy well-being with correlation between quantitative results and prognostic value
4. Easily tested, inexpensive, and with quickly obtainable results

Human chorionic gonadotropin (hCG) has been the traditional pregnancy substance measured. It fits these requirements only partially by being relatively unique to pregnancy in women in the reproductive years, having a serum half-life of 20 to 36 hours [56], and being critical for maintenance of the corpus luteum [21].

Historically, pregnancy testing was based on a biologically induced change in animals exposed to urine from pregnant women [1]. Although it has now been proven that many normal tissues retain the capacity to produce hCG [9], the only significant sources of biologically active hCG in women of reproductive age are pregnancy or neoplasm, usually trophoblastic in origin [10]. Many problems of sensitivity (the ability to detect low levels of hCG when present) and specificity (the ability to discern when no hCG is present) were associated with the original animal testing systems.

Development of immunoassay techniques in the 1960s led to improvements in sensitivity [70] (Table 4-1). Based on the ability of a protein molecule such as hCG to cause an antibody response when injected into an appropriate animal, immunoassay test systems changed pregnancy testing from an extended laboratory test to an office procedure. All total animal bioassay systems are time consuming, expensive, and

Table 4-1. Assays for human chorionic gonadotropin

Test	End point	Time involved (hr)	Approximate sensitivity (IU/ml)
Ascheim-Zondek (1927)	Hemorrhagic follicles and corpora lutea in immature mice (urine)	120	3–5
Friedman (1931)	Ovulation in rabbits (urine)	24–46	3–5
Kupperman (1947)	Hyperemia in rat ovaries (serum)	2	3–5
Latex slide test (1962)	Immunologic agglutination of latex particles on a slide (urine)	(2 minutes)	3–5
Hemagglutination (1960)	Inhibition of hemagglutination reaction (urine)	2	0.75
Latex inhibition tube test (1980)	Immunologic flocculation of beta subunit specific latex particle in a tube (urine)	1.5	0.250
Radioimmunoassay (1968)	Competitive binding of labeled antigen (serum)	24–48	0.010
Beta subunit radioimmunoassay (1972)	Competitive binding of labeled antigen with beta subunit specific antibody	3–6	0.003
Radioreceptorassay (1974)	Binding of hCG-LH to specific sites on bovine corpora lutea	1	0.001

relatively nonspecific; immunoassay testing is easy, reproducible, inexpensive, and fast. Though hampered by interference of nonspecific substances such as protein and various drugs, the cost efficiency and accuracy of immunotesting with the now-familiar latex flocculation slide tests and hemagglutination inhibition tube tests make it the most used technique of pregnancy diagnosis [19].

The development of radioimmunoassay techniques (RIA) in 1968 made possible one further improvement in testing. The structural similarity of human luteinizing hormone (hLH) and hCG hampered early pregnancy testing due to a lack of specificity [50]. Human luteinizing hormone and hCG are both quaternary glycoprotein structures composed of two alpha and two beta chains. The structural dissimilarity is only in the beta chains. The beta chain of hCG has a unique carboxyl terminal group composed of 28 to 30 aminoacids not present in the hLH beta chain [56]. Early RIA techniques were based on antibody developed to the whole hCG molecule. In 1972 Vaitukaitis et al. [68] described an RIA testing system based on a beta subunit specific antibody, which permitted measurement of hCG in the presence of hLH. With this added specificity hCG measurement is possible as early as 8 days after ovulation (Fig. 4-1). The problems of time and expense with any RIA technique are well balanced by specificity and sensitivity, when such precision is needed. Radioimmunoassay techniques represent a major laboratory procedure requiring a gammacounter, skilled personnel, and attention to detail for reproducible results.

The new generation of immunoassay tube tests use a beta hCG specific antigen covalently bonded to latex particles to improve sensitivity and specificity of urine testing [19] (Table 4-1). The macroflocculation end point is unmistakable, so the other favorable elements of immunoassay, mainly reproducibility and ease, are maintained. As with all immunoassay techniques, only the presence of an hCG-like molecule is verified; no assessment of biologic activity can be made.

Saxena et al. [61] in 1974 developed an hCG testing system based on radioreceptor techniques (RRA). Radioreceptor techniques measure the presence of a molecule as it binds actively in vitro to a specific receptor site. In the case of hCG, binding to bovine corpora lutea membrane is assessed. Since hCG and hLH bind to the same receptor site with similar avidity, the only way to differentiate between them is to routinely set the negative end point of the test high, as in the commercially available Biocept-G RRA test (Table 4-2). The advantage of being able to follow the LH surge of ovulation induction and early pregnancy with the same test system is useful only when menstrual cycle timing is known [62]. The disadvantages of RRA testing are similar to RIA systems in terms of equipment and laboratory personnel. Receptor tests are not faster to run than current qualitative RIA procedures [54].

The antibody used in most clinical hCG RIA testing is raised against the entire beta subunit of hCG, not just the specific 28 to 30 unique aminoacid tail piece, which has proven poorly antigenic [49]. Most antisera detect both intact hCG molecules as well as the beta subunit of hCG. While only the intact molecule is biologically active, the production of beta hCG chain appears to be the rate-limiting step [67]. After the first trimester variable and increasing quantities of free alpha chains can

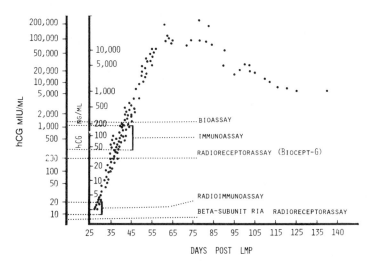

Fig 4-1. Normal beta subunit hCG radioimmunoassay pregnancy curve with comparative sensitivities of various pregnancy tests indicated (1 ng = 5.7 mIU/ml). (From F. R. Batzer. Hormonal evaluation of early pregnancy. *Fertil. Steril.* 34:1, 1980. Reproduced with permission of the publisher, The American Fertility Society.)

be detected simultaneously with a constant level of intact hCG molecule [8] (Fig. 4-2). The significance of this in terms of pregnancy evaluation and monitoring of trophoblastic diseases is only beginning to be appreciated [69]. Trophoblastic tumors have been shown to secrete variable ratios of free subunits. Thus, RRA testing, which measures only biologically intact hCG molecules, may have certain disadvantages [63]. Discrepancies between immunologic and biologic measurements of hCG can be explained on this basis [67].

WHICH TEST TO CHOOSE?

The choice of specific test depends on the clinical situation and is easily made if early pregnancy hCG production is understood (see Fig. 4-1).

Following fertilization in the ampullary portion of the tube, the blastocyst moves toward the uterus for implantation about 72 to 80 hours after ovulation [20]. Secretion of hCG-like material by rabbit blastocysts and other animal embryos before implantation has been described [28]. Preimplantation hCG production has been suggested in humans as measured by RRA 4 days after fertilization [61]. Such embryonic signals would help explain the immediate changes of maternal endocrine function that occur in the conception cycle, resulting in prevention of corpus luteum regression [30]. In gen-

eral, hCG is detected 9 to 12 days after the hLH peak [52] or 8 to 11 days after induced or spontaneous ovulation [11, 15, 45], by which time implantation has occurred.

Properly timed exogenous hCG or hLH can extend and increase progesterone production from the corpus luteum, postponing the onset of menses, but only for a finite period of time [27]. Except for a difference in serum half-life (20–36 hours for hCG [56] as opposed to approximately 50 minutes for hLH) [43], the two molecules are indistinguishable in terms of this biologic effect. Antisera to the unique beta subunit piece also failed to neutralize this biologic activity of hCG [49]. The markedly prolonged half-life of hCG due to the additional sugar moieties increases its potency during this crucial period despite its low level. Measurable levels of hCG in IUD wearers [7] and the high rate of subclinical abortion found in normal populations attempting to conceive [23, 51] support hCG's appearance as diagnostic of fertilization and attempted implantation.

Once detected, levels of hCG double at a predictable rate of 1.2 to 2.2 days during the first 30 days postovulation [5, 11, 16, 50]. Peak values of hCG occur during the first trimester of pregnancy, decreasing to maintenance levels of 10 percent or less during the remainder of the pregnancy, about 5,000 mIU per milliliter (Fig. 4-2).

The early presence of hCG and its predictable exponential rise in normal pregnancy have led to evaluation of pregnancy well-being by hCG quantification [12]. Single estimates of hCG are indicative only of the presence or absence of viable trophoblastic tissue, dependent on the sensitivity and specificity of the test used for accuracy in this diagnosis. Early immunologic test-

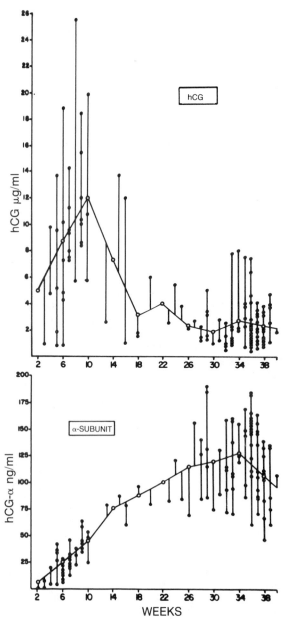

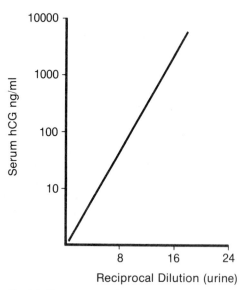

Fig. 4-3. Regression analysis of urinary and ($r = 0.99$) serum hCG titers in successful pregnancies during the first 30 days following ovulation (From S. L. Corson, F. R. Batzer, and S. Schlaff. A comparison of serial quantitative serum and urine tests in early pregnancy. *J. Reprod. Med.* 26:611, 1981.)

Fig. 4-2. Levels of hCG determined by RRA *(upper panel)* and alpha subunit determined by hCG alpha RIA *(lower panel)* in sera from 124 normal pregnant women. The closed circles represent each individual determination. The open circles represent the mean of determinations obtained from subjects studied within 4 consecutive weeks. (From R. Benveniste and A. Scommegna. Human chorionic gonadotropin α-subunit in pregnancy. *Am. J. Obstet. Gynecol.* 141:952, 1981.)

ing was variably predictive of pregnancy outcome [46]. This is understandable when a minimum sensitivity of 750 mIU per milliliter for most immunoassay systems and interference of other substances (e.g., protein, blood) are considered [22]. Using the newer generation of immunoassay tube tests, set to measure 250 mIU per milliliter, positive urine results have been recorded when serum beta hCG RIA values were as low as 23 ng per milliliter, and as early as day 12 to 14 after ovulation [18].

There are few data on simultaneous prospective serum and urinary testing. Marshall et al. [50] recorded the parallel nature of urinary and serum pregnancy curves in early pregnancy. Reporting on simultaneous measurement of urinary hCG by mouse uterine weight bioassay and serum hCG by hLH-hCG RIA, a linear rise for 3 weeks following ovulation was noted. Corson, Batzer, and Schlaff [19] reported similar linearity using a urinary beta subunit specific hCG latex agglutination immunoassay technique and serum beta hCG RIA (Fig. 4-3).

Since most on-the-spot pregnancy testing is performed on urine, an appreciation of the potential differences between urine and serum test systems and of confounding substances is imperative. If hCG is injected intramuscularly, only about 20 percent of it will be excreted in a form biologically and antigenically

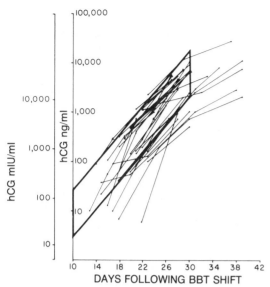

Fig. 4-4. Serial beta hCG RIA values during the first 30 days of successful pregnancies in 38 pregnancies. The solid line encloses the 95 percent confidence limits in successful pregnancies. (From F. R. Batzer et al. Serial β-subunit human chorionic gonadotropin doubling time as a prognosticator of pregnancy outcome in an infertile population. *Fertil. Steril.* 35:307, 1981. Reprinted with permission of the publisher, The American Fertility Society.)

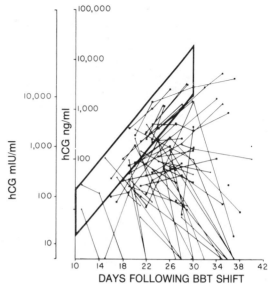

Fig. 4-5. Serial beta hCG RIA values in 53 patients who aborted spontaneously. Twenty-six patients had a negative slope. Five patients with a normal slope aborted in the second trimester. The solid line encloses the 95% confidence limits in successful pregnancies. (From F. R. Batzer et al. Serial β-subunit human chorionic gonadotropin doubling time as a prognosticator of pregnancy outcome in an infertile population. *Fertil. Steril.* 35:307, 1981. Reprinted with permission of the publisher, The American Fertility Society.)

recognizable as intact hormone [57]. Sialic acid moieties that prolong hCG serum half-life are changed in excreted hCG forms [24]. In addition, urinary measurement represents the excretion of a substance over time balanced against the secretory rate. The milieu of urine, especially protein, has always been known to affect urinary testing, increasing the false positive rate [22].

The concept of hCG doubling time, introduced by Marshall et al. [50], has been utilized as a prognostic index [5, 16]. Normal gestational growth is associated with doubling times of 1.2 to 2.2 days [5, 16, 48, 50], correlating with the doubling time of trophoblastic cell number [11]. (Doubling time is computed by dividing the logarithm of 2 by the slope of the line derived from serial hCG values.)

The concept of doubling time is practical as well as predictive. It obviates the need for ovulation dating to avoid false identification of a low-for-date value. Each patient becomes her own control with ovulation timing for subsequent ultrasound and serum testing calculated on that basis, not patient recall. It is available as a predictive index long before other specific diagnostic pregnancy changes have occurred, anatomic [34] and hormonal [66]. It increases predictive accuracy for

successful pregnancies [39] and especially for pregnancies with low-for-date values [5] (Figs. 4-4 and 4-5). When applied to tube macroflocculation immunoassay urine testing in a semiquantitative technique, it proved equally useful with impressive immediacy of results within the office setting [19].

OTHER PLACENTAL AND STEROID HORMONES

Part of the totipotential nature of the trophoblast is its secretion of a variety of different substances, many of which appear to be pregnancy specific. Use of the basic principles of immunology have permitted the isolation of several new placental proteins, including human placental lactogen [33], pregnancy-specific beta$_1$ glycoprotein [13], pregnancy-associated plasma protein A, and others [41]. Though their functional roles in pregnancy are unknown, their usefulness will probably be as indicators of placental function, not pregnancy diagnosis.

Steroid hormones secreted in huge quantities during pregnancy are present as a continuum through the normal menstrual cycle [58]. Though much emphasis has been placed on their measurement for pregnancy prognosis, early values are not diagnostic of pregnancy [71]. The wide range of "normal" makes diagnostic criteria difficult to define until the fifth and eighth week of fetal gestation when estradiol and progesterone, respectively, are consistently above those of the normal menstrual cycle [66] (Fig. 4-6). The concomitant rise in prolactin is secondary to the rise in estrogens [3] in early pregnancy.

ULTRASOUND

Ultrasonic examination provides the anatomic dimension of early pregnancy growth and detection. Its widespread application in all obstetric care has provided rapid quantification of in vivo information. Recent increases in the resolution of sonographic equipment have augmented precision, but present limitations of the technology still make hormonal testing the definitive evaluation of the presence of growing trophoblastic tissue [63].

The sonographic landmarks of early pregnancy can be seen as three progressive changes. During the first 26 days postovulation definitive changes of trophoblastic function cannot be visualized. A decidual reaction can be seen within the uterus as evidenced by loss of the central uterine cavity echo and increasing echoes within the endometrium [59].

Between 26 and 36 days postovulation a definitive gestational sac should be discernible. The presence of a growing gestational sac relates to the beta hCG level in a linear fashion, as both are functions of the trophoblast (Fig. 4-7). Its absence in the presence of a positive and increasing beta hCG RIA should raise the suspicion of an ectopic gestation [40]. The concept of a "critical level" of beta hCG, above which a gestational sac should be visualized within the uterus in a normal pregnancy, has proven most useful. This critical level as described appears to be about 1000 ng per milliliter [6] (1 ng = 5.7 mIU/ml) or 6000 mIU per milliliter [35,38]. While ultrasound is most useful in ruling out ectopic pregnancy by demonstration of an intrauterine sac, it must be coupled with beta hCG RIA testing during this early period to be accurate, even when the exact duration of pregnancy is known [36]. Other ultrasonic criteria for early pregnancy failure during this period include a poorly defined sac, small-for-date sac, abnormal intrauterine echoes, low implanted sac, growth failure, or double sac [31].

By 8 menstrual weeks or 45 days postovulation, fetal heart motion (FHM) should be present [2]. Fetal heart motion is consistent with continued pregnancy beyond the first trimester in more than 95 percent of cases despite symptomatology [6, 35] (Fig. 4-8). Should there be

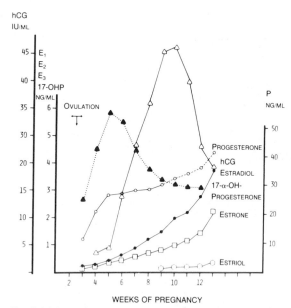

WEEKS OF PREGNANCY

Fig. 4-6. Mean plasma values of hCG, P, 17-OHP, and unconjugated E_1, E_2, and E_3 for 10 normal patients followed weekly from the third to the thirteenth week of pregnancy. Arrow indicates the presumed time of ovulation. Weeks of pregnancy = weeks from LMP. (From D. Tulchinsky and C. J. Hobel. Plasma human chorionic gonadotropin, estrone, estradiol, estriol, progesterone, and 17 α-hydroxyprogesterone in human pregnancy. *Am. J. Obstet. Gynecol.* 117:884, 1973.)

any question as to the date of conception, as often happens when bleeding complicates early pregnancy, serial studies should be obtained.

ECTOPIC PREGNANCY

Low hCG values do not distinguish between ectopic pregnancy and impending abortion. Only a negative quantitative serum beta hCG RIA rules out significant trophoblastic tissue growth [60] except in certain cases of neoplastic disease [69]. The results of the usual immunologic urinary testing are negative or equivocal in more than 50 percent of ectopic pregnancies [60]. But the increased sensitivity of the new generation urinary macroflocculation tube tests seems to be very adequate, detecting hCG in more than 85 percent of patients with ectopic gestation, according to one study [14]. While low beta hCG levels were once considered diagnostic of ectopic pregnancy [44], use of serial values and a critical level of beta hCG in conjunction with ultrasound is now the appropriate approach to clinically subtle cases

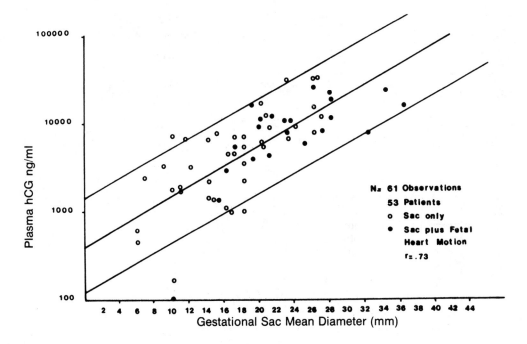

Fig. 4-7. Simultaneous measurement of plasma hCG and gestational sac mean diameter (GSMD) in 53 pregnancies (61 observations) during the first 42 days postovulation. The lines represent the linear regression ± 2 S.E.M. in these successful pregnancies (r = 0.73). Open circles indicate the presence of a gestational sac only, while solid circles indicate simultaneous fetal heart motion (FHM). (From F. R. Batzer et al. Landmarks during the first forty-two days of gestation demonstrated by the β-subunit of human chorionic gonadotropin and ultrasound. *Am. J. Obstet. Gynecol.* 146:973, 1983.)

[6, 37, 38] (see discussion in section on Ultrasound). Prospective application of these techniques will minimize tubal damage, helping to preserve fertility in already compromised patients and to decrease significant morbidity and mortality.

WHAT DOES A POSITIVE PREGNANCY TEST MEAN?

The meaning of a positive pregnancy test depends not only on the type, sensitivity, and specificity of the test used, but also on when it is obtained clinically. The question becomes one of which test to use when. In the routine office setting, when the patient is relatively sure of her menstrual history, a rapid slide test backed up by a macroflocculation tube test should be adequate. Posi-

tive results are easier to rely on than negative ones for complete diagnosis, even with the new generation tube tests. When there is an emergency room question and time is critical, one of the semiquantitative RIA tests is essential in the face of negative immunologic testing, if results can be obtained rapidly enough. This is where the new enzyme-linked immunoabsorbent assay (ELISA) tests will prove invaluable (see discussion in section on New Techniques): test time is 1 hour; hands-on technician time is 5 minutes; the positive end point is clear; sensitivity is 25 to 50 mIU per milliliter; and no special laboratory training or equipment is needed. Cost effectiveness is excellent with only one additional positive and negative control tube necessary with each test.

If at this point uncertainty still exists about pregnancy location, simultaneous ultrasound and quantitative RIA testing may provide the answer. If the hCG value is above the critical level and no intrauterine sac is visualized, an ectopic pregnancy must be suspected until proven otherwise. If the value is less than the critical value and a watchful approach is possible, the studies are repeated and calculated on the basis of the hCG doubling time concept (about 2+ days). If the value does not rise appropriately, either a miscarriage is predicted or an ectopic pregnancy is present. Most ectopic pregnancies will not present serious dif-

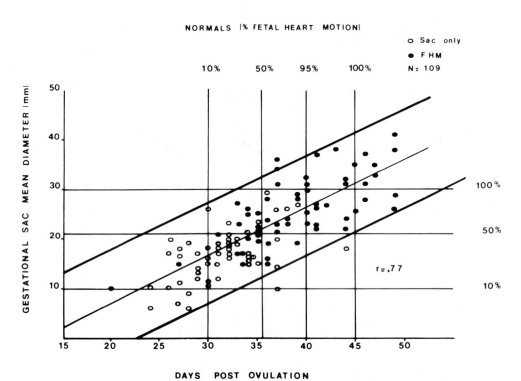

Fig. 4-8. Growth of gestational sac mean diameter (GSMD) during the first 50 days postovulation in 109 observations (71 pregnancies). The diagonal lines represent the mean ± 2 S.E.M. in these successful pregnancies ($r = 0.77$). Open circles indicate the presence of a gestational sac only, while solid circles indicate simultaneous fetal heart motion (FHM). The vertical and horizontal grids indicate the increasing percentage of cases in which FHM was noted; the vertical grid by days postovulation, the horizontal grid by GSMD. (From F. R. Batzer et al. Landmarks during the first forty-two days of gestation demonstrated by the β-subunit of human chorionic gonadotropin and ultrasound. *Am. J. Obstet. Gynecol.* 146:973, 1983.)

ficulty before 30 days postovulation, by which time this question will be resolved.

Close inspection of the regression of urinary hCG following first-trimester pregnancy termination is self-explanatory [17] (Fig. 4-9). Considering a half-life of 48 hours for hCG following induced pregnancy termination, immunoassay pregnancy testing may still be positive at 1 week and sensitive beta hCG RIA tests may remain positive for up to 3 months [17, 47]. Here also, serial application of a sensitive test will help provide the appropriate diagnosis. The test chosen depends on the needs of the patient and the physician. Choice of an overly sensitive test following spontaneous or induced abortion may actually confuse rather than clarify.

With the plethora of tests available (Table 4-2), the most practical one for routine office application would appear to be the macroflocculation immunoassay tube test for many reasons including office convenience, cost, clear end point, reproducibility, and rapidity of results. It is important to note that urine stored in a refrigerator will give reproducible urinary pregnancy results up to 1 week [18]. Freezer storage, however, may give spurious results.

A recent comparison of the five available over-the-counter urinary pregnancy tests, all hemagglutination inhibition immunoassays, reported a low false positive rate for most [26]. Sensitivity is set to measure hCG levels usually present at about 2 weeks past the missed menses to avoid the problem of a questionable end point or false positive result. There are newer tests on the horizon that will evaluate pregnancy well-being by measuring compounds other than hCG, but it is doubt-

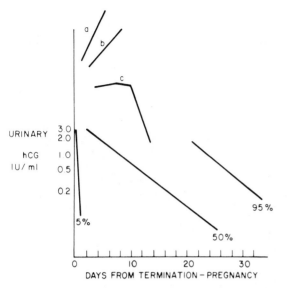

Fig. 4-9. The spontaneous regression of urinary hCG following termination of pregnancy in the first trimester, shown with confidence intervals. Cases with spotting or bleeding and persistently positive pregnancy tests are best followed by serial hCG determinations (made on dilutions of urine). Rapidly increasing levels may be seen in choriocarcinoma (line *a*); less rapidly increasing levels may be seen with hydatidiform mole (line *b*); intact intrauterine pregnancies may also appear as line *b;* and incomplete abortions may appear as line *c,* with a rapid decline of hCG levels as tissue is completely expelled. (From S. L. Corson [ed.]. Early pregnancy diagnosis. *J. Reprod.Med.* [Suppl. 26], 1981.)

ful that they will replace hCG immunoassay testing for routine diagnosis in the near future.

NEW TECHNIQUES FOR PREGNANCY EVALUATION

Monoclonal Antibodies

Problems with antibody production have made specific hCG measurement difficult due to the similar chemical composition of hCG and the other glycoproteins. Synthetic and native hCG-derived beta hCG chains or C terminal peptides have proven to be poorly immunogenic or poorly reactive with native hormones. Re-

cently introduced techniques of monoclonal antibody production of predefined specificity by hybrid cell lines have provided a unique approach to this problem [42]. This technique permits the creation of a single antibody to the specific components of the hCG molecule beta subunit and other confirmational components of the hCG molecule. Eventually a more specific antibody for pregnancy testing may be routinely used, once easy production is possible [32, 65].

Enzyme-linked Immunoabsorbent Assay (ELISA)

The technique of enzyme-linked immunoabsorbent assay has recently been applied to hCG measurement [25, 29]. While RIA or RRA systems have been extensively utilized for measurement of biologic substances because of their accuracy and sensitivity, they have several drawbacks, including nuclear waste, expense, sophisticated equipment, and unstable and short-lived radiosotopes. The recent development of enzyme immunoassay and receptor assay systems, in which an enzyme is utilized for antigen labeling instead of a radioactive marker, has circumvented some of these problems. The advantages of such a technique include greater stability of enzyme-antigen conjugates, simpler equipment for measurement of enzyme activities, and no nuclear waste products or problems. The enzyme yields a color-change reaction with an appropriate substrate, which is measurable and often directly visible. Eventually these techniques will provide the basis of future do-it-yourself qualitative pregnancy tests.

Rosette Inhibition Test

Originally reported by Morton and others [53], measurement of an early pregnancy factor (EPF) by the Rosette Inhibition Test has been difficult to duplicate and controversial. Based on the detection of a modification of maternal lymphocyte activity, the theoretic basis of the test is very plausible. Early suppression of the maternal immune system would seem essential for pregnancy nidation and viability. Early pregnancy factor is active before placental production of hCG begins at the time of implantation. Its usefulness as a test in humans is hampered by the involved lengthy mechanics of the test at present [64].

These are the three newest test concepts on the horizon. However, the rampant growth of data from in vitro fertilization–embryo transfer programs will undoubtedly soon provide more hints as to what allows or disrupts the process of fertilization, nidation, and growth of a pregnancy.

Table 4-2. Comparative data on pregnancy tests

Home pregnancy tests

Kit	Acu-Test	Answer	Daisy 2	e.p.t.	Predictor
Manufacturer	J. B. William Co., Inc.	Diagnostic Testing, Inc.	Ortho Pharmaceutical Corp.	Warner-Lambert Co.	Whitehall Laboratories
Method	Hemagglutination inhibition	Hemagglutination inhibition	Hemagglutination inhibition	Hemagglutination inhibition	Hemagglutination inhibition
Indicator particle	Coated red blood cells	Coated red blood cells	Coated red blood cells	Coated red blood cells	Coated red blood cells
End point	Positive—ring at bottom of test tube Negative—no ring	Positive—ring at bottom of test tube Negative—no ring	Positive—ring at bottom of test tube Negative—no ring	Positive—ring at bottom of test tube Negative—no ring	Positive—ring at bottom of test tube Negative—no ring
Sensitivity (IU/ml)[a]	0.4–0.8	1.0	0.6–0.8	0.5–1.0	0.6–0.9
Earliest detection	9 days from missed period	9 days from missed period	6 days from missed period	9 days from missed period	9 days from missed period
% overall accuracy claimed	97%	96%	97.3%	99.5%	98.94–99.73%
Reagents	Ready to use	Ready to use	Ready to use	Ready to use	Ready to use
Amount/specimen	0.5 ml/urine	2 drops/urine	2 drops/urine	3 drops/urine	0.1 ml/urine
Equipment	All included	All included	All included	All included	All included
Reaction time	2 hours	2–4 hours	1 hour	2 hours	2–3 hours
Interfering substances	Detergent Sunlight Heat	Detergent Urine cloudy, pink, red, or has strong odor Menopausal women Certain diseases or medications	Detergent Sunlight Heat Urine cloudy, pink, or red Certain conditions specific to individual	Detergent Sunlight Heat	Detergent Sunlight Heat
Vibration interference	Yes	Yes	Yes	Yes	Yes

Slide tests

Kit	Sensi-Slide	Prognosis	UCG-Slide Test	Dap Test Macro	Pregnosticon Dri-Dot
Manufacturer	Roche Diagnostics	Roche Diagnostics	Wampole Laboratories	Wampole Laboratories	Organon Diagnostics
Indicator particle	Latex covalent bonded	Latex covalent bonded	Coated latex adsorptive bond	Coated latex adsorptive bond	Coated latex
End point	Positive—milky white Negative—agglutination	Positive—milky white Negative—macroagglutination	Positive—milky white Negative—macroagglutination	Positive—macroagglutination Negative—milky white	Positive—milky green Negative—macroagglutination

Slide tests

Kit	Sensi-Slide	Pregnosis	UCG-Slide Test	Dap Test Macro	Pregnosticon Dri-Dot
Sensitivity	0.8 IU hCG/ml	1.5–2.5 IU hCG/ml	2 IU hCG/ml	2 IU hCG/ml	1–2 IU hCG/ml
Earliest detection	At time of missed period	5 days from missed period	5 days from missed period	4 days from missed period	5 days from missed period
% overall accuracy claimed	98.4%	97.3%	97%	—	98.6%
Specimen preparation	None	None	First morning void	Filtering of urine is crucial to test accuracy	None
Rotation	Gentle	Vigorous	Slow, gentle rocking necessary to prevent breakup of agglutination	Gentle	Slow and gentle to prevent breakup of agglutination
Interference	Protein	None	Blood/protein/bacteria	Low specific gravity/prozone effects	Blood/drugs/protein/detergent
Readability	Easy-to-read large particles	Easy-to-read large particles	Fine particles; may be hard to read; needs light for interpretation	Hard to read	Easy-to-read agglutination
Stability	24 months	24 months	18 months	24 months	36 months
Storage	Refrigerate at 2–8°C	Refrigerate at 2–8°C	Refrigerate at 2–8°C	Refrigerate at 2–8°C	Room temperature

Slide tests

Kit	Pregnosticon Slide Test	Gravindex 90	Pregnate	Pregna β-Slide	β-Clone hCG Assay
Manufacturer	Organon Diagnostics	Ortho Diagnostics	Fisher Scientific	International Diagnostics	Monoclonal Antibodies, Inc.
Indicator particle	Coated latex	Coated latex adsorptive bond	Coated latex adsorptive bond	Coated latex adsorptive bond	Latex covalent bonded
End point	Positive—milky white Negative—macroagglutination	Positive—milky white Negative—agglutination	Positive—milky white Negative—agglutination	Positive—greenish mixture Negative—agglutination	Positive—milky white Negative—agglutination
Sensitivity	1–2 IU hCG/ml	3.5 IU hCG/ml	2–4 IU hCG/ml	2 IU hCG/ml	0.5 IU hCG/ml
Earliest detection	5 days from missed period	No claim	No claim	No claim	No claim
% overall accuracy claimed	98.6%	98%	98.4%	99.5%	98.5%
Specimen preparation	None	None	None	Centrifuge if turbid	Centrifuge or filter if turbid

Table 4-2 (continued)

Slide tests

Kit	Pregnosticon Slide Test	Gravindex 90	Pregnate	Pregna β-Slide	β-Clone hCG Assay
Rotation	Gentle	Slow and gentle to prevent breakup of ag-glutination	Gentle	Gentle	Gentle
Interference	Protein/blood	Drugs/protein specific grav-ity/detergent	None	Blood/protein/bacteria	None
Readability	Easy-to-read ag-glutination	Direct light source needed; parti-cles readability biggest problem	Fine particles	Green color is hard to read; requires high intensity lamp	Easy-to-read ag-glutination
Stability	12 months	12 months	18 months	12 months	12 months
Storage	Refrigerate at 2–8°C	Refrigerate at 2–8°C	Refrigerate at 2–8°C	Refrigerate at 2–8°C	Refrigerate at 2–8°C

Tube tests

Kit	Sensi-Tex	Placentex	UCG-Test	UCG-Quik Tube	UCG-Lypho-Test
Manufacturer	Roche Diagnos-tics	Roche Diagnos-tics	Wampole Diag-nostics	Wampole Diag-nostics	Wampole Labora-tories
Method	Indirect aggluti-nation inhibi-tion	Indirect aggluti-nation inhibi-tion	Hemagglutina-tion inhibition	Hemagglutina-tion inhibition	Hemagglutination inhibition
Indicator particle	Latex, covalent-bonded	Latex, covalent-bond-ed	Coated red blood cell	Coated red blood cell	Coated red blood cell
End point	Positive—milky white Negative—floc-culation	Positive—milky white Negative—floc-culation	Positive—ring Negative—mat	Positive—ring Negative—mat	Positive—ring Negative—mat
Sensitivity	0.25 IU hCG/ml	1.0 IU hCG/ml	Undiluted—0.5 IU hCG/ml Diluted—1.3 IU hCG/ml	1.0 IU hCG/ml	0.5–1.0 IU hCG/ml
Earliest detection	At or before missed period	4 days from missed period	4 days from missed period	4 days from missed period	4 days from missed period
% overall accu-racy claimed	99.2%	98.1%	98%	98%	98%
Procedure	Specimen/anti-gen mix/heat-ing block	Specimen/anti-gen mix/heat-ing block	Dilute 2 tubes/antibody/specimen/an-tigen/shake	Control/pa-tient/speci-men/ 2 tubes	Specimen/antigen mix/rack
Reagents	Ready to use	Ready to use	Ready to use	Lyophilized; must be re-constituted	Lyophilized; must be reconstituted

Tube tests

Kit	Sensi-Tex	Placentex	UCG-Test	UCG-Quik Tube	UCG-Lypho-Test
Specimen/amount	Urine/1 ml	Urine/1 ml	Urine (first morning void)/1 ml undiluted, 0.25 ml diluted, or serum/1 ml	Urine (first morning void)/0.1 ml	Urine (first morning void)/0.1 ml
Specimen preparation	Filter or centrifuge if turbid	Filter or centrifuge if turbid	Filter or centrifuge if turbid	Filter or centrifuge if turbid	Filter or centrifuge if turbid
Equipment	Heating block	Heating block	Tubes/rack	Rack	Rack
Setup time	60 seconds	60 seconds	4–5 minutes	5 minutes	5 minutes
Reaction time	90 minutes	Positives—90 minutes Negatives—60 minutes	2 hours	Positives—1 hour Negatives—2 hours	1 hour
Interfering substances	High levels of protein	High levels of protein	Blood/protein/bacteria/drugs/LH/detergent/hygroscopic	Blood/protein/bacteria	Blood/protein/bacteria
Vibration interference	None	None	Probable	Probable	Probable
Readability	Flocculation extremely easy to read	Flocculation extremely easy to read	Rings (inconclusive)	Rings	May be hard to read; atypical rings
Storage	Refrigerate at 2–8°C	Refrigerate at 2–8°C	Refrigerate at 2–8°C	Refrigerate at 2–8°C	30°C

Tube tests

Kit	β-Neocept	Pregnosticon with Accusphere Reagents	Gravindex 90	Pregna-β
Manufacturer	Organon Diagnostics	Organon Diagnostics	Ortho Diagnostics	International Diagnostics
Method	Hemagglutination inhibition	Hemagglutination inhibition	Hemagglutination inhibition	Hemagglutination inhibition
Indicator particle	Coated red blood cell	Coated red blood cell	Coated red blood cell	Coated red blood cell
End point	Positive—ring Negative—mat	Positive—ring Negative—mat	Positive—ring Negative—mat	Positive—ring Negative—mat
Sensitivity	0.15 IU hCG/ml	0.6–0.9 IU hCG/ml (exact sensitivity stated on package)	0.5 IU hCG/ml	0.4–0.8 IU hCG/ml
Earliest detection	At or before missed period	4 days from missed period	4–7 days from missed period	4 days from missed period
% overall accuracy claimed	99–100%	98.9%	98.5%	98%

Table 4-2 (continued)

Tube tests

Kit	β-Neocept	Pregnosticon with Accusphere Reagents	Gravindex 90	Pregna-β
Procedure	Specimen/buffer/shake	Specimen/buffer/shake	Control patient tubes/antibody/specimen/shake/antigen/shake/rack	Specimen/buffer/mix/rack
Reagents	Ready-to-use	Ready-to-use	Lyophilized; must be reconstituted	Prefilled tube
Specimen/amount	Urine/0.05 ml	Urine/0.1 ml	Urine/1 drop	Urine/2 drops
Specimen preparation	None (filter or centrifuge if turbid)	None (filter or centrifuge if turbid)	Filter or centrifuge if turbid	Filter or centrifuge if turbid
Equipment	Rack	Rack	Rack	Rack
Setup time	60 seconds	60 seconds	5 minutes	4 minutes
Reaction time	60 minutes (or less)	120 minutes (or less)	1½ hours	2 hours
Interfering substances	Hygroscopic/detergent/LH/heat block/sun/protein/drugs/bacteria	Heat/sun/LH/detergents/protein/drugs/bacteria/hygroscopic	Protein/drugs	Drugs/protein/bacteria
Vibration interference	Probable	Very probable	Very probable	Probable
Readability	Easy to read—rings	Easy to read—rings	Rings; frequently inconclusive	Rings; may be hard to read
Storage	Refrigerate at 2–8°C	Room temperature	Refrigerate at 2–8°C	Room temperature

Radioassays

Kit	Roche β-hCG RIA	Beta-Tec	Radioimmunoassay of Human Chorionic Gonadotropin (hCG) Beta Subunit Specific	Concep-7-β-HCG
Manufacturer	Roche Diagnostics	Wampole Laboratories	Cambridge Nuclear	Leeco Diagnostics
Kit size	100	125	100	
Sensitivity	2 mIU hCG/ml (25 mIU hCG/ml qual) serum; 100 mIU hCG/ml urine	30 mIU hCG/ml (range: 3–50 mIU hCG/ml) (qual/quant)	50 mIU hCG (qual); 15 mIU hCG (quant)	30 mIU hCG/ml serum; 100 mIU hCG/ml urine
Manual assay steps	6 pipette 1 dispense Decant	4 pipette 1 dispense Aspirate	6 pipette 1 dispense Decant	6 pipette 1 dispense Decant
Incubation time/temperature	30 minutes room T 15 minutes room T	30 minutes 37°C + 80 minutes room T	1 hour 37°C + 10 minutes room T	30 minutes 37°C
Centrifugation	10 minutes at 1,500 g	15 minutes at 1,600 g	30 minutes at 1,500 g	20 minutes at 1,500 g
Specimen/volume	Serum/plasma (no gross lipidemia hemolysis or turbidity) 200 μl; urine 100 μl	Serum (no gross hemolysis, lipidemia or turbidity) 50, 100, 200, 300, 500 μl	Serum/plasma (no gross hemolysis) 200 μl	Serum/plasma 0.5 ml (no gross hemolysis); urine 0.5 ml (centrifuge if cellular or crystalline)

Radioassays

Kit	Roche β-hCG RIA	Beta-Tec	Radioimmunoassay of Human Chorionic Gonado-tropin (hCG) Beta Subunit Specific	Concep-7-β-HCG
Special equipment required	Gamma counter	37°C water bath Ice water bath Gamma counter	Refrigerated centrifuge Gamma counter	37°C water bath Gamma counter
Control provided	1 positive	None	2 positive	Serum: 1 negative, 1 positive Urine: 1 negative, 1 positive
Storage	2–8°C	2–8°C	2–8°C	2–8°C
Stability (shelf life)	52 days	6 weeks	See vial	6 weeks

Radioassays

Kit	HCG-β Radioimmunoassay Kit	HCG-β Radioimmunoassay Kit	Beta-hCG RIA	Beta-CG Pregnancy Assay Monitor
Manufacturer	BIO-RIA	BIO-RIA	Monitor Science Corporation	Science Corporation
Kit size	125,250	125	150	60
Sensitivity	6 mIU hCG/ml	20 mIU hCG/ml	5 mIU hCG/ml	40 mIU hCG/ml
Manual assay steps	5 pipette 1 dispense Decant	5 pipette 1 dispense Decant/aspirate	6 pipette Aspirate	4 pipette 1 dispense Aspirate/decant
Incubation time/temperature	12–24 hours room T 6–24 hours room T	2–6 hours room T 5 minutes room T	2 hours 37°C + 2 hours 37°C + 2 hours 37°C or overnight 2–8°C	45 minutes room T 10 minutes room T
Centrifugation	15–30 minutes at 1,250 g refrigerated	15 minutes at 1,250 g refrigerated	15 minutes at 1,500 g at 2.8°C	10 minutes at 1,500 g
Specimen/volume	Serum/plasma (no heparin) 100 μl (2), 200 μl (2)	Serum/plasma (no heparin) 100 μl (2), 200 μl (2)	Serum/plasma (no heparin, gross hemolysis) 100 μl (2), 100 μl (2)	Serum/plasma (no heparin, gross hemolysis) 100 μl (1)
Special equipment required	Refrigerated centrifuge Gamma counter	Refrigerated centrifuge Gamma counter	Refrigerated centrifuge 37°C water bath Gamma counter	Gamma counter
Control provided	1 positive	1 positive ± 5 mIU hCG/ml	None	1 negative 1 positive
Storage	2–4°C	2–4°C	2–8°C	2–8°C
Stability (shelf life)	4 weeks (23 days)	1 month	8–10 weeks	8–10 weeks

Table 4-2 (continued)

Radioassays

Kit	Chorio SHure	Chorio-Quant	RIA-Nate	β-hCG Radioimmunoassay Kit
Manufacturer	NML Laboratories	NML Laboratories	Mallinckrodt Nuclear	Becton Dickinson Immunodiagnostics
Kit size	100	100	50	100
Sensitivity	40 mIU hCG/ml serum; 80 mIU hCG/ml urine	30 mIU hCG/ml (serum-qual); 60 mIU hCG/ml (urine-qual); 5 mIU hCG/ml (serum-quant)	25 mIU hCG/ml serum; 100 mIU hCG/ml urine	Serum: 30 mIU hCG/ml (qual); 2.8 mIU/ml (quant); urine: 100 mIU hCG/ml
Manual assay steps	4 pipette 1 dispense Decant	4 pipette 1 dispense Decant	4 pipette 1 dispense Decant	4 pipette 1 dispense Decant
Incubation time/temperature	15 minutes 37°C + 30 minutes 37°C + 10 minutes room T	15 minutes 37°C + 30 minutes 37°C + 10 minutes room T	1 hour room T	35 minutes room T (qual) or 30 minutes room T + 90 minutes room T (quant)
Centrifugation	10 minutes (1,000 to 1,500 g)	10 minutes (1,000 to 1,500 g)	30 ± 5 minutes at 1,500 to 2,000 g or 45 minutes at 1,000 g	20 minutes at 1,500 g or 30–40 minutes at 1,000 g
Specimen/volume	Serum/plasma 200 μl; urine 100 μl	Serum/plasma 200 μl; urine 100 μl	Serum 200 μl (no gross hemolysis or lipidemia); urine 100 μl	Serum/plasma 200 μl; urine 100 μl
Special equipment required	Gamma counter 37°C water bath	Gamma counter 37°C water bath	Gamma counter	Gamma counter 37°C water bath (optional)
Control provided	1 negative	Qualitative; 0 standard used for negative control	None	Serum: 1 negative, 1 positive Urine: 1 negative, 1 positive
Storage	2–8°C	2–8°C	2–8°C	2–8°C
Stability (shelf life)	6 weeks	6 weeks	14 days (frozen standard 15°C)	See vial

Radioassays

Kit	Preg-Stat	β III hCG-Beta	RSL hCG β-subunit kit	Biocept-G[b]
Manufacturer	Sereno Laboratories	Sereno Laboratories	Radioassay Systems Laboratories	Wampole Laboratories
Kit size	75	125	100	30
Sensitivity	25 mIU hCG/ml	3–4 mIU hCG/ml (25–30 mIU hCG/ml qual; 1–2 mIU hCG/ml 45 minutes quant)	40 mIU hCG/ml (< 0.5 ng hCG/ml; 2.5 mIU hCG/ml is stated as negative for hCG)	200 mIU hCG/ml

Radioassays

Kit	Preg-Stat	β III hCG-Beta	RSL hCG β-subunit kit	Biocept-G[b]
Manual assay steps	4 pipette 1 dispense Decant	5 pipette Decant	4 pipette Aspirate/decant	2 pipette Aspirate/decant
Incubation time/temperature	30 minutes room T	2 hours room T	1 hour 37°C (qual) 2 hours 37°C (quant)	30 minutes 37°C
Centrifugation	15 minutes at 1,600–3,000 g room T	15 minutes at 1,500–3,000 g room T	10–15 minutes at 2,300–2,500 g	15 minutes at 2,000–5,000 RPM
Specimen/volume	Serum/plasma (no gross hemolysis or lipidemia) 100 μl	Serum/plasma (no gross hemolysis or lipidemia) 100 μl	Serum 100 μl	Serum (no hemolysis or gross lipidemia; must be refrigerated) 100 μl (2)
Special equipment required	Gamma counter	Gamma counter	Water bath 37°C centrifuge Gamma counter	Ice water bath 37°C water bath Gamma counter
Control provided	1 positive 1 negative	1 negative 1 positive	1 negative 1 positive	None
Storage	2–8°C	2–8°C	4–8°C	2–8°C
Stability (shelf life)	30 days	See vial	8 weeks	5 weeks

ELISA tests

Kit	ModEL Urine hCG Assay	ModEL Serum hCG Assay	Sensi-Chrome
Manufacturer	Monoclonal Antibodies, Inc.	Monoclonal Antibodies, Inc.	Roche Diagnostics
Kit size	100	50	25/100
Sensitivity	50 mIU hCG/ml (urine)	25 mIU hCG/ml (serum)	50 mIU hCG/ml
Manual assay steps	3 pipette 4 wash/decant	4 pipette 4 wash/decant	1 pipette 1 wash
Incubation time/temperature	5 minutes room T 20 minutes room T 30 minutes room T	60 minutes room T 20 minutes room T	15 minutes 5 minutes
Centrifugation	None	None	None
Specimen/volume	Urine 50, 300, 500 μl (4 ml or wash bottle)	Serum 50, 300, 500 μl (4 ml or wash bottle)	Urine 0.5 ml
Special equipment	None	None	Vortex
Control provided	Negative control 50 mIU/ml calibrator	Negative control 25 mIU/ml calibrator	None (color chart)
Storage	2–8°C	2–8°C	2–8°C
Stability: Lyophilized Reconstituted	1 year 8–16 weeks	1 year 8 weeks	As per expiration date

[a]According to manufacturer.
[b]Radioreceptor assay.

REFERENCES

1. Albert, A., and Berkson, J. A clinical bio-assay for chorionic gonadotropin. *J. Clin. Endocrinol. Metab.* 11:805, 1951.
2. Anderson, S. G. Management of threatened abortion with real-time sonography. *Am. J. Obstet. Gynecol.* 55:259, 1980.
3. Barberia, J. M., et al. Serum prolactin patterns in early human gestation. *Am. J. Obstet. Gynecol.* 121:1107, 1975.
4. Batzer, F. R. Hormonal evaluation of early pregnancy. *Fertil. Steril.* 34:1, 1980.
5. Batzer, F. R., et al. Serial β-subunit human chorionic gonadotropin doubling time as a prognosticator of pregnancy outcome in an infertile population. *Fertil. Steril.* 35:307, 1981.
6. Batzer, F. R., et al. Landmarks during the first forty-two days of gestation demonstrated by the β-subunit of human chorionic gonadotropin and ultrasound *Am. J. Obstet. Gynecol.* 146:973, 1983.
7. Beling, C. G., Cederqvist, L. L., and Fuchs, F. Demonstration of gonadotropin during the second half of the cycle in women using intrauterine contraception. *Am. J. Obstet. Gynecol.* 125:855, 1976.
8. Benveniste, R., and Scommegna, A. Human chorionic gonadotropin α-subunit in pregnancy. *Am. J. Obstet. Gynecol.* 141:952, 1981.
9. Borkowski, A., and Muquardt, D. Human chorionic gonadotropin in the plasma of normal, nonpregnant subjects. *N. Engl. J. Med.* 301:298, 1979.
10. Braunstein, G. D., et al. Ectopic production of human chorionic gonadotropin by neoplasmas. *Ann. Intern. Med.* 78:39, 1973.
11. Braunstein, G. D., et al. Secretory rates of human chorionic gonadotropin by normal trophoblast. *Am. J. Obstet. Gynecol.* 115:447, 1973.
12. Braunstein, G. D., et al. First-trimester chorionic gonadotropin measurements as an aid in the diagnosis of early pregnancy disorders. *Am. J. Obstet. Gynecol.* 131:25, 1978.
13. Braunstein, G. D., et al. Interrelationships of human chorionic gonadotropin, human placental lactogen, and pregnancy-specific β₁-glycoprotein throughout normal human gestation. *Am. J. Obstet. Gynecol.* 138:1205, 1980.
14. Braunstein, G. D., and Asch, R. H. Predictive value analysis of measurements of human chorionic gonadotropin, pregnancy specific β₁-glycoprotein, placental lactogen, and cystine aminopeptidase for the diagnosis of ectopic pregnancy. *Fertil. Steril.* 39:62, 1983.
15. Catt, K. J., Dufau, M. L., and Vaitukaitis, J. L. Appearance of hCG in pregnancy plasma following the initiation of implantation of the blastocyst. *Clin. Endocrinol. Metab.* 40:537, 1975.
16. Chartier, M., et al. Measurement of plasma human chorionic gonadotropin (hCG) and β-hCG activities in the late luteal phase: Evidence of the occurrence of spontaneous menstrual abortions in infertile women. *Fertil. Steril.* 31:134, 1979.
17. Corson, S. L. (Ed.). Early pregnancy diagnosis. *J. Reprod. Med.* (Suppl. 26), 1981.
18. Corson, S. L., and Batzer, F. R. Early urinary pregnancy testing: Correlation with serum beta-HCG radioimmunoassay. *J. Reprod. Med.* 27:725, 1982.
19. Corson, S. L., Batzer, F. R., and Schlaff, S. A comparison of serial quantitative serum and urine tests in early pregnancy. *J. Reprod. Med.* 26:611, 1981.
20. Croxatto, H. B., et al. Studies on the duration of egg transport by the human oviduct. *Am. J. Obstet. Gynecol.* 132:629, 1978.
21. Csapo, A. I., and Pulkkinen, M. Indispensability of the human corpus luteum in the maintenance of early pregnancy: Luteectomy evidence. *Obstet. Gynecol. Surv.* 33:69, 1978.
22. Duenhoelter, J. H. Pregnancy tests—evaluating and using them. *Contemp. Obstet. Gynecol.* 19:239, 1982.
23. Edmonds, D. K., et al. Early embryonic mortality in women. *Fertil. Steril.* 38:447, 1982.
24. Good, A., et al. Molecular forms of human chorionic gonadotropin in serum, urine and placental extracts. *Fertil. Steril.* 28:846, 1977.
25. Hamada, K., et al. Simultaneous competitive enzyme immunoassay for human chorionic gonadotropin. *Endocrinol. Jpn.* 25:515, 1978.
26. Hanlon, J. T., et al. An evaluation of the sensitivity of five home pregnancy tests to known concentrations of human chorionic gonadotropin. *Am. J. Obstet. Gynecol.* 144:778, 1982.
27. Hanson, F. W., Powell, J. E., and Stevens, V. C. Effects of hCG and human pituitary LH on steroid secretion and functional life of the human corpus luteum. *J. Clin. Endocrinol. Metab.* 32:211, 1971.
28. Haour, F., and Saxena, B. B. Detection of a gonadotropin in rabbit blastocyst before implantation. *Science* 185:445, 1974.
29. Hashimoto, M., and Kawaoi, A. Development of an enzyme-linked receptor assay (ERA) for hCG. *Endocrinol. Jpn.* 24(3):307, 1977.
30. Heap, R. B., Flint, A. P., and Gadsby, J. E. Role of embryonic signals in the establishment of pregnancy. *Med. Bull.* 35:129, 1979.
31. Hellman, L. M., Kebayashi, M., and Cromb, E. Ultrasonic diagnosis of embryonic malformations. *Am. J. Obstet. Gynecol.* 115:615, 1973.
32. Hussa, R. O. Clinical utility of human chorionic gonadotropin and subunit measurements. *Obstet. Gynecol.* 60:1, 1982.
33. Josimovich, J. B. Human Placental Lactogen. In F. Fuchs and A. Klopper (eds.), *Endocrinology of Pregnancy* (2nd ed.). Hagerstown, Md.: Harper & Row, 1977. P. 191.
34. Jouppila, P. Clinical and ultrasonic aspects in the diag-

nosis and follow-up of patients with early pregnancy failure. *Acta Obstet. Gynecol. Scand.* 59:495, 1980.

35. Jouppila, P., Huhtaniemi, I., and Tapanainen, J. Early pregnancy failure: Study by ultrasonic and hormonal methods. *Obstet. Gynecol.* 55:42, 1980.

36. Jouppila, P., Tapanainen, J., and Huhtaniemi, I. Plasma hCG and ultrasound in suspected ectopic pregnancy. *Eur. J. Obstet. Gynecol. Reprod. Biol.* 10:3, 1980.

37. Kadar, N., Caldwell, B. V., and Romero, R. A method of screening for ectopic pregnancy and its indications. *Obstet. Gynecol.* 58:162, 1981b.

38. Kadar, N., DeBore, G., and Romero, R. Discriminatory hCG zone: Its use in the sonographic evaluation for ectopic pregnancy. *Obstet. Gynecol.* 58:156, 1981a.

39. Karow, W. G., and Gentry, W. C. Corpus luteum function during pregnancies of previously infertile women. *Obstet. Gynecol.* 48:603, 1976.

40. Kelly, M. T., Santos-Ramos, R., and Duenhoelter, J. H. The value of sonography in suspected ectopic pregnancy. *Obstet. Gynecol.* 53:703, 1979.

41. Klopper, A. The New Placental Proteins: Their Role in Pregnancy. In J. R. Givens (ed.), *Endocrinology of Pregnancy.* Chicago: Year Book, 1981.

42. Kofler, R., Berger, P., and Wick, G. Monoclonal antibodies againt human chorionic gonadotropin (hCG): 1. Production, specificity, and intramolecular binding sites. *Am. J. Reprod. Immunol.* 2:212, 1982.

43. Kohler, P. O., Ross, G. T., and Odell, W. D. Metabolic clearance and production rates of human luteinizing hormone in pre- and postmenopausal women. *J. Clin. Invest.* 47:38, 1968.

44. Kosasa, T., et al. Early detection of implantation using a radioimmunoassay specific for human chorionic gonadotropin. *J. Clin. Endocrinol. Metab.* 36:622, 1973a.

45. Kosasa, T. S., et al. Measurement of early chorionic activity with a radioimmunoassay specific for human chorionic gonadotropin following spontaneous and induced ovulation. *Fertil. Steril.* 25:211, 1974.

46. Kunz, J., and Keller, P. J. HCG, HPL, oestradiol, progesterone and AFP in serum in patients with threatened abortion. *Br. J. Obstet. Gynaecol.* 83:6401, 1976.

47. Lau, H. L., et al. The appearance and disappearance of urinary hCG determined by simple immunoassays and radioimmunoassays. *Adv. Plann. Parenthood* 16:45, 1981.

48. Lenton, E. A., Neal, L. M., and Sulaiman, R. Plasma concentrations of human chorionic gonadotropin from the time of implantation until the second week of pregnancy. *Fertil. Steril.* 37:773, 1982.

49. Louvet, J. P., et al. Absence of neutralizing effect of antisera to the unique structural region of human chorionic gonadotropin. *J. Clin. Endocrinol. Metab.* 39:1155, 1974.

50. Marshall, J. R., et al. Plasma and urinary chorionic gonadotropin during early human pregnancy. *Obstet. Gynecol.* 32:760, 1968.

51. Miller, J. F., et al. Fetal loss following implantation: A prospective study. *Lancet* 1:554, 1980.

52. Mishell, D. R., et al. Initial detection of human chorionic gonadotropin in serum in normal human gestation. *Am. J. Obstet. Gynecol.* 102:110, 1968.

53. Morton, H., Rolfe, B., and Clunie, G. J. A. An early pregnancy factor detected in human serum by the rosette inhibition test. *Lancet* 1:394, 1977.

54. Post, K. G., et al. A rapid, centrifugation-free radioimmunoassay specific for human chorionic gonadotropin using glass beads as solid phase. *J. Clin. Endocrinol. Metab.* 50:169, 1980.

55. Robinson, H. P. The diagnosis of early pregnancy failure by sonar. *Br. J. Obstet. Gynaecol.* 82:849, 1975.

56. Ross, G. T. Clinical relevance of research on the structure of human chorionic gonadotropin. *Am. J. Obstet. Gynecol.* 129:795, 1977.

57. Ross, G. T. Human Chorionic Gonadotropin and Maternal Recognition of Pregnancy. In *Maternal Recognition of Pregnancy* (Ciba Foundation Symposium 64). Excerpta Medica, 1979. Pp. 191–208.

58. Ross, G. T., et al. Pituitary and gonadal hormones in women during spontaneous and induced ovulatory cycles. *Recent Prog. Horm. Res.* 26:1, 1970.

59. Sakamoto, C., and Nakano, H. The echogenic endometrium and alternations during menstrual cycle. *Int. J. Gynaecol. Obstet.* 20:255, 1982.

60. Sandvei, R., Stoa, K. F., and Ulstein, M. Radioimmunoassay of human chorionic gonadotropin β-subunit as an early diagnostic test in ectopic pregnancy. *Acta Obstet. Gynecol. Scand.* 60:389, 1981.

61. Saxena, B. B., Hasan, S. H., and Haour, F. Radioreceptor assay of human chorionic gonadotropin: Detection of early pregnancy. *Science* 184:793, 1974.

62. Saxena, B. B., et al. Radioreceptorassay of luteinizing hormone-human chorionic gonadotropin in urine: Detection of the luteinizing hormone surge and pregnancy. *Fertil. Steril.* 28:163, 1977.

63. Seppala, M., et al. Improved diagnosis of pregnancy-related gynaecological emergencies by rapid human chorionic gonadotropin beta-subunit. *Br. J. Obstet. Gynaecol.* 88:138, 1981.

64. Smart, Y. C., et al. Validation of the rosette inhibition test for the detection of early pregnancy in women. *Fertil. Steril.* 37:779, 1982.

65. Stenman, U. H., et al. Monoclonal antibodies to chorionic gonadotropin: Use in a rapid radioimmunoassay for gynecologic emergencies. *Obstet. Gynecol.* 59:375, 1982.

66. Tulchinsky, D., and Hobel, C. J. Plasma human chorionic gonadotropin, estrone, estradiol, estriol, progesterone, and 17-α-hydroxyprogesterone in human pregnancy. *Am. J. Obstet. Gynecol.* 117:884, 1973.

67. Vaitukaitis, J. L. Changing placental concentrations of hu-

man chorionic gonadotropin and its subunits during gestation. *Clin. Endocrinol. Metab.* 38:755, 1974.

68. Vaitukaitis, J. L. Human Chorionic Gonadotropin. In F. Fuchs and A. Klopper (eds.), *Endocrinology of Pregnancy* (2nd ed.). Hagerstown, Md.: Harper & Row, 1977. P. 63.

69. Wehmann, R. E., et al. Fetus, placenta, and newborn: Improved monitoring of gestational trophoblastic neoplasia using a highly sensitive assay for urinary human chorionic gonadotropin. *Am. J. Obstet. Gynecol.* 140:753, 1981.

70. Wide, L. An immunological method for the assay of human chorionic gonadotropin. *Acta Endocrinol.* (Copenh.) 41:1, 1962.

71. Yoshimi, I., et al. Corpus luteum function in early pregnancy. *Am. J. Obstet. Gynecol.* 117:884, 1973.

72. Zondek, B., and Goldberg, S. Placental function and foetal death. *Br. J. Obstet. Gynaecol.* 64:1, 1957.

II. Surgical Methods

5. First-Trimester Abortion Technology

Andrew M. Kaunitz
David A. Grimes

Because induced abortion is a frequently used and controversial means of fertility control as well as a social issue of great importance, this procedure has been studied intensively. As a result, more is known about the morbidity and mortality associated with induced abortion than that associated with any other surgical procedure. In reviewing the technology of first-trimester abortion we will emphasize preventing morbidity and mortality associated with this method of fertility control.

The term *first-trimester* is not consistently defined. More importantly, in abortion practice the term is not clinically useful because pregnancy should be viewed as a continuum [15]. For the purpose of this chapter, however, we will use the term to refer to pregnancies of up to 12 menstrual weeks' gestation.

INCIDENCE OF FIRST-TRIMESTER ABORTION IN THE UNITED STATES

First-trimester abortion is one of the surgical procedures most commonly performed in this country. In 1980 1,162,249 abortions performed up to 12 menstrual weeks' gestation were reported to the Centers for Disease Control (CDC), representing 90 percent of all abortions performed that year [17]. Suction or sharp curettage accounted for 99 percent of these first-trimester procedures. Fifty-six percent of these curettage procedures were performed up to 8 menstrual weeks' gestation, 30 percent at 9 to 10 weeks, and 14 percent at 11 to 12 weeks [17].

PREOPERATIVE EVALUATION

As with any surgical procedure, preoperative evaluation of the patient is important. The history can identify relevant gynecologic problems such as uterine leiomyomata; medical conditions such as asthma or rheumatic heart disease; and sensitivities to medications commonly administered to women having abortions.

The physical examination should cover the heart, lungs, abdomen, and pelvis. The pelvic examination should be performed after the patient empties her bladder, since a full bladder may distort bimanual examination of the uterus. The examination should assess the size and position of the uterus as well as the adnexal structures. Rectovaginal examination may be especially helpful when the uterus is posterior or midposition or when the patient is obese. If the size of the uterus is unclear, ultrasonography may help clarify whether an intrauterine gestation is present, the position of the uterus, and the gestational age. Existing data, however, do not support the routine preoperative use of ultrasonography for first-trimester abortion patients.

A uterus smaller than expected (on the basis of menstrual history) should alert the physician to several possibilities: The woman may not be pregnant, she may have had an incomplete or missed abortion, or she may have an ectopic pregnancy. The physician should repeat the pelvic examination and pregnancy test. Ultrasonography or laparoscopy, as well as serial quantitative hCG determinations, may be required to establish the diagnosis.

A uterus larger than expected should alert the physician to other possibilities. For example, the pregnancy may be more advanced than the menstrual history indicates. The physician should establish the gestational age with ultrasonography; then the physician and the patient must decide whether to proceed and, if so, determine the appropriate procedure and setting. If the uterus is tender, asymmetric, or substantially larger than the menstrual history indicates it should be, leiomyomata, adnexal cysts, or hydatidiform moles may be present.

The selection of routine preoperative laboratory tests for women undergoing abortion must balance the medical usefulness of each test with the expense and inconvenience involved. Routine Rh determinations, urinalyses, and hematocrits are appropriate.

Culturing the cervix for gonorrhea is also a common practice, because of the increased risk of postabortion infection for women whose preoperative gonorrhea cultures are positive [12]. In one study 10,453 women were cultured for cervical gonorrhea before undergoing first-trimester abortion; 0.6 percent had positive cultures [34].

Depending on the laboratory used, results of a culture may not be available for several days. In deciding whether an abortion should be delayed until the results are available, the physician must weigh the risks associated with performing an abortion on the occasional patient with asymptomatic cervical gonorrhea against the risks associated with delaying the procedure for all patients.

Syphilis serology and cervical cytology may be appropriate as screening tests. Since these tests, however, do not directly improve the safety of abortion procedures, individual circumstances should govern their use.

It is not medically necessary to perform an antibody screen on abortion patients. Few Rh-negative abortion patients are already sensitized; and unnecessary administration of Rh-immune globulin is inexpensive and associated with negligible risk. Therefore, it is appropriate to treat Rh-negative women having first-trimester abortions with 50 μg of Rh-immune globulin without assessing antibody status.

CURETTAGE TECHNIQUES

Curettage techniques for performing first-trimester abortions can be categorized in two ways: sharp-curettage or suction-curettage procedures. While sharp curettage was the principal means of abortion in the United States before suction curettage became widely available, suction curettage is safer [66]. In addition, suction curettage can be performed more rapidly and with less cervical dilation than sharp curettage.

Although the definitions of suction curettage and menstrual regulation overlap, we will use the term *menstrual regulation* to refer to abortions performed early in gestation and requiring minimal or no cervical dilation. *Suction curettage* will be used to refer to suction-curettage abortions that require cervical dilation and that are performed later in the first trimester.

History

The use of aspiration to evacuate the endometrial cavity dates back to a Russian physician who reported this technique in 1927 [69]. Chinese physicians reported using this technique in 1958 [64]. The use of suction curettage to perform first-trimester abortion became widespread in Europe during the 1960s [42, 71]; in the United States suction curettage has been the primary method of performing first-trimester abortion since the early 1970s [17].

Menstrual Regulation

Transcervical aspiration of a gestation up to 50 days after the onset of the last menses has been called *menstrual regulation*. The terms *menstrual extraction, menstrual aspiration, menstrual induction,* and *minisuction* are synonymous with menstrual regulation. The simplicity, safety, and efficacy of this procedure have been well documented [70]. A flexible plastic cannula 4 to 6 mm in diameter (e.g., the Karman cannula) is commonly used to perform menstrual regulation [41]. The Karman cannula (Fig. 5-1) features a blunt tip with two apertures on the side; several versions of this cannula are marketed. The blunt tip may reduce the risk of uterine perforation, and the apertures act as small curets. With proper care and sterilization with either glutaraldehyde or ethylene oxide, this type of cannula can be reused several times. Cannulas should be inspected before each use and discarded if any defect is noted, as the tip has been known to break off in the uterus.

Some self-locking syringes designed specifically for menstrual regulation have a valve that permits the creation of a vacuum before beginning the procedure (Fig. 5-1). Alternative vacuum sources include foot-operated,

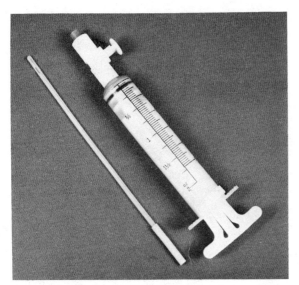

Fig. 5-1. Karman cannula and self-locking syringe used in menstrual regulation. (Courtesy International Projects Assistance Services, Chapel Hill, N.C.)

hand-operated, water-operated, and electric vacuum pumps.

Menstrual regulation has often been performed without positive confirmation of pregnancy. Before 1979 urine pregnancy tests could not reliably detect pregnancy until 6 menstrual weeks' gestation. In addition, some women do not want to know if they are pregnant at the time of menstrual regulation. In a study of 500 cases of menstrual regulation [5], for instance, histologic examination of the curettings failed to demonstrate pregnancy in 35 percent. New and more sensitive pregnancy tests have improved the ability to diagnose early pregnancy; perhaps their availability will decrease future unnecessary procedures.

Before beginning the procedure, the physician performs a bimanual examination to confirm the size and position of the uterus. The physician exposes the cervix with a vaginal speculum, cleanses the cervix and upper vagina with an antiseptic solution, and grasps the cervix with a tenaculum. Paracervical anesthesia can be used for the tenaculum placement and uterine evacuation; most physicians, however, find the use of anesthesia unnecessary. If dilation is required, smaller cannulas (e.g., 4- or 5-mm diameter) can be used as dilators [63]. The suction cannula itself is used to determine the direction of the endometrial cavity; the use of sounds or dilators is rarely necessary.

The physician gently advances the cannula toward the fundus and then attaches the vacuum source. As suction is applied, blood and tissue begin to flow.

When this flow decreases, the surgeon both rotates the cannula and uses it in scraping fashion. The grating sensation of bare endometrium and the flow of blood-tinged bubbles signal the completion of the procedure. This procedure can take from 1 to 10 minutes, depending on physician experience, patient discomfort, and gestational age.

If a syringe is used as a vacuum source, it may be removed from the cannula to reactivate the vacuum if necessary. Some investigators feel that withdrawing the cannula and replacing it in the endometrial cavity increases the risk of infection. Air must never be expelled from a syringe attached to the cannula lest air embolization occur.

Complications from menstrual regulation are infrequent and usually minor. Data collected from 21 countries [23] indicate an overall incidence rate of 3.9 percent for major complications from menstrual regulation; immediate major complications included hypotension, fever, cervical lacerations, acute infections, anesthetic reactions, uterine perforation, and excessive blood loss (in no case requiring transfusion). These immediate major complications occurred overall in 0.85 percent of the women in this study. Most of the major complications, however, were delayed and included failed procedures, subacute infections, bleeding, and undiagnosed ectopic pregnancies.

Incomplete abortions are more commonly reported in connection with menstrual regulation than with abortion performed later in the first trimester. Fortney's data [23], however, dispute earlier assertions that incomplete abortions are more likely with earlier than later menstrual regulation procedures. Other investigators have reported that the failure rate for menstrual regulation declines with increasing physician experience [4] and with the use of 5-mm or 6-mm rather than 4-mm cannulas [4, 63].

Suction Curettage Later in the First Trimester

The term *suction curettage* refers to dilation of the cervix and evacuation of the uterine contents up to 12 weeks' gestation. The terms *vacuum curettage* and *vacuum aspiration* are synonymous with suction curettage.

After emptying her bladder, the woman is assisted to the operating table. The dorsal lithotomy position is usually used. Shaving is not necessary, nor are sterile drapes, gowns, caps, and masks. "No touch" technique, in which the portions of the sterile instruments introduced into the uterus are not touched or contaminated, can be used rather than the full sterile technique. Either local or general anesthesia can be used for first-trimester abortions; techniques and safeguards are discussed later in this chapter.

After bimanual pelvic examination to confirm uterine

size and position, the physician inserts a speculum to expose the cervix. Although a weighted speculum is commonly used in performing abortions under general anesthesia, this type of instrument may be uncomfortable for women who are awake. Most physicians operating with local anesthesia employ a standard-length bivalve speculum, such as the Pederson or Graves. Stubblefield [64], however, recommends the use of a shorter speculum, such as the Moore modification of the Graves speculum, thus permitting the physician to pull the cervix closer to the introitus, making suction curettage easier and safer to perform.

The physician cleanses the cervix and vagina with an antiseptic solution and places a tenaculum forceps on the cervix. Some physicians prefer the use of an "atraumatic" tenaculum but this instrument may be more likely to lacerate the cervix if it pulls off. If the single-tooth tenaculum is applied in a vertical fashion with one tooth of the tenaculum inside the cervical canal, the tenaculum may be less likely to pull out of the cervix and cause a laceration.

The tenaculum may be placed on either the anterior or posterior portion of the cervix. Posterior placement of the tenaculum may be particularly helpful if the uterus is retroverted. If local anesthesia is used, placing a 1-ml to 2-ml wheal of anesthetic on the ectocervix before applying the tenaculum spares the patient the uncomfortable pinch she might otherwise feel.

The use of metal sounds before cervical dilation is controversial—a thin, rigid uterine sound may easily perforate a pregnant uterus. Although some physicians use the sound to determine the direction of the endocervical canal, many avoid the use of metal sounds completely. A small dilator may be a better probe than the traditional metal sound.

Firm traction on the cervix with the tenaculum straightens the axis of the uterus and makes dilation safer. Physicians in the United States have traditionally used either Hegar dilators, which are blunt with a rounded tip, or Pratt dilators, which are tapered and curved. When Hulka [38] measured the force required for cervical dilation, more force was needed to use Hegar dilators as compared with Pratt dilators. Physicians who prefer Hegar dilators should consider using dilators that increase in diameter by one-half mm rather than 1 mm.

Dilation is probably the most dangerous part of suction curettage, because perforation of the uterus occurs more commonly during dilation than during curettage. Although some physicians match the dilation to the number of weeks' gestation (e.g., 8 menstrual weeks' gestation = 8 mm dilation), less dilation may suffice. For example, a 10-mm cannula inserted through a cervix dilated to 10 mm can evacuate a 12-week pregnancy. The likelihood of perforation [8] or permanent damage to the cervix [39] may increase when the cervix is dilated to more than 10 mm.

Some physicians have questioned whether to use flexible or rigid suction cannulas in first-trimester abortions. A study of 1,099 suction curettage abortions compared flexible and rigid plastic suction cannulas [52]; no differences in the complication rates for these two types of cannulas were found. The use, therefore, of either flexible or rigid suction cannulas in suction-curettage abortions is acceptable.

The suction cannula should be advanced beyond the internal os but not to the level of the fundus. The physician attaches the suction cannula to the vacuum apparatus and turns it on (in the United States suction curettage generally is performed with an electric vacuum pump). Amniotic fluid and tissue should appear in the suction tubing; the physician should remove as much of the products of conception as possible by rotating the suction cannula in the lower uterine segment. Vigorous back and forth motion of the cannula is unnecessary and may increase the risk of perforation.

As the procedure nears completion, the physician notes the appearance of bubbles, a gritty feeling of the cannula against the uterus, and the uterus clamping down on the cannula. A sharp metal curet can be introduced into the uterus to ensure thorough emptying; afterwards, the suction cannula can be introduced into the uterus a final time.

NONSURGICAL METHODS OF CERVICAL DILATION

Because both acute and long-term postabortion complications may be related to cervical dilation, investigators are searching for improved methods of cervical dilation [57]. Several are described here.

Laminaria

Laminaria tents are produced from the hydroscopic seaweeds *Laminaria digitata* or *L. japonicum*. These tents were previously difficult to sterilize and therefore were shunned by physicians in the United States, who felt they caused infections. However, laminaria now receive gamma radiation, which eliminates potential pathogens except for spores.

Laminaria are available in several sizes, individually wrapped and threaded with strings. In their dry state they resemble smooth wooden sticks. Stubblefield [65] prefers to use the *L. japonicum* species and has assembled a list of American suppliers.

After performing a bimanual examination, the physician inserts a speculum, cleanses the cervix, and grasps the laminaria tents with a sterile forceps. The physician should place the laminaria just past the internal os. Shallow placement of the tent may result in its expulsion from the cervix. Enough tents are placed to fit snugly inside the cervix. The physician then holds a folded or rolled gauze sponge against the cervix with a forceps and maintains this pressure as the speculum is removed. Although laminaria tents can be placed 3 to 6 hours preoperatively, some physicians insert them 1 day before the abortion.

To remove the tents, the physician inserts a speculum and places traction on the strings attached to the laminaria. If the removal is difficult, the physician should try to dislodge one tent by twisting it out. In first-trimester abortion proper placement of one or more laminaria usually results in at least 8 mm of cervical dilation; suction curettage is possible in many such patients without the use of rigid dilators.

Laminaria appear to cause cervical dilation through a direct dehydrating effect on the cervix [67] and by provoking the release of endogenous prostaglandins that effect uterine cramping and cervical dilation [76]. The latter effect may explain the transient cramps many women experience after laminaria are inserted.

Few large series have been published comparing complications of suction curettage in regard to the use of laminaria. In their study of 800 suction-curettage abortions Hale and Pion [31] found that the use of laminaria was associated with a 12-fold decrease in the risk of cervical lacerations.

Gold and colleagues [25] reported on complications following 29,760 suction-curettage abortions, 11 percent of which involved the use of laminaria. Rates of postoperative fever were the same for the laminaria and rigid-dilator groups, but uterine perforation was significantly less common ($p < .05$) in the laminaria group. Surprisingly, cervical lacerations were more common in the laminaria group, but this difference was not statistically significant.

In both of these studies laminaria may have been used preferentially when difficulty with cervical dilation was anticipated; complication rates in these studies are therefore difficult to interpret. Too few patients were included in a recent randomized study of laminaria use to allow valid comparison of complication rates [76].

Because cervical dilation with laminaria occurs slowly, their use entails additional inconvenience for patients and physicians. Until more data are available, individual preference should determine the use of laminaria in first-trimester abortions.

Prostaglandins

The search for atraumatic methods of cervical dilation has recently focused on prostaglandins. Dingfelder and his colleagues [21] used an electronic force monitor to study prostaglandin $F_{2\alpha}$ ($PGF_{2\alpha}$) and prostaglandin E_2 (PGE_2) in regard to dilation during first-trimester abortions. Prostaglandins and placebos were administered as vaginal suppositories 3 hours before abortion. Compared with women in the placebo group, women in the group receiving $PGF_{2\alpha}$ were found to have cervices that were less resistant during dilation with rigid dilators. In fact, many of the women receiving $PGF_{2\alpha}$ dilated enough to allow suction curettage without the use of rigid dilators or anesthesia. PGE_2 produced less cervical dilation than $PGF_{2\alpha}$, but more dilation than the placebo.

Other randomized studies [48, 74] have confirmed the ability of prostaglandins to dilate the cervix in first-trimester abortions. However, all these studies have reported nausea, vomiting, and painful uterine cramping as a consequence of prostaglandin use. Dingfelder's series is representative; 60 percent of the PGE_2 group experienced at least one episode of emesis, 45 percent of the $PGF_{2\alpha}$ group had diarrhea, and, overall 10 percent of the prostaglandin-treated group experienced severe painful uterine cramping. Investigators continue to develop and test prostaglandin analogues in the hope of improving efficacy and reducing side effects.

Osmotic Dilators

Bhiwandiwala [10] has devised a new dilator that she terms the "osmotic dilator." This device is a thin tent made of polyvinyl sponge and impregnated with magnesium sulfate. It is inexpensive to manufacture and easy to sterilize. Unpublished reports suggest that this new dilator produces substantial cervical softening and dilation more rapidly than laminaria. Ongoing clinical trials are evaluating this new device.

PROSTAGLANDINS AS ABORTIFACIENTS IN THE FIRST TRIMESTER

Since prostaglandins stimulate uterine contractions and dilate the pregnant cervix, these compounds have been investigated as abortifacients. Analogues of $PGF_{2\alpha}$ and PGE_2 given intramuscularly [9] and vaginally [14, 49, 72] have been evaluated in studies of women having first-trimester abortions. Five to 15 percent of these women experienced incomplete or failed abortion. In addition, most experienced severe uterine pain and/or gastrointestinal side effects [24].

Although prostaglandins with fewer side effects are currently being developed and evaluated [19], prostaglandins have not yet achieved the safety and effectiveness of suction curettage for first-trimester abortion.

ANESTHESIA FOR FIRST-TRIMESTER ABORTIONS

Although local and general anesthesia are both commonly used for first-trimester abortions in the United States, local anesthesia appears to be used more often. These two forms of anesthesia are associated with different risks and benefits.

Grimes and associates [26] studied complications associated with 54,155 first-trimester abortions; two-thirds of the patients received local anesthesia, while the remainder received general anesthesia. Although overall rates of major complications were similar for both groups of women, differences in rates of specific complications were noted.

Rates of uterine perforation and hemorrhage, intraabdominal hemorrhage, and cervical trauma were higher for the group of women receiving general anesthesia. Local anesthesia, however, was associated with higher rates of convulsions and postoperative fever. Perhaps physicians operating with local anesthesia use a gentler technique, which results in lower rates of perforation. Since postoperative fever may be caused by retained tissue, less vigorous curettage under local anesthesia may explain the higher rates of fever for this group of women.

Because general anesthesia requires more personnel and equipment for its administration than local anesthesia, it is more expensive. Many women choose general anesthesia, however, to minimize pain during their abortions.

Peterson and associates [58] compared the risk of death associated with first-trimester abortions in regard to whether local or general anesthesia was used. These investigators found that abortions performed under general anesthesia were associated with an overall two-to fourfold increase in the risk of death when compared with abortions performed under local anesthesia.

Little attention has been focused on the choice of anesthetic agents. Lidocaine, a commonly used agent, is an amide and is metabolized more slowly than ester anesthetics. Chloroprocaine, an ester anesthetic, is rapidly hydrolyzed by plasma pseudocholinesterase. Because the relatively large quantities of local anesthetics used in performing first-trimester abortions may result in toxic levels, chloroprocaine may be the preferred agent for abortions [27]. Maximum recommended doses are 800 mg for chloroprocaine and 300 mg for lidocaine. The maximum doses are lower for persons of less than average weight; unless a vasoconstrictor is used, the dose of lidocaine should in no case exceed 2 mg per pound.

A recent study measured plasma lidocaine levels during paracervical block for suction curettage; 90 to 100 mg of lidocaine was administered to each of the 49 women [7]. In no case did plasma lidocaine levels approach toxic levels, emphasizing the safety of paracervical block when appropriate doses of anesthetic are used.

At a given dose of local anesthetic, less toxicity occurs when epinephrine is combined with the anesthetic [59]. Epinephrine combined with local anesthetics has also subjectively been reported to lower the blood loss during second-trimester abortions [22]. In the absence of a contraindication to using sympathomimetic agents, therefore, chloroprocaine with dilute epinephrine is an excellent choice for local anesthesia in first-trimester abortions. A 1% or 2% solution of chloroprocaine is appropriate. To prepare an anesthetic solution with dilute epinephrine (e.g., 1:200,000), 0.15 ml of 1:1,000 epinephrine is added to 30 ml of local anesthetic.

Although no injection technique precludes the possibility of intravascular injection, the physician should attempt to avoid this possibility by withdrawing from the syringe before injecting the anesthetic. Initial signs of local anesthetic toxicity include apprehension, dizziness, paresthesia, blurred vision, ringing in the ears, and tremors. These symptoms may progress rapidly to convulsions [27]. (The prevention and treatment of local anesthetic toxicity have been discussed elsewhere.)

During the administration of local anesthesia or manipulation of the cervix, some women may experience vasovagal syncope. Because vasovagal reactions include trembling, convulsive movements, and grand mal seizures with apnea, these reactions may be hard to distinguish from local anesthetic toxicity. A recent publication [56] details the recognition and treatment of vasovagal syncope and emphasizes the role of cardiopulmonary resuscitation in severe cases.

Several techniques can be used to administer paracervical local anesthesia; the use of a 20-gauge spinal needle attached to a finger-grip handle syringe is convenient. Some physicians inject anesthetic into the uterosacral ligaments, although this may be more painful than other techniques. Anesthetic can be injected just below the cervicovaginal mucosa at the 3 and 9 o'clock positions or at the 3, 5, 7, and 9 o'clock positions. A useful technique is to place the needle just over the site selected and then ask the patient to cough; this maneuver "pops" the mucosa over the needle tip and may decrease the discomfort associated with placing the needle. This technique also helps to obtain appropriate submucosal placement of the medication.

McKenzie and Shaffer [50] have described the use of a jet-injector to administer local anesthesia in first-trimester abortions. While this method is quick and can provide anesthesia using less agent than conventional techniques, its expense may limit its use to settings where large numbers of procedures are performed.

All these techniques can provide anesthesia adequate

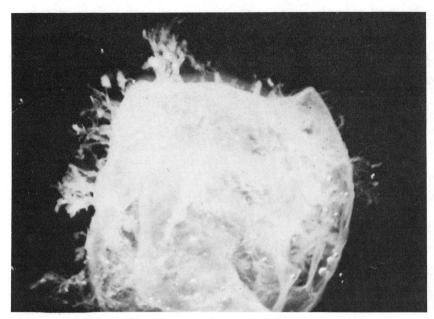

Fig. 5-2. Trophoblastic tissue floating in water. (× 8.) (Courtesy Milton Danon, M.D., Parkmed, New York, N.Y.)

for cervical dilation. However, because paracervical anesthesia does not anesthetize the endometrial cavity, some patients find the curettage painful.

No aspect of administering local anesthesia during first-trimester abortions is more important than the physician-patient interaction during the procedure. A calm, sensitive, and unhurried physician who talks to the patient throughout the procedure can do much to make the woman more comfortable.

EXAMINING PRODUCTS OF CONCEPTION

Examining the products of conception is an important but frequently ignored component of first-trimester abortion procedures. Specimens should be removed from the collection bag, rinsed, and allowed to float in a shallow dish with a small amount of water. If the specimen is held over a light, trophoblastic tissue will appear white, with a fine, frondlike appearance; decidua will look darker and more shaggy and irregular in texture (Figs. 5-2 and 5-3).

Trophoblastic villi may be hard to identify in specimens obtained as a result of abortions performed early in the first trimester. If no villi are seen grossly, the specimen should be viewed under a dissecting microscope or hand-held lens. Floating the specimen in

white vinegar blanches villi white and facilitates their recognition.

Fetal parts can be identified in the abortion specimen at 8 weeks' gestation and beyond; Stubblefield [64] finds it helpful to measure the length of the fetal foot to corroborate gestational age. If fetal parts are identified and no gross hydropic changes are noted in the trophoblastic tissue, there is no medical indication for submitting the tissue for histopathologic analysis [2]. When no fetal parts or villi are identified, the physician must assume that an ectopic pregnancy is present until this diagnosis is excluded. Differential diagnosis in this setting includes false-positive pregnancy tests, unrecognized early spontaneous abortion, uninterrupted intrauterine gestation, uterine anomaly, and extrauterine pregnancy. One management approach is the following [65]:

1. Repeat the pregnancy test with a sensitive, 2-hour tube urine test. Draw a blood specimen for a serum pregnancy test.
2. Reexamine the patient.
3. Reexamine the specimen and obtain a frozen section (if available) and a permanent section to be reviewed expeditiously by a pathologist.
4. If the 2-hour urine pregnancy test is positive and the physician suspects a continued intrauterine pregnancy, a second curettage is appropriate.

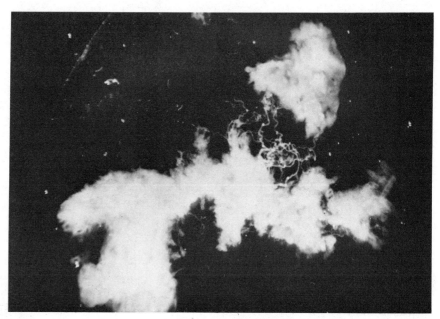

Fig. 5-3. Decidual tissue floating in water. (× 8.) (Courtesy Milton Danon, M.D., Parkmed, New York, N.Y.)

5. If the pregnancy test is positive and the physician does not suspect a continued intrauterine pregnancy, the woman should have ultrasonography done. If ultrasonography fails to reveal an intrauterine pregnancy, examination under anesthesia, repeat curettage, and laparoscopy may be indicated.
6. If the pregnancy test is negative, an ectopic pregnancy is unlikely. If the pelvic examination is normal, the woman may be permitted to go home if she is accompanied by a responsible adult. These women should be alerted to symptoms of ectopic pregnancy, given a 24-hour telephone number, and scheduled for a 1-week return visit. Blood should be sent for a quantitative serum pregnancy test specific for the beta subunit of human chorionic gonadotropin (hCG).

During the 1-week visit the physician reviews the results of the serum pregnancy test and pathology report and reexamines the woman. On the basis of this evaluation, the physician should be able to decide whether to hospitalize her or to continue to follow her for presumed unrecognized spontaneous abortion or false-positive initial pregnancy test. The combined use of serial quantitative hCG assays in clinically stable women with suspected ectopic pregnancies may allow more precise diagnosis and expeditious management [40].

POSTOPERATIVE CARE

Immediate Postoperative Monitoring

During the immediate postoperative period life-threatening complications may occur. Examples of these include pulmonary aspiration of gastric contents in women awakening from general anesthesia and hypovolemic shock associated with uterine perforation. Because most first-trimester abortions are performed on outpatients, supervision of their recovery is particularly important. Early recognition and treatment of acute postoperative complications require trained personnel and careful monitoring. Resuscitation equipment and personnel trained in its use are vital. A physician should be readily available whenever a woman is in the recovery room. In preparation for emergencies, non-hospital facilities should establish a system for the rapid transportation of women to a nearby hospital.

COMPLICATIONS OF FIRST-TRIMESTER ABORTIONS

Abortion complications can be grouped temporally into three categories [3]: immediate, delayed, and late. Immediate complications are those that develop within 3 hours of the procedure. Delayed complications develop thereafter and up to 28 days after the abortion. Late complications occur after 28 days. This section emphasizes clinical recognition and management of specific first-trimester abortion complications in each of these categories.

Immediate Complications

HEMORRHAGE

Reports of uterine hemorrhage from abortion are difficult to interpret because of inconsistent definitions and unreliable means of estimating volume blood loss. The best index of clinically significant blood loss from abortion may be the use of blood transfusion. Although physicians' indications for administering blood vary, hemorrhage requiring transfusion is considered serious enough to outweigh its cost and hazards. A study of 54,155 suction-curettage abortions found a transfusion rate of 0.6 per 100 abortions [26].

In first-trimester abortions use of local rather than general anesthesia has been associated with lower transfusion rates [26]. Intraoperative oxytocic agents have been noted to decrease measured blood loss during suction curettage [44, 45].

Hern [33] has detailed the management of hemorrhage during suction curettage. Upon encountering heavy bleeding, the physician should remove the speculum and put digital pressure bilaterally over the area of uterine vessels. Intravenous fluids with oxytocin and a parenteral ergot preparation should be administered. These maneuvers may control the bleeding.

Next, a ring forceps should be placed into the uterus to remove any remaining placental tissue. The largest curet the cervix can accommodate is then introduced and used to both empty and explore the uterus. If no perforation is discovered, the uterus appears empty, and heavy bleeding persists, the most likely cause is either atony or a cervical laceration.

The physician may be able to determine whether the problem is atony or laceration by placing a suction curet into the uterine cavity. If blood is flowing from the fundal portion of the uterus, atony is the likely cause. If no bleeding is noted until the curet is withdrawn to the internal os, a cervical laceration is the probable cause. Regardless of the etiology of the uterine bleeding, uterine massage and continued administration of oxytocic agents are appropriate in this setting.

If hemorrhage from uterine atony persists, prostaglandins may be used. Prostaglandins have been used effectively to treat postpartum atony [32].

Continued heavy bleeding from the lower uterus or endocervix suggests a laceration of the descending branch of the uterine artery; diagnosis and treatment of this life-threatening injury are discussed in a recent publication [6].

COAGULOPATHY

Acquired coagulopathy associated with suction curettage is extremely rare, occurring in about 8 per 100,000 cases (CDC unpublished data). Coagulopathy should be suspected when persistent uterine bleeding is accompanied by bleeding from venipuncture or at other sites. If a sample of blood collected in a glass tube fails to clot after 5 minutes, a coagulation disorder may be present. The hematocrit, platelet count, fibrinogen, prothrombin and partial thromboplastin time, and fibrin degradation products should be determined. Transfusion of fresh frozen plasma or cryoprecipitate is appropriate treatment for coagulopathies during first-trimester abortion.

ACUTE HEMATOMETRA

Acute postabortal hematometra is readily treatable. This clinical entity has also been called the postabortion or "redo" syndrome [55]. Because diagnostic criteria for this entity vary, reports of its incidence among suction-curettage patients have been inconsistent, ranging from approximately 0.2 to 1 per 100 abortions [55, 61]. Patients with postabortion hematometra usually note the onset of severe and progressive lower abdominal cramping within 2 hours of their abortion. Vaginal bleeding is less than usual, and pelvic examination reveals a distended and markedly tender uterus. Neither hypotension nor anemia is present. Prompt reevacuation of the uterus can usually be performed without anesthesia or dilation and results in the evacuation of clotted and liquid blood. Rapid relief of symptoms follows.

When a significant amount of fetal or placental tissue at recurettage is found, the diagnosis should be retained products of conception, not postabortion hematometra. An oxytocic agent is administered at recurettage. Although many physicians routinely administer ergot drugs to women after abortion, the usefulness of this practice has not been established. Intravenous oxytocin, which decreases uterine bleeding during suction curettage and causes fewer side effects than ergot compounds [44, 45], may be a more appropriate agent for the prophylaxis of postabortion hematometra when such prophylaxis is deemed necessary.

PERFORATION OF THE UTERUS

Perforation of the uterus is a worrisome but, fortunately, infrequent complication of curettage abortion. Recent studies of suction-curettage abortions report perforation rates of approximately 0.2 per 100 procedures [8, 26].

Many of the reported risk factors for uterine perforation during suction curettage involve the use of specific types of instruments; uterine sounds [54], dilators or curets greater than 10 mm in diameter [8], and rigid dilators [25] may increase the risk of uterine perforation. Also, use of general rather than local anesthesia increases the risk of this complication [26].

The sudden onset of generalized abdominal pain during suction curettage or persistent (sometimes transient or delayed) postabortion vaginal bleeding are less specific but common features of perforation.

Perforation through the uterine fundus may cause little bleeding; evaluation and management of such cases may require diagnostic laparoscopy only. In Berek's series [6], however, 80 percent of abortion-related perforations were located in the cervix or lower uterine segment. This type of injury is particularly treacherous, as it frequently is associated with lacerations of the uterine artery.

The abortion should be discontinued as soon as perforation is suspected. Shock, hemorrhage, extensive instrumentation of the uterus after perforation, or the presence of bowel or fat among the curettings are indicators for prompt laparotomy. In their absence, laparoscopy may be appropriate. During laparoscopy the site of perforation and extent of bleeding can be determined. Hematomas should be observed for increasing size, and the bowel and bladder should be inspected. If appropriate, the abortion can be completed under laparoscopic guidance. However, laparotomy must be performed immediately if uncontrolled bleeding, bowel or urinary-tract injury, or an expanding hematoma become apparent during the laparoscopy. When uterine perforations are managed in this fashion, few women sustaining such perforations during suction-curettage abortions require laparotomy [43].

CERVICAL INJURY
Cervical trauma is a relatively common and occasionally serious complication of first-trimester abortion. In larger studies of suction-curettage abortions the incidence of cervical injury has ranged from 0.18 [8] to 0.96 per 100 abortions [26]. These rates must be cautiously interpreted, however, because of the lack of consistent definitions and the wide range of potential damage. For example, both a superficial cervical tear caused by a tenaculum as well as a laceration of the descending branch of the uterine artery related to a cervical perforation may be classified as cervical injuries.

Cervical injury during suction curettage usually occurs during dilation [75]. Cervical lacerations are commonly related to use of a tenaculum. Such lacerations can usually be managed by applying direct pressure with gauze for several minutes, although suturing is occasionally required. Penetrating cervical lacerations caused by dilators may extend into the uterine vasculature. Damage to the internal os related to dilation may cause problems in subsequent pregnancies. Cervical

synechiae and stenosis are rare complications of curettage abortions [30] and may be associated with amenorrhea.

EMBOLISM
Three types of potentially lethal emboli may occur during or after abortions: thrombus, air, and amniotic fluid. Although reliable incidence figures for these complications are not available, all gynecologic surgery entails some risk of thromboembolism. Air embolism is rare; a fatal case was related to improper attachment of the suction tubing to the exhaust port of a suction machine [53]. Since all 15 cases of fatal amniotic-fluid embolism in women undergoing abortion between 1972 and 1978 occurred at 14 or more weeks' gestation [29], the risk of fatal amniotic-fluid embolism from first-trimester abortion appears negligible.

Delayed Complications

RETAINED PRODUCTS OF CONCEPTION
Retained products of conception following an induced abortion may result in infection, bleeding, or both. This complication, however, is uncommon. A recent large study of abortion morbidity following suction curettage reported 0.61 cases of retained products of conception per 100 abortions [26].

Women with retained products of conception often report cramping and heavy bleeding, which may be accompanied by fever. Although these problems usually occur within 1 week of the abortion, delayed presentation can occur. It may be difficult to distinguish between retained products of conception and infection. Repeat suction curettage is appropriate treatment.

INFECTION
Infection, frequently related to retained tissue, is the most common delayed complication of first-trimester abortions. Because of the lack of uniform definitions and diagnostic criteria, incidence rates for postabortion infections are difficult to interpret. However, fever provides a relatively objective measure of the frequency of infectious morbidity. The incidence of temperature 38°C or higher for 1 or more days after suction curettage has been reported to be 0.75 per 100 abortions [26]. Several risk factors for postabortion infection have been identified, including advanced gestational age, untreated endocervical gonorrhea [12], use of local rather than general anesthesia [26], and the use of instillation techniques of abortion. A large prospective sequential study of first-trimester abortions has suggested that the routine administration of oral tetracycline for 4 days, starting just before the procedure, reduces the postabortion infection rate [35]. Two other studies [11, 47] support the prophylactic use of tetracycline for first-

trimester abortion. A recent randomized study conducted in Denmark [62] evaluated the use of intramuscular penicillin G with oral pivampicillin in preventing infections after first-trimester abortions: This study found that the benefits of prophylactic therapy were limited to those women with a history of pelvic inflammatory disease.

Uterine tenderness, fever, and excessive bleeding occurring 3 to 7 days postoperatively are the hallmarks of postabortion infection. The organisms responsible for postabortion infections are similar to those causing gynecologic infection in women who are not pregnant. Guidelines published by the Centers for Disease Control [16] concerning antibiotic therapy for pelvic inflammatory disease are applicable in treating postabortion infections. Prompt recurettage is indicated in women with postabortion infections and should not be reserved for those patients who have failed to respond to antibiotic therapy.

Although 12 women died of sepsis following legal abortion in the United States during 1975 to 1977 [28], when treated with aggressive antibiotic therapy and prompt recurettage, few women develop life-threatening postabortion infections. (Ledger [46] has recently reviewed the diagnosis and treatment of life-threatening postabortion infections.)

Late Complications

Compared with information about the immediate and delayed complications of legal abortion, information about late complications is limited. Because many years may elapse before long-term morbidity after abortion is observed and because the possible adverse sequelae may be rare, studies to determine any late complications must be rigorously designed to avoid possible bias. One or more of the following methodologic weaknesses have characterized many such studies: (1) inadequate documentation or confirmation of abortion histories for either the study or the control group; (2) inadequate information about the abortion procedure being studied as a potential risk factor; (3) failure to report or control for potentially confounding variables common to both the index abortion (risk factor under study) and the late complication being investigated; examples of such variables include marital and socioeconomic status, history of smoking, and history of pelvic infection.

The differences in the study designs as well as the discrepancies in conclusions from studies conducted in a variety of countries make the subject of late complications an unresolved issue. In their review of the international literature Hogue and colleagues [37] analyzed the methodologies and findings of more than 100 studies of late effects of induced abortion.

SECONDARY INFERTILITY
Because uterine synechiae have been related to induced abortion, concern has been expressed over the ability of women having induced abortions to conceive later. A case-control study in Greece [68] reported a 3.4-fold increase in the risk of subfecundity for women who had had abortions. Abortion, however, is illegal in Greece, and the results of this study cannot be generalized to legal abortion. Studies in Japan [60], Yugoslavia [36], and the United States [20] have not demonstrated decreased fertility among women who have had abortions.

SPONTANEOUS ABORTION
Cervical incompetence, considered by some to be a potential risk of induced abortion, may result in pregnancy wastage through spontaneous abortion or premature deliveries. A multicenter study sponsored by the World Health Organization [73] indicated that spontaneous abortion was, in fact, more common among women with previous abortions; however, the most important factor in determining increased risk was the method of abortion.

While a lower risk of spontaneous abortion was associated with the use of small-caliber cervical dilation and suction curettage, a higher risk was associated with the use of larger-caliber dilation and sharp curettage. A recent publication [18] presents perhaps the most sophisticated study available on the subject of spontaneous abortion following induced abortion. This study did not find an increase in the frequency of either first- or second-trimester fetal loss among women with prior induced abortions.

ECTOPIC PREGNANCY
Prior tubal infection is a major risk factor for extrauterine pregnancy. Because postabortion infection occurs in approximately 1 percent of women (see previous discussion), induced abortion has been scrutinized as a possible risk factor for subsequent ectopic pregnancy. In summarizing the available data, Hogue and colleagues [37] concluded that if there is an increased risk of ectopic pregnancy following induced abortion, it is confined to those women experiencing infections.

PREMATURITY
As previously stated, cervical incompetence associated with induced abortion might be expected to result in an increased risk of premature deliveries. Hogue and colleagues [37] noted that while some studies reported an increased risk of prematurity in women with a history of induced abortion, others reported no such increased risk. As with spontaneous abortions, the extent of dilation and the method of uterine evacuation may be the most important factors.

Without treatment, the frequency of Rh sensitization among Rh-negative women following induced abortion is approximately 4 percent [51]; sensitization occurs more frequently in late rather than early abortions. The American College of Obstetricians and Gynecologists [1] has recommended that unsensitized Rh-negative, D^u-negative women undergoing abortion at less than 13 weeks' gestation receive 50 μg of Rh-immune globulin. By following this recommendation, providers of abortion services can help prevent subsequent hemolytic disease of the newborn.

MORTALITY

The death-to-case rate for legal abortion is remarkably low. In the United States from 1972 to 1980 the risk of death associated with abortions performed up to 12 weeks' gestation was only 1.1 per 100,000 procedures [17]. As with morbidity, delay in performing the abortion is the principal factor affecting mortality in first-trimester abortions. Table 5-1 shows that the risk of dying approximately doubles for each 2 weeks of delay after 8 menstrual weeks' gestation. Prompt action by women obtaining abortions and by their physicians can do much to lower the morbidity and mortality associated with this procedure.

Anesthesia and analgesia are the main causes of death associated with first-trimester legal abortion (Table 5-2); most deaths attributed to one of these two causes are due to general anesthesia. Other common causes of death from legal abortion are hemorrhage, infection, and embolism. These data underscore the joint responsibility of the physician and anesthetist to ensure the safe provision of abortion services.

PREVENTING COMPLICATIONS

Avoiding delay is of paramount importance in preventing complications. Women expressing ambivalence about continuing their pregnancies should receive expert counseling as soon as possible. If abortion is elected, prompt service is important.

Use of local rather than general anesthesia may reduce rates of hemorrhage, uterine trauma, and mortality. Toxic levels of local-anesthetic agents should be avoided by using doses of anesthetic appropriate to body weight. Pratt and other tapered dilators allow the cervix to be dilated with less force than Hegar dilators and therefore may reduce rates of cervical trauma. Nonsurgical methods of cervical dilation in first-trimester abortion are promising but await further technical development and clinical evaluation.

Suction curettage is associated with lower rates of uterine injury and hemorrhage than sharp curettage. Curets should be advanced into the uterus only as far as necessary for completion of the procedure.

Table 5-1. Death-to-case rate for legal abortions by weeks of gestation, United States, 1972–1980

Weeks of gestation	Deaths[a]	Abortions[b]	Rate[c]	Relative risk[d]
≤8	19	4,073, 472	0.5	1.0
9–10	31	2,382,516	1.3	2.6
11–12	25	1,197,915	2.1	4.2
13–15	20	419,767	4.8	9.6
16–20	55	430,907	12.8	25.6
≥21	14	91,343	15.3	30.6
Total	164	8,595,920	1.9	

[a] Excludes deaths from ectopic pregnancy.
[b] Based on distribution of 6,108,658 abortions (71.1% with weeks of gestation known).
[c] Deaths per 100,000 abortions.
[d] Based on index rate of 0.5 per 100,000 abortions performed at ≤8 menstrual weeks' gestation.
Source: Abortion Surveillance 1979–1980. Atlanta: Centers for Disease Control. May 1983.

Table 5-2. Causes of death from legal abortion at ≤12 weeks' gestation, United States, 1972–1980

Cause of death	Number	Percent
Anesthesia/analgesia	27	35
Hemorrhage	13	17
Infection	12	15
Embolism	12	15
Other	14	18
Total	78	100

Routine inspection of the products of conception can help raise the level of suspicion of ectopic gestations in women undergoing first-trimester abortion procedures. Staff providing postoperative care should be skilled in recognizing and treating immediate complications.

Treatment of preexisting gonorrhea and the use of prophylactic antibiotics appear to lower rates of post-abortion infection. The intraoperative use of oxytocic agents may help prevent uterine hemorrhage, and the administration of Rh-immune globulin to Rh-negative patients will help prevent Rh sensitization.

Induced first-trimester abortion is one of the most frequently performed operations on women—and one of the safest. In the United States fewer than 1 woman per 100 suffers a major complication from abortion, and the death-to-case rate of 1.1 deaths per 100,000 first-trimester abortions is extremely low. Emerging data on the long-term effects of first-trimester abortions appear reassuring. Insights gained through epidemiologic studies of abortion can make this procedure even safer.

REFERENCES

1. American College of Obstetricians and Gynecologists. The selective use of rho (D) immune globulin. *Technical Bulletin* 61, 1981.
2. American College of Obstetricians and Gynecologists. *Standards for Obstetric-Gynecologic Services* (5th ed.). Washington, D.C.: American College of Obstetricians and Gynecologists, 1982.
3. Andolsek, L., et al. The safety of local anesthesia and outpatient treatment: A controlled study of induced abortion by vacuum aspiration. *Stud. Fam. Plann.* 8:118, 1977.
4. Atienza, M. F., et al. Menstrual extraction. *Am. J. Obstet. Gynecol.* 121:490, 1975.
5. Bendel, R. P., William, P. P., and Butler, J. C. Endometrial aspiration in fertility control: A report of 500 cases. *Am. J. Obstet. Gynecol.* 1215:328, 1976.
6. Berek, J. S., and Stubblefield, P. G. Anatomic and clinical correlates of uterine perforation. *Am. J. Obstet. Gynecol.* 135:181, 1979.
7. Blanco, L. J., Reid, P. R., and King, T. M. Plasma lidocaine levels following paracervical infiltration for aspiration abortion. *Obstet. Gynecol.* 60:506, 1982.
8. Bozorgi, N. Statistical analysis of first trimester pregnancy terminations in an ambulatory surgical center. *Am. J. Obstet. Gynecol.* 127:763, 1977.
9. Brenner, P. F., et al. Termination of early gestation with intramuscular (15s)-15 methyl prostaglandin $F_{2\alpha}$ *Contraception* 11:279, 1975.
10. Brenner, W. E. and Zuspan, K. Synthetic laminaria for cervical dilation prior to vacuum aspiration in midtrimester pregnancy. *Am. J. Obstet. Gynecol.* 143:475, 1983.
11. Brewer, C. Prevention of infection after abortion with a supervised single dose of oral doxycycline. *Br. Med. J.* 281:780, 1980.
12. Burkman, R. T., et al. Untreated endo-cervical gonorrhea and endometritis following elective abortion. *Am. J. Obstet. Gynecol.* 126:648, 1976.
13. Burkman, R. T., Atienza, M. F., and King, T. M. Culture and treatment results in endometritis following abortion. *Am. J. Obstet. Gynecol.* 128:556, 1977.
14. Bygdeman, M., et al. Early pregnancy interruption by 15 (s) 15 methyl prostaglandin $F_{2\alpha}$ methylester. *Obstet. Gynecol.* 48:221, 1976.
15. Cates, W., Jr., and Grimes, D. A. The Trimester Threshold for Pregnancy Termination: Myth or Truth? In M. J. N. C. Keirse et al. (eds.), *Second Trimester Termination*. The Hague, Holland: Leiden University Press, 1982. Pp. 41–51.
16. Centers for Disease Control. Sexually transmitted diseases: Treatment guidelines. *M.M.W.R.* 31:435, 1982.
17. Centers for Disease Control. Abortion Surveillance 1979–1980. May, 1983.
18. Chung, C. S., et al. Induced abortion and spontaneous fetal loss in subsequent pregnancies. *Am. J. Public Health* 72:548, 1982.
19. Csapo, A. I., et al. Menstrual induction in preference to abortion (Letter to the Editor). 1:90, 1980.
20. Daling, J. R., Sapdoni, L. R., and Emanuel, I. Role of induced abortion in secondary infertility. *Obstet. Gynecol.* 57:59, 1981.
21. Dingfelder, J. R., et al. Reduction of cervical resistance by prostaglandin suppositories prior to dilation for induced abortion. *Am. J. Obstet. Gynecol.* 122:25, 1975.
22. Finks, A. A. Mid-trimester abortion. *Lancet* 1:263, 1973.
23. Fortney, J. A., and Laufe, L. E. Menstrual Regulation. In J. J. Sciarra, G. I. Zatuchni, and J. J. Speidel (eds.), *Risks, Benefits and Controversies in Fertility Control*. Hagerstown, Md.: Harper & Row, 1978. Pp. 274–281.
24. Gail, L. J. The use of prostaglandins in human reproduction. *Popul. Rep.* [G]. No. 8, 1980.
25. Gold, J., et al. The Safety of Laminaria and Rigid Dilators for Cervical Dilation Prior to Suction Curettage for First Trimester Abortion: A Comparative Analysis. In F. Naftolin and P. G. Stubblefield (eds.), *Dilation of the Uterine Cervix*. New York: Raven, 1980. Pp. 363–370.
26. Grimes, D. A. et al. Local versus general anesthesia: Which is safer for performing suction curettage abortions? *Am. J. Obstet. Gynecol.* 135:1030, 1979.
27. Grimes, D. A. and Cates, W., Jr. Deaths from paracervical anesthesia used for first-trimester abortion. *N. Engl. J. Med.* 295:1397, 1976.
28. Grimes, D. A., Cates, W., Jr., and Selik, R. M. Fatal septic abortion in the United States, 1975–1977. *Obstet. Gynecol.* 57:739, 1981.
29. Guidotti, R. J., Grimes, D. A., and Cates, W., Jr. Fatal amniotic fluid embolism during legally induced abortion, United States, 1972 to 1978. *Am. J. Obstet. Gynecol.* 141:257, 1981.
30. Hakim-Elahi, E. Postabortal amenorrhea due to cervical stenosis. *Obstet. Gynecol.* 48:723, 1976.
31. Hale, R. W., and Pion, R. J. Laminaria: An underutilized clinical adjunct. *Clin. Obstet. Gynecol.* 15:829, 1972.
32. Hayashi, R. H., Castillo, M. S., and Noah, M. N. Management of severe post-partum hemorrhage due to uterine atony using an analogue of prostaglandin $F_{2\alpha}$. *Obstet. Gynecol.* 58:426, 1981.
33. Hern, W. M. First Trimester Abortion: Complications and Their Management. In J. J. Sciarra (ed.), *Gynecology and Obstetrics*. Philadelphia: Harper & Row, 1982. Pp. 1–8.
34. Hodgson, J. E. and Portmann, K. C. Complications of 10,453 consecutive first-trimester abortions: A prospective study. *Am. J. Obstet. Gynecol.* 120:802, 1974.
35. Hodgson, J. E., et al. Prophylactic use of tetracycline for first trimester abortions. *Obstet. Gynecol.* 45:574, 1975.
36. Hogue, C. J. R. Low birth weight subsequent to induced abortion. *Am. J. Obstet. Gynecol.* 123:675, 1975.

37. Hogue, C. J. R., Cates, W., Jr., and Tietze, C. The effects of induced abortion on subsequent reproduction. *Epidemiol. Rev.* 4:66, 1982.

38. Hulka, J. F., et al. A new force monitor to measure factors influencing cervical dilatation for vacuum curettage. *Am. J. Obstet. Gynecol.* 120:166, 1974.

39. Johnstone, F. D., et al. Cervical diameter after suction termination of pregnancy. *Br. Med. J.* 1:68, 1976.

40. Kadar, N., Caldwell, B. V., and Romero, R. A method of screening for ectopic pregnancy and its indications. *Obstet. Gynecol.* 58:162, 1981.

41. Karman, H., and Potts, M. Very early abortion using syringe as a vacuum source. *Lancet* 1:1051, 1972.

42. Kerslake, D., and Casey, D. Abortion induced by means of the uterine aspirator. *Obstet. Gynecol.* 30:35, 1967.

43. Lauersen, N. H., and Birnbaum, S. Laparoscopy as a diagnostic and therapeutic technique in uterine perforations during first-trimester abortions. *Am. J. Obstet. Gynecol.* 117:522, 1973.

44. Lauersen, N. H., and Conrad, P. Effect of oxytocic agents on blood loss during first-trimester suction curettage. *Obstet. Gynecol.* 44:428, 1974.

45. Lauritz, J. B., Paull, J. D., and McInnes, M. Oxytocin: Oxytocic of choice in first trimester. *Med. J. Aust.* 2:319, 1980.

46. Ledger, W. J. Septic Abortion and Septic Pelvic Thrombophlebitis. In G. R. G. Monif (ed.), *Infectious Disease in Obstetrics and Gynecology.* Philadelphia: Harper & Row, 1982. Pp. 415–434.

47. London, R. S., et al. Use of doxycycline in elective first trimester abortion. *South. Med. J.* 71:672, 1978.

48. MacKenzie, I. Z., and Fry, A. Prostaglandin E$_2$ pessaries to facilitate first trimester aspiration termination. *Br. J. Obstet. Gynaecol.* 88:1033, 1981.

49. Marrs, R. P., et al. Termination of early gestation with (15s)-15-methyl prostaglandin F$_{2\alpha}$ methyl ester vaginal suppositories. *Contraception* 24:617, 1981.

50. McKenzie, R., and Shaffer, W. L. A safer method for paracervical block in therapeutic abortions. *Am. J. Obstet. Gynecol.* 130:317, 1978.

51. McMaster Conference on Prevention of Rh Immunization. *Vox Sang.* 56:50, 1979.

52. Miller, E. R., et al. First trimester abortion by vacuum aspiration: Interphysician variability. Presented to the 104th annual meeting, American Public Health Association. Miami Beach, Fla., Oct. 17, 1976.

53. Munsick, R. A. Air embolism and maternal death from therapeutic abortion. *Obstet. Gynecol.* 39:688, 1972.

54. Nathanson, B. N. Management of uterine perforations suffered at elective abortion. *Am. J. Obstet. Gynecol.* 1054, 1972.

55. Nathanson, B. N. The postabortal pain syndrome: A new entity. *Obstet. Gynecol.* 41:739, 1973.

56. Naulty, J. S., and Ostheimer, G. W. CPR for vasovagal syncope. *Contemp. Obstet. Gynecol.* 18:21, 1981.

57. Ott, E. R. Cervical dilation. *Popul. Rep.* [F]. No. 6, 1977.

58. Peterson, H. B., et al. Comparative risk of death from induced abortion at 12 weeks' gestation performed with local versus general anesthesia. *Am. J. Obstet. Gynecol.* 141:763, 1981.

59. Ritchie, J. M., and Cohen, P. J. Cocaine, Procaine and Other Synthetic Local Anesthetics. In L. S. Goodman, and A. Gilman (eds.), *The Pharmacological Basis of Therapeutics* (5th ed.). New York: Macmillan, 1975. Pp. 379–403.

60. Roht, L. H., and Aoyama, H. Induced abortion and its sequelae: Pre-maturity and spontaneous abortion. *Am. J. Obstet. Gynecol.* 120:868, 1974.

61. Sands, R. X., Burnhill, M.S., and Hakim-Elahi, E. Postabortal uterine atony. *Obstet. Gynecol.* 43:595, 1974.

62. Sonne-Holm, S., et al. Prophylactic antibiotics in first trimester abortions: A clinical controlled trial. *Am. J. Obstet. Gynecol.* 139:693, 1981.

63. Stim, E. M. Minisuction: An office abortion procedure. *Adv. Plann. Parent.* 9:1, 1974.

64. Stubblefield, P. G. Current technology for abortion. *Curr. Prob. Obstet. Gynecol.* 2:1, 1978.

65. Stubblefield, P. G. Surgical Techniques for First Trimester Abortion. In J. J. Sciarra (ed.), *Gynecology and Obstetrics.* Philadelphia: Harper & Row, 1982. Pp. 1–8.

66. Tietze, C., and Lewit, S. Joint program for the study of abortion (JPSA): Early medical complications of legal abortion. *Stud. Fam. Plann.* 3:97, 1972.

67. Tokarz, R. D., Williford, J. F., and Soderstrom, R. M. Mobility of fluid as a factor in acute therapeutic dilation of the human cervix. *Adv. Plann. Parent.* 16:22, 1981.

68. Trichopoulos, D., et al. Induced abortion and secondary infertility. *Br. J. Obstet. Gynaecol.* 83:645, 1976.

69. Van der Vlugt, T., and Pitrow, P. T. Uterine aspiration techniques. *Popul. Rep.* [F]. No. 3, 1973.

70. Van der Vlugt, T., and Pitrow, P. T. Menstrual regulation update. *Popul. Rep.*[F]. No. 4, 1974.

71. Vojta, M. A. A critical review of vacuum aspiration: A new method for the termination of pregnancy. *Obstet. Gynecol.* 30:28, 1967.

72. Wan, L. S., Stiber, A. J., and Tarkel, J. Termination of very early pregnancy by vaginal suppositories-(15s)-15-methyl prostaglandin F$_{2\alpha}$ methyl ester. *Contraception* 24:603, 1981.

73. World Health Organization Task Force on the Sequelae of Abortion. The Association of Induced Abortion with Adverse Outcome in Subsequent Pregnancy. In J. J. Sciarra, G. I. Zatuchni, and J. J. Speidel (eds.), *Risks, Benefits and Controversies in Fertility Control.* Hagerstown, Md.: Harper & Row, 1978. Pp. 368–389.

74. World Health Organization Task Force on Prostaglandins for Fertility Regulation. Vaginal administration of 15-methyl-PGF$_{2\alpha}$ methyl ester for preoperative cervical dilation. *Contraception* 23:251, 1981

75. Wulff, G. J. L., Jr., and Freiman, S. M. Elective abortion: Complications seen in a freestanding clinic. *Obstet. Gynecol.* 49:351, 1977.

76. Ye, B. L., Yamamoto, K., and Tyson, J. E. Functional and biochemical aspects of laminaria use in first trimester pregnancy termination. *Am. J. Obstet. Gynecol.* 142:36, 1982.

6. Induced Abortion in the Midtrimester

Phillip G. Stubblefield

INDICATIONS

Abortion is safer the earlier in pregnancy it is performed [11]. Now pregnancy can be diagnosed by sensitive hormonal tests even before the expected menstrual period is missed. Why then is there any need for induced abortion in the midtrimester? Formerly, delays of many weeks were common, as women searched for a provider, underwent extensive physical and psychological testing, and were passed on by an abortion committee. These procedural delays were made unnecessary by the U.S. Supreme Court in 1973 when it legalized abortion throughout the land. However, legality did not mean availability, and a substantial proportion of women seeking abortion still cannot find it promptly. With each year following legalization the proportion of abortions performed in the midtrimester declined, and most recently only 10 percent of U.S. abortions are performed after 12 menstrual weeks [11]. The patient factor most associated with late abortion is *youth* [10]: In 1980 24.6 percent of abortions for women under age 15 were midtrimester, while 14 percent of abortions for women 15 to 19 and only 6.7 percent of abortions for women 30 to 34 were midtrimester procedures [11]. Another important subgroup are those with medical indications, as when prenatal diagnosis reveals a fetal defect or when there is a serious maternal health risk from pregnancy. In our own experience, perhaps not well represented in the literature, an important group of women seeking abortion in the midtrimester are those with serious psychopathology [6].

As fully reviewed by Bracken and Kasl [6], the reasons for delay are complex and are not the same for all women. Some, especially young women, are slow to acknowledge that the pregnancy exists, others are truly ambivalent as to whether they should seek abortion or continue their pregnancy, and many experience serious difficulties in finding abortion services at a price they can pay.

The proportion of abortions performed after 12 weeks has not fallen in the past 3 years. This may be in part the unfortunate result of stringent requirements in some areas for parental permission that delay minor women from obtaining abortions until the pregnancy is more advanced.

THE EVOLUTION OF TECHNIQUES

Technology for midtrimester abortion has changed markedly in the past decade in the United States. It was formerly taught that transcervical instrumental evacuation of the uterus should never be attempted after 12 menstrual weeks. Women who sought abortion in the midtrimester were either treated by hysterotomy, a major surgical procedure, or by instillation of hypertonic saline through amniocentesis. Safe amniocentesis is difficult before 16 menstrual weeks, and as a result the concept of a "gray zone" developed; women who requested abortion at 13 to 15 weeks were regularly delayed until 16 to 20 weeks and then treated by saline infusion. During the 1970s prostaglandins became available as an alternative to hypertonic saline. Another important direction was the development of the combination of intraamniotic urea and low doses of prostaglandin. Many groups found ways to improve the efficacy of such labor-inducing abortifacient agents.

However, the most important change was the realization, largely brought about by the publications of the Centers for Disease Control, that instrumental evacuation through the cervix, was, in fact, the procedure of choice for most of the midtrimester [20]. By the end of the decade an important change had occurred, away from saline infusions or major abdominal surgery and toward variations of dilatation and evacuations (D&E). By 1980 D&E procedures were more common than amnioinfusion, even at 16 to 20 weeks, and amnioinfusion was favored only for those procedures done at or after 21 weeks [11].

In Asia and in northern Europe other labor-inducing techniques are used to cause abortion in the midtrimester. One of the more widely used is the rivanol-catheter method. A rubber urinary catheter is inserted transcervically into the extrauterine space. The antiseptic sodium rivanol is injected through the catheter, and oxytocin is given intravenously. Fetal expulsion generally occurs within 48 to 72 hours. Another method, favored in Japan, is to place laminaria tents in the cervix to produce dilatation, then insert a rubber balloon called a *metreurynter* into the lower uterine cavity, and attach a weight to the balloon to provide traction while intravenous oxytocin is given [53].

PRESENT MIDTRIMESTER TECHNIQUES

Dilatation and Evacuation (D&E)

ALTERNATIVE TECHNIQUES

Several techniques have been used for the transcervical instrumental evacuation of the uterus [54]. These differ primarily in the preparatory steps that precede the evacuation. Bierer and Steiner [4] used forcible dilatation followed by laminaria insertion under general anesthesia and repeated this over 2 to 3 days until wide cervical dilatations were obtained before evacuating the uterus with "long, strong" forceps under general anesthesia. Slome [48] performed the first step of forcible dilatation and laminaria placement under paracervical block with lidocaine and epinephrine and added needle

aspiration of the amniotic fluid; the uterine evacuation was performed under general anesthesia the following day. Davis [13] reported a more invasive first-day procedure with no laminaria: After forcible dilatation under general anesthesia the membranes were ruptured, the umbilical cord pulled down and out, and an antibiotic cream placed in the vagina with packs; on the second day additional forcible dilatation was carried out, and the macerated fetus then extracted.

The most influential of early D&E practitioners was Finks. He reported 2,000 D&E cases in 1973 [15]. He thoroughly infiltrated the cervix with local anesthetic containing epinephrine 1:200,000, using a 1½ inch needle inserted into the cervix to its full length at four sites, and then performed forcible dilatation carefully and slowly. Subsequently, the pregnancy was evacuated with long forceps. Finks' one-stage technique has been widely adopted by other physicians, among them Van de Bergh [59] in Holland and Peterson in the United States [41].

Hanson [24] further perfected the laminaria technique. Multiple small Japanese laminaria were used. Forcible dilatation of the cervix and general anesthesia were avoided. Cases of less than 16 weeks' gestation were evacuated after 5 hours. Laminaria were left in place overnight for gestations beyond 16 weeks. The amniotic fluid was aspirated with a 12-mm cannula and vacuum, and the pregnancy was evacuated with ring forceps (Forrester) while the operator maintained firm pressure on the uterine fundus with one hand. Barr [2] developed a similar technique but used forcible dilatation before placing the laminaria.

Hern [25], influenced by the Japanese use of laminaria, developed his own technique, utilizing multiple sets of laminaria. One laminaria was inserted on the first day and replaced with several the following morning. That afternoon these were removed and replaced with a third set, which were left in place overnight. The abortion was performed the next morning under local anesthesia in an office surgery, 41 hours or so after placement of the first laminaria. DeLee [14] used a somewhat simpler approach, with two sets of laminaria placed on successive days, followed by evacuation on the third day. Darney [12] and Stubblefield [54] have also used this technique.

Presently most United States practitioners use either a one-stage procedure with forcible dilatation of the cervix or they employ a two-stage procedure with multiple small laminaria placed the first day followed by extraction on the next day.

Choice among these alternative techniques becomes more important as gestational age advances. As we have demonstrated, pregnancies at 13 and 14 menstrual weeks are readily evacuated with the 12-mm vacuum cannula routinely used at 12 weeks [56]. The

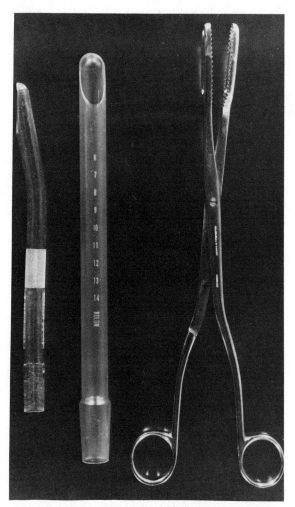

Fig. 6-1. Instruments used for midtrimester uterine evacuation: 12- and 16-mm vacuum cannula, Sopher forceps.

cervix is usually fairly easily dilated with tapered dilators such as Pratt's or Denniston's sufficient for insertion of the 12-mm cannula. However, unless routine ultrasound is practiced, the gestation sized preoperatively as 14 weeks can easily turn out to be 16, requiring larger instruments and a larger cervical diameter. For this reason, we very strongly advise routine use of laminaria tents for D&E after 13 weeks.

MEANS FOR EVACUATION

Most practitioners of D&E use any of several heavy long forceps to evacuate the pregnancy and utilize a vacuum cannula only as an adjunct to rupture the fetal membranes and drain the fluid initially and as a final step to ensure complete evacuation of all placental tissue. Instruments useful for uterine evacuation are shown in Figure 6-1. The ideal forceps would be strong enough to crush fetal tissue but light enough to transmit sensation to the operator's hand for careful control. Forrester forceps are favored by some, and certainly these provide excellent "feel," but they are too light and short for the more advanced gestations. The longer, stronger Sopher and Bierer forceps are very useful but do not allow the same control. Recently Hern has introduced a new forceps of his own design, which appears to approach the ideal.*

We have found that large-bore vacuum cannulas and collection systems are a great help in the early midtrimester [56]. The 16-mm vacuum system allows evacuation of pregnancies through 16 weeks by the vacuum technique and thus might allow the surgeon experienced with first trimester procedures to extend his range safely into the early midtrimester.† At 17 weeks and beyond, even the 16-mm vacuum system is inadequate and becomes only a useful adjunct to forceps extraction. A detailed description of uterine evacuation is provided by Hern in his monograph [25].

CHOICE OF LAMINARIA

There are two species of laminaria in medical use: *Laminaria digitata*, which come from Scandinavia, and *L. japonicum*, from Japan. We much prefer the Japanese laminaria, as they are small and tapered and retain their integrity after swelling. The laminaria digitata become soft and gelatinous as they swell, easily become entrapped in the cervical canal, and often fragment with removal by forceps. In early midtrimester pregnancies one medium laminaria japonicum left in place overnight will produce a mean cervical calibration of 12.1 mm, while two such laminaria tents yield a mean of 14.1 mm [53]. Still greater dilatation is achieved by more laminaria and is also related to an increase in gestational age. We have compared one versus two sets of laminaria tents before evacuation and concluded that in pregnancies at 17 to 19 weeks the greater dilatation and greater ease for the surgeon afforded by the more prolonged treatment were not worth the cost to the patient of the additional day's delay [57]. However, Darney [12] has reported that two sets of laminaria were especially helpful after 19 weeks. Certainly Hern's series [26] in which multiple sets of laminaria were used provides a standard of safety for late midtrimester D&Es that none have surpassed. We have recently modified our own technique and now insist on two successive sets of laminaria, each in place overnight,

*Hern forceps available through V. Mueller, Inc., Linden, N.J.
†16-mm vacuum systems available through Rocket of London, Inc., of Branford, Conn. and Medispec of Lafayette, Calif.

before evacuation on the third day, when pregnancy has progressed to 20 weeks or beyond.

After 20 weeks, even with wide dilatation from multiple sets of laminaria, evacuating the fetus is more difficult. For this reason Hern [25] has advocated intraamniotic infusion of urea, followed by surgical evacuation of the fetus after labor has begun. Finks [16] has revived Davis' two-stage procedure with intentional rupture of the membranes and cutting of the umbilical cord on day 1 and has reported safe D&E abortion to 26 weeks.

CHOICE OF ANESTHETIC
First-trimester abortion is safer if performed under local as opposed to general anesthesia. General anesthesia increases the risk for major perforation, visceral injury, hemorrhage, hysterectomy, and death [19]. We suspect that this decreased morbidity is partly because the awake patient signals her discomfort when the operator pushes too hard with an instrument. On occasion when perforation has occurred, the patient's complaint of upper abdominal pain has stopped the operator from further instrumentation and prevented serious injury to the bowel. No such comparison statistics exist for midtrimester D&E, but we would expect a proportionally even greater advantage for avoiding general anesthesia in the midtrimester when the uterus is large, soft, and easily perforated. We think that this is the reason that most United States experts insist on avoiding full general anesthesia in the midtrimester. Intravenous sedation with short-acting analgesic-anxiolytic combinations provides an important measure of comfort for the patient. For years we have used the combination of fentanyl, 0.05 to 0.10 mg, and diazepam, 5 to 10 mg, without complication. These are always given very slowly, never as a bolus. If the patient seems oversedated after the procedure, naloxone is administered prophylactically.

PROPHYLACTIC ANTIBIOTICS
Though still controversial in first-trimester abortion and of unproven value in the midtrimester, prophylactic antibiotics are widely used with D&E, especially when laminaria are utilized.

EPINEPHRINE AND VASOPRESSIN AS ADJUNCTS
Early practitioners of D&E advised the use of epinephrine 1:200,000 mixed with the paracervical anesthetic as a means for reducing blood loss [15]. No randomized controlled trial has been performed, but Koplik [36] has reported that epinephrine use speeds patient recovery after first-trimester abortion, and it is commonly used for D&E. The 1:100,000 concentration commercially available mixed with 1% lidocaine is too strong. We use equal parts of plain 1% lidocaine and 1% lidocaine with

epinephrine to produce the desired concentration of both agents: epinephrine 1:200,000 in lidocaine 1%. Some prefer to use chloroprocaine because of its rapid inactivation if inadvertently injected intravascularly and add the desired epinephrine concentration themselves. Great caution is required to avoid errors in epinephrine dosages: Overdose can produce immediate, life-threatening pulmonary edema.

Glick [17] advised the use of Pituitrin injected paracervically to reduce bleeding with D&E. Pituitrin is a mixture of oxytocin and vasopressin. Vasopressin is used in gynecologic surgery to reduce bleeding from cervical conization or from myomectomy. It produces profound local vasoconstriction and also uterine contraction, but it is an extremely potent hypertensive agent. Again, though no controlled trial exists, experts such as Peterson [42] are convinced that vasopressin is of great value with D&E. It must be used with caution. The 20-unit ampule should be diluted in 60 cc or so of local anesthetic solution, so that at most a total of 10 units is given at multiple sites with the paracervical block. It should not be used in women with heart disease or any degree of hypertension.

UTEROTONIC AGENTS
All agree that intravenous or intracervical oxytocin is helpful with D&E, but there is controversy as to the time of administration. Some give it throughout the procedure while others wait until the uterus is empty, feeling that earlier use and resultant uterine contractions make it more difficult to locate retained fetal parts. Ergot preparations are routinely given intramuscularly after the procedure. The benefit of 0.1 mg intramuscular ergot in reducing postabortal hematometra in the first trimester has been reported by Sands and colleagues [47], but no such study exists for the midtrimester.

Recently the 15 methyl analogue of prostaglandin $F_{2\alpha+}$ has been licensed in the United States for midtrimester abortion.* This drug has proved of tremendous value in managing postpartum hemorrhage and probably would be of benefit as an adjunct with D&E.

COMMON D&E PROBLEMS AND THEIR MANAGEMENT
Although in the skilled hands of experts serious complications have been infrequent, the potential for life-threatening damage to the patient is definitely present with D&E procedures. Attention to small details of technique that may prevent complications is therefore extremely important.

---

*Prostin 15 M. Upjohn Company, Kalamazoo, Mich.

Laminaria Difficulties. If more than one or two medium-sized Japanese laminaria cannot be inserted without difficulty, it may be that the gestational age is, in reality, only 12 or 13 weeks and the small number of laminaria will suffice. However, if reexamination of the uterus confirms a more advanced gestational age, one can resort to two sets of laminaria. The first set of laminaria is left in place overnight; the following morning these are removed and replaced with an additional six or eight medium-sized Japanese laminaria. By late afternoon of the second day, sufficient dilatation will have been achieved to allow the procedure to be readily performed.

Most patients will experience some cramping discomfort with the insertion of laminaria. When four or five medium-sized laminaria are inserted, it is helpful to have the patient remain lying on the table for 15 or 20 minutes after insertion to avoid syncope. Some patients experience extreme degrees of pain associated with vomiting after laminaria insertion. In such a case it is best to remove one or two laminaria if several had been inserted. The patient's discomfort will then usually subside, and she can be allowed to go home. Most women who have only one or two laminaria inserted will experience minimal discomfort through the evening after insertion. However, when four or five tents are used, patients will report significant cramping and menstrual-like pain, and an analgesic medication should be offered. Occasionally, the membranes may be ruptured with laminaria insertion; the laminaria should be left in place, prophylactic antibiotic used, and the procedure performed the next day as planned.

Occasionally, and especially in the young primigravid patient, the internal os of the cervix is quite resistant to dilatation; the laminaria will be indented by the cervix, balloon out above the internal os, and thus become very difficult to remove. This problem is most likely when a single large laminaria has been used, for if multiple smaller tents are inserted, one can always be removed and then the others. Especially with *L. digitata*, the tents will become quite soft and may fragment with attempts at removal; this is avoided by using laminaria of the *japonicum* species. If the laminaria cannot be removed with persistent gentle effort, it is best to stop. Some authors have advocated inserting a small dilator alongside the entrapped laminaria. However, this is very likely to perforate the uterus. It is preferable to abandon efforts at removal and wait another 6 hours. During this time the cervix will soften and dilate further, and removal of the laminaria will become easy.

Inability to Complete the Procedure. It is not uncommon to find that the fetal calvarium has remained in the uterus after the abortion procedure was thought to have been completed. If gentle efforts at extraction fail, it is best

not to persist. Intravenous oxytocin is begun, and the patient is allowed to wait for 2 hours. By this time uterine activity will have pushed the retained tissue down to the level of the internal os where it can be easily extracted without further anesthesia.

Accurate estimation of gestational age is difficult in the midtrimester. We recommend frequent use of ultrasound if the pregnancy is thought to be beyond 16 menstrual weeks. Once the abortion procedure is commenced and the membranes ruptured, if the operator then perceives that the pregnancy may be too far advanced, gestational age can be confirmed by measuring the length of the fetal foot. According to Streeter [52], a fetal foot length of 26.8 mm corresponds to 18 menstrual weeks; 30.7 mm, 19 weeks; 33.3 mm, 20 weeks; and 35.2 mm, 21 weeks. If multiple laminaria tents have been used and the cervix is widely dilated, a surgeon familiar with midtrimester curettage procedures can satisfactorily extract a pregnancy up to 20 or 21 weeks. Beyond this, we feel that the procedure should be abandoned unless the surgeon routinely performs more advanced D&E procedures. The patient can be treated with intravenous oxytocin or systemic prostaglandins and prophylactic antibiotics; the curettage procedures can be resumed after 24 hours have elapsed to allow for fetal maceration.

Systemic Prostaglandins

Two prostaglandins are available in the United States for systemic administration to produce abortion: vaginal suppositories of PGE_2 and the 15 methyl analogue of prostaglandin $F_{2\alpha}$ (Prostin 15 M) by intramuscular injection. Both are highly effective, are easy to administer, and can be used at any gestational age. PGE_2 is given as a 20-mg vaginal suppository every 3 hours. In a large group of midtrimester patients the mean time from start of treatment to fetal expulsion was 13.4 hours, with about 90 percent of patients aborting by 24 hours [58]. The process takes a little longer with Prostin 15 M. When 250 mcg is given intramuscularly every 2 hours, the mean times to abort are 15 to 17 hours, with 80 percent aborting by 24 hours [45]. Side effects are significant with both methods. The prostaglandins directly stimulate the smooth muscle of the gastrointestinal tract. With intramuscular Prostin 15 M, 83 percent experienced vomiting and 71 percent experienced diarrhea in one large trial [45]. There is somewhat less vomiting and diarrhea when PGE_2 is used: 39 percent had vomiting and 25 percent had diarrhea in the trial cited earlier, and half the patients had neither side effect [58]. With PGE_2, however, temperature is elevated by direct central effect of the drug: About one-third of patients will have more than 1°C elevation of temperature and fevers of 40°C are not uncommon, although life-threatening pyrexia has only rarely been encountered. This is not a problem with Prostin 15 M, which actually lowers the temperature slightly. Prostaglandins can cause bronchospasm and constriction of the coronary arteries. Myocardial infarction was reported in one hypertensive woman with a fetal death in utero who was treated with PGE_2 [50]. One death has also been reported [35]. These systemic prostaglandins were especially attractive as means for abortion at 13 to 15 weeks, avoiding the need to delay the abortion until 16 weeks for amnioinfusion. Robbins and Surrago [46] have reported that D&E is superior to vaginal PGE_2 at 13 to 15 weeks. When considering abortion at 16 weeks and beyond, the systemic prostaglandins have to be compared to medications given by the intrauterine route with amniocentesis. Intrauterine administration is associated with fewer side effects, and as intrauterine methods were available before systemic prostaglandins, they are more often favored. Vaginal PGE_2 and Prostin 15 M, however, are very important as adjuncts to intrauterine methods. Often patients who fail to abort from saline infusion or intraamniotic prostaglandin will go on to abort after only one or two doses of either PGE_2 or Prostin 15 M and will thus be spared operative intervention [38].

Intrauterine Prostaglandin

The first prostaglandin approved in the United States was $PGF_{2\alpha}$ by intraamniotic infusion. Intraamniotic $PGF_{2\alpha}$ has some advantages over amnioinfusion of hypertonic saline: The abortion process is faster, there is no direct adverse effect on blood coagulation as there is with hypertonic saline, and an accidental intravascular injection is much less likely to be fatal. Unfortunately, many more patients will require a second intraamniotic dose with $PGF_{2\alpha}$ than with the saline, and more of the abortions will be incomplete. Gastrointestinal side effects are more common, and importantly, the prostaglandin is not directly toxic to the fetus. Transient fetal survival occurs in 7 to 10 percent of cases, presenting ethical problems of great magnitude. Intraamniotic prostaglandin was initially hailed as safer than saline, but as documented by the CDC, problems of failed abortion, retained tissue, infection, and bleeding were more common with prostaglandin than with saline [19]. In our own institution we felt that life-threatening complications should be less likely with prostaglandin and persevered in efforts to make it work better. We found, as did others, that overnight pretreatment with laminaria tents improved the results. The mean times from abortion were reduced from 29 hours to 14 hours, 82 percent of patients aborted by 24 hours, and many fewer required a second intraamniotic infusion [55]. Because abortion was complete within 1 hour in only half

of our cases, we outfitted a treatment room with a uterine aspirator and performed routine curettage aided by low-dose intravenous sedation, whether apparently complete or not. This brought our rates of retained tissue and infection to low levels [53]. We learned to manage failed prostaglandin abortions by D&E, as advocated by Burkeman [7], or by systemic prostaglandins when they became available and thus no longer needed to resort to hysterotomy for failed abortion.

We demonstrated that treatment with antiemetics markedly reduced the vomiting from prostaglandin without prolonging the time to abortion [33].

Prostaglandin and Hypertonic Saline

Another approach to augmenting $PGF_{2\alpha}$ has been the addition of 50 cc of 20% NaCl as reported by Borten [5]. This does add the possible hazard of intravascular injection of saline but improves efficacy and appears to reduce the incidence of fetal survival, at least for cases prior to 20 weeks. Kerenyi et al. [35] combined 150 to 200 ml of 20% saline with 20 mg of $PGF_{2\alpha}$. This method would be preferred, especially for abortions after 20 weeks.

Urea and $PGF_{2\alpha}$

Hypertonic urea by intraamniotic injection is a better choice than hypertonic saline: Accidental intravascular injection is much less hazardous, and while virtually all saline-treated patients develop a subclinical disseminated intravascular coagulopathy, only one-third of urea-treated patients will exhibit coagulation changes [9]. Urea by itself is very slow to produce abortion; it must be augmented. Formerly this was done with high-dose intravenous oxytocin, but the addition instead of low-dose $PGF_{2\alpha}$ has made this the method of choice for late midtrimester abortion when a labor-induced method is preferred. Eighty grams of urea are instilled into the amniotic sac along with 5.0 mg of $PGF_{2\alpha}$. The mean time to abortion is 17.5 hours, and 80 percent will abort by 24 hours [8]. Combinations with higher doses of prostaglandin and oxytocin will work faster but add greater risk for rupture of the cervix, a potential problem with all the labor-induction methods [51]. An important consideration in choosing urea, especially for abortions at 20 to 24 weeks, is that fetal survival appears to be quite rare.

Hypertonic Saline

Amnioinfusion of hypertonic saline continues to be the most common method for late midtrimester abortion in the United States. The usual technique is to perform amniocentesis, remove some amniotic fluid, and then instill 200 cc of 20 to 23% NaCl through connector tubing and gravity flow from a single-dose bottle of commercially prepared pyrogen-free solution. Authorities vary in the amount of amniotic fluid they remove. Mean times from instillation to abortion are 33 to 35 hours [3, 37].

Case reports have documented the occasional occurrence of disastrous complications from saline infusion, such as cardiovascular collapse, hypernatremia associated with cerebral edema, acute renal failure, and amniotic fluid embolism. Nevertheless, the main problems of saline abortion—failed abortion, incomplete abortion, and retained tissue associated with hemorrhage and infection—are common to other midtrimester methods that attempt to induce labor.

Intravenous administration of oxytocin improves the efficacy and reduces the rate of occurrence of the problems of infection, retained placenta, blood loss, and failed abortion but adds other hazards. The mean interval from instillation to fetal abortion is reduced to 25 to 26 hours if an oxytocin infusion of 17 to 67 mU per milliliter is begun within 8 hours of saline instillation, but not if the oxytocin infusion is delayed beyond this critical interval [3]. Higher rates of oxytocin infusion will shorten the mean injection-to-abortion interval still more, to 20 to 21 hours, but add more hazards. Kerenyi et al. [35] used 100 to 200 mU per minute and reported the occurrence of two uterine ruptures and "a few" cases of annular detachment of the cervix when the high oxytocin infusion rate was used. Even at modest infusion rates oxytocin places the patient at risk for water intoxication, especially if treatment is continued for 24 hours without interruption. Use of high-dose oxytocin also appears to increase the risk for serious disseminated intravascular coagulopathy (DIC).

Laminaria and Hypertonic Saline

Treatment with laminaria tents will shorten the interval to abortion but appears to increase the risk of infection when utilized with saline [49]. This is very much in contrast to the experience with vacuum curettage [18], D&E [1, 24, 25], and prostaglandins, where infectious complications with laminaria use have been very rare [55]. We believe that the risk of infection in saline treatment is increased by laminaria use and suspect that this is the result of (1) tissue destruction by the saline and (2) relatively prolonged times from treatment to abortion, which allow time for bacterial multiplication in the extraamniotic space.

Where high-dose oxytocin has been added to the regimen so that the interval to abortion is short, as reported by Hachamovitch et al. [23], infection has been uncommon. Hachamovitch inserted multiple laminaria tents into the cervix, instilled intraamniotic saline 2 to 3 hours later, and then started oxytocin intravenously at 417 to 555 mU per minute after another 2 hours. He reported a mean time from instillation to abortion of only 12.5 hours, and complications were minimal. These excellent results require replication by others, but we caution that uterine rupture, cervicovaginal fistula, and cervical evulsion can occur even when laminaria are used.

Transient fetal survival is highly unlikely in pregnancies of less than 24 weeks' gestation provided a full dose of intraamniotic saline is given, but it has been reported after 24 weeks. We strongly advise routine ultrasound before any abortion after 20 weeks because of the difficulty in being sure of gestational age from menstrual data and clinical examination alone.

Common Problems with Labor-Induction Methods

Difficulties in performing amniocentesis diminish with practice. If a bloody tap is encountered, the tip of the needle is either too superficial or too deep and within the wall of the uterus or the placenta. If blood initially drawn into the needle gives way to clear fluid after repositioning the needle, it is reasonable to proceed with amnioinfusion. Fortunately, with the wide availability of ultrasound, it is no longer necessary to labor with a difficult amniocentesis. The problem may be one of a uterine anomaly, large fibroids, undiagnosed fetal death, a smaller gestation than anticipated, or perhaps an ovarian cyst and no pregnancy at all. All are readily demonstrated by good ultrasound.

Water intoxication in the patient receiving oxytocin would be heralded by the development of maternal edema, weight gain, headache, and clouding of the sensorium in association with reduction of urine output. In normal women cessation of oxytocin infusion usually results in clinical improvement in a short time. The problem is prevented by administering oxytocin by infusion pump in a small volume of balanced electrolyte solution (Ringer's lactate) or normal saline. Even more important is to allow the patient a 2-hour rest off oxytocin every 12 hours.

Excessive bleeding at the time of fetal expulsion or thereafter may indicate retained tissue, or it may indicate disseminated intravascular coagulopathy (DIC). Blood should be drawn for crossmatch, coagulation studies, and fibrin split products. An additional tube is kept at bedside and allowed to clot under observation. The uterus is then explored with a sponge stick under local anesthesia to confirm that there is no retained tissue and to rule out cervical laceration. Blood is given as needed, and if there is evidence of DIC and bleeding continues, fibrinogen (cryoprecipitate), fresh frozen plasma, and platelet concentrates are given.

Retained placenta is common with prostaglandin abortion and less common with urea and saline methods. The patient remains at risk for bleeding until the abortion is completed, and as time passes, her chance of developing endometritis also increases. We prefer to intervene if the placenta has not passed within 2 hours after fetal expulsion. Experienced physicians can readily accomplish this using minimal intravenous sedation in a treatment room setting; full anesthesia or an operating room should not be necessary. The bulk of the placenta is removed with ring forceps, and a large sharp curet and 12-mm vacuum cannula are used alternately to complete the procedure.

Failed abortion is a special concern with all the labor-induction methods. All these methods appear to produce results similar to those shown in Figure 6-2 for our laminaria-PGF$_{2\alpha}$ method. That is, 90 percent or so of patients abort fairly promptly, and the remaining 10 percent take much longer. When should we intervene with another method? When the only possible intervention was hysterotomy, a major surgical procedure, it was worth waiting for abortion from the primary method. However, now that the systemic prostaglandins are available, we think it advisable to move on to a secondary method after a predetermined time limit is reached. In our practice if a woman has not aborted by 24 hours or if membranes have ruptured and uterine activity has ceased, vaginal prostaglandin is administered. With abortions less than 20 weeks' gestation vaginal evacuation of the pregnancy is a safe and relatively easy procedure; this approach has been advocated by several authorities, and we fully concur [7]. In the 1980s labor-induction abortions are most often reserved for use at 20 to 24 weeks. Vaginal evacuation after 20 weeks is more difficult, but because the many hours of labor will have compacted the fetal parts into the lower uterine segment and dilated the cervix, the experienced physician, properly equipped with strong ovum forceps, can accomplish safe evacuation in most cases. The more advanced the gestation, the longer we would persist with systemic prostaglandin before resorting to instrumental evacuation [38].

Uterine rupture has been reported with all the intraamniotic methods, but most cases also involved augmentation with oxytocin [21]. We have had two uterine ruptures in several thousand cases treated with laminaria and intraamniotic PGF$_{2\alpha}$. Both were older multigravidas treated with high-dose oxytocin after failing to abort from the prostaglandin alone [43]. In our experience previous cesarean section has not been associated with uterine rupture as a special hazard, but we suggest that oxytocin be avoided or limited to low infusion rates in such cases. Young primigravida women are at risk for a different kind of trauma, *cervical rupture*, or cervicovaginal fistula. In these cases the vigorous

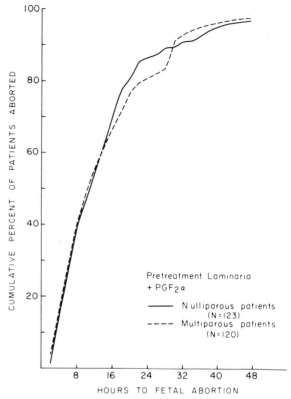

Fig. 6-2. Cumulative percent of patients aborted versus time. Laminaria pretreatment overnight, followed by intraamniotic prostaglandin F$_{2\alpha}$. (From P. G. Stubblefield, D. Kayman, and L. O. Burns. unpublished data, 1979.)

uterine contractions against an unyielding cervix produce a spontaneous tear in the lower uterine segment, usually posterior, with resultant expulsion of the pregnancy through a fistula behind the cervical os. Overnight pretreatment with laminaria tents greatly reduces the risk for this problem but does not eliminate it altogether. Cervical rupture is seen with intraamniotic PGF$_{2\alpha}$, urea-PGF$_{2\alpha}$, and saline augmented with high-dose oxytocin, but not when vaginal PGE$_2$ is used alone. These tears are repaired vaginally, after debriding the devitalized tissue. Repair is best accomplished with a few 0 chromic sutures placed through all layers: cervical epithelium, cervical stroma, and vaginal mucosa.

Disseminated intravascular coagulopathy is well known as a hazard of hypertonic saline and can also occur with intraamniotic urea. Less well known is that DIC is rarely seen as a complication of D&E procedures [39]: A recent study from the Centers for Disease Control [31] reported an incidence of only 8 of 100,000 with first-trimester vacuum curettage, 191 of 100,000 with midtrimester D&E, and 658 of 100,000 with amnioinfusion of hypertonic saline [31].

Extraamniotic PGF$_{2\alpha}$, Laminaria, and Oxytocin

Hodgson [27] developed a combination method for midtrimester abortion by intrauterine administration of prostaglandin into the extraamniotic space. First the cervix was dilated by overnight treatment with multiple laminaria tents. Then a Foley-type urinary catheter was placed through the cervical canal into the extraamniotic space. After two test doses of 0.5 mg each, two more doses of 2.0 mg PGF$_{2\alpha}$ were given through the catheter (total dose, 5 mg), and then a continuous infusion of 3.7 mg per hour was given by electric infusion pump. The mean time from start of PGF$_{2\alpha}$ to abortion was 12.3 hours with 85 percent aborting by 24 hours. Prophylactic tetracycline was used, and there was only one infectious complication of 300 patients treated. There were no instances of even transient fetal survival and no cervical trauma, suggesting distinct advantages of this method over other prostaglandin regimens.

CHOICE OF MIDTRIMESTER METHODS

Dilatation and evacuation is easily performed at 13 to 15 weeks by a surgeon with some first-trimester experience, especially if laminaria or osmotic dilators are used first. Resident physicians on our service have consistently been able to terminate 16-week pregnancies safely by D&E under the following conditions: overnight placement of multiple laminaria japonicum tents, use of 16-mm vacuum cannula system, local anesthesia augmented with intravenous sedation, good nursing support, and direct hands-on supervision by a small group of experienced faculty [1]. We therefore see little indication for any procedure other than D&E before 17 weeks, although we would argue that D&E should always be done under the conditions described above. The best present alternative to D&E in the early midtrimester is vaginal prostaglandin E$_2$, but Robins and Surrago [46] have shown D&E to be safer and more effective than PGE$_2$.

After 16 weeks there are many alternatives. None is truly satisfactory; each has its own constellation of possible complications. When the entire second trimester is considered, D&E methods appear safer [20, 30], but as noted by Kafrissen et al. [30] in their recent comparison of D&E and urea-prostaglandin F$_{2\alpha}$, the advantage of D&E is for procedures at 13 to 16 weeks. For procedures done after 16 weeks the risks for major complications and death are comparable. Patient preference cannot be ignored. Kaltreider et al. [32] have demonstrated

that the psychological impact of D&E is less for the patient than is that of amnioinfusion abortion. Our preference is to offer, up to 20 weeks, D&E under local anesthesia after overnight placement of laminaria tents. For procedures at 20 to 21 weeks we presently use the three-stage procedure with two sets of laminaria tents but refer the patient for saline-prostaglandin when abortion is required after this. While we feel that for the usual operator, infusion methods are best at the end of the midtrimester, we note that several skilled practitioners do offer D&E up to 24 weeks. The lowest complication rate is that achieved by Hern [26] for his combination method of multiple stages of laminaria and intraamniotic injection of urea followed by a D&E procedure after labor is initiated.

FETAL DEATH IN UTERO

In our opinion fetal death in utero can be managed as one would manage a primary abortion at the same gestational age. We use D&E techniques after overnight placement of laminaria tents through 21 weeks and then resort to vaginal PGE$_2$ suppositories. Beyond 24 weeks we advise against the use of the full-dose suppositories because of the potential for overstimulation of the third-trimester uterus that might result in uterine rupture. In these cases we cut the suppositories into pieces and administer one-quarter of a suppository (5 mg) at hourly intervals until fetal expulsion occurs.

LATE SEQUELAE OF MIDTRIMESTER ABORTION

Epidemiologic data generated from the last decade have largely laid to rest concerns that first-trimester abortion is a significant hazard for later reproduction [28]. Nonetheless, we are concerned for the reproductive futures of women who have had forcible wide dilatation of the cervix for midtrimester abortion. We have shown that the cervix recovers completely after laminaria dilatation, as noted by calibrations done 2 weeks postabortally [57]. However, Johnstone [29] noted persistent wide cervical diameters in first-trimester patients dilated forcibly beyond 10 mm. Spontaneous losses have been reported to follow D&E with forcible dilatation [44], and increased rates of prematurity have also been observed [41]. The cervical rupture that can be seen with PGF$_{2\alpha}$ and with saline or urea augmented with high-dose oxytocin also concerns us. For these reasons we strongly advocate the use of laminaria rather than forcible dilatation for D&E, and we would avoid high-dose oxytocin to augment infusion methods. Continued surveillance of pregnancies subsequent to midtrimester abortion is needed until the issues concerned with late sequelae are fully resolved.

THE UPPER LIMIT FOR MIDTRIMESTER ABORTION

The public, pregnant women, and their doctors and nurses become progressively more troubled by abortion as gestational age advances. Infants liveborn at 24 weeks and weighing more than 600 grams occasionally survive, provided they are afforded neonatal intensive care, and at 26 weeks half of liveborns will survive with neonatal intensive care. Therefore, in our opinion 23 completed weeks should be the usual outer limit for induced abortion, except in the instance of late discovery of serious fetal abnormality. Ultrasound should be routinely used at 20 weeks and beyond in order to reduce the risk of inadvertently attempting an abortion at or after 24 weeks. When such procedures are necessary at an advanced gestational age because of serious threat to maternal health, we must also consider the welfare of the fetus. Often an additional delay and the use of steroids administered to the mother will improve chances for fetal survival after cesarean section although at the price of greater maternal risk. Given the sensitive nature of such interventions, each case must be managed individually for maximal benefit to both patients: mother and fetus.

REFERENCES

1. Altman, A., et al. Midtrimester abortion by laminaria and vacuum evacuation (L&E) on a teaching service: A review of 789 cases. *Adv. Plann. Parent.* 16:1, 1981.
2. Barr, M. M. Midtrimester abortion at 12–20 weeks by dilatation and evacuation method under local anesthesia. *Adv. Plann. Parent.* 13:16, 1978.
3. Berger, G. S., and Edelman, D. A. Oxytocin administration, instillation to abortion time, and morbidity associated with saline instillation. *Am. J. Obstet. Gynecol.* 121:941, 1975.
4. Bierer, I., and Steiner, V. Termination of pregnancy in the second trimester with the aid of laminaria tents. *Med. Gynecol. Sociol.* 6:9, 1971.
5. Borten, M. Use of combination prostaglandin F_2 and hypertonic saline for midtrimester abortion. *Prostaglandins* 12:625, 1976.
6. Bracken, M.D., and Kasl, S.V. Delay in seeking induced abortion: A review and theoretical analysis. *Am. J. Obstet. Gynecol.* 121:1008, 1975.
7. Burkeman, R. T., et al. The management of midtrimester abortion failures by vaginal evacuation. *Obstet. Gynecol.* 49:233, 1977.
8. Burkeman, R. T., et al. Hyperosmolar urea for elective midtrimester abortion: Experience in 1913 cases. *Am. J. Obstet. Gynecol.* 131:10, 1978.
9. Burnett, L. S., et al. Intra-amniotic urea as a midtrimester abortifacient: Clinical results and serum and urinary changes. *Am. J. Obstet. Gynecol.* 121:7, 1975.
10. Cannon-Bonventre, K. Educational methodologies to decrease second trimester abortions. American Institutes for Research, Cambridge, Mass. Contract 200-77-0701, Centers for Disease Control.
11. Centers for Disease Control. Abortion Surveillance 1980, January, 1983.
12. Darney, P. D. Midtrimester abortion under ultrasound guidance. Post Graduate course, National Abortion Federation, Tampa, Fla., Jan. 31, 1983.
13. Davis, G. Midtrimester abortion. *Lancet* 2:1926, 1972.
14. DeLee, S. T. Termination of pregnancy in the midtrimester using a new technique. *Int. J. Surg.* 61:545, 1976.
15. Finks, A. I. Midtrimester abortion. *Lancet* 1:263, 1973.
16. Finks, A. I. Therapeutic abortion: Dilatation and evacuation in late midtrimester: Technical details for safety. Paper presented to the symposium Abortion: Spontaneous and Induced. Maui, Hawaii, Oct. 10–15, 1982.
17. Glick, E. Personal communication, Oct. 4, 1980.
18. Gold, J., et al. The Safety of Laminaria and Rigid Dilators for Cervical Dilatation Prior to Suction Curettage for First Trimester Abortion: A Comparative Analysis. In F. Naftolin and P. G. Stubblefield (eds.), *Dilatation of the Uterine Cervix: Connective Tissue Biology and Clinical Management.* New York: Raven, 1980. Pp. 363–372.
19. Grimes, D. A., et al. Midtrimester abortion in intra-amniotic prostaglandin F_2: Safer than saline? *Obstet. Gynecol.* 49:612, 1977.
20. Grimes, D. A., et al. Midtrimester abortion by dilatation and evacuation: A safe and practical alternative. *N. Engl. J. Med.* 296:1141, 1977.
21. Grimes, D. A., et al. Fatal uterine rupture during oxytocin-augmented, saline-induced abortion. *Am. J. Obstet. Gynecol.* 130:591, 1978.
22. Grimes, D. A., et al. Local versus general anesthesia: Which is safer for performing suction curettage abortion? *Am. J. Obstet. Gynecol.* 135:1030, 1979.
23. Hachamovitch, M., Bracken, M. B., and Simons, H. Saline instillation abortion with laminaria and megadose oxytocin. *Am. J. Obstet. Gynecol.* 135:327, 1979.
24. Hanson, M. S. D&E midtrimester abortion preceded by laminaria. Paper presented to the 16th annual meeting of the Association of Planned Parenthood Physicians. San Diego, Calif., Oct. 26, 1978.
25. Hern, W. M. Midtrimester abortion. *Obstet. Gynecol. Annual* 10:375, 1981.
26. Hern, W. M. Outpatient second trimester D&E abortion through 24 menstrual weeks' gestation. *Adv. Plann. Parent.* 16:7, 1981.
27. Hodgson, J. E. Three hundred late midtrimester abortions

induced by extra-amniotic PGF$_{2\alpha}$ and intracervical laminaria tents. *Adv. Plann. Parent.* 14:61, 1979.

28. Hogue, C. J., Cates, W., Jr., and Tietze, C. The effects of induced abortion on subsequent reproduction. *Epidemiol. Rev.* 4:66, 1982.

29. Johnstone, F. D., et al. Cervical diameter after suction termination of pregnancy. *Br. Med. J.* 1:68, 1976.

30. Kafrissen, M. E., et al. A comparison of intra-amniotic instillation of hyperosmolar urea and prostaglandin F$_{2\alpha}$ vs dilatation and evacuation for midtrimester abortion. *J.A.M.A.* In press, 1984.

31. Kafrissen, M. E., et al. Coagulopathy and induced abortion: Rates and relative risks. *Am. J. Obstet. Gynecol.* 147:344, 1983.

32. Kaltreider, N. B., Goldsmith, S., and Margolis, A. J. The impact of midtrimester abortion techniques on patients and staff. *Am. J. Obstet. Gynecol.* 135:235, 1979.

33. Kaul, A. F., Federschneider, J. M., and Stubblefield, P. G. A controlled trial of antiemetics in abortion by PGF$_{2\alpha}$ and laminaria. *J. Reprod. Med.* 20:213, 1978.

34. Kerenyi, T. D. Personal communication, Jan., 1979.

35. Kerenyi, T. D., Mandelaman, N., and Sherman, D. H. Five thousand consecutive saline abortions. *Am. J. Obstet. Gynecol.* 116:593, 1973.

36. Koplik, L. On the use of epinephrine to reduce the morbidity of abortion performed under local anesthesia. Paper presented to the 18th annual meeting of the Association of Planned Parenthood Physicians. Denver, Oct. 3, 1980.

37. Laurenson, N. H., and Schulman, J. D. Oxytocin administration in midtrimester saline abortion. *Am. J. Obstet. Gynecol.* 115:420, 1973.

38. Lauersen, N. H., and Wilson, K. H. The effects of intramuscular injections of 15 (S)-15 methyl prostaglandin F$_{2\alpha}$ in failed abortions. *Fertil. Steril.* 28:1044, 1977.

39. Osathandonh, R., et al. Coagulopathy associated with midtrimester D&E. *Adv. Plann. Parent.* 16:1, 1981.

40. Patterson, S. P., White, J. H., and Reaves, E. M. A maternal death associated with prostaglandin E$_2$. *Obstet. Gynecol.* 54:123, 1979.

41. Peterson, W. Dilatation and Evacuation: Patient Evaluation and Surgical Techniques. In G. I. Zatuchni, J. J. Sciarra, and J. J. Speidel (eds.), *Pregnancy Termination: Procedures, Safety and New Developments.* Philadelphia: Lippincott/Harper, 1979.

42. Peterson, W. D & E evolution of technique. Paper presented to the National Abortion Federation Post Graduate course. San Francisco, Calif., Sept. 21, 1981.

43. Propping, D., Stubblefield, P. G., and Golub, J. Uterine rupture following midtrimester abortion by laminaria, prostaglandin F$_{2\alpha}$ and oxytocin: Report of two cases. *Am. J. Obstet. Gynecol.* 128:689, 1977.

44. Richardson, J. A., and Dixon, G. Effects of legal termination on subsequent pregnancy. *Br. Med. J.* 1:1303, 1976.

45. Robins, J., and Mann, L. I. Second generation prostaglandins: Midtrimester pregnancy termination by intramuscular injection of a 15-methyl analog of prostaglandin F$_{2\alpha}$. *Fertil. Steril.* 27:104, 1976.

46. Robins, J., and Surrago, E. J. Early midtrimester pregnancy termination: A comparison of dilatation and evacuation and intravaginal prostaglandin E$_2$. *J. Reprod. Med.* 27:415, 1982.

47. Sands, R. X., Burnhill, M. S., and Hakim-Elahi, E. Postabortal uterine atony. *Obstet. Gynecol.* 43:595, 1974.

48. Slome, J. Termination of pregnancy. *Lancet* 2:881, 1972.

49. Smith, R. G., Palmore, J. A., and Steinhoff, P. G. The potential reduction of medical complications from induced abortion. *Int. J. Gynaecol. Obstet.* 15:337, 1978.

50. Southern, E. M., et al. Vaginal prostaglandin E$_2$ in the management of fetal intrauterine death. *Br. J. Obstet. Gynaecol.* 85:437, 1978.

51. Strauss, J. H., et al. Laminaria use in midtrimester abortions induced by intra-amniotic prostaglandin F$_{2\alpha}$ with urea and intravenous oxytocin. *Am. J. Obstet. Gynecol.* 134:260, 1979.

52. Streeter, G. L. Weight, sitting height, head size, foot length, and menstrual age of the human embryo. *Contrib. Embriol.* (Carnegie) 11:157, 1920.

53. Stubblefield, P. G. Current technology for abortion. *Curr. Prob. Obstet. Gynecol.* 2:1, 1978.

54. Stubblefield, P. G. Midtrimester Abortion by Curettage Procedures: An Overview. In J. E. Hodgson (ed.), *Abortion and Sterilization: Medical and Social Aspects.* London: Academic, New York, Grune & Stratton, 1981. Pp. 277–296.

55. Stubblefield, P. G., et al. Laminaria augmentation of intra-amniotic PGF$_{2\alpha}$ for midtrimester pregnancy termination. *Prostaglandins* 10:413, 1975.

56. Stubblefield, P. G., et al. A randomized study of 12 mm vs. 15.9 mm vacuum cannulas in midtrimester abortion by laminaria and vacuum curettage. *Fertil. Steril.* 29:512, 1978.

57. Stubblefield, P. G., Altman, A. M., and Goldstein, S. P. Randomized trial of one versus two days of laminaria treatment prior to late midtrimester abortion by uterine evacuation: A pilot study. *Am. J. Obstet. Gynecol.* 143:481, 1982.

58. Surrago, E. J., and Robins, J. Midtrimester pregnancy termination by intravaginal administration of prostaglandin E$_2$. *Contraception* 26:285, 1982.

59. Van der Bergh, A. S. The Bloemenhoveklinick. Abortion procured in the second trimester of pregnancy. *Med. Contact* 48:1555, 1974.

7. Female Sterilization

Carl J. Levinson
Herbert B. Peterson

TRENDS

Over the past decade voluntary female sterilization has become increasingly important as a method of fertility control. By 1980 more than 60 million women had undergone sterilization worldwide [39]. Surveys indicate that sterilization is the most common method of fertility control in the United States; an estimated 5 million women aged 15 to 44 have undergone sterilization in U.S. hospitals from 1970 to 1980 [50]. During that time the mean age of sterilization was 30 years. With respect to timing of the procedure, there has been a general trend away from the postpartum toward interval sterilization; this occurred with a concurrent increase in the utilization of laparoscopy. The introduction of the laparoscope also has resulted in a dramatic reduction in the length of hospital stay required for sterilization and has promoted an increase in ambulatory sterilization.

INDICATIONS AND CONTRAINDICATIONS

In general, women and sugeons are no longer beset by a series of complicated rules restricting sterilization. The procedure is both legal and available in all 50 states. There are virtually no mandatory indications. However, there are certain situations in which sterilization may be deemed the best method of contraception: when the individual is totally incapable of understanding and managing the circumstances of life; when pregnancy may have a deleterious effect on a psychiatric problem; when pregnancy would tax already abnormal cardiac and pulmonary and renal functions to the extent of being life-threatening; or when genetic evaluation has indicated a high risk of fetal abnormality. Other than the above, sterilization is basically an *elective* procedure. For various reasons a woman may decide that she has no desire for future childbearing. The nulligravida may seek freedom from ever bearing children. A multigravida may decide that the present number of children is adequate. Those in the latter phase of the reproductive era may consider it unfair to a child to be reared by elderly parents. The reasons are manifold, personal, and of significance to the individual. The physician must counsel the patient with respect to her decision. Patient and physician must agree that the procedure should be performed.

Absolute medical contraindications are virtually nonexistent. In certain instances federal government regulations or laws proscribe the performance of sterilization in minors or in mentally incompetent persons incapable of giving informed consent. Some regulations mandate a waiting period between consent and performance of the procedure, which may be up to 30 days.

The physician should have serious reservations about performing a sterilization in a teenager and strong concerns about sterilizing a nulligravida and should be probing in all other cases.

Laparotomy is contraindicated if all forms of anesthesia are contraindicated. Laparotomy should not be performed if there is a simpler and safer method available.

Laparoscopy is contraindicated in the presence of advanced cardiovascular or respiratory disease, acute peritonitis, intestinal obstruction, or an acute surgical abdomen. Marked obesity and previous surgery are relative contraindications. Minilaparotomy is contraindicated in the face of acute pelvic infection or peritonitis. Truly marked obesity may be a relative contraindication; the same is true for marked abdominal adhesions.

Culdoscopy and culpotomy have few contraindications. Culdoscopy cannot be performed if the patient cannot tolerate an anesthetic or the knee-chest position. Culpotomy and culdoscopy are contraindicated in the face of an obscured cul-de-sac owing to endometriosis, chronic pelvic inflammatory disease (PID), or massive pelvic adhesions. Both procedures are contraindicated when acute pelvic infection is present.

Hysteroscopy and the blind forms of intrauterine sterilization are contraindicated in the following sets of circumstances: in the presence of acute pelvic infection; during pregnancy; in the presence of unexplained abnormal uterine bleeding; in the face of potential genital malignancy; or where there is suspected trauma of the uterine cavity. It is relatively contraindicated in the face of a marked stenosis of the cervix.

COUNSELING

All patients requesting sterilization must be counseled. The process should be objective and straightforward. If the physician has specific viewpoints, these should be expressed and made known to the patient. Wherever possible, the couple should be seen together. Such counseling should include:

The consequences of their decision
Evaluation of the patient's emotional status
Review of the motive for sterilization
Answers to all questions to the reasonable satisfaction of the patient
Reassurance and support

It is important to speak to the patient at the appropriate level of understanding. The counseling physician must provide information on the following:

Alternative means of contraception
The possibility of sterilization of the partner
A general review of the methods available
The method suggested by the physician and the reason for it
The site of the operative procedure
The timing of the procedure
The choice of the anesthetic
The immediate alternatives to the failure of the chosen procedure (e.g., the performance of a laparotomy in the event of a failed laparoscopy)
The permanent nature of the procedure
The failure rate as evidenced by general statistics for the particular procedure
A general review of the technical aspects of the procedure
What the results of the procedure will be (e.g., what happens to the egg? What about menstruation? Any change in sexuality?)
Preoperative instructions
Risks of the operative procedure (preferably presented in written form)
Postoperative manifestations and potential complications
Format for hospitalization
Review of financial considerations
Signing of appropriate consent forms

TECHNIQUES

At one time it was easy to distinguish contraception from sterilization in that the former was considered to be temporary while the latter was considered to be irreversible. Since this distinction is no longer quite so clear, sterilization is often referred to as permanent contraception. Even as sterilization is being performed, both patient and physician may be considering the statistics with respect to *reversal* of sterilization. Certainly this is unrealistic at the present time. There is no doubt that a simple, safe, and effective reversible type of sterilization is desirable, but none has yet been devised. Reversal is possible but unreliable.

Sterilization procedures are used throughout the world. For many years *hysterectomy* was used as a technique. This is still occasionally true today, but the decade from 1970 to 1980 gave rise to a marked increase in female sterilization by *tubal occlusion* as a result of new techniques that were safer and simpler and could be performed in a variety of settings with less expense. Of these, laparoscopy is more prevalent in the developed countries, while minilaparotomy is more widely used in underdeveloped nations. *Vasectomy* has remained the stable technique for male sterilization.

In conjunction with the development of new mechanical techniques, a new attitude toward sterilization became evident, concurrent with the women's liberation movement, one goal of which is to establish parity between men and women. As they perceived that childbearing was no longer their prime motivation in life, some women sought freedom from the concerns (and often fears) of pregnancy. They sought out careers and entered the work force. Sterilization, along with contraception, was viewed as a means of protection that would enable one to expand lifestyles.

The 1960s brought with it a remarkable change in attitude toward the performance of sterilization. Only two decades ago, in the early 1960s, sterilization committees existed in most hospitals. In some institutions these committees represented the only hope for a woman seeking the procedure. Their judgment, often based on a formula related to age and parity, translated into the performance of few sterilizations. For this reason and often for religious considerations hysterectomy was used to provide "permanent contraception." Over the course of the decade these original concepts were overturned and replaced by more liberal ones, allowing the decision to be reached by the patient with or without the consent of her husband. However, human mores are never static: In recent years certain proscriptions have resulted from financial and legal considerations.

Hysterectomy Technique

As indicated above, hysterectomy has been used as a form of female sterilization. However, it is not generally considered to be appropriate for this purpose unless there are other indications. These other indications should (by themselves) be sufficient for the performance of the hysterectomy (recurrent bleeding, symptomatic uterine prolapse, leiomyomata, endometriosis, chronic PID, etc.). The less hysterectomy is used as a form of sterilization, the better. It is a major surgical procedure involving a rather high morbidity and complication rate. Morbidity is estimated at 29 percent for the abdominal approach and 43 percent for the vaginal route [27]. This is particularly true when performed in association with a cesarean section (cesarean hysterectomy); there is no elective indication for hysterectomy as a sterilizing procedure in the puerperal state.

Tubal Occlusion Technique

The fallopian tube is far from a simple structure. Until the recent advent of in vitro fertilization and embryo transplant, the tube was absolutely necessary for human procreation. Not only does it serve as a conduit for egg, sperm, and embryo but it facilitates movement of these structures in the appropriate directions and provides a hospitable and supportive environment en route. Nevertheless, it has no known function other than that of reproduction. In addition to these factors, the tube is readily accessible and relatively small and can be altered surgically without significant blood loss. The concept of tubal occlusion is the basis of most surgical techniques for sterilization.

There is a fine review of the history of tubal sterilization by Sciarra [43]. The operation is 150 years old, having first been reported in 1834 as a means of preventing further obstetric complications in patients with contracted pelves [6]. It was not until almost 50 years later (1880) that a tubal ligation was performed at the time of cesarean section. The next historic milestone was the performance of the Madlener procedure [31] in 1910. Contributions have subsequently been made by Irving [24] in 1924, Pomeroy [5] in 1930, Aldridge [1] in 1934, Kroener [26] in 1935, and Uchida [51] in 1946.

There are several routes to the performance of tubal occlusion:

1. Abdominal
   a. Laparotomy
   b. Minilaparotomy
   c. Laparoscopy
2. Vaginal
   a. Culdoscopy
   b. Culdotomy
3. Intrauterine
   a. Hysteroscopy

ABDOMINAL

Laparotomy. Traditional laparotomy is not a procedure of choice for sterilization. The length of the incision (even low transverse) leads to increased hospital stay and potential increased morbidity and discomfort. A conventional laparotomy should be reserved for those patients requiring surgical procedures in addition to tubal sterilization.

Minilaparotomy. The minilaparotomy has become exceedingly popular in the last decade, particularly in underdeveloped countries. The procedure can be done under general or local anesthesia (as described by Penfield [35]). Under ideal circumstances the uterus will be anteverted, the patient is thin, and the procedure is rapidly performed. Despite its name, the procedure should be evaluated as for any laparotomy, and strict aseptic technique should be utilized. The bladder must be empty. An intrauterine manipulator and a dorsal lithotomy position often facilitate anteversion of the uterus, thereby bringing the tubes closer to the abdomi-

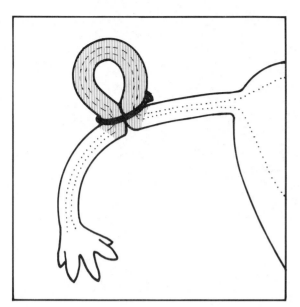

Fig. 7-1. The Madlener technique.

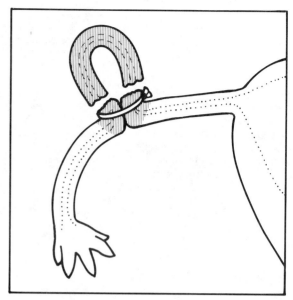

Fig. 7-2. The Pomeroy technique.

nal wall. A small 3-cm transverse suprapubic incision is made, after which the anterior rectus fascia is incised, the rectus muscles separated, and the posterior fascia and peritoneum incised. Using appropriate retractors and manipulators, each tube is brought into the incision and identified. The tube is then occluded by the method of choice. The abdominal wall is closed in layers.

Contraindications to minilaparotomy include a fixed retroverted uterus and massive obesity. Two advantages attributed to the minilaparotomy procedure are the small incision and the short length of time required for the procedure. Occasionally, the incision must be extended and a longer time is required. The experience and technical skill of the operator appear to be paramount in resolving these issues.

Minilaparotomy requires fundamental surgical techniques, surgical skill and experience, and adherence to all basic surgical principles. Under local anesthesia with an experienced surgeon, this procedure may be the safest form of female sterilization.

The following special techniques have been developed. The techniques described by Pomeroy, Irving, Aldridge, Uchida, and Cook, as well as excision techniques, all require laparotomy or minilaparotomy. Although the choice of technique varies with geographic location, the Pomeroy technique has become the standard by which the success of all sterilizations is measured.

THE MADLENER TECHNIQUE. The Madlener technique [31] (Fig. 7-1) is infrequently used but is presented because of its historic interest and its comparable nature to the Pomeroy technique and the Falope ring technique. In the manner of Madlener, a loop in the midportion of the tube is developed, the base of the loop is crushed, and the crushed area is ligated with a *nonabsorbable* suture. Failure rates were high [45], presumably because of the development of fistula and recanalization. The similarity to the Falope ring technique should be noted; it has not yet been explained why the latter is so much more successful.

THE POMEROY TECHNIQUE. In the Pomeroy technique [5] (Fig. 7-2) a loop of tube is developed in the midportion of the tube. However, the tube is not crushed. Instead, the base is ligated with an *absorbable* suture, the upper portion of the loop is excised, and (depending on individual variations) the ends of the tubes may be retied separately or cauterized. The proximal and distal segments of the tube often separate when the suture material has disintegrated, adding to the efficiency of the procedure. The failure rate is 1 to 4 per thousand [45] with more failures resulting from postpartum tubal ligations than interval procedures. Such failures may be the result of fistula formation or recanalization.

THE IRVING TECHNIQUE. As originally described and as often used, the Irving technique [24] (Fig. 7-3) is associated with cesarean section. The principle is ingeniously simple. The tube is divided in its isthmic portion. The proximal segment is then buried between the leaves of the broad ligament. Under these circum-

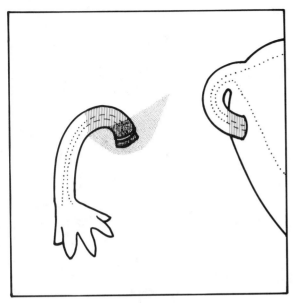

Fig. 7-3. The Irving technique.

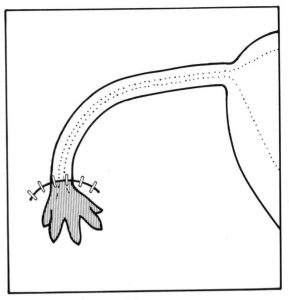

Fig. 7-4. The Aldridge technique.

stances, fistula formation and recanalization are theoretically impossible. Indeed, failures are virtually unknown.

THE ALDRIDGE TECHNIQUE. The Aldridge procedure [1] (Fig. 7-4), described 50 years ago, is most appealing because of its potential reversibility. No part of the tube is destroyed. Instead, the distal end of the tube (ampulla and fimbria) are buried into a newly created opening of the peritoneum. The tube is theoretically kept in place by several sutures between tubal serosa and peritoneum. The failure rate was unacceptable [16] and the technique rarely utilized. However, there has been a resurgence of interest recently [15].

EXCISION OF ALL OR SEGMENTS OF THE TUBE. Complete excision of the tube (Fig. 7-5) is obviously a successful technique for sterilization. However, it is rarely used since it involves a full laparotomy and interference with blood supply and is technically more complicated. It may, however, be performed in conjunction with other surgical procedures such as ectopic pregnancy or removal of a neoplastic ovary.

Excision of the midportion of the tube is essentially the performance of a Pomeroy procedure. It is rarely performed.

Resection of the cornua is occasionally performed. However, it is not popular or frequently used for a variety of reasons: This region of the uterus is extremely vascular, and hemorrhage is a major risk; interference with the blood supply to the ovary is a real risk; and technical skill for hemostasis is required.

Excision of the *distal* end of the tube, either the fimbria or fimbria and distal ampulla, was described by Kroener. This portion is excised after suture ligation for hemostasis. The amount of tube removed varies, making the exact success of the procedure difficult to evaluate. This fact is of significance in discussion of reversibility. The more ampulla that remains, the more likely the success of distal salpingostomy. Although the failure rate is low [26], the procedure is occasionally complicated by the formation of hydrosalpinx.

THE UCHIDA TECHNIQUE. For over a quarter of a century Uchida [51] has used a sterilization technique (Fig. 7-6) in an extremely large personal series of cases (over 20,000 cases) with virtually no failures. The technique carries some of the principles of the Irving procedure. An epinephrine-saline solution (1:1,000) is injected into the subserosal layer of the tube. Thus, the muscularis and mucosa are separated. The serosa is incised, a segment of tube is removed, the distal end of the tube is ligated, and the proximal portion ligated and buried. The procedure is simple and rapidly performed by those familiar with the technique.

THE COOK TECHNIQUE. Another variation of the Irving technique was described by Cook (Fig. 7-7). The tube is incised, and the proximal end is ligated and then buried in the round ligament. The distal end is ligated but not buried. There is relatively little blood loss in the region of the round ligament, thereby making it more acceptable than burial into the myometrium. It can be performed as an interval procedure. The failure rate is

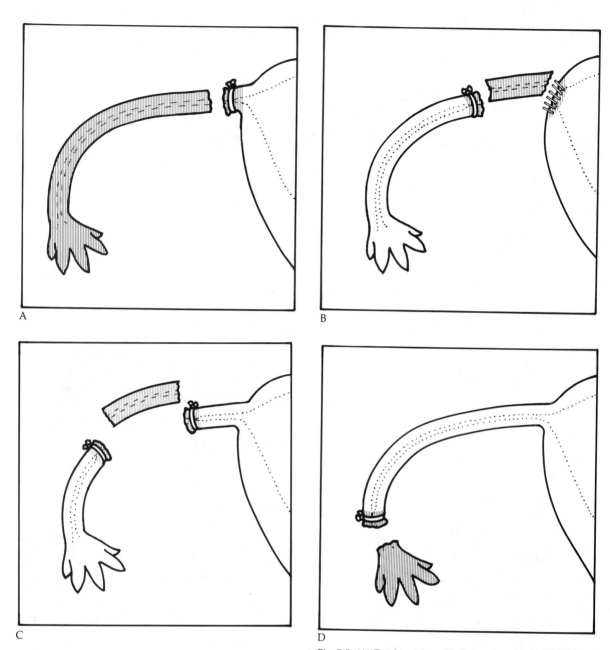

Fig. 7-5. (A) Total excision. (B) Cornual excision. (C) Midexcision. (D) Fimbrial excision.

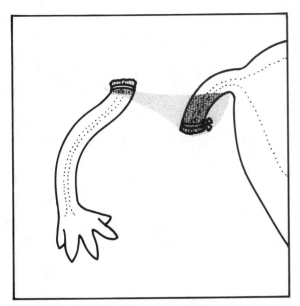

Fig. 7-6. The Uchida technique.

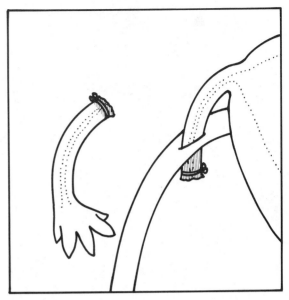

Fig. 7-7. The Cook technique.

similar to that of other procedures, 1 to 4 per thousand [43].

Laparoscopy. Laparoscopy has become exceedingly popular (particularly in developed countries) in the past decade. This technique uses fiberoptic illumination along with insufflation, allowing for distention of the abdomen with nonexplosive gases, providing greater visibility and safety.

Preceded by many decades by peritoneoscopy, modern laparoscopy was developed primarily by Palmer [34] in France, Steptoe [48] in England, and Frangenheim [18] in Germany during the 1960s. It gained widespread acceptance in the United States in the early 1970s. It is a procedure made successful by technical improvements and operator experience.

The procedure of laparoscopy is adequately described in a number of available publications [37, 48]. The contraindications of massive obesity, severe cardiopulmonary disease, and bowel obstruction must be observed. The procedure can be performed under local anesthesia, but usually general anesthesia is used, including intubation for controlled respiration. The Verress needle is used with a puncture site at the umbilicus through which carbon dioxide is insufflated, usually 2 to 3 liters. A modfication of this procedure is the performance of "open laparoscopy" as described by Hasson [20] in which an incision is made in the umbilicus and entry is made into the abdomen under direct vision.

Once insufflation is completed, a trocar and sheath are thrust into the peritoneal cavity in the midline and in the direction of the sacral hollow. The trocar is removed and replaced by the laparoscope. The laparoscope is attached by means of a fiberoptic cord to the light source. With adequate insufflation, a good light source, and a clear endoscope, visualization should be excellent. The procedure should be preceded by emptying of the bladder and the use of the Trendelenburg position to allow bowel to fall from the pelvis into the upper abdomen.

Visualization usually is adequate with laparoscopy performed as described above. Occasionally vision is poor owing to retroversion of the uterus or the presence of bowel in the pelvis. One of two techniques may be used to overcome these problems. Before starting the laparoscopy, an intrauterine cannula may be placed; this may be manipulated to bring the uterus forward, thereby facilitating visualization of the tubes and ovaries. Another approach is to perform a second puncture in the midline in the suprapubic area with a 3-mm or 6-mm sheath, allowing the entry of a probe or other operative instruments. (It is our firm conviction that this *double-puncture technique* allows for better visualization and easier manipulation, thereby promoting patient safety.) Through the second puncture, instruments can be inserted, which may manipulate, grasp, band, clip, or coagulate.

The procedure is terminated by removal of all the instruments, allowing the escape of as much gas as possible, and a simple closure of the small incisions. It

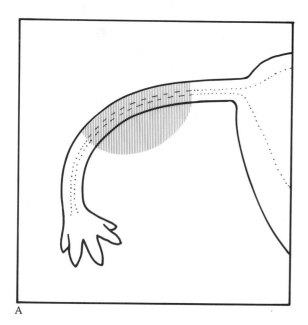

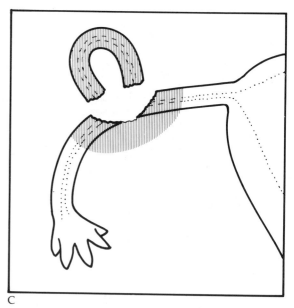

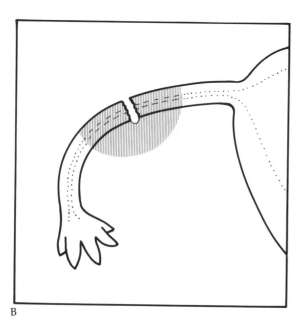

Fig. 7-8. (A) Unipolar electrosurgery. (B) Unipolar-cut electrosurgery. (C) Unipolar-snare electrosurgery.

is the preference of the authors to use subcuticular 4-0 absorbable sutures.

UNIPOLAR ELECTROSURGERY. The purpose of applying electrosurgery (Fig. 7-8) to the fallopian tube is to destroy the architecture with subsequent scarring resulting in closure. This can be performed by the application of a unipolar current. This current is transmitted to the tube by means of a pair of tongs, which can be introduced through a second puncture or in a channel adjacent to the laparoscope; the latter is the operating laparoscope or the one-puncture technique. The current is usually applied to the thin midportion (isthmus) of the tube; however, the injury can be transmitted more medially or distally, as the experience of the operator indicates.

The original use of high voltage generators with unipolar technique resulted in certain complications. The current is introduced at the level of the tube but has to travel through the patient's body to the ground plate (dispersive electrode), which is attached to the patient's buttock or thigh. The most tragic problem is "bowel burn" resulting in necrosis of the bowel wall, development of vague abdominal symptoms in 2 to 6 days, followed by a classic acute abdomen necessitating bowel resection. The problem of bowel burn can be obviated almost completely by the use of bipolar current.

Several variations were introduced with the original

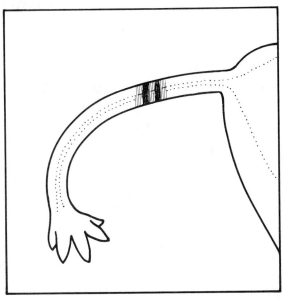

Fig. 7-9. Bipolar electrosurgery.

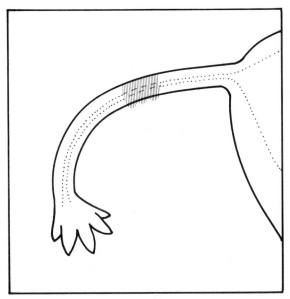

Fig. 7-10. Thermocoagulation.

use of unipolar current. Some felt that transection of the tube was necessary after it had been electrosurgically destroyed. Several studies have indicated that this is not true [46, 55]. It was also felt, originally, that it was necessary to remove a segment of the tube as a pathologic specimen, primarily for medicolegal reasons. This proved both unwise and impractical, since it required more technical skill, it resulted in increased intraoperative bleeding, and the charred specimen was relatively unidentifiable.

BIPOLAR ELECTROSURGERY. A marked improvement in patient safety developed with the use of the bipolar electrosurgical technique (Fig. 7-9). Although high frequency current is used, the tongs applied to the tubes carry the current down one tong, through the tissue, and up the other, thereby minimizing passage of current through the body. The injury is limited mainly to the portion of the tube grasped beneath the tongs, with little involvement of adjacent tissue. With a few careful considerations, the bipolar technique is eminently successful and safe: The instruments must be used with compatible electrosurgical units; the tube must be properly grasped; and adequate electric current must be allowed to pass. Bowel burns will be the result of inadequate surgical skill rather than instrument failure.

THERMOCOAGULATION. Thermocoagulation (Fig. 7-10) has been more popular in Europe, particularly Germany, than in the United States. Although electric current is used, the system requires only 4 to 5 volts. The current produced is minimal but serves to heat an ele-

ment; this element in turn burns or "cooks" that portion of the tube with which it is in contact. Special equipment has been designed to determine the length of passage of current and the heat to which the element is brought; it even produces an audible signal to indicate the phase of the cycle. Excellent reports have been published by Semm [44], but large-scale studies are not available.

ELECTROCAUTERY. The Waters Company has devised another instrument (Fig. 7-11) based primarily on the principle of heat application in order to cause destruction of the tube. The element in this case is a metal hook, which may be heated by a battery. The hook serves to engage the tube, which is pulled into a surrounding sheath. It is within the sheath that the tube is coagulated and cut. Extensive data regarding efficiency are not available.

FALOPE RING. After the initial successes reported using electrosurgical techniques for sterilization with the laparoscope, the inevitable occurred: Reports of complications accumulated and were subsequently published. Burns, particularly bowel burns, were among the most devastating and insidious in onset, usually resulting in peritonitis requiring laparotomy; they were difficult to explain and therefore malpractice prone. In the pursuit of a better way, mechanical occlusive devices were developed. The first of these was the ring or band (the Falope ring) devised by Yoon [54] (Fig. 7-12). The ring may be applied through a minilaparotomy or through a single-puncture or double-puncture laparoscopic tech-

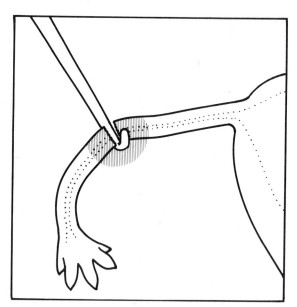

Fig. 7-11. Electrocauterization.

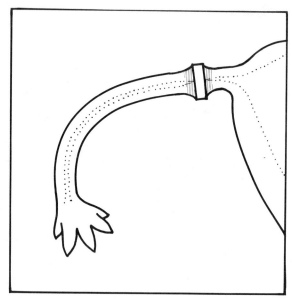

Fig. 7-13. Clip.

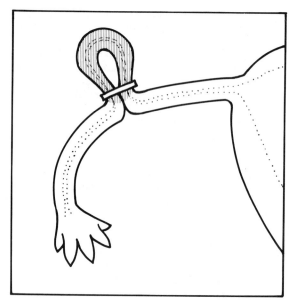

Fig. 7-12. The Falope ring.

nique. Special equipment has been devised for each. The basic equipment consists of three segments: an inner pair of tongs, a middle cylinder, and an outer cylinder. A small band (ring) made of Silastic is placed on the projecting tip of the middle cylinder. The tongs are extruded to lift up the thinnest portion of the tube. Once the tube has been brought within the middle cylinder, the outer cylinder is pushed downward to extrude the ring onto the base of the knuckle of tube. With reasonable care, the device is simple and safe to use. Extreme caution must be exercised where the tube is markedly thickened or bound down by adhesions. The Falope ring technique is physically similar to the Madlener technique; however, the results are considerably better. Long-term broadly collected data indicate a most acceptable failure rate of 2 to 4 per thousand [12].

CLIPS. Three clips (Fig. 7-13) are currently in use, all named after the original designer: Hulka, Bleier (Secuclip), and Filshie. The Hulka clip is the most widely used in the United States whereas the Bleier clip has been used extensively in Germany and the Filshie clip in Great Britain. The principle is the same. A clip is inserted into an applicator. The applicator is devised to enter a sheath by closing the jaws but not locking them. Once inside the abdomen, the jaws are opened and the clip applied across the isthmic portion of the tube. The width of the clip is 3 to 4 mm, thereby damaging a rather small portion of tube (in consideration of potential reversibility). The nonhinged ends of the clip interlock, thereby producing a permanent, nonmovable grasp of the fallopian tube. The Hulka clip is made of plastic but covered by a gold-plated stainless steel spring to maintain it in the closed position. Interlocking grooves on the inner surface serve to eliminate dead space and discourage slippage. The Bleier (Secuclip) clip is even simpler in design, composed entirely of plastic. The applicator holds the clip in place until it is properly placed around the tube, after which it is closed. Long-term studies are not available in the United States. The Filshie clip is similar in consistency and design. However, the inner surface is lined with silicone, which tends to spread, thereby eliminating any dead space caused by necrosis of tissue within the clip.

All clips have the disadvantage of requiring fairly sophisticated applicators. An occasional disadvantage is the necessity to push the tube ahead of it in setting up the appropriate site for application of the clip; this is not always easily performed. All clips have the advantage of minimal tubal destruction while providing reliable occlusion until complete vascular necrosis occurs in the segment encompassed.

VAGINAL

Culdoscopy. Culdoscopy is a procedure that was popular in the 1960s before the introduction of laparoscopy. The technique consists of the introduction of a telescopic instrument into the peritoneal cavity through an incision into the posterior vaginal fornix. This requires the patient to be in the knee-chest position. In this manner bowel falls away from the pelvis towards the diaphragm. There are numerous difficulties with the technique. Before the introduction of the fiberoptic light system, light was provided by a bulb at the end of the culdoscope, which had the potential of causing thermal injury. The position is an awkward one, particularly when performed under general anesthesia, requiring much in the way of a support system. There is little distention of the abdomen other than the air that enters through the vaginal incision. This air is more irritating than carbon dioxide. Visualization is difficult, and the image inverted. All in all, it is a difficult procedure and has largely been abandoned in favor of laparoscopy.

Culdotomy. Culdotomy is a technique preferred by some individuals. The patient may be in the dorsal lithotomy or knee-chest position. An incision is made in the posterior cul-de-sac, much in the same manner as the beginning of a vaginal hysterectomy. Long instruments are needed. Much of the success of the procedure depends on the experience and technical skill of the operator since, as in most vaginal procedures, more surgical dexterity is required. Various instruments have been devised for bringing the tubes into the colpotomy

incision, where they may be occluded by one of several methods.

The cul-de-sac is normally extremely thin and readily entered. A mobile uterus and tube allow easy access to the tube. The incision is easily closed, and the postoperative course is usually benign. Problems are apt to develop if the surgeon is inexperienced, if the vagina is infected or improperly cleansed, if the uterus or tubes are fixed by PID or endometriosis, or if there is inadequate competent help. The rate of serious pelvic infection appears to be higher as it is with most procedures performed vaginally when compared with the same procedures performed abdominally [45].

INTRAUTERINE

Hysteroscopy. Hysteroscopy is a technique whereby an endoscopic instrument is introduced into the uterine cavity through the transcervical approach. It is an old technique that has become revitalized by the availability of fiberoptic light systems, newer distending media, and other newer instrumentation (see Chap. 9).

SPECIAL ASPECTS

Timing of the Procedure

Initially almost all sterilizations were performed at the time of delivery, the first being performed at cesarean section. Since 1970 there has been a shift toward interval sterilization. There are advantages and disadvantages in timing the procedure to coincide with the end of a pregnancy; these certainly vary from individual to individual but some general statements may be made.

POSTABORTION

Some women who request elective abortion also desire permanent sterilization. Recent studies [2, 11] suggest that this procedure in conjunction with first-trimester abortion has a low complication rate, whether it is performed by laparoscopy or by minilaparotomy. It is still debatable whether complication rates for abortion and sterilization performed concurrently are greater than the additive risks of two separate procedures. Available evidence would suggest that complication rates for the concurrent procedures are certainly not appreciably greater. Another consideration is the psychologic sequelae following concurrent procedures. Cheng [9] reports the results of a WHO Task Force study on the sequelae of abortion; it suggests that 2 to 10 percent of women sterilized at abortion might have subsequently changed their minds about the sterilization if given the opportunity. He further reported that 4 percent of the women who desired sterilization at abortion but instead decided on interval sterilization became pregnant before the subsequent sterilization. Obviously, any decision regarding sterilization at the time of induced abortion requires weighing individual concerns as well as aggregate medical and psychologic risks. Recently the CDC [36] reported that a nationwide surveillance of abortion deaths showed that the risk of dying from an abortion/sterilization is more than 3 times increased if done by hysterotomy or hysterectomy. It was thus concluded that, unless there are additional gynecologic indications for these procedures, the extra risks of performing hysterectomy do not appear to be justified.

POSTPARTUM

Until very recently most women undergoing sterilization did so shortly after vaginal delivery. The major advantage of this timing was convenience, since the procedure did not appreciably prolong hospitalization. These postpartum procedures have not been studied extensively as have the newer surgical approaches. Studies of safety and efficiency that have been performed do not allow for detailed comparison with interval laparoscopy or minilaparotomy, since there are numerous differences in study methodology [25]. Still, abundant data exist to suggest that postpartum procedures are both safe and effective. Shepherd [45], in an extensive review of the literature to 1974, determined that morbidity rates for postpartum tubal ligation range from 1 to 21 percent with a median of 13 percent. (These figures are higher than morbidity rates for interval procedures.) In those studies reviewed, the interval between delivery and sterilization (up to 5 days, which was the maximum length studied) did not affect the incidence of febrile morbidity. Shepherd noted that postpartum procedures carried statistically greater morbidity than did those interval procedures reviewed. It is not known whether differences in morbidity are attributable to the recent pregnancy. It is also unknown whether the morbidity of vaginal deliveries followed shortly by sterilization is greater than that for two separate procedures. It is not certain whether regret is more likely if the procedure is performed postpartum.

Sterilization failures will be discussed later in this chapter; studies addressing postpartum sterilization failures are hampered by methodologic limitations: patients lost to follow-up, variations in the length of observation, etc. Given these limitations, Shepherd's review of 17 studies, covering a variety of tubal occlusion techniques, showed reported failure rates ranging from .04 to 1 percent.

INTERVAL

The timing of a sterilization procedure during the interval phase means that it is not done in relationship to pregnancy (delivery or abortion). This permits the health and well-being of a child to be determined before a permanent form of contraception is introduced. The procedure may be done by laparoscopy or minilaparotomy.

In 1970 fewer than 1 percent of such sterilizations in United States hospitals were performed by laparoscopy, and the average length of stay was 7 days [12]. With the advent of laparoscopy, outpatient sterilization became a reality. Several large studies [20, 22, 33] have demonstrated that interval sterilization by laparoscopy is, in general, a safe operation. Complication rates are discussed later in this chapter, but the overall complications are few, and major morbidity is most infrequent. The convenience of interval laparoscopy was noteworthy in a prospective multicenter study conducted by the CDC [13]; the overwhelming majority of patients did not require an overnight hospital stay, and the average return to normal activities was 4 to 14 days.

Minilaparotomy is preferred for women seeking sterilization in much of the world because of its simplicity and the fact that complicated technical equipment is not necessary. Vitoon [52] in Thailand described the procedure generally accepted today as minilaparotomy. His procedure was a modified Pomeroy technique for tubal occlusion, operating through a 2-cm transverse abdominal incision, which could be performed on an outpatient basis using local anesthesia. The International Fertility Research Program [39] in an international study suggested that minilaparotomy compared favorably with interval laparoscopic sterilization in terms of safety and efficacy.

In-Hospital or Other Setting

The vast majority of tubal sterilizations in the United States are performed in hospitals. There has been a recent trend toward performing this procedure in outpatient surgical units that are hospital based. As indicated before, much of this trend is a result of the popularity of laparoscopy. In the years from 1975 to 1978 135,000 women in the United States had hospital-based outpatient sterilizations of which 89 percent were by laparoscopy [13].

There are also non-hospital-based centers for such surgery. These freestanding surgicenters have become increasingly popular. In 1980 3 percent of tubal sterilizations in the United States were performed in such freestanding facilities [13] (these include surgical centers and private offices). The stated advantage of such units is that they can offer the same procedure at far less cost with greater convenience. It is of concern as to whether appropriate safety can be provided in such settings in the event of hemorrhage or shock. The complications of laparoscopy and minilaparotomy that occur during inpatient sterilizations can presumably occur when the same procedure is performed on an outpatient basis.

Life-threatening events such as anesthetic problems and major vessel hemorrhage are of particular concern. Penfield [35] has offered suggestions for decreasing the risks of outpatient sterilization, which include the use of local anesthesia and either open laparoscopy or minilaparotomy in order to avoid major vessel lacerations. The need for backup hospital service is obvious, and he suggests that transfers should be possible in less than 10 minutes.

Comments on Reversibility

Detailed discussion of sterilization reversal is covered elsewhere in this book. At this point, the authors enter a few philosophical comments. The consideration of reversibility (conceptually) is recent. When the number of female sterilization procedures increased markedly in the early 1970s, the accent was on the performance of a safe and effective procedure, *effective* meaning the absence of failures. Sterilizations were once restricted according to age and parity. With the performance of more sterilization procedures in younger women along with changes in emotional, social, and cultural factors, it was inevitable that there would be an increased need to provide a safe and effective means of reversal. At least one study [21] showed convincingly that more patients would undergo sterilization if an effective means of reversal were available.

In addition to the younger age of the patient and the frequency with which the procedure is performed, there are specific elements leading to requests for reversal; these include divorce and subsequent remarriage, a simple change of mind within the same family (for emotional or economic reasons), the death of a child, or a change in lifestyle. Any of these factors may have validity for the individual couple. Since there are probably 1 million sterilizations annually in the United States, if only 1 in 100 wishes to regain the capacity for childbearing, then 10,000 individuals might seek reversals. Sterilization counseling is essential and must be thorough. The low rate of reversal requests would seem to indicate that sterilization counseling is reasonably well done. Young women oriented toward careers especially need to understand their situations. At the time of counseling the sterilization procedure must be presented as permanent. Simultaneously, the physician might consider special aspects of the individual patient. For example a young patient could be sterilized with a technique that minimally damages the tube, such as the clip. Using this device, there will be minimal destruction of tissue and minimal interference with the blood supply, and the ampulla and fimbria will not be affected.

Both the patient and the physician have responsibility with respect to sterilization procedures. The patient is responsible for careful consideration of the initial request. The physician must counsel wisely and adequately, depending on the life situation of the couple or individual. The individual must have ample time to reflect on her decision in the light of the counseling. The most appropriate method must be selected for each individual, a method that involves maximum safety, maximum efficacy, and maximum potential for reversibility, where indicated.

COMPLICATIONS

Types

Studies addressing the safety of sterilization operations are difficult to compare. Overall, major complications attributable to sterilization are infrequent, a fact consistently shown by national and international studies. In a nationwide surveillance of tubal sterilization, the CDC [36] has determined that deaths are rare; the case fatality rate in the United States is approximately 4 per 100,000 procedures. Complications of general anesthesia were the leading cause of death; sepsis and hemorrhage were the other important causes. (These were the findings in a review of 29 deaths during the period 1977–1981, including sterilizations performed by laparoscopy or laparotomy. Many of these deaths were considered preventable.)

LAPAROSCOPY

Complications of laparoscopic sterilization are infrequent, occurring in less than 4 percent of cases. These are consistent findings of several national and international studies. The American Association of Gynecologic Laparoscopists (AAGL) [38] reported that in 1979 major complications occurred in only 1.8 per 1,000 cases. (Major complications are defined as those requiring laparotomy for correction.) Such complications included bowel burns, penetrating injuries, and injury to major and minor abdominal and pelvic vessels. The Royal College of Obstetricians and Gynaecologists [7] reported 4.06 complications per 1,000 procedures (including 3 deaths) in 30,000 laparoscopic sterilizations; the complications were of the same nature as in the AAGL survey cited above. The CDC [12] is currently conducting an ongoing prospective multicenter study in the United States, the Collaborative Review of Sterilization (CREST). To date, the complication rate is 1.7 per 100 procedures. Complications were defined as unintended major surgery, transfusions, febrile morbidity, life-threatening event, rehospitalization, or death. The risk for general anesthesia was 4 times greater than that for local anesthesia when adjustment was made for such variables as obesity, history of PID, history of prior abdominal surgery, and history of pulmonary disease. The study appears to confirm the overall impression that complications of general anesthesia are the leading cause of death from laparoscopic sterilization.

Various laparoscopic techniques were compared in a study performed by the International Fertility Research Program (IFRP) [3], which evaluated 24,000 procedures in 27 countries. Complications occurred in 17 per 1,000 procedures; the most significant were bowel injuries and vessel lacerations. Surgical complications were categorized by patient characteristics, surgical approach, and tubal occlusion techniques; no important difference was found in any of these three categories. The Hulka-Clemens spring clip had the lowest surgical complication rate in each category.

Less serious complications of laparoscopic sterilization occurred more frequently than the life-threatening episodes. These included omental emphysema, uterine perforation, cervical laceration, bladder injury, wound infection, and pelvic inflammatory disease. Nevertheless, as stressed earlier, overall complication rates are low, and major complications are infrequent.

MINILAPAROTOMY

There are few large studies regarding the safety of minilaparotomy. The IFRP [33] reviewed over 5,000 modified Pomeroy minilap sterilizations; there was a surgical complication rate of 0.79 percent. Most of these were uterine perforations or bladder injury. The study suggests that complications of minilaparotomy are infrequent and that life-threatening complications are rare.

Prevention of Complications

TRAINING

It is important that the operating surgeon be experienced. Such experience can be derived in a variety of ways. In the early 1970s there were formal courses in laparoscopy; this has now become the province of the residency training program. Residents should have specific training in techniques of laparoscopy, open laparoscopy, and minilaparotomy because it may be necessary to use any of these on a given occasion in the practice of gynecology.

The training can be begun with a formal course on nonliving models. This is customarily followed by observation and then assisting. The training of the assistant surgeon in laparoscopy is facilitated if a double eyepiece can be attached to the laparoscope so that both the operator and the assistant can view simultaneously. The resident must understand the basic components of the equipment, how to manage equipment failures, indications and contraindications, and nuances of the technique. Once this has been mas-

tered, the resident may then be allowed to perform the procedure under the direct observation of an experienced physician acting as first assistant. It has been clearly shown that the performance of 50 to 100 such procedures prepares the operator sufficiently to proceed independently. The complication rate drops considerably if the operator has performed more than 200 procedures [23].

PATIENT SELECTION

A sterilization procedure is, by and large, an elective procedure. There is no reason to perform it at a time when the patient may be jeopardized. Therefore, it is well to understand the contraindications to laparotomy and laparoscopy.

Class IV cardiac patients are best treated with minilaparotomy under local anesthesia. Such severe disease is generally considered a contraindication for laparoscopy. Acute peritonitis or bowel distention are also contraindications. Patients who have had multiple previous abdominal surgical procedures are at high risk. For these patients, a minilaparotomy or open laparoscopy may prove to be safer than traditional laparoscopy. The operator must proceed with caution. Abdominal hernias are a relative contraindication to any of the abdominal procedures. Marked obesity is a relative contraindication, although several studies have indicated that both laparotomy and laparoscopy can be performed in these patients. At the opposite end of the spectrum, great care must be exercised in entering the abdomen of the extremely thin patient, since the distance between the skin and the promontory of the sacrum may be very short. Either scalpel or trocar can damage the iliac or sacral vessels. As indicated earlier, patients with symptomatic uterine disease may be better served by hysterectomy than by tubal sterilization.

EQUIPMENT

The equipment necessary for laparotomy or minilaparotomy is traditional. Minilaparotomy requires smaller instruments, small retractors, and a uterine elevator. These should be readily available.

Laparoscopy, on the other hand, requires highly sophisticated technical equipment. It is beyond the realm of this work to go into great detail, but a few comments are necessary. Most insufflators are calibrated to deliver approximately 1 liter per minute. All valves and connections must be airtight. The pressure gauge must be monitored at all times. The intraabdominal pressure should be no more than 10 mm Hg above the starting pressure. The light source should be checked for shorts and grounded. Extra bulbs must be available. The authors recommend the use of a 300-watt (photo) bulb, since it provides much better light than a 150-watt bulb. The light cord should be checked frequently; frequent bending will impair light transmission. Numerous excellent laparoscopes are available. The laparoscope should be in good working order and checked frequently for cracks. It should be certain that the trocars and laparoscopes fit the trocar sleeve properly. Trocars should have sharp points. Gaskets must be in the proper working order, not torn or worn. Verress needles should be sharp and the spring mechanism in good working order. An intrauterine cannula for manipulation of the cervix and uterus is often necessary to view the posterior wall of the uterus, tubes, and ovaries as well as the cul-de-sac.

PROCEDURE

Entry into the abdomen by means of the open laparoscopy or minilaparotomy technique must be made with the same care as any laparotomy. All patients undergoing pelvic surgery must be catheterized before the procedure. Special care must be taken with laparoscopy. The patient must be properly insufflated, generally with 2 to 3 liters of gas. Entry with the trocar through the umbilical site should be directed at the sacral hollow, in the midline (if penetrated, the uterus will forgive; the iliac vessel will not). Correct penetration can be checked by "feel," observance of the intrauterine pressure, and direct visualization. The authors strongly recommend the double-puncture technique so that manipulations of the sterilizing instrument and the visualizing instrument are separate.

The major serious complication from unipolar coagulation for sterilization has been bowel burns. These can be minimized by adherence to a few basic principles. The pneumoperitoneum must be good. The patient must be properly relaxed by the anesthetic. The electric equipment must be intact and in good working order. The patient must be properly grounded. Bowel should be displaced toward the diaphragm. The tube must be easily visualized and separate from adjacent structures. The sleeve should be made of metal (not fiberglass) as recommended by Soderstrom [47]. Bipolar coagulation for sterilization is less complicated and has fewer risks. These can be virtually eliminated if the bipolar forceps are cleansed properly. The forceps and the generator must be properly matched. It should be impossible to put the bipolar forceps into the unipolar mode. The power should be kept off until such time as the operator is ready to apply it. Local anesthetic dripped on the tube will prevent immediate postoperative pain. It is not necessary (with unipolar or bipolar coagulation) to excise a segment of tube; risk is increased with such excision, no further information is obtained, and it is not required for the medicolegal purposes.

Risks with the *Falope ring* can likewise be minimized. The tube should be grasped at its thinnest portion. All motions should be slow and deliberate. Only the tube and not the mesosalpinx should be grasped. As the tongs are brought into the central cylinder, the entire instrument should be pushed forward so as not to put the mesosalpinx on an undue stretch. The rings should not be applied if the wall of the tube is markedly thickened or if the tube is bound down by excessive adhesions. Again, application of a local anesthetic fluid will prevent immediate postoperative pain.

Applications of the *clip* may occasionally be difficult if the tube is markedly thickened or if the tube is particularly pliable. Care must be taken to place the clip across the entire tube. The clip applicator must be mechanically correct and the clip properly seated into the jaws of the applicator. This should be tested several times before entry into the abdomen. It is probably easier to apply the clip through a second puncture. A dropped, unretrievable clip or ring may be allowed to reside in the abdominal cavity with little risk of acute or chronic complication.

SPECIAL COMPLICATIONS

Failures

The goal of all sterilization procedures is to provide an effective method with safe techniques. Effectiveness is measured in "failure rates." Since the number of failures is difficult to establish, failure rates are often skewed. A large number of physicians may do a small number of cases each, and the failure rate among these occasional operators is frequently high. Series are rarely published from such individuals, so none of this information appears in the literature. On the other hand, experienced physicians with large series will report the results, often with extremely low failure rates. Series derived from the compilation of material at various centers performed under different circumstances by physicians with a wide variety of experiences give a panoramic view of the failure rate. Wherein lies the truth? The answer is somewhere between the unpublished high failure rates (assumed) and the published glowing reports, and reasonably close to the broad series.

There is remarkable consistency in the presence of *luteal phase pregnancy*. Several reports [3, 29] of different methods provide similar statistics with an average rate of 2.0 to 2.5 per 1,000. These cases could be eliminated by operating only in the proliferative phase, insisting on a reliable form of contraception or perhaps routine D&C at the time of sterilization. Even so, such failures would occur.

It is quite possible to *fail to make proper identification* of the fallopian tube and mistakenly sterilize an adjacent structure. Such structures are readily available, particularly the round ligament and the ovarian ligament. This is more likely to occur during a laparoscopic approach or a minilaparotomy and less likely with the vaginal approach. In a laparoscopic series pregnancy resulting from sterilization of the wrong pelvic structure averaged one pregnancy per 1,000 [3].

The most distressing type of pregnancy following sterilization is that which occurs from a *technical failure*. Apparently the procedure is properly performed, yet a pregnancy results. As might be anticipated, the rate of failure ranges considerably in reported series. Nevertheless, when such series [3, 7, 38] are collated, the difference is not so great as might be expected. Technical failures following laparoscopic sterilization may be the result of fistula formation, recanalization, or improper technique. Fistula formation is more likely to occur when there are areas of necrosis such as occur with extensive electrosurgical damage. Recanalization may occur with the clip if application is improper or with the electrical technique if the burn is inadequate. Improper technique may occur with any method: the electrosurgical burn may not be adequate; the clip may be improperly placed or inadequately closed; an attempt may be made to place the ring on a tube that is too thick or scarred by adhesions, resulting in inadequate encircling of the tube.

Loffer and Pent [30] identify a true failure rate of 0.9 to 6.0 per 1,000 sterilizations. The IFRP [3] studied over 24,000 procedures performed in 27 countries in an international study in which life-table techniques were used to account for variations in patient follow-up. The 12-month failure rate per 1,000 procedures was as follows: electrocoagulation 2.3; Silastic band 4.4; and Rocket clip 1.9.

There are few large studies of the efficacy of minilaparotomy sterilization. The IFRP study showed a failure rate of 3 per 1,000 at 12 months, using a modified Pomeroy technique.

It should be noted that time is a factor in consideration of failures. The more time that elapses, the higher the failure rate may be. Cheng [9] (Singapore) reported a large series composed primarily of postpartum laparotomy sterilizations. The study is significant in that the pregnancy rate at the end of 2 years was almost twice that noted at 1 year. He also indicated that most failures occur within 2 years after sterilization.

The existing data for sterilization failures are limited and imperfect. It is obvious that certain techniques are best suited to certain individuals and that great experience increases the efficiency of any technique. The overall failure rates are comparable, generally ranging from 1 to 8 per 1,000 procedures. Experience would indicate that surgeons should continue to use those techniques with which they are the most familiar and comfortable, provided the procedure is both safe and efficient.

Posttubal Ligation Syndrome

If the posttubal ligation syndrome does indeed exist, it encompasses a potpourri of symptoms including irregular bleeding, pelvic pain, change in sexual habits, increased need for subsequent gynecologic surgery, and abnormal endocrine manifestation. The problem is not a frivolous one, since there are between 500,000 and 1 million sterilizations done annually in the United States. If the incidence is only 10 percent, this would indicate 50,000 to 100,000 gynecologic problems annually [8, 32, 42, 49].

Numerous studies have been reported regarding the posttubal ligation syndrome. Most of the early studies were retrospective reviews, screening previously sterilized women for symptoms and then reporting the data collected. Often these reports ignored such pertinent facts as the increasing age of the patient, the number of years since the operative procedure, the type of surgery, the menstrual status of the patient before surgery, and the use of oral contraceptives just before the sterilization procedure. Consideration was not given to the concept that older women and their older gynecologists might view somewhat differently the uterus of a sterile woman and one that was potentially fertilizable. In many instances the number of cases was extremely small. The data collected in numerous studies with respect to menstrual function following tubal sterilization vary in objectivity. Women with abnormal menses following sterilization frequently have had a similar pattern before the procedure, often masked by the use of oral contraceptives.

A more modern control study was reported by Bhiwandiwala [3, 4] in a multicenter prospective study examining cycle regularity, amount of flow, dysmenorrhea, intermenstrual bleeding, and duration of flow. While there was a slight increase in menstrual pain among women who had unipolar electrosurgery, there was no change in the prevalence of abnormal menstrual findings for any of the other groups.

With respect to abnormal endocrine findings, the cornerstone study was done by Radwanska, Berger, and Hammond [40] and reported in 1979. They studied 40 women with normal menstrual cycles who had been sterilized by laparoscopic electrosurgery and Pomeroy procedures. These women were requesting reversal of sterilization. As part of the evaluation preoperatively, progesterone levels were obtained in the midluteal phase, 5 to 10 days before the onset of the menses. The sterilized group had a mean progesterone of 9.4 ng per milliliter compared with 17.4 ng per milliliter in a control group of 24 normal women with infertile male partners. It was surprising, then, that neither Gomel [19] nor Winston [53] found abnormal menstrual patterns in women requesting reversal of sterilization. This latter clinical observation was supported by the findings of Corson et al. [10], who studied hormone levels (estrogen and progesterone) in four groups: (1) patients sterilized by bipolar electrosurgery, (2) patients sterilized by Falope ring, (3) patients who had undergone hysterectomy with ovarian conservation, and (4) normal control patients. All the women were asymptomatic and had regular menstrual patterns (except the hysterectomy group). No significant difference in hormone levels was found in any group, allowing the investigators to conclude that neither tubal sterilization nor hysterectomy had any adverse effect on ovarian steroidogenesis.

An interesting study was done by El Minawi [17] who did phlebograms on patients who were going to undergo sterilization procedures by a variety of methods and compared them with postoperative phlebograms done 3 months after the procedure. The major changes consisted of increased quantity and tortuosity of the venous system. The greatest x-ray changes were found with unipolar electrosurgery, the least changes with the Uchida technique. Sterilization by bipolar electrosurgery, Pomeroy technique, and the Falope ring caused intermediate changes.

The conclusions are that previous studies regarding the presence of a posttubal ligation syndrome have had important methodologic limitations that may have biased results. Although the results are conflicting, there appear to be indications that there is no strong evidence for such a syndrome. The more destructive type of sterilization procedures may indeed result in vascular changes that interfere with subsequent ovarian function. The extent of the problem is magnified by the large number of patients undergoing such procedures annually. However, several recent studies [4, 28] would appear to refute the existence of a syndrome. The validity of these studies is enhanced by the presence of well-documented menstrual histories before sterilization.

Ectopic Pregnancy

The ectopic pregnancy rate has doubled in the past decade; thus, this problem is an important health concern. (Ectopic pregnancies are the leading cause of maternal death in black women [41].)

Tubal sterilization does not increase the risk of a woman having an ectopic pregnancy. In fact, a report from the CDC gives evidence that occlusion of the tubes decreases the absolute risk of a woman having an ectopic pregnancy, since it so markedly decreases the risk of her becoming pregnant at all. However, should a woman become pregnant after tubal sterilization, there is a good likelihood that this pregnancy will lodge in the tube—that is, the relative risk is increased. In the AAGL 1979 survey [38], 33 percent of failures reported were ectopic pregnancies. In the review of Loffer and Pent [29], ectopic pregnancies ranged from 14 to 90 percent.

It would be of great interest to determine which technique increases susceptibility to ectopic pregnancy. However, there are insufficient data to make such an evaluation. Overall evidence appears to suggest that electrocoagulation procedures are slightly more effective in preventing intrauterine pregnancy than are mechanical techniques. However, should a pregnancy occur, there is a slightly increased possibility of ectopic pregnancy. This is supported by the AAGL survey [38]: Failure after electrocoagulation resulted in 30 to 50 percent ectopic pregnancies; failure after mechanical techniques resulted in 20 percent ectopic pregnancies. A CDC study [14] supports this concept. The presumed but not yet proven theory is that fistula formation is more common following electrocoagulation because of extensive tubal destruction. The mechanism is one of sperm exiting from the proximal open stump and entering the fimbriated end of the tube, causing ectopic pregnancy in the distal stump.

In summary, tubal sterilization does *not* result in an increased number of ectopic pregnancies, and it is not yet known which, if any, techniques predispose to this complication.

REFERENCES

1. Aldridge, A. H. Temporary surgical sterilization with subsequent pregnancy. *Am. J. Obstet. Gynecol.* 27:741, 1934.
2. Amin, H. K., and Neuwirth, R. S. Further experiences with laparoscopic sterilization concomitant with vacuum curettage for abortion. *Fertil. Steril.* 24:593, 1973.
3. Bhiwandiwala, P. P., Mumford, S. D., and Feldblum, P. J. A comparison of different laparoscopic sterilization occlusion techniques in 24,439 procedures. *Am. J. Obstet. Gynecol.* 144:319, 1982.
4. Bhiwandiwala, P. P., Mumford, S. D., and Feldblum, P. J. Menstrual pattern changes following laparoscopic sterilization with different occlusion techniques: A review of 10,004 cases. *Am. J. Obstet. Gynecol.* 145:684, 1983.
5. Bishop, E., and Nelms, W. F. A simple method of tubal sterilization. *N.Y. State J. Med.* 30:214, 1930.
6. Blunell, J. In T. Castle (ed.), *The Principles and Practice of Obstetrics.* Washington: Duff-Green, 1834.
7. Chamberlain, G., and Brown, J. C. (eds.) *Gynaecological Laparoscopy: The Report of the Working Party of the Confidential Enquiry into Gynaecological Laparoscopy.* London: The Royal College of Obstetricians and Gynaecologists, 1978.
8. Chamberlain, G., and Foulkes, J. Late complications of sterilization by laparoscopy. *Lancet* 2:878, 1975.
9. Cheng, M. C. E., et al. Sterilization failures in Singapore: An examination of ligation techniques and failure rates. *Stud. Fam. Plann.* 8:109, 1977.
10. Corson, S. L., et al. Hormonal levels following sterilization and hysterectomy. *J. Reprod. Med.* 26:363, 1981.

11. Courey, N. G., and Cunanan, R. G. Combined laparoscopic sterilization and pregnancy termination. *J. Reprod. Med.* 10:291, 1973.

12. DeStefano, F., et al. Complications of interval laparoscopic tubal sterilization. *Obstet. Gynecol.* 61:153, 1983.

13. DeStefano, F., et al. Demographic trends in tubal sterilization. *Am. J. Pub. Health* 72:480, 1982.

14. DeStefano, F., et al. Risk of ectopic pregnancy following tubal sterilization. *Obstet. Gynecol.* 60:326, 1982.

15. Droegemueller, W., Chvapil, M., and Christian, C. D. Modified Aldridge Procedure. In J. J. Sciarra, G. I. Zatuchni, and J. J. Speidel (eds.), *Reversal of Sterilization*. Hagerstown, MD.: Harper & Row, 1978.

16. Edwards, I. E., and Hakanson, E. Y. Changing status of tubal sterilization. *Am. J. Obstet. Gynecol.* 115:347, 1973.

17. El Minawi, M., Mashhor, N., and Reda, M. S. Pelvic venous changes after tubal sterilization. *J. Reprod. Med.* 28:641, 1983.

18. Frangenheim, H. Coelioscopie inder unterbauch chirugie. *Dtsch. Med. Wochenschr.* 43:109, 1965.

19. Gomel, V. Profile of women requesting reversal of sterilization. *Fertil. Steril.* 30:39, 1978.

20. Hasson, H. M. Open laparoscopy: A report of 150 cases. *J. Reprod. Med.* 12:234, 1974.

21. Hoffman, J. J. Sterilization Reversal: Assessment of Demand and Results. In I. Brosens and R. Winston (eds.), *Reversibility of Female Sterilization*. London: Academic, 1978.

22. Hulka, J. F., Fishbourne, J. I., and Mercer, J. P. Laparoscopic sterilization with a spring clip. *Am. J. Obstet. Gynecol.* 116:715, 1973.

23. Hulka, J. F., et al. Complications Committee of the AAGL: Second Annual Report, 1973. In J. M. Phillips (ed.), *Gynecological Laparoscopy*. New York: Grune & Stratton, 1974.

24. Irving, F. C. A new method of insuring sterility following cesarean section. *Am. J. Obstet. Gynecol.* 8:335, 1924.

25. Keith, L., et al. Postpartum laparoscopy for sterilization. *J. Int. Fed. Obstet. Gynecol.* 8:145, 1970.

26. Kroener, N. F., Jr. Surgical sterilization by fimbriectomy. *Am. J. Obstet. Gynecol.* 104(2):247, 1969.

27. Ledger, W. J., Reite, A., and Headington, J. T. The surveillance of infection of an inpatient gynecology service. *Am. J. Obstet. Gynecol.* 113:662, 1972.

28. Liebermann, B. A., et al. Menstrual patterns after laparoscopic sterilization using the spring-loaded clip. *Br. J. Obstet. Gynaecol.* 85:376, 1978.

29. Loffer, F. D., and Pent, D. Indications, contraindications, and complications of laparoscopy. *Obstet. Gynecol. Surv.* 30:407, 1975.

30. Loffer, F. D., and Pent, D. Pregnancy after laparoscopic sterilization. *Obstet. Gynecol.* 55:643l, 1980.

31. Madlener, M. Uber sterilisierende operationen an den tuben. *Zentralbl. Gynakol.* 14:78, 1881.

32. Muldoon, M. J. Gynaecological illness after sterilization. *Br. Med. J.* 1:84, 1972.

33. Mumford, S. D., Bhawandiwala, P. P., and Chi, I. C. Laparoscopic and minilaparotomy female sterilisation compared in 15,167 cases. *Lancet* 2:1066, 1980.

34. Palmer, M. R. Essais de sterilisation tubaire coelioscopique par electro coagulation isthmique. *B Fed. Soc. Gynecol. Obstet.* 14:298, 1962.

35. Penfield, A. J. *Female Sterilization by Minilaparotomy or Open Laparoscopy*. Baltimore: Urban & Schwarzenberg, 1980.

36. Peterson, H. B., et al. Mortality risk associated with tubal sterilization in United States hospitals. *Am. J. Obstet. Gynecol.* 143:125, 1982.

37. Phillips, J. M. *Laparoscopy*. Baltimore: Williams & Wilkins, 1977.

38. Phillips, J. M., et al. 1979 AAGL Membership Survey. *J. Reprod. Med.* 26:529, 1981.

39. Population Information Program. *Reversing female sterilization. Pop. Rep.* [C]. No. 8, 1980.

40. Radwanska, E., Berger, G. S., and Hammond, J. Luteal deficiency among women with normal menstrual cycles seeking reversal of sterilization. *Obstet. Gynecol.* 54:189, 1979.

41. Rubin, F. L. et al. Ectopic pregnancy in the United States. *J.A.M.A.* 249:1725, 1983.

42. Sacks, S., and Lacrois, G. Gynecologic sequelae of postpartum tubal ligation. *Obstet. Gynecol.* 19:22, 1962.

43. Sciarra, J. J., Zatuchni, G. I., and Speidel, J. J. *Reversal of Sterilization*. Hagerstown, Md.: Harper & Row, 1978.

44. Semm, K. *Atlas of Gynecologic Laparoscopy and Hysteroscopy*. Philadelphia: Saunders, 1977.

45. Shepherd, M. K. Female contraceptive sterilization. *Obstet. Gynecol. Surv.* 29:739, 1973.

46. Soderstrom, R. M. Laparoscopic Sterilization: A Comprehensive Review. In J. M. Phillips (ed.), *Gynecological Laparoscopy: Principles and Techniques*. New York: Grune & Stratton, 1974.

47. Soderstrom, R. M. Safeguards in laparoscopy: Education, equipment, care, and electron control. *Contemp. Obstet. Gynecol.* 11:95, 1978.

48. Steptoe, P. C. *Laparoscopy in Gynecology*. Edinburgh and London: Livingston, 1967.

49. Stock, R. J. Evaluation of sequelae of tubal ligation. *Fertil. Steril.* 29:169, 1978.

50. Surgical Sterilization Surveillance. Centers for Disease Control, March, 1981.

51. Uchida, H. Uchida tubal sterilization. *Am. J. Obstet. Gynecol.* 121:153, 1975.

52. Vitoon, O. Suprapubic minilaparotomy. *Contraception* 10:251, 1974.

53. Winston, R. M. L. Tubal Anastomosis for Reversal of Sterilization in 45 Women. In I. Brosens and R. M. L. Winston (eds.), *Reversibility of Female Sterilization*. London: Academic, 1978.

54. Yoon, I. B. Silicone Ring. In J. M. Phillips (eds.), *Laparoscopy*. Baltimore: Williams & Wilkins, 1977.

55. Yuzpe, A. A., et al. Laparoscopic tubal sterilization by the "burn only" technique. *Obstet. Gynecol.* 49:106, 1977.

8. Female Sterilization Reversal

Stephen L. Corson

Over 60 million women throughout the world currently utilize tubal sterilization for continuing contraception [30]. Best estimates are that close to 1 million women are sterilized annually in the United States. Even after adequate counseling as to the irreversible nature of surgery, patients do, in fact, inquire about tubal reconstitution. All presently accepted procedures are designed as permanent forms of contraception, but techniques currently under evaluation may offer reversible surgical sterilization (see Chap. 9). Advances in techniques of reversal procedures leading to improved pregnancy rates have been made known to the public through news media. This knowledge, coupled with a climbing incidence of divorce and remarriage, has served to increase the demand for tubal reconstruction. Given the mobility of the population, it is difficult to estimate actual numbers. Depending on exclusion policies related to age and parity governing sterilization guidelines in various localities, the actual rate for reversal *request* probably lies between 0.1 and 1.0 percent.

What is the profile of patients requesting reversal of sterilization? Winston [36] reported on 103 patients from Hammersmith Hospital. The mean age at sterilization was 26.7 years. In retrospect 78 (75.7%) were unhappily married at the time of sterilization, and 81 cited remarriage as the reason for the reversal request. The mean of term pregnancies in the entire group was 3.1. Gomel [14] reported on 100 consecutive patients seeking sterilization reversal. Fully 89 percent were 30 years or under with a mean of 2.39 children per patient when sterilized. Fifty-three patients were not in a stable marital relationship at the time of sterilization. A change in marital status was the precipitating factor in requesting restoration of fertility in 63 percent. Crib death (7%) and family tragedies (4%) were the next highest reasons. Purely psychologic factors accounted for 6 percent and desire for more children 10 percent.

These figures support the premise that the woman most apt to subsequently apply for sterilization reversal is unhappily married and a mother of two or more children at the time of sterilization. Gynecologists have been most concerned about single, never pregnant or never delivered, comparatively young women seeking sterilization. These women, in fact, rarely desire reversal.

TUBAL ANATOMY AND PHYSIOLOGY

The paired organs described by Fallopius as ending with a trumpet-like flare serve as much more than passive conduits for spermatozoa and oocytes passing in opposite directions. Within the framework of this chapter we shall review briefly the structure and functions

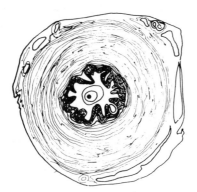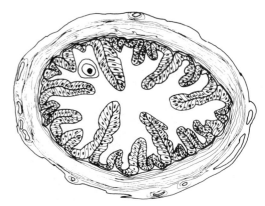

Fig. 8-1. Cross sections through the tube, showing the narrow lumen, thick-walled isthmus versus the wide lumen and redundant mucosa of the ampulla.

of the tube; an excellent book has been written on the subject by Pauerstein [26]; a more recent text chapter by Eddy [10] is also recommended as an additional source of more detailed information.

The normal human tube varies between 6 and 15 cm in length with a mean of about 11 cm. Starting proximally, the intramural or interstitial portion of the tube is that portion contained within the uterine wall. It is usually 1.0 to 3.5 cm in length with a lumen of 150 to 400 μm. In addition to the usual circular and longitudinal muscular coats, an additional longitudinal layer derived from the uterus envelops this portion of the tube. The course of the tube through the myometrium is usually not linear and may be quite tortuous. No histologically demonstrable uterotubal junction can be identified.

The isthmic portion, usually 2 to 3 cm in length, is next. The extra muscle layer becomes attenuated, and in cross section a structure with a thick wall and narrow lumen is seen. Its lining is mainly populated by secretory cells, which produce mucin in increased amounts near the time of ovulation. Human data show that the isthmus is not a prerequisite for fertility [27, 37].

The ampulla measures 5 to 8 cm with a lumen progressing from less than 2 mm proximally to more than 1 cm distally. Its flared end known as the infundibulum contains the projections called *fimbria* that are vital to ovum pickup. Mucosal folding is marked while the muscular coats are thin. The appearance in cross section is quite distinct from the isthmus (Fig. 8-1).

The blood supply to the tube comes from the uterine artery proximally and the ovarian artery distally. A rich collateral arcade of vessels in the broad ligament sends off "feeders" segmentally (Fig. 8-2).

FUNCTION

Sperm Transport

In spite of the fact that well over 100 million sperm may be deposited in the vagina with each ejaculation, the barriers of the cervix, the uterotubal junction, and the isthmus serve to dramatically lower the actual number reaching the ampulla. Sperm have been demonstrated to enter the tube as early as 30 minutes after cervical contact [32]. Therefore, an active tubal transport mechanism must be postulated, since the intrinsic speed of spermatozoan motility cannot explain this finding. Given that cilia beat toward the uterus, this is even more amazing. The segmental contractions of the tube, which change in frequency and amplitude with hormonal changes during the cycle, must play a key role in sperm transport as well as in propulsion of the passive oocyte.

Capacitation

Fresh sperm in seminal plasma penetrate oocytes poorly. Removal of sperm from the seminal plasma and resuspension and incubation in physiologic salt/albumin solutions allow for capacitation in in vitro fertilization programs [13]. Under normal conditions this complex set of reactions occurs in the tube. Capacitation involves the destabilization of the plasma membrane enveloping the sperm head. An acrosomal reaction then ensues, which releases from the sperm enzymes that aid in dissolving the corona radiata and zona pellucida around the oocyte. How long sperm maintain the ability to fertilize remains unknown. Motile sperm have been recovered from the tube 85

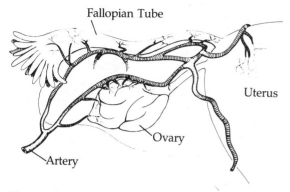

Fallopian Tube

Uterus

Ovary

Artery

Fig. 8-2. Blood supply of the tube, showing ovarian and uterine arcade.

hours after coitus [1]. In our own practice pregnancy has occurred not infrequently following an isolated coital episode or insemination 3 to 4 days before actual ovulation.

Secretory Activity

Increasing estrogen levels stimulate secretory activity, which is most marked in the isthmus by an outpouring of mucus. The tubal fluid changes in composition according to the menstrual cycle. It is presumed that these changes within the tubal milieu bear heavily on the status of the oocyte and early embryo.

Ciliary Function

Although women with altered cilia function may be fertile [6, 19], there is little doubt that ciliary activity in conjunction with tubal contraction is of major importance in oocyte transport. Cilia beat toward the uterus and are most dense in the outer ampulla. Reversal of an ampullary segment in the rabbit, causing a reversed ciliary beat, prevents oocyte transfer across that segment [11].

Ovum Pickup and Transport

Muscles in the mesosalpinx and especially the fimbria ovarica contract at the time of ovulation to bring the fimbria into better contact with the ovary. The infundibulum with its dense population of cilia sweeps over the ovary and comes into contact with the sticky cumulus mass surrounding the oocyte. Rabbit experiments have demonstrated the importance of fimbria in egg capture [5]. Only recently, with careful surgical eversion of the remaining endosalpinx, has it been possible to achieve reasonable results with fimbriectomy sterilization reversal in humans [25]. Under normal cir-

cumstances the oocyte is fertilized in the ampulla and resides at the isthmic-ampullary junction for about 72 hours [12]. Transit time through the isthmus is another 8 hours. Pregnancies following various types of tubal implantation procedures prove that this normal sequence can be abrogated.

PREOPERATIVE ASSESSMENT

Although the only real indicator of fertility is pregnancy, the potential of the couple about to embark on a program of sterilization reversal needs to be studied before any operative procedure.

The Male

A properly performed semen analysis has been used as a routine indicator of male reproductive performance, which, even if historically positive, does not obviate the need for seminal testing. While each laboratory establishes its own norms, in general a volume of 2 to 5 ml with a concentration in excess of 20 million per ml is usually acceptable. More than 60 percent of the sperm should have motility of satisfactory quality, and normal morphology on a stained specimen should exceed 60 percent. Testing should be performed after 2 to 4 days of sexual abstinence. The WHO guidebook on seminal testing is an excellent reference [3]. A new, easily employed method of quantifying sperm motility in standardized bovine mucus (Penetrak*) may be used as an adjunct.

The Female

HISTORY

The previous reproductive history with special attention to ease of conception and outcome can furnish much in the way of data helpful in counseling the individual patient. The operative note and pathology report dealing with the sterilization should be reviewed. As pointed out by Taylor and Leader [34], however, 27 percent of patients assessed endoscopically following Pomeroy sterilization were deemed inoperable.

OVULATORY FUNCTION

Generally speaking, the basal body temperature (BBT) chart can serve as an accurate assessment of ovulatory function. More expensive alternatives include luteal phase endometrial biopsy and serum progesterone determinations. Although some authors [2, 28, 29] report altered luteal function following sterilization, others [9, 24] have not confirmed these results. Moreover, the high term pregnancy rates with absence of increased

*Syva Co., Palo Alto, Calif. 94304.

early abortion achieved with reversal argues against a major luteal defect as a significant factor.

Altered ovulatory function of a subtle nature is not surprising in women in the mid-thirties and older, the time when reproductive efficiency begins to wane. Obviously anovulatory women can be given trial courses of ovulation induction before surgery, but they must realize that any demonstrable ovulatory defect lowers their overall success expectancy. Each surgeon must decide on absolute and relative contraindications to surgery. Age of the female is only one of these considerations.

POSTCOITAL TESTING

The postcoital test is a nonstandardized procedure showing poor correlation with actual pregnancy rates. Although it may be of some help, especially in cases where seminal quality is marginal, a good result is more meaningful than a poor one. If performed, it should be timed to coincide with expected ovulation according to the BBT record.

TUBAL ASSESSMENT

It is our belief that hysterosalpingography should be performed before any intended tubal restoration. First, unsuspected endometrial lesions such as submucous myoma may be disclosed. Second, and more important, information concerning the proximal tubal segment can be gleaned. This is of special importance in laparoscopic electric sterilizations, since demonstration of dye in the intramural portion of the tube or beyond suggests that some sort of direct anastomosis will be possible as opposed to an implantation procedure, which has a lower success rate.

LAPAROSCOPY

No patient should have laparotomy as an elective procedure for sterilization reversal without the benefit of endoscopic evaluation. In order to minimize anesthesia risk, cost, and patient logistics, we customarily perform the laparoscopic examination at the same time as the intended reversal. This may not be possible in all institutions because of allotment of operating room time. As Taylor and Leader [34] showed, 27 percent of patients with Pomeroy procedures were rejected laparoscopically for repair. Often the finding is one of very short distal segments. In other cases disruption of the blood supply has caused fimbrial degeneration. Subclinical pelvic infection may have resulted in dense pelvic adhesions. Laparoscopic electric procedures may result in complete absence of any recognizable tube. When all is said and done, however, the burden of the decision falls on the surgeon. Adherence to rigid criteria will produce excellent statistical results; a more liberal approach, however, will produce more births.

Although classified as elective major surgery, the morbidity is low because most patients are young healthy women. Any major complication is unexpected and particularly disastrous. Thus, the process by which patients are chosen for surgery demands great thought and attention to both physical factors and emotional needs and often seems more difficult than the surgery itself.

TYPES OF STERILIZATION USUALLY PERFORMED AND EASE OF REVERSAL

The variations of tubal sterilization techniques are discussed in Chapter 7. I shall not discuss the unique challenges posed by each as encountered at the time of reversal but instead consider three of the more commonly performed operations vis-à-vis reversal.

Before laparoscopic methods of sterilization became popular, most operations were performed by the Pomeroy laparotomy technique or one of its modifications (Irving, Uchida). This technique is still popular, especially when performed in the immediate postpartum state. Instrumentation facilitating minilaparotomy has brought about renewed interest in tubal ligation as a safe outpatient alternative to laparoscopic methods.

The amount of tube removed and the location of the defect thus formed can vary tremendously from side to side as well as between patients. A small piece of isthmic resection offers the best prognosis for restoration of fertility for a number of reasons: First, the isthmus is less critical than the ampulla for fertility; second, the thick muscular walls permit excellent and accurate coadaptation; and third, the surgeon encounters segments of equal diameter.

Often, however, one finds that the isthmic-ampullary junction has been removed or that the ampulla was the actual site of resection, leaving widely separated isthmic and infundibular portions to be connected. There are a number of methods for dealing with this problem. Sutures can be taken in the broad ligament to bring the ends closer together and to lessen the tension on the anastomotic line. The inequality of the tubal diameters can be managed by a number of approaches as shown in Figure 8-3. The smaller diameter can be incised at the antimesosalpingeal border and enlarged. The smaller segment can be telescoped into the larger, but the curb thus formed may cause an impediment to egg transfer, increasing the risk of ectopic pregnancy. Another criticism of this maneuver is juxtaposition of isthmic muscularis to ampullary mucosa. One can refrain from complete removal of the scar tissue from the distal stump so as to keep the lumen small, but this move may also impede tubal motility. Yet another method is based on cutting the proximal portion on a

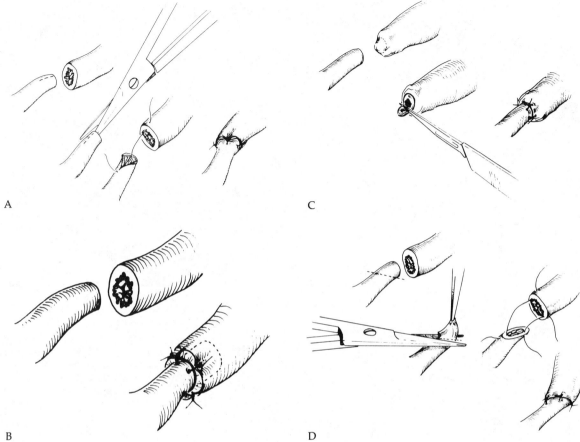

A

C

B

D

Fig. 8-3. Anastomosis of segments with unequal diameters. (A) Incision of smaller segment at the antimesosalpingeal border. (B) Telescoping smaller segments into larger. (C) Reduction of larger lumen by limiting excision of fibrous scar. (D) Tangential preparation of narrow segment.

tangent to increase the area there. Doing this causes the muscular layers to be anastomosed on an angle, which is also less than totally desirable. Therefore, while a Pomeroy sterilization might seem at first to be the most favorable type to reverse, this often is not the case.

Kroener fimbriectomy procedures are often performed through a culpotomy approach in women with some degree of pelvic relaxation. Generally speaking, loss of fimbriae is associated with poor return of fertility, even when tubal patency has been restored.

Laparoscopic sterilization began as unipolar procedures with or without tubal resection. The end result, in either case, was loss of considerable tubal length as a result of avascular necrosis far exceeding the visual area

of damage seen at the initial episode. Although the isthmus was the primary site, spread of current often caused severe vascular changes within the intramural portion and loss of ampullary tube as well. The advent of bipolar methods changed this dramatically and reduced the spread of current into the vascular arcade of the mesosalpinx. Patients sterilized in this fashion are usually good candidates for reversal.

Occlusive methods of sterilization, such as use of a clip or Silastic band, were popularized laparoscopically, although now they are often done by minilaparotomy. The persistent antifertility effect depends on avascular necrosis of the segment compressed and not on simple continued mechanical occlusion of the lumen. The area of damage, including changes in the adjacent tube, is often as small as 3 to 6 mm. Therefore, these patients can expect high (70–80%) rates of pregnancy following tubal repair, so long as no other negative fertility factors are present.

RESULTS OF STERILIZATION REVERSAL

Evaluation of sterilization reversal rates gleaned from the literature is not an easy task. The major problem is that most authors report the number of patients operated as opposed to the number screened. Thus, a surgeon with liberal prerequisites would be expected to produce a pregnancy rate inferior to that of a surgeon employing more rigid criteria (e.g., a cut-off of age 36 versus age 39).

The final results depend more on the skill of the surgeon than on the type of procedure employed or the diameter of the suture used. Traumatic surgery performed with the microscope will not equal results obtained with gentle technique in the absence of magnification.

It is in the area of sterilization reversal that microsurgery has achieved gynecologic legitimacy. Semantics, however, have clouded the issue. Does the use of magnifying loupes qualify as true microsurgery? Is there a minimum suture diameter to be considered in the definition? The results and discussion that follow are confounded by these and other variables. As a practical example, how does one best code a patient who conceives after an isthmo-isthmic anastomosis on one side and an isthmo-ampullary on the other; should she be dropped from consideration entirely?

Perhaps the best data come from surgeons who compare their own results with macro- and microtechniques assuming no change in criteria used for patient selection. It is my personal conviction that once the operator has mastered the technique of operating through a microscope, results will improve as a result of gentle tissue manipulation alone.

Magnification with directed lighting allows for more accurate approximation of the segments with the finest needles and suture easily handled. Inspection of the mucosa under the microscope permits complete removal of fibrotic tissue and avoidance of small blood vessels.

One of the pioneers in microsurgical tubal reversals is Robert Winston from Hammersmith in London. Table 8-1 is reproduced from one of his publications [38]. The data clearly show that operations confined to the cornual and isthmic areas have the best prognosis for reasons previously mentioned. Of 126 patients operated, 73 conceived with only three ectopic pregnancies noted.

Victor Gomel [15], another leader in microsurgical tubal surgery, has reported similar results. Of 118 patients operated, 76 (64.4%) achieved at least one intrauterine pregnancy; only one ectopic pregnancy was noted. In a subgroup of 47 patients with at least 18 months following repair, the pregnancy rate was 80.8 percent. In the entire series the mean time to conception was 10.2 months, with the longest interval being 40 months.

Rock et al. [31] addressed specifically a group of patients seeking reversal of unipolar cauterization sterilization. Twenty-five of 48 patients (52%) conceived, with a 36 percent liveborn rate. They noted that 71 percent had associated tubal disease such as endometriosis or proximal hydrosalpinx. Peterson et al. [27] in 1977 described a new implantation technique designed to cope with short distal segments and extensive cornual damage. This posterior implantation resulted in pregnancy in 50 percent of the first 16 patients. Levinson [21] subsequently reported a larger series in which this technique was employed; the pregnancy rate was 75 percent (18 of 24) in patients previously sterilized by laparoscopic cautery technique (Fig. 8-4).

Grunert et al. [16] summarized the results of tubal anastomosis following sterilization according to macro- and microtechniques (Table 8-2). The superiority of the microsurgical approach seems obvious. On the other hand, Jones and Rock [20] reported a series of 12 patients with 10 pregnancies using what they termed macrosurgical techniques. It should be noted, however, that they employed magnifying loupes and 6-0 suture.

What are the essentials of surgical technique as applied to tubal surgery? Quite simply, the key factors are gentle handling of tissue, meticulous hemostasis, and accurate coadaptation with the minimal suture (size and number) necessary to deal with tension on the joint. Use of the microscope allows the surgeon to better meet these goals, since it is the eye and not the hand that is the limiting factor in this type of surgery.

My own technique, similar to that employed by both Winston and Gomel, is outlined below.

Cycle Timing

The follicular phase is most desirable because of tubal mucosal proliferation and avoidance of a corpus luteum subject to bleeding when retracted or handled.

Magnification

Because Doctor Batzer and I usually operate together as a two-person team, we prefer a Zeiss OPMI-6 or OPMI-7 microscope with opposed heads. A hand control for the microscope in a sterile plastic bag is preferred to a foot control. A microscope with a long multipointed arm or a ceiling mount allows operator comfort. For single-operator cases a converted colposcope affords an inexpensive alternative with excellent optics and lighting [8].

Preparation

We believe that an intrauterine instrument for dye perfusion is preferable to a Buxton clamp arrangement.

Table 8-1. Results of tubal anastomosis for reversal of sterilization

	Cornu-isthmus	Isthmus-isthmus	Cornu-ampulla	Isthmus-ampulla	Ampulla-ampulla	Miscel-laneous	Total
Number of operations	17	16	26	27	19	21	126
Number of pregnancies	12	12	14	17	8	10	73
Number of ectopic pregnancies			1	2		(1)	3
Pregnancy rate	71%	75%	54%	63%	42%	48%	58%

Source: From R. M. L. Winston, Microsurgery of the fallopian tube: From fantasy to reality. *Fertil. Steril.* 34:521, 1980. Reprinted with permission of the publisher, The American Fertility Society.

Table 8-2. Results of tubal anastomosis by macro- and microtechniques

Author	Macrosurgery			Microsurgery		
	No.	Intrauterine pregnancy	Ectopic pregnancy	No.	Intrauterine pregnancy	Ectopic pregnancy
Williams	5	0	0			
Seigler & Perez	46	17	0			
Wheeless	1	0	0			
McCormick & Torres	14	4	3			
Hodari, Vibhasiri, & Isaac	13	8	1			
Diamond	12	3	3	28	16	2
Wilson				3	2	0
Winston				126	73	3
Gomel				118	76	1
Daniell				16	10	2
Grunert, Drake, & Takaki				37	21	1
Total	91	32(35%)	7(8%)	328	198(60%)	9(3%)

Source: From G. M. Grunert, T. S. Drake, and N. K. Takaki, Microsurgical reanastomosis of the fallopian tubes for reversal of sterilization. *Obstet. Gynecol.* 58:148, 1981. Reprinted with permission of The American College of Obstetricians and Gynecologists.

The latter is bulky, and I have never been happy about transfundal needling to reach the endometrium. We use a HUI or HUMI* apparatus for this purpose with sterile intravenous tubing brought up to a syringe on the abdominal drapes. Dilute indigo carmine dye is employed. A Foley catheter is placed in the urinary bladder. The vagina is packed, especially posteriorly in the vault, to elevate the uterus into the abdominal cavity; this avoids traction on adnexal structures during the operation.

A Pfannestiel incision is usually adequate, particularly in multigravid women with a relaxed anterior wall. Alternatively a Czerny modification, that of nick-

ing the rectus muscle at its pubic insertion with repair upon closing the abdomen, gives quite adequate exposure. A plastic wound drape manufactured by 3M keeps blood from entering the abdomen. The Kirschner four-bladed retractor affords excellent exposure. Through judicious choice of lateral blade sizes, pressure on the femoral nerve and great vessels is avoided; nevertheless, tension should be relaxed from time to time, especially if the operating time is prolonged. Soaking wet sponges, woven to reduce lint content, are used for bowel retraction and to pack the cul-de-sac of Douglas in order to form a platform for the adnexae. This pack is covered with Silastic rubber cut to fit around the back of the uterus in order to present a smooth surface. Irrigation is performed throughout the

*National Catheter Co., Argyle, N.Y. 12809.

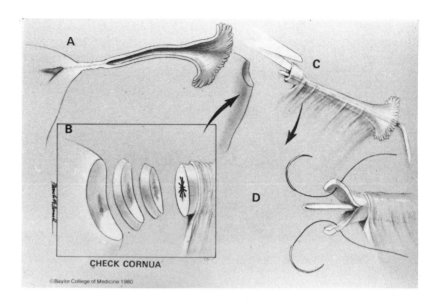

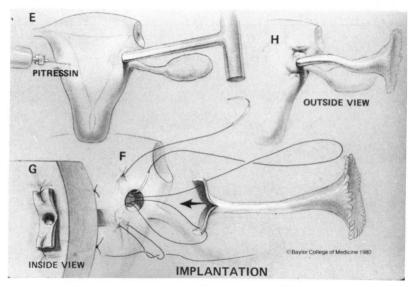

Fig. 8-4. Technique of posterior implantation of tube into uterus. (Reprinted with permission from C. Levinson. Implantation procedures for intramural obstruction. *J. Reprod. Med.* 26:347, 1981.)

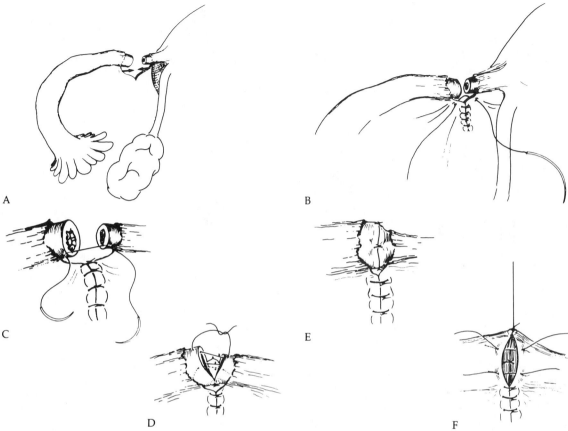

Fig. 8-5. (A and B) Approximation of trimmed stumps via sutures in broad ligament. (C and D) First layer of approximation with extramucosal sutures, 6 o'clock. (E and F) Serosal sutures to relieve tension on first suture line and to create a smooth surface.

procedure with warm lactated Ringer's solution containing epinephrine 1:400,000 and 5,000 units of heparin per liter.

Anesthesia

We have employed general anesthesia, spinal, and continuous epidural anesthesia without a preference, leaving the choice to the anesthesiologist after discussion with the patient.

Surgical Technique

Microsurgical forceps, unratcheted needle drivers, and scissors are used. An electric needle with a hand control attached to a low-voltage generator is employed for cutting and coagulation. We have employed the carbon dioxide laser as well without an apparent difference in pregnancy rate. Neurosurgical bipolar forceps are also used for hemostasis. Glass or quartz rods or Teflon probes are used for retraction and tissue handling. A Hoffman tubal clamp attached to the mesosalpinx is used in cases where the defect is especially long in order to oppose the segments before suturing. Double armed 8-0 Vicryl suture is used for the primary anastomosis and serosal supporting sutures. We have also employed 9-0 nylon material. Tissues are kept moist by use of a syringe with a plastic tip (an Intracath). Sponges are *never* used on pelvic serosal surfaces.

Figure 8-5 shows the basic repair. The stumps are trimmed back under microscopic inspection until healthy mucosa is encountered. The broad ligament is approximated to reduce tension. The six o'clock suture is taken first, as an exit bite through the muscularis avoiding the mucosa, by each operator seated on either side of the table. This is a key point; it facilitates the surgery tremendously and avoids awkward suturing positions. The twelve o'clock suture follows, with the three and nine o'clock afterward. A splint is not used except transiently if the cornua is involved. Serosal sutures complete the procedure. With this approach we consistently can perform the entire operation within 2 to 2½ hours.

Adjuvants

We use prophylactic antibiotics started intravenously on call to the operating room and for 24 hours thereafter. Doxycycline is our current choice. As mentioned above, a specialized irrigation is used with epinephrine to suppress bleeding from small vessels and heparin to avoid fibrin deposition. We do not employ intraperitoneal high molecular weight dextran or steroids by any route in these cases, although we do advocate the use of these agents in operations for chronic inflammatory conditions such as endometriosis and salpingitis. We do not use hydrotubation.

Follow-up

Routine hysterosalpingography is performed at 6 months if the patient has not conceived. At that time additional studies are performed as necessary.

FACTORS AFFECTING OUTCOME

We have alluded to the myriad of factors that affect fertility in general. Here consideration is given to more specific items. Tubal length is certainly one of the things to be considered.

Boeckx and Winston [7] studied the effect of tubal shortening in the rabbit. Fully 50 percent conceived after total isthmic resection, but there were no pregnancies when 70 percent or more of the ampulla was removed. McComb and Gomel [22] found a similar effect in rabbits. Beyth and Winston [4], using the rabbit, obtained pregnancy in 15 of 16 animals subjected to fimbriectomy (distal 2 cm). An interesting serendipitous discovery was that of impeded ovulatory function on the operated side. Other authors have commented on the importance of tubal length. Silber and Cohen [33] noted no pregnancy in women where reanastomosed segments were less than 3 cm. Three of seven conceived with 3 to 4 cm of tube, and all 11 with more than 4 cm conceived. Henderson [18] reported pregnancy in 10 of 16 of those with tube 6 cm or longer but only in 1 of 7 with a length 5 cm or less. A unique method of dealing with specific anatomic problems was reported by Haney [17], whose patient conceived after anastomosis of segments of contralateral tubes connected posteriorly to the uterus.

The importance of atraumatic handling of tissues has been demonstrated by Margara [23], who covered rabbit ovaries with a single cell layer of peritoneum. Corpora lutea decreased on the grafted side, and only 30 percent of the eggs that did escape the ovary were captured by the tube.

Vasquez et al. [35] have demonstrated with electron microscopy that flattening and deciliation following sterilization appear to be related to increasing duration of time.

THE FUTURE

An increasing number of in vitro fertilization (IVF) programs have been established, with pregnancy rates close to 20 percent. Once the number of facilities becomes sufficient to cope with the large numbers of never-pregnant infertile women with irreparable tubal disease, women seeking sterilization reversal will become more eligible for consideration as patients in these clinics.

Newer methods of sterilization such as the hysteroscopic approach described by Cooper in Chapter 9 may offer truly reversible sterilizations without major surgery to the tube. Until that time we must fully counsel our patients before sterilizing operations. We should also attempt to perform these procedures with as little tubal damage as possible consistent with no loss of efficacy of the sterilizing procedure itself—a goal more easily stated than achieved.

REFERENCES

1. Algren, M. Sperm transport to and survival in the human fallopian tube. In C. J. Pauerstein (ed.), *Seminar on Tubal Physiology and Biochemistry. Gynecol. Obstet. Invest.* 6:306, 1975.
2. Alvarez-Sanchez, F., et al. Pituitary-ovarian function after tubal ligation. *Fertil. Steril.* 36:606, 1981.
3. Belsey, M. A., et al. (eds.), *Laboratory Manual for the Examination of Human Semen and Semen-Cervical Mucus Interaction.* Geneva: World Health Organization, 1980.
4. Beyth, Y., and Winston, R. M. L. Ovum capture and fertility following microsurgical fimbriectomy in the rabbit. *Fertil. Steril.* In press, 1984.
5. Blandau, R. J. Gamet Transport: Comparative Aspects. In E. S. E. Hafez and R. J. Blandau (eds.), *The Mammalian Oviduct.* Chicago: University of Chicago Press, 1969. P. 129.
6. Bleau, G., Richer, C. L., and Bosquet, D. Absence of dynein arms in cilia of endocervical cells in a fertile woman. *Fertil. Steril.* 30:362, 1978.
7. Boeckx, W. D., and Winston, R. M. L. Unpublished data.

8. Corson, S. L. An inexpensive operating microscope. *Obstet. Gynecol.* 54:518, 1979.

9. Corson, S. L., Batzer, F. R., and Levinson, C. Hormonal patterns following sterilization and hysterectomy. *J. Reprod. Med.* 26:363, 1981.

10. Eddy, C. A. Physiology of the Fallopian Tube. In J. V. Reyniak and N. H. Lauersen (eds.), *Principles of Microsurgical Techniques in Infertility.* New York: Plenum, 1982. P. 116.

11. Eddy, C. A., et al. The role of cilia in fertility: An evaluation by selective microsurgical modification of the rabbit oviduct. *Am. J. Obstet. Gynecol.* 132:814, 1978.

12. Edwards, R. G., Bavister, B. D., and Steptoe, P. C. Early stages of fertilization in vitro of human oocytes matured in vitro. *Nature* 221:1307, 1970.

13. Fishel, S. B., and Edwards, R. G. Essentials of Fertilization. In R. G. Edwards and J. M. Purdy (eds.), *Human Conception In Vitro.* London: Academic, 1982. P. 157.

14. Gomel, V. Profile of women requesting reversal of sterilization. *Fertil. Steril.* 30:39, 1978.

15. Gomel, V. Microsurgical reversal of female sterilization: A reappraisal. *Fertil. Steril.* 33:587, 1980.

16. Grunert, C. M., Drake, T. S., and Takaki, N. K. Microsurgical reanastomosis of the fallopian tubes for reversal of sterilization. *Obstet. Gynecol.* 58:148, 1981.

17. Haney, A. F. Utilization of contralateral fallopian tube segments in tubal reanastomosis. *Fertil. Steril.* 37:701, 1982.

18. Henderson, S. R. Reversal of female sterilization: Comparison of microsurgical and gross surgical techniques for tubal anastomosis. *Am. J. Obstet. Gynecol.* 139:73, 1981.

19. Jean, Y., et al. Fertility of a woman with nonfunctional ciliated cells in the fallopian tubes. *Fertil. Steril.* 31:349, 1979.

20. Jones, H. W., Jr., and Rock, R. A. On the reanastomosis of fallopian tubes after surgical sterilization. *Fertil. Steril.* 29:702, 1978.

21. Levinson, C. J. Implantation procedures for intramural obstruction. *J. Reprod. Med.* 26:347, 1981.

22. McComb, P., and Gomel, V. The influence of fallopian tube length on fertility in the rabbit. *Fertil. Steril.* 31:673, 1979.

23. Margara, R. In preparation.

24. Meldrum, D. R. Microsurgical tubal reanastomosis: The role of splints. *Obstet. Gynecol.* 57:613, 1981.

25. Novy, M. J. Reversal of Kroener fimbriectomy sterilization. *Am. J. Obstet. Gynecol.* 137:198, 1980.

26. Pauerstein, C. J. *The Fallopian Tube: A Reappraisal.* Philadelphia: Lea & Febiger, 1974.

27. Peterson, E. P., Musich, J. R., and Behrman, S. J. Uterotubal implantation and obstetric outcome after previous sterilization. *Am. J. Obstet. Gynecol.* 128:662, 1977.

28. Radwanska, E. J., Berger, G. S., and Hammond, J. Luteal deficiency among women with normal menstrual cycles requesting reversal of tubal sterilization. *Obstet. Gynecol.* 54:189, 1979.

29. Radwanska, E., Headley, S. K., and Dmowski, P. Evaluation of ovarian function after tubal sterilization. *J. Reprod. Med.* 27:376, 1982.

30. Reversing female sterilization. *Popul. Rep.* [C]. vol. VIII, No. 5, 1980.

31. Rock, J. A., et al. Tubal anastomosis following unipolar cautery. *Fertil. Steril.* 37:613, 1982.

32. Rubinstein, B. B. Sperm survival in women. *Fertil. Steril.* 2:15, 1951.

33. Silber, S. J., and Cohen, R. Microsurgical reversal of female sterilization: The role of tubal length. *Fertil. Steril.* 33:598, 1980.

34. Taylor, P. J., and Leader, A. Reversal of female sterilization. How reliable is the previous operative report? *J. Reprod. Med.* 27:246, 1982.

35. Vasquez, G., et al. Tubal lesions subsequent to sterilization and their relation to fertility after attempts at reversal. *Am. J. Obstet. Gynecol.* 138:86, 1980.

36. Winston, R. M. L. Why 103 women asked for reversal of sterilisation. *Br. Med. J.* 2:279, 1977.

37. Winston, R. M. L. Microsurgical tubocornual anastomosis for reversal of sterilization. *Lancet* 1:284, 1977.

38. Winston, R. M. L. Microsurgery of the fallopian tube: From fantasy to reality. *Fertil. Steril.* 34:521, 1980.

9. Hysteroscopic Sterilization

Jay M. Cooper

Voluntary sterilization has become the most prevalent method of fertility regulation, and its use is widespread in both developed and developing countries.

HISTORY OF FEMALE STERILIZATION

Although 200 techniques of female sterilization have been described, tubal sterilization is a relatively new operation [2]. A wide range of transcervical techniques for female sterilization have been suggested since the initial attempt in 1849 by Friorep [14], who passed a nitric acid–coated probe through a woman's cervix to chemically stricture the tubal ostia.

The use of the hysteroscope for direct visual approach to the tubal ostia for the purpose of sterilization was initially suggested by Mickulicz-Radecki and Freund [42] in 1927. They performed "blood-less tubal sterilizations" in experimental animals.

Schroeder [39] in 1934 performed intramural sterilization of the tubes by electrocoagulation under direct hysteroscopic visualization in two patients. The electro-probe was inserted into the tubal ostia, and an electric current was initiated. Intensity of the current required for coagulation was determined by the warmth of the uterus as felt transabdominally by a hand placed over the lower abdomen.

After Schroeder's [39] report in 1934 hysteroscopic sterilization procedures were rarely performed. However, in the early 1970s there appeared to be a renewed interest in a viable hysteroscopic sterilization technique as evidenced by the convention of a workshop in Minneapolis, Minnesota, in 1973 sponsored by the Program for Applied Research on Fertility Regulation (PARFR) [40]. Twenty of the world's experts in gynecologic endoscopy addressed the major questions regarding the safety and efficacy of hysteroscopic sterilization. Additionally, there were concerns regarding the difficulty of learning to use this technique, as well as the cost, complexity, and maintenance of the equipment necessary to perform hysteroscopic sterilization.

HYSTEROSCOPIC TECHNIQUES AND INSTRUMENTATION (TABLE 9-1)

Pantaleoni [26] introduced hysteroscopy as an examination method for discovery of intrauterine diseases in 1869. Utilizing a kerosene lamp for a light source, he performed his first examination on a 60-year-old woman whose bleeding had resisted all therapy and found polyplike growths (Table 9-1). The 1970 publication of Edström and Fernström [10] describing the use of high molecular weight dextran as a distending

Table 9-1. Historic developments in hysteroscopic technique and instrumentation

Author	Year	Contribution	Reference
Pantaleoni	1869	Identified intrauterine polyps in examining a 60-year-old woman with abnormal bleeding	26
Heineberg	1914	Introduced irrigating system with inflow and outflow channels to improve intrauterine visualization	18
Rubin	1925	Carbon dioxide distention of uterine cavity	37
Mickulicz-Radecki and Freund	1927	Suggested hysteroscopically directed tubal sterilization Biopsy-taking ability	42
Norment	1920	Rubber balloon filled with air for uterine distention	25
Silander	1963	Rubber balloon filled with water for uterine distention	43
Menken	1968	Utilized viscous solution (polyvinyl pyrrolidine) of polymer mixtures for uterine distention	24
Edström and Fernström	1970	Utilized 32% dextran 70 for uterine distention	10
Norment and Sikes	1970	Utilized 5% dextrose in water for uterine distention	25
Lindemann	1976	Utilized calibrated equipment for safe, effective CO_2 uterine distention	23
Porto and Serment	1973		27
Brueschke	1977	Steerable hysteroscope	1

medium marked the beginning of modern hysteroscopy.

Three currently utilized media for uterine distention include high molecular weight dextran, dextrose 5% in water, and carbon dioxide gas. Dextrose 5% in water simply and easily achieves uterine distention. It is rapidly absorbed from the peritoneal cavity, and it is particularly safe for the purposes of uterine distention. A major disadvantage is that the liquid medium mixes well with blood, which may result in obscured vision.

Although pioneered by Rubin [37] in 1925, carbon dioxide gas insufflation for uterine distention did not become practical until Lindemann and Mohr [23] and Porto and Serment [27] separately introduced a safe, reliable technique (Fig. 9-1). Because of the possibility of gas intravasation and secondary hypercarbia, careful monitoring of gas delivery into the uterine cavity is essential.

High molecular weight dextran (32% dextran 70 in dextrose [Hyskon*]) has the advantage of high viscosity (molecular weight 70,000) and biodegradability. It is electrolyte free and electrically nonconductive. It provides excellent visualization because it is nonmiscible with blood. The disadvantage of this distending medium is the possibility of allergic or anaphylactic reaction, because the substance is a polysaccharide with antigenic potential. As well, immediate cleansing of the hysteroscope with hot water is essential to avoid

*Pharmacia, Inc., Piscataway, N.J.

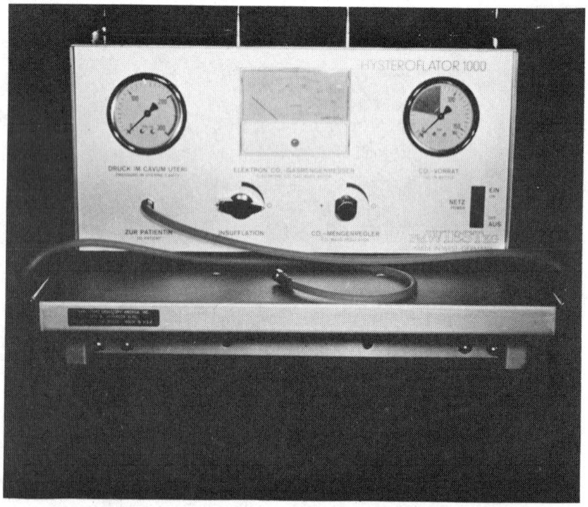

Fig. 9-1. Hysteroflator for safe carbon dioxide distention.

hardening and crystallization of the material within the instrument.

The present-day hysteroscope is a modified version of the cystoscope (Fig. 9-2). It consists of (1) a telescope 4 to 6 mm in diameter with a fore-oblique lens system; (2) a metallic sheath approximately 7 mm in diameter, for introduction of the telescope, with separate operating channels for the distending medium; (3) a fiberoptic bundle for transmission of external light; and (4) addi-

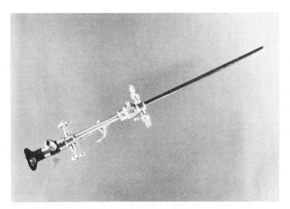

Fig. 9-2. Storz 7-mm operating hysteroscope.

tional ancillary instruments for intrauterine manipulation or surgical intervention, including atraumatic catheters, probes, forceps, scissors, cutting loops, and electrodes.

Several fundamental elements are standard to most hysteroscopic procedures. The patient is placed in the dorsolithotomy position, and the vagina and cervix are washed with an antiseptic solution. Although general anesthesia can be utilized, hysteroscopy is easily performed utilizing local anesthesia administered in a paracervical block. The endocervical canal and uterine cavity are carefully sounded, and, if necessary, endocervical dilatation is accomplished with tapered dilators. Examination of the uterine cavity is initiated after the hysteroscope has been inserted to the level of the internal os. Advancing the telescope toward the tubal ostia, the cornual regions are carefully examined. Determination of tubal patency is easily accomplished by advancing an atraumatic catheter to the tubal ostia and attempting to pass a small amount of methylene blue dye solution.

Recent or ongoing uterine, cervical, or adnexal infections as well as pregnancy are the two major contraindications to the performance of hysteroscopy. Pelvic infections that have not been adequately treated can be exacerbated by the hysteroscopic procedure. Though rare, complications of hysteroscopy can occur and should be appropriately managed. Uterine perforation of the lower uterine segment during cervical dilatation or of the fundus on insertion of the hysteroscope too far beyond the internal cervical os is a recognized complication.

Medium-related complications are infrequent but are unique for each of the distending media. These include allergic and anaphylactic reactions to dextran or hypercarbia, acidosis, and cardiac arrhythmias if intravasation of carbon dioxide occurs.

HYSTEROSCOPIC STERILIZATION TECHNIQUES

Whether ''blind'' or hysteroscopically directed, transcervical sterilization procedures can be divided into three categories based upon the mechanism of tubal occlusion. Sterilization can be effected by (1) destruction of the interstitial portion of the oviduct by thermal energy (electrocoagulation or cryosurgery); (2) injection techniques for the delivery of sclerosing substances or tissue adhesives; and (3) mechanical occlusive devices or plugs to block the oviduct [41].

Electrocoagulation Techniques

Quinones and his coworkers have had the greatest experience utilizing electrocoagulation techniques. Dextrose 5% in water was utilized for distention of the endometrial cavity at approximately 100 mm of mercury.

Between April 1972 and June 1977 Quinones and his coworkers [41] performed 1,284 hysteroscopic tubal electrocoagulation procedures, with an overall bilateral tubal occlusion rate of 80 percent. Patients utilized either oral contraception or intrauterine devices (IUDs) until a hysterosalpingogram was performed 2 to 14 weeks postoperatively to confirm tubal occlusion. No pregnancies occurred in 513 patients with hysterosalpingographic evidence of bilateral occlusion who were followed for 1 year. Six pregnancies were reported overall, three occurring in the interstitial tubal segment. After a careful analysis of the cases in which the procedure failed to occlude the tubes, Quinones found the following variables to be important: (1) the phase of the menstrual cycle: Identification of the tubal openings was easier in the 4 to 5 days following the last day of menstruation; (2) the type of electrodes used: Better results were obtained in cases performed with a Silastic-tipped cylindrical electrode; (3) size of electrode: Most of the failures (52.9%) occurred with electrodes that were the thinnest (4 and 5 French units; numbers 6 and 7 French units were preferable); (4) the coagulating current and the length of time used: A current of 25 watts for 8 seconds appeared most reliable; and (5) the amount of the tube destroyed: Adequate tissue destruction was dependent on the length of the electrode introduced into the intramural portion of the tube. No one factor was responsible for the high failure rate. For some failed procedures two or three of the variables mentioned were present. Of the 423 patients followed for 5 years in whom bilateral tubal occlusion was demonstrated, after one or two procedures 16 (3.8%) later became pregnant [29]. Two of these pregnancies were ectopic.

Utilizing the hysterosalpingogram to document

Table 9-2. Mechanical tubal occlusive devices

Device/clinical investigator	Animal studies	Human studies	Present status	Reference
Polymer flock ITD/Richart et al.	Monkey	None	No active clinical trials	35
Metal alloy ITD/Richart et al.	Monkey	None	No active clinical trials	35
Claw device/Popp	None	None	No active clinical trials	41
Hydrogel-nylon P-Block/Brundin	None	35 women	Ongoing clinical trials	2
Ceramic plug/Craft	8 rabbits	15 women	No active clinical trials	7
Polyethylene UTJD/Hosseinian et al.	Baboon	33 women	Ongoing clinical trials	19, 20
Preformed silicone rubber plug/				
Sugimoto	None	32 women	Ongoing clinical trials	41
Porto	None	Uncertain	Uncertain	41
Nylon ITD/Hamou	Limited	57 women	Ongoing clinical trials	16
Formed-in-place silicone plug/				
Erb/Reed	Limited rabbit studies	365 women	Ongoing multicenter clinical trials	11–13, 31–34
Cooper/Houck		415 women		3–5, 21

ITD = intratubal device; UTJD = uterotubal junction blocking device.

sterility after hysteroscopic tubal coagulation, other investigators had similar experiences. Lindemann and Mohr [22] found at least one patent tube in 33 of 124 women 12 weeks postoperatively. Rimkus and Semm [36] found at least one patent tube in 61 percent of 49 patients undergoing a tubal coagulation procedure. Two perforations with the cauterizing probe occurred, and five of the 49 patients subsequently conceived.

In another study ten collaborators from the United States, Thailand, West Germany, India, and Singapore reported the results of procedures performed in 584 women [8]: 186 (35.5%) were considered failures either because of incomplete blockage of the tubes or subsequent pregnancies. Successful bilateral tubal occlusion could be demonstrated in only 57 percent of the women. Second sterilization procedures were undertaken in 27 percent of the patients; 16 percent had a third sterilization procedure, and 3 percent continued to show tubal patency despite a third attempt at sterilization. Fifty-nine pregnancies (23.7%) were reported in the 249 cases that were not tested for tubal patency. Of the 345 women who had hysterosalpingographic evidence of tubal occlusion, 3.2 percent conceived.

In the total population there were 25 major complications (3.2%). These involved tubal and cornual ectopic pregnancies; excessive uterine bleeding and perforations; acute and prolonged endometritis with pain, bleeding, and fever; and bowel damage with resultant peritonitis. One patient died as a result of this last complication.

This collaborative report had a sobering effect upon clinical investigators who just 3 years earlier had enthusiastically attended the PARFR meetings that had examined the great potential for hysteroscopic sterilization.

Hysteroscopic Injection of Chemicals

Quinones attempted hysteroscopically controlled quinacrine infusion in the tubal ostia [28]. However, the failure rate was so high in an initial group of 60 patients that the technique was abandoned.

Hysteroscopically Directed Placement of Intratubal Mechanical Devices

Many experimental designs of tubal plugs have been described (Table 9-2). Brundin [2] has for several years worked to develop a hydrogelic tubal blocking device fixed on a firm nylon skeleton (Fig. 9-3). The hydrogel is a polymeric compound of polyvinyl pyrrolidine and methylacrylate. Two nylon "wings" are incorporated into the design to prevent expulsion immediately after plug placement, allowing for hydratization to occur following plug insertion.

Between September 1981 and April 1982 oviductal

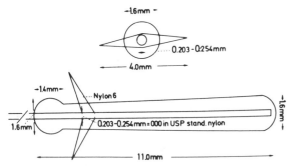

Fig. 9-3. Diagrammatic representation of Brundin's hydrogelic plug.

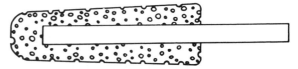

Fig. 9-4. Diagrammatic representation of Craft's ceramic plug.

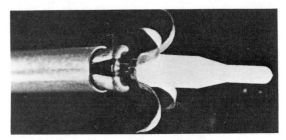

Fig. 9-5. Hosseinian's polyethylene plug.

occlusion with the Mark 7 P-block was attempted in 35 women in an outpatient setting. All subjects were pretreated with terbutaline 0.25 mg before the administration of a paracervical block containing mepivacaine hydrochloride. Carbon dioxide was utilized for uterine distention. Application of both devices required 10 to 15 minutes. The patients reported negligible discomfort, and there have been no significant intraoperative or postoperative complications.

Bilateral tubal occlusion was possible in only 15 of the 35 women on the first attempt. Reasons given for failure of plug placement included anatomic factors such as narrowed tubal orifices or sharply bent intramural tubal segments. Four women conceived, in each case within 2 months of plug insertion. No tubal pregnancies have been reported. Hysterosalpingograms are planned to evaluate the incidence of tubal closure in cases where the plugs were successfully placed. A change in the size of the device to accommodate a narrower tubal orifice is planned.

Ceramic Plugs

Craft [7] evaluated the tubal occlusive properties of ceramic plugs in a limited number of studies utilizing rabbits and human volunteers (Fig. 9-4). Fifteen human subjects had attempts at plug placement at hysteroscopy with Hyskon utilized for uterine distention under general anesthesia immediately before hysterectomy performed for gynecologic disease. Ten women had successful bilateral plug placement. In the remaining five cases satisfactory plug placement was impossible secondary to technical problems preventing proper alignment of the introducer with the tubal ostia. One uterine perforation was encountered.

Craft felt that improvements in hysteroscopic instrumentation with some provision for endoscope steerability were required to increase the accuracy of

insertion. There has been little recent investigation of the ceramic plug device.

Polyethylene Plug

Hosseinian et al. [19] designed a polyethylene plug that measured approximately 10 mm in length with a diameter of 1 mm at the tip and 2 mm at the base. Four metallic spines are attached to the base of the plug by an assembly screw (Fig. 9-5); these function to fit the plug in place by penetrating the adjacent myometrium. A specially designed instrument, inserted through the operating channel of the hysteroscope, is used to place the devices.

Before initiating human studies, 21 procedures were successfully completed in baboons. The animals were allowed to mate, and successful contraception for 8 consecutive months was recorded. Eight of 15 baboons conceived after hysteroscopic removal of the device, achieving a total of 12 pregnancies.

Hysteroscopic placement of the devices was undertaken in 33 human volunteers for a period of up to 6 months. No adverse side effects were observed during the 6 months of observation. Effective closure was achieved in 91 percent of the tubes; one pregnancy occurred. After removal of the plugs from 20 women, 90 percent of the tubes showed tubal patency. All these women subsequently underwent hysterectomy. Histologic studies showed moderate tissue reaction around the anchoring spines. Distention of the tubal lumen and flattening of the endosalpinx were also observed [19].

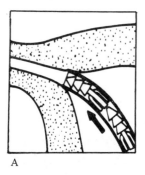
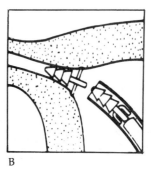
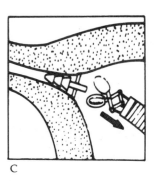

A   B   C

Fig. 9-6. Diagrammatic representation of placement of Sugimoto's preformed silicone plug.

Preformed Silicone Plugs

Sugimoto [44], after having considerable experience with electrocoagulation of the tubal ostia, turned to evaluation of a mechanical blocking device of his own design (Fig. 9-6). The intratubal device (ITD) is made of silicone rubber and is packed in advance into an introducer made of Teflon tubing 1.5 mm in diameter. An obturator wire pushes the plug out of the introducer into the tubal ostia under direct hysteroscopic visualization. When 32 patients underwent hysterosalpingograms before undergoing hysterectomy, bilateral tubal occlusion was confirmed if the devices had been exactly fitted [41]. No long-term follow-up studies have appeared in the literature regarding this seemingly promising technique.

Nylon Intratubal Device

Hamou [16] has recently initiated human trials of nylon plugs placed in the tubal ostia with the use of the colpomicrohysteroscope [15]. The device is made of surgical nylon, is inert, and is radiopaque. Placement of the device is accomplished during an outpatient visit, utilizing no anesthesia. Carbon dioxide is utilized for uterine distension.

The device has an open loop at each extremity to prevent migration within the tube or into the uterine cavity. Each loop has an elastic "memory." Once the distal portion is in the tubal isthmus, it will expand (Fig. 9-7). The midpiece, measuring 23 mm in length and 1 mm in diameter, is flexible and permits negotiation of the interstitial portion of the tube. Removal of the plug is easily effected by traction on the proximal loop.

To this date 57 patients have had the procedure attempted. Successful plug placement was accomplished in 49 (86%) at the initial attempt. Three patients had a unilateral ITD inserted with intrauterine bleeding impairing visualization of the opposite tubal ostia. These

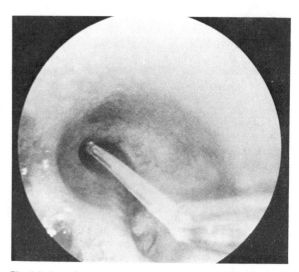

Fig. 9-7. Introduction of Hamou's nylon intratubal device.

patients had repeat procedures 1 month later and had a successful device placement.

Fifty-one patients who had a successful procedure underwent repeat hysteroscopy one month following the initial attempt. In 46 cases both devices remained properly in place. In three cases a unilateral device was found expelled into the uterine cavity, and two patients lost an ITD during subsequent menstruation. Each of these patients had a repeat procedure to replace the expelled device; however, in three cases expulsion recurred.

Side effects appear to be minimal, although one patient required plug removal soon after the procedure because of unremitting pelvic pain. There have been no reports of intrauterine or ectopic pregnancies in patients wearing these devices.

Formed-In-Place Silicone Rubber Plug

Corfman and Taylor [6] were the first to suggest occlusion of the oviducts with silicone rubber. Soon after, several investigators [17, 30] carried out experiments infusing catalyzed viscous silicone rubber into the uteri of animals. A research and development program to design a system and application technique for a nonincisional method blocking the fallopian with medical-grade silicone rubber was initiated by Robert Erb in 1971 [11]. Prototype instruments were developed for the mixing and delivery of high-viscosity silicone to the fallopian tubes by hysteroscopic techniques. Effective instillation of oviductal plugs was accomplished initially in New Zealand white rabbits by direct visualization. Subsequent studies with extirpated human uteri indicated that custom-fitted oviductal plugs could be instilled effectively [12].

Under hysteroscopic control, catalyzed liquid silicone polymer flows into the oviduct through a silicone rubber obturator tip positioned at the tubal ostium (Fig. 9-8). The formed-in-place plug becomes bonded to the obturator tip. The resulting flexible structure is larger in diameter at both ends than it is in the isthmus and thus remains in place to achieve tubal occlusion.

Erb postulated that the formed-in-place plug would have the following advantages: (1) It is not deliberately destructive or adhesive to the tubal tissues, and (2) its occluding member does not force the tissue to conform to its shape but rather assumes the shape of the tubal lumen [12]. The initial human study consisted of nine prehysterectomy patients who had plug instillation immediately before the surgical removal of the uterus and fallopian tubes. Histologic examination of the fallopian tubes revealed no abnormalities related to the instillation of the plugs. Clinical trials in human subjects desiring sterilization began in 1978 [21, 31–33, 35].

The specialized instruments developed for this procedure include (1) the guide assembly with obturator tip (Fig. 9-8); (2) the mixer-dispenser syringe; and (3) the fluid-flow actuator pump (Fig. 9-9).

The guide assembly catheter, composed of two concentric polyvinyl catheters, is passed through the operating channel of the hysteroscope and conveys the liquid silicone composition to the tubal ostium through the obturator tip. It also allows for the remote separation of the obturator tip from the cured silicone in the catheter guide assembly. The premolded obturator tip, made of Dow-Corning Silastic 382 medical-grade elastimer (75%) and spherical silver powder (25%), is positioned at the end of the catheter guide assembly. It accomplishes a sealing action at the tubal ostium, preventing escape of the liquid silicone during its infusion into the tubal lumen. The basic obturator tip is approximately 2 mm in diameter and 5 mm in length; however,

E-1   E-2   E-3   E-4   R-1   C-1

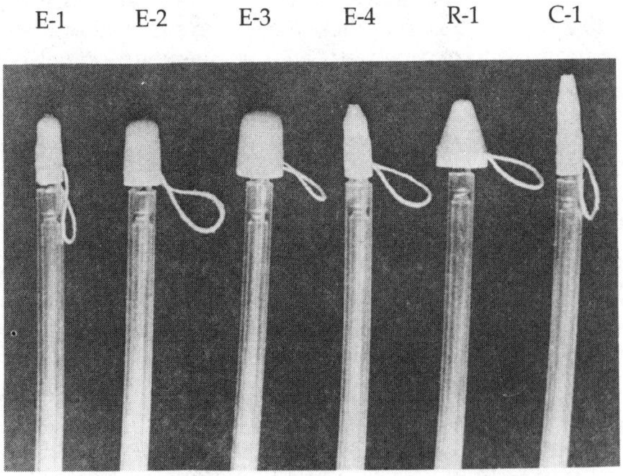

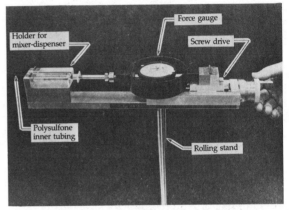

Fig. 9-8. Alternate obturator tips available for use in formed-in-place silicone plug procedure.

Fig. 9-9. Fluid-flow actuator pump utilized for infusing silicone for tubal occlusion procedure.

alternate obturator tip sizes and configurations are available to accommodate variations in anatomy at the uterotubal junction (Fig. 9-8). A retrieval loop is imbedded into the obturator tip to allow for possible removal of the plug.

The non-air-entraining mixer-dispenser allows one to mix thoroughly a small quantity of catalyst (stannous octoate) with the very viscous silicone material in a short time (35 seconds) without introducing any air.

The fluid-flow actuator is used to effect flow of the catalyzed silicone composition through the guide assembly into the tubal ostia. This cannot be accomplished by direct manual handling of the mixer-dispenser syringe because of the high viscosity of the fluid (about 10,000 times the viscosity of water).

The procedure is accomplished in an office setting utilizing paracervical block anesthesia. A standard operating hysteroscope with a 4-mm diameter operating channel is utilized. Hyskon is used to distend the endometrial cavity. A single roentgenogram is obtained following the procedure. Because the silicone material is silver impregnated, the plugs are radiopaque and are easily seen and evaluated on the roentgenogram.

No two patients will have identical plugs, owing to the unique method in which the plugs are formed. However, there are valid hysteroscopic and radiologic characteristics that allow appropriate categorization of plugs (Fig. 9-10). The major characteristic of a normal plug is a "dumbbell" configuration with continuity between a thick obturator tip at the ostium; a thinner isthmic portion, and a bulbous distal portion (Fig. 9-11).

Of the 415 women who had an attempted tubal occlusion procedure in one series [5], 328 had a "successful" procedure in which normal plugs were placed, a "satisfactory" postprocedure roentgenogram demonstrating normal plugs, and a "satisfactory" postprocedure roentgenogram at 3 months.

Unremitting tubal spasm was responsible for an unsuccessful procedure in 24 of the 415 patients (5.8%). Intrauterine blood or fragments obscuring clear visualization of tubal ostia prevented a successful tubal occlusion procedure in 30 of 415 patients (7.2%). Inability to achieve parallel axis between the catheter and the tubal ostia resulted in a failed procedure in 17 of 415 patients (4.1%).

There have been no major complications. Hospitalization or additional surgery as a result of the sterilization procedure has been unnecessary. There have been no intrauterine or tubal pregnancies in the group of 328 patients who had normal plugs placed and who had a normal 3-month postprocedure roentgenogram.

In almost every case there is hysteroscopic or radiologic evidence that clearly distinguishes the normal from the abnormal plug. Correct interpretation of the roentgenogram of the pelvis is the determining factor (Fig. 9-11), minimizing the need for more expensive and time-consuming hysterosalpingography.

PROBLEMS COMMON TO ALL HYSTEROSCOPIC STERILIZATION TECHNIQUES

Regardless of the techniques employed, all hysteroscopic sterilization techniques must cope with or overcome several common problems.

Uterotubal spasm is often found at the time of hysteroscopy. Unfortunately, in the majority of cases the etiology remains unclear. It is impossible to accurately predict those patients in whom spasm will be a prob-

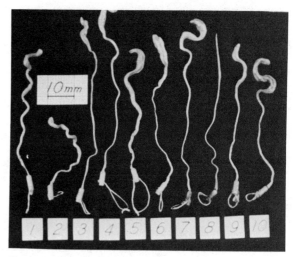

Fig. 9-10. Variations of normal formed-in-place plugs. All are normal except for number 8.

lem. In most cases it is temporary in nature with spontaneous remission allowing for proper tubal obturation. Smooth muscle relaxants, beta mimetic agents, and anti-prostaglandin medications have all been suggested as having a beneficial effect in either preventing or alleviating tubal spasm [2, 5, 21].

Inadequate intrauterine visualization resulting from mucus, blood, and endometrial fragments is another common problem experienced by the hysteroscopist. Visualization of the tubal ostia is clearly superior during the proliferative phase of the menstrual cycle. An aid available to the hysteroscopist is the use of suction aspiration of the endometrial cavity with a plastic tubing inserted through the operating channel of the hysteroscope. Judicious use of this technique can dramatically improve intrauterine visualization.

Unsuspected intrauterine pathology can be expected to be found in a small percentage of women desiring sterilization who are free of gynecologic complaints [4]. Polyps, intramural myomata, synechiae, and uterine structural abnormalities can sometimes interfere with clear visualization, thereby preventing the performance of a successful sterilization procedure.

Of paramount importance in achieving clear intrauterine visualization is the distending medium utilized. Increased endometrial vascularity and edema as well as significant transtubal flow of carbon dioxide into the peritoneal cavity with diaphragmatic irritation make carbon dioxide less desirable for a procedure of longer duration. Similarly, for longer procedures 5% dextrose in water appears not to be as effective in allowing clear visualization. Because Hyskon has the unique

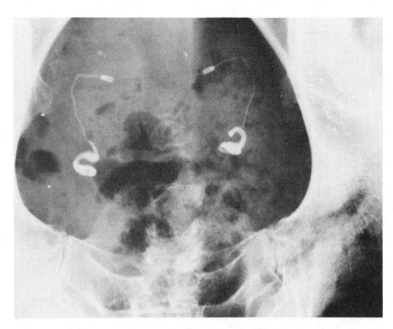

Fig. 9-11. Roentgenogram showing two normally formed, normally placed formed-in-place silicone plugs.

property of being immiscible with blood, it has been used for uterine distention in patients undergoing procedures lasting as long as 80 minutes.

Maintenance of adequate intrauterine distention is of major importance in achieving visualization and obturation of tubal ostia. This is often difficult in cases where the cervix is patulous. Escape of the distending medium allows for collapse of the endometrial cavity, making proper visualization difficult or impossible.

Inability to obtain proper alignment between the instrument responsible for tubal obturation and the tubal ostia is another common problem in all hysteroscopic sterilization procedures (Fig. 9-12). Brueschke and his coworkers [1] developed a steerable fiberoptic hysteroscope by utilizing an imaging fiberoptic bundle instead of a rigid lens system as found in rigid hysteroscopes (Fig. 9-13). The distal tip of the hysteroscope is flexible so that it can be moved transversely across an arc of 180 degrees without moving the entire instrument. It has the additional advantages of being electrically insulated as well as completely sealed to allow for total immersion in water or sterilizing solutions. Disadvantages of the instrument are its weight (1.5 lb) and its limited vision when compared with standard rigid hysteroscopes. Although adequate, vision is inferior to that possible with nonflexible endoscopes, which make use of rigid lenses rather than an imaging fiberoptic bundle.

These disadvantages resulted in the instrument receiving minimal use after 1977.

PRACTICAL CONSIDERATIONS LIMITING THE DEVELOPMENT OF HYSTEROSCOPIC STERILIZATION TECHNIQUES

A clear knowledge of the anatomy and function of the oviduct is helpful in appreciating the difficulty in designing a reliable hysteroscopic sterilization procedure.

The length of the oviduct varies from 6 to 15 cm. On the basis of its anatomy, the oviduct is divided into the infundibulum, ampulla, isthmus, and intramural segment. The diameter of the tubal lumen undergoes a reduction of up to 95 percent from 2 cm at the fimbrial ostium to 100 microns in the interstitial segment [9]. The thickness of the myosalpinx is greatest in areas where the luminal diameter is smallest. This relationship reaches an extreme at the level of the intramural segment, in which a threadlike lumen is surrounded by a massive thickness of muscle. The constricted lumen and limited compliance of the intramural segment of the oviduct offer additional barriers to effective sterilization techniques. When nonviscous materials are used, spillage into the peritoneal cavity with resulting chemical peritonitis is difficult to avoid. If viscous or rapidly

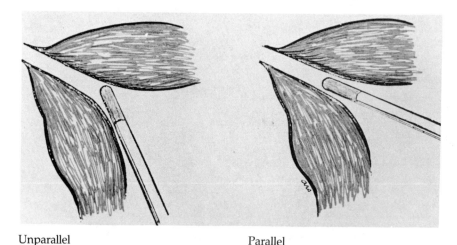

Unparallel   Parallel

Fig. 9-12. Schematic illustration of parallel and lack of parallel axis between catheter and tubal ostia.

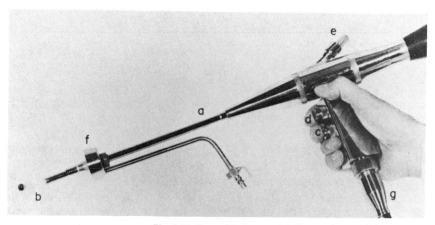

Fig. 9-13. Brueschke's steerable hysteroscope.

polymerizing material is used to achieve sterilization, unacceptably high intrauterine pressures may be required to allow these substances to pass into the tubal lumen. Rapid injection at high pressure could lead to embolization of the material into the vasculature surrounding the oviductal lumen.

During periods of spontaneous muscle activity or vascular distention, the intramural tubal lumen may be physiologically narrowed and resistant to the passage of material. Attempts to force material through this area under pressure might induce spasm and edema [9].

The ampulla with its thin myosalpinx is highly compliant. It may be passively distended 3 to 4 times its normal diameter without a concomitant increase in in-

traluminal pressure. In contrast, the isthmus and intramural segments, with thick myosalpinx, are less compliant. To be effective, occlusive intraluminal material or devices should totally occlude the lumen and remain in place. Tubal compliance works against this.

Hysteroscopic procedures, which are designed to damage and destroy the functional integrity of the intramural oviductal lumen, depend on sufficient tissue destruction to allow replacement by nonfunctional scar tissue, which occludes the lumen. The anatomy of the oviduct tends to minimize trauma and to promote healing. The oviduct, particularly the intramural segment, is surrounded by a rich vasculature. This minimizes trauma induced by thermal energy and also supports rapid healing, regrowth, and restoration of function with minimal scarring.

In severely traumatized oviducts chronic inflammation may lead to the reestablishment of patency through delayed formation of tubouterine fistulas. Such an explanation would substantiate the higher than anticipated number of tubal pregnancies following cauterization of the intramural tubal segment [9].

Reversibility of hysteroscopic sterilization is contingent upon the extent of tubal destruction. Techniques that achieve sterilization by means of thermal or chemical cauterization discourage the potential for reversibility because of the extensive tissue insult necessary to prevent tissue regeneration. However, intraluminal plugs may offer promise of reversibility. If such devices totally occlude the lumen without inducing significant damage, removal might result in reestablished fertility without the need for major surgical repair [9].

FUTURE OF HYSTEROSCOPIC STERILIZATION PROCEDURES

The ideal sterilization procedure should be safe as well as effective. It should be applicable to ambulatory patients with the use of local anesthesia or without anesthesia, since many of the complications that relate to sterilization procedures are complications that occur with the use of anesthetic agents. It should be socially and personally acceptable; it should be inexpensive and applicable to large numbers of patients; and it should be potentially reversible in the event of a change in desire for fertility potential on the part of the patient [41]. A sterilization procedure that fulfills all these requirements has not yet been developed. Theoretically, hysteroscopic sterilization techniques have a clear advantage over traditional sterilization approaches because they can be accomplished without major surgery or general anesthesia. For this reason there is a renewed interest in developing a highly efficacious and safe hysteroscopic method of tubal closure.

Recent attention has focused on the concept of mechanically blocking or occluding the oviducts with intratubal devices. Hosseinian's UTJD [19, 20], Hamou's ITD [15, 16], and Erb's formed-in-place silicone plug [11–13] seem to be the most promising of these newer occlusive designs. Although this technique appears to be both safe and effective, significant limitations exist that may prevent or delay widespread application and acceptance of this promising procedure. One major disadvantage is the need for sophisticated equipment and technology. Another limitation is the time demand on the physician and the assistant: The average procedure requires 70 to 90 minutes of assistant time and 30 to 50 minutes of physician time. An additional concern is the

potential for inadvertent disruption of "normal" plugs at the time of the diagnostic dilatation and curettage, should this be indicated at some later date. Preceding the dilatation and curettage with a diagnostic hysteroscopy might obviate this potential.

Undoubtedly, one of the major reasons for the increased interest in hysteroscopic sterilization is the potential for later reversibility, but there has been no clinical experience in human subjects with the purposeful reversal of the tubal occlusion procedure with formed-in-place plugs. The potential of a new technology, such as reliably reversible sterilization, cannot be accurately predicted. The increasing use and current popularity of essentially irreversible sterilization suggests, however, that the impact of an easily reversible technique would be even greater.

Hysteroscopic sterilization techniques will not likely be as universally applicable as are traditional sterilization procedures, most particularly laparoscopic sterilization. Unsuspected intrauterine or tubal pathology, unremitting tubal spasm, laterally positioned tubal ostia, and endometrial bleeding or fragmentation contribute to the possibility of an unsuccessful procedure. Improvements in instrumentation and technique as well as the identification of medications to prevent or control tubal spasm are reasonable future expectations. However, the application of hysteroscopic sterilization procedures to more than 90 percent of an unselected patient population is unrealistic.

REFERENCES

1. Brueschke, E. E., Saneveld, L. J. D., and Wilbands, G. D. A Steerable Hysteroscope and Mechanical Tubal Occlusive Devices. In J. J. Sciarra, W. Droegemueller, and J. J. Speidel (eds.), *Advances in Female Sterilization Techniques.* Hagerstown, Md.: Harper & Row, 1976.

2. Brundin, J. Hydrogel Tubal Blocking Device: P-Block. In G. I. Zatuchni, et al. (eds.), *Female Transcervical Sterilization.* Philadelphia: Lippincott, 1983.

3. Cooper, J. M., and Houck, R. M. Study Protocol, Criteria, and Complications of the Silicone Plug Procedure. In G. I. Zatuchni, et al. (eds.), *Female Transcervical Sterilization.* Philadelphia: Lippincott, 1983.

4. Cooper, J. M., Houck, R. M., and Rigberg, H. S. The incidence of intrauterine abnormalities found at hysteroscopy in patients undergoing elective hysteroscopic sterilization for abnormal uterine bleeding. *J. Reprod. Med.* 128:659, 1983.

5. Cooper, J. M., Houck, R. M., and Rigberg, R. S. Hysteroscopic tubal occlusion with formed-in-place silicone plugs: A clinical study. *Obstet. Gynecol.* 62:587, 1983.

6. Corfman, P. A., and Taylor, H. C. An instrument for

transcervical treatment of the oviduct and uterine cornua. *Obstet. Gynecol.* 27:880, 1966.

7. Craft, I. Utero-Tubal Ceramic Plugs. In J. J. Sciarra, W. Droegemueller, and J. J. Speidel (eds.), *Advances in Female Sterilization Techniques.* Hagerstown, Md.: Harper & Row, 1976.

8. Darabi, K. F., Roy, K., and Richart, R. M. Collaborative Study on Hysteroscopic Sterilization Procedures: Final Report. In J. J. Sciarra, G. I. Zatuchni, and J. J. Speidel (eds.), *Risks, Benefits, and Controversies in Fertility Control.* Hagerstown, Md.: Harper & Row, 1978.

9. Eddy, C. A., and Pauerstein, C. J. Anatomic and Physiologic Factors Affecting the Development of Transcervical Sterilization Techniques. In G. I. Zatuchni, et al. (eds.), *Female Transcervical Sterilization.* Philadelphia: Lippincott, 1983.

10. Edström, A., and Fernström, I. The diagnostic possibilities of modified hysteroscopic technique. *Acta Obstet. Gynecol. Scand.* 49:327, 1970.

11. Erb, R. A. Apparatus and Method for the Hysteroscopic Nonsurgical Sterilization of Females. United States Patent 4,245,623, 1981.

12. Erb, R. A. Silastic Tubal Plugs: Instruments and Technique. In G. I. Zatuchni, et al. (eds.), *Female Transcervical Sterilization.* Philadelphia: Lippincott, 1983.

13. Erb, R. A., and Reed, T. P. Hysteroscopic oviductal blocking with formed-in-place silicone rubber plugs: Method and apparatus. *J. Reprod. Med.* 23:65, 1979.

14. Friorep, R. Zur Vorbengung der Nothwendigkeit des Kaiserschnitts und der Perforation. Notiz Gerburtshilfe Natur-Uno Heilkd 11:9, 1849.

15. Hamou, J. Hysteroscopy and microhysteroscopy with a new instrument: The micro-hysteroscope. *Acta Eur. Fertil.* 12:1, 1981.

16. Hamou J. Hysteroscopic Tubal Occlusion with Nylon Intratubal Device. Presented to the American Association of Gynecologic Laparoscopists, Annual Meeting, San Diego, 1982.

17. Hefnawi, F., Fuchs, A. R., and Laurence, A. A. Control of fertility by temporary occlusion of the oviduct. *Am. J. Obstet. Gynecol.* 99:421, 1967.

18. Heineberg, A. Uterine endoscopy: An aid to precision in the diagnosis of intra-uterine disease. *Surg. Gynecol. Obstet.* 18:513, 1914.

19. Hosseinian, A. H., Lucero, S., and Kim, M. H. Hysteroscopic Implantation of Utero-Tubal Junction Blocking Devices. In J. J. Sciarra, W. Droegemueller, and J. J. Speidel (eds.), *Advances in Female Sterilization Techniques.* Hagerstown, Md.: Harper & Row, 1976.

20. Hosseinian, A. H., and Morales, W. A. Clinical Application of Hysteroscopic Sterilization Utilizing Utero-Tubal Junction Blocking Devices. In G. I. Zatuchni, et al. *Female Transcervical Sterilization.* Philadelphia: Lippincott, 1983.

21. Houck, R. M., and Cooper, J. M. Hysteroscopic tubal oc-

clusion with formed-in-place silicone plugs: A clinical study. *Obstet. Gynecol.* 60:641, 1982.

22. Lindemann, H. J., and Mohr, J. Tuben Sterilisation Per Hysteroskop. *Sex. Med.* 3:122, 1974.

23. Lindemann, H. J., and Mohr, J. CO_2 hysteroscopy: Diagnosis and treatment. *Am. J. Obstet. Gynecol.* 124:129, 1976.

24. Menken, F. S. Eine Neves Verfahren Mit Vorrichtung Zur Hysteroskopie. *Endoscopy* 3:200, 1971.

25. Norment, W. B., and Sikes, H. Fiber-optic hysteroscopy: An improved method for viewing the interior of the uterus. *N.C. Med. J.* 31:251, 1970.

26. Pantaleoni, D. Cited by T. Silander in Hysteroscopy through a transparent rubber balloon in patients with carcinoma of the uterine endometrium. *Acta Obstet. Gynecol. Scand.* 42:284, 1963.

27. Porto, R., and Serment, H. Pneumo-hysteroscopie. *Gaz. Med. France* 80:4985, 1973.

28. Quinones, R., Alvarado, A., and Ley, E. Hysteroscopic sterilization. *Int. J. Gynaecol. Obstet.* 16:27, 1976.

29. Quinones, R., Gallegos, L., and Ley, E. Personal communication, 1982.

30. Rakshit, B. Attempts at chemical blocking of the fallopian tube for female sterilization. *J. Obstet. Gynecol. India* 20:618, 1970.

31. Reed, T. P., and Erb, R. A. Hysteroscopic oviductal blocking with formed-in-place silicone rubber plugs: II. Clinical studies. *J. Reprod. Med.* 23:69, 1979.

32. Reed, T. P., and Erb, R. A. Tubal occlusion with silicone rubber: An update. *J. Reprod. Med.* 25:25, 1980.

33. Reed, T. P., and Erb, R. A. Hysteroscopic Female Sterilization with Formed-In-Place Silicone Rubber Plugs. In J. M. Phillips (ed.), *Endoscopic Female Sterilization: A Comparison of Methods.* Downey, Calif. American Association of Gynecologic Laparoscopists, 1982.

34. Reed, T. P., Erb, R. A., and Demaeyer, J. Tubal occlusion with silicone rubber: Update 1980. *J. Reprod. Med.* 26:534, 1981.

35. Richart, R. M., et al. Evaluation of polymer flock and metal alloy intratubal device in pig-tailed monkeys. *Contraception* 18:459, 1978.

36. Rimkus, B., and Semm, K. Hysteroscopic sterilization: A routine method? *Int. J. Fertil.* 22:121, 1977.

37. Rubin, I. C. Uterine endoscopy, endometroscopy with the aid of uterine insufflation. *Am. J. Obstet. Gynecol.* 10:313, 1925.

38. Schneider, T. Problem of the tubal sphincter. *A.J.R.* 48:527, 1942.

39. Schroeder, C. Uber den Avsbau und die Leistungen der Hysteroskopie. *Arch. Gynecol.* 156:407, 1934.

40. Proceedings of The Program For Applied Research on Fertility Regulation, Minneapolis, Minnesota. In J. J. Sciarra, J. C. Butler, and J. J. Speidel (eds.), *Hysteroscopic Sterilization.* New York: Intercontinental Medical Books, 1974.

41. Sciarra, J. J. Hysteroscopic Approaches for Tubal Closure.

In G. I. Zatuchni, M. H. Labbok, and J. J. Sciarra (eds.), *Research Frontiers in Fertility Regulation.* Hagerstown, Md.: Harper & Row, 1980.

42. Siegler, A. M., and Grunebaum, A. The 100th anniversary of tubal sterilization. *Fertil. Steril.* 34:610, 1980.

43. Silander, T. Hysteroscopy through a transparent rubber balloon. *Surg. Gynecol. Obstet.* 114:125, 1962.

44. Sugimoto, O. Hysteroscopic Sterilization by Electrocoagulation. In J. J. Sciarra, J. C. Butler, and J. J. Speidel (eds.), *Hysteroscopic Sterilization.* New York: Intercontinental Medical Books, 1974.

45. Sweeney, W. J. The interstitial portion of the uterine tube: Its gross anatomy, course, and length. *Obstet. Gynecol.* 19:3, 1962.

10. Vasectomy

Joseph E. Davis

Vasectomy, or more exactly, vas sectioning and occlusion, has become a popular elective procedure for permanent male contraception in the United States, Asia, and parts of Europe. Though cultural barriers to its acceptance currently exist in other parts of the world, vasectomy has been introduced into Africa, Latin America, and the Middle East. In spite of predictions that men would not accept the procedure for fear of lost masculinity or castration, reports indicate that when properly presented, men in all societies welcome the procedure when their concern for limitation of family size and economic and educational advancement outweighs their desire for more children, and where concern for risks of maternal morbidity and female contraceptive method failure are overriding considerations.

As with many other contraceptive methods for which popularity and acceptance preceded thorough scientific understanding of effects and sequelae, so the effects of vasectomy on the proximal genital tract have come under scrutiny by serious investigators only in the past 10 years. Prospective studies of vasectomized and matched controls have not revealed significant differences in chemical or endocrine parameters. Epidemiologic studies to date have revealed no increased tendency toward vascular disease or heart attack in vasectomized men as compared with age-matched controls [15, 16, 29, 38–40].

Although the techniques for female sterilization have become increasingly simpler and safer, vasectomy has nonetheless been extremely popular in the United States since 1965. It is estimated that more than 250,000 men have the operation yearly. According to the Association for Voluntary Sterilization, more than 5 million men in the United States have had a vasectomy.

As the demand for voluntary male and female sterilization has grown, governments have begun to remove the remaining legal restrictions. In 1972 United States courts struck down the last state law prohibiting sterilization. Since then, the poor have been able to obtain free or inexpensive operations through Medicaid or state health funds. The only restriction on the use of government money for sterilization is that the person involved must give informed consent, be 21, and be legally competent.

In most countries of the industrialized world sterilization is legal or unregulated. Sterilization is a government-sponsored family planning method in Thailand and the Philippines. The only nations where sterilizations are still prohibited or difficult to obtain are located in sub–Sahara Africa and the Arab world.

The First International Conference on Vasectomy (see Appendix 10-1) was held in Colombo in October 1982 under the sponsorship of Sri Lanka's Ministry of Plan Implementation and the World Federation of Health Agencies for the Advancement of Voluntary

Surgical Contraception. The conference, attended by 67 people from 24 countries, produced a plan of action that states that "vasectomy is one of the safer and most effective methods of contraception and is even safer and more widely deliverable than female methods of sterilization." The highest vasectomy rate is found in the United States, where about 17 percent of married men aged 35 to 44 have had a vasectomy, but interest in vasectomy is growing worldwide among both consumers and providers of services.

The long-term health effects of vasectomy prompted considerable discussion. A 1975 report of the atherosclerotic effect of vasectomy in cynomolgus monkeys gave rise to widespread concern, and the acceptance of vasectomy decreased as a result [2]. The Colombo conference reviewed several published and unpublished reports on research to determine if this effect occurs in man; all have produced negative results, and the conference found in these reports "reassuring evidence that long-term ill effects are not associated with vasectomy" [15, 16, 24, 30, 39, 40].

The process leading to a decision for or against vasectomy appears to be remarkably similar in different countries, including the United States, Bangladesh, Australia, Mexico, and Brazil. Not all men are good candidates for vasectomy. Those who make poor candidates are often unable to distinguish between their own perceptions of satisfactory sexual performance and the ability to impregnate. Vasectomy may be accepted intellectually but not emotionally, and emotional rejection can be a bar to an honest appraisal of this birth-control method. Managers of services—vasectomists and counselors—may also fail to make this distinction. Most participants at the Colombo conference felt that uncertainty among providers could, in part, explain why in many countries vasectomy is not more generally available and that this factor should be considered when program staffs are selected and trained.

Studies and experience from countries in every region of the world show that men will accept vasectomies despite commonly held assumptions about male attitudes or about the effect of perceived religious prohibitions. Local demand for vasectomy can best be assessed by attitude surveys and by asking men what specific services they seek. The most important factor in a man's decision to accept vasectomy is contact with men who have undergone this procedure and are satisfied with it. Programs should exploit this fact. Thorough counseling and postoperative reassurance seem to be two of the most important ways to ensure satisfaction.

The conference found that when vasectomy is made available in centers of excellence in those areas where vasectomy is thought to be unacceptable, demand can be surprisingly high. For example, the men-only Propater Clinic in Sao Paulo, Brazil, had done 1,500 vasectomies in 19 months and is now performing 150 procedures a month. Yet the clinic has, to date, been advertised only by word-of-mouth. Data from this center indicate that about half of the men were poor and had completed 6 or fewer years of school. Forty-seven percent of the men had one or two living children; over two-fifths had at least one unwanted child, and 28 percent stated that their wives had already had at least one abortion.

The conference concluded that, while monitoring and research should continue, vasectomy is one of the safest and most effective methods of fertility control and should be made easily available as a part of health and family planning services everywhere.

In the late 1890s the clinical uses of vasectomy were explored by surgeons in conjunction with operations on the prostate. Ochsner performed such operations in 1897 and reported in the *Journal of the American Medical Association*, April 22, 1899, that no change whatever had been noted in the sex lives of his patients following successful vasectomies. Although the operation gained in popularity over the years, it was the consensus among physicians that a vasectomy, once done, was irreversible. However, in 1945 an accidental vasectomy during a hernia repair led to the first attempt to rejoin the vas. Following this attempt, other surgeons reported cases of vasovasotomy with return of sperm to the ejaculate, even when the vasectomy had been performed several years earlier. Perhaps this is one reason why the popularity of vasectomy for contraception has increased sharply in the past decades.

The Association for Voluntary Sterilization estimates that 75 percent of all voluntary sterilizations performed in the United States during 1970 were vasectomies, which represented a considerable upward trend in male sterilization from 10 years earlier when 60 percent of all voluntary sterilizations were performed on the female [41].

Most men in the United States requesting vasectomies are over age 30, have two or three children, and have utilized other forms of contraception. Some couples have found other methods inconvenient, while others may have suffered ill effects related to oral contraceptives, pelvic infections associated with uterine devices, or the psychologic and/or economic consequences of contraceptive failure, necessitating abortions or continued unplanned pregnancies.

Whereas failure rates of temporary methods of contraception are additive year by year, the 0.1 percent chance of recanalization decreases after the first year of vasectomy to virtually zero, making it, along with closure of the female tubes, the most effective method of permanent contraception [44].

BIOLOGY OF THE VAS

Anatomy

The vas deferens is easily palpable in the scrotum as a portion of the spermatic cord. It is about 35 cm in length and extends from the tail of the epididymis to the prostate, where it forms, together with the duct of the seminal vesicle, the ejaculatory duct.

The vas deferens is composed of three layers of smooth muscle: the outer and inner longitudinal and middle circular layers. It is capable of powerful peristaltic motion. The lumen of the vas, like the tubules of the epididymis, is lined with epithelium lying on the basement membrane arranged with submucosal and longitudinal folds. There is a thick sheet of connective tissue exterior to the muscle layer. The vas deferens may be divided into five portions: (1) the sheathless epididymal portion contained within the tunica vaginalis, (2) the scrotal portion, (3) the inguinal division, (4) the retroperitoneal or pelvic division, and (5) the ampulla. The portion of the vas of clinical interest for vasectomy is generally the midscrotal area.

The blood supply of the vas deferens arises from the deferential artery, a branch of the inferior vesicle artery and an important collateral circulation mechanism for the testicle. It is also an important artery in terms of possible hemorrhage following vasectomy if it is not carefully separated from the sheath of the vas or suitably ligated or coagulated.

Histology

The human vas deferens is a firm tubular structure about 3 to 4 mm in diameter. It is composed of epithelial mucosa, surrounded by a thick muscular wall and adventitia. Collagen fibers are found interspersed in the muscle layers. The epididymis has two concentric smooth muscle layers that turn into three at the junction of the vas deferens. In turn, these muscle layers are surrounded by adventitia, which contains small branches of the inferior spermatic nerve and blood vessels.

The epithelium and lamina propria of the vas deferens are folded into 8 to 12 longitudinal ridges. The epithelium, which is pseudostratified, is composed predominantly of tall, thin principal cells extending from the base to the lumen and small, round pyramidal basal cells. The principal cells have long stereocilia on their luminal surfaces. Scanning microscopy has revealed that the vas mucosa is carpeted with microvilli, which appear particularly tortuous in man.

Innervation and Theories of Sperm Transport

Innervation of the vas consists of short adrenergic postganglionic neurons [8]. The nerves of the testis (i.e., the superior spermatic nerves) arise from the renal plexus and the intermesenteric nerves and travel in association with the testicular arteries, whereas the inferior spermatic nerves arise from the hypogastric plexus and course around and along the vas deferens to innervate the epididymis. In man the middle spermatic nerves arise from the hypogastric ganglia, whereas innervation to the testis is generally by classic long neurons. At the junction of the epididymis and the vas deferens the amount of adrenergic innervation increases. Histologic and pharmacologic studies indicate both adrenergic and cholinergic components. Adrenergic fibers are found in both longitudinal and circular muscles; these fibers are most likely the motor supply of the vas muscle.

Studies of the physiology and structure of the vas deferens indicate that generally the vasa from most species respond similarly. Stimulation of the hypogastric nerve causes the isolated duct to contract longitudinally. If the vas is bathed in noradrenaline, the intensity of the contraction increases [37]. If the tissue has been previously exposed to reserpine, the contractions diminish unless the nerve is again exposed to noradrenaline. Phentolamine blocks contractions. Exposure to guanethidine or bethanidine, which especially affect the short adrenergic neurons, greatly reduces or abolishes contractions. Thus, the pharmacologic evidence as well as the histochemical studies support adrenergic innervation [3].

The mechanism of sperm transport through the vas deferens is still not totally understood. The heavy smooth muscle layers equip the vas deferens for vigorous peristalsis. It is hypothesized that spermatic fluid could be transported by (1) pressure exerted by the epididymis, (2) peristalsis of the walls of the vas deferens, and (3) active contraction at ejaculation of the wall of the vas deferens constricting the lumen. A combination of these propulsion mechanisms is probable.

Though different theories are currently under consideration, the sequence of events in sperm transport probably include (1) continuous movement of spermatozoa through the cauda epididymis and vas deferens owing to peristalsis caused by contractions of the smooth muscle, (2) emission that involves a coordinated contractile wave from the epididymis to the urethra, (3) strong adrenergically caused contractions of the wall that push the majority of the sperm of each ejaculate through the vas deferens, and (4) propulsion of the sperm to the ampulla and urethra by short, powerful, adrenergically mediated contractions of possibly the cauda epididymis and certainly the vas deferens.

CONTRAINDICATIONS TO VASECTOMY

Although vasectomy is a simple operation that can be performed almost anywhere, the more removed the setting is from medical backup, the more important it is to screen out men who are at the highest risk of complications.

The major physical contraindications to vasectomy are local infections and systemic blood disorders. Local infections, which can prevent normal healing, are easily recognized and should be eradicated before the operation is performed. Other local conditions that make vasectomy more difficult to perform include inguinal hernia or previous surgery for hernia or orchiopexy, hydrocele, varicocele, preexisting scrotal lesions, or a thick, tough scrotum.

Systemic blood disorders that call for special precautions would include any disease (e.g., hemophilia) that interferes with normal blood clotting. In such cases the technique used should minimize tissue trauma, and emergency backup facilities should be available. The therapeutic use of anticoagulants may require some precautions. Other systemic diseases, such as diabetes or hypertension, are not contraindications to vasectomy but hospitalization in these cases may be advisable.

There is no physiologic basis for an adverse psychologic response to vasectomy. Although there is a paucity of reliable information on the subject, the available literature suggests that a normal, sexually well-adjusted male will experience no significant psychologic changes following elective sterilization if he understands what he can expect during and after the procedure and if he is given the opportunity to express his fears and have his questions answered in advance [13]. When psychologic problems do occur postoperatively, they usually stem from preoperative attitudes and conditions generally related to poor screening.

For the man with serious neuroses or sexual maladjustments, vasectomy may not be advisable. If professional counseling is available, vasectomy candidates with suspected emotional problems should be interviewed and evaluated individually. Tests measuring psychologic adjustment indicate that postoperative problems can usually be traced to preoperative ones [43, 44].

PREOPERATIVE COUNSELING AND PREPARATION

A patient's request for vasectomy must be made voluntarily and must be accompanied by written, educated, and informed consent. The operative permission must include statements that the man seeking sterilization was given (1) a fair explanation of the surgical procedure; (2) a description of the attendant discomforts and risks; (3) a description of the benefits to be expected; (4) an explanation concerning appropriate alternative methods of family planning and the effect and impact of the proposed sterilization, including the fact that it must be considered to be an irreversible procedure; (5) an offer to answer any inquiries concerning the procedure; and (6) information that the individual is free to withhold or withdraw consent to the procedure at any time before the sterilization.

In the counseling process special attention must be paid to the fact that sterility is not guaranteed, to the immediate physical effects of the procedure, and to the possible long-range psychologic reactions. Counseling may be done by a trained nonphysician; however, a physician must assume the responsibility for the content of the material provided by the counselor to the patient, for ascertaining that such counseling has been done before the performance of the procedure, for seeing that all the patient's questions have been satisfactorily answered, and for assuring that informed consent has been obtained.

Consent of the spouse is not required by law, but the inclusion of the spouse in the counseling and decision-making process is recommended when feasible. While there should be no rigid guidelines regarding the waiting period between the interview and the performance of the procedure, the physician should use his judgment based on evaluation of the patient (preferably the couple) as to a reasonable period in which the patient can reflect upon his decision. In general, a 2- to 3-week period is adequate, but this should be determined individually. The interview should include a general history, system review, attention to previous genital surgery, and any adverse reactions to drugs. Ideally, the patient should receive a complete physical examination following the interview. Attention should be paid to genital anomalies and individual characteristics such as associated hydrocele, undescended or retractile testes, scars, or thick scrotum, so that the surgeon may be prepared to manage them intraoperatively. In some instances the procedure may be best performed in the hospital under anesthesia. The patient should be instructed that the hair from the base of the penis extending onto the scrotum will require shaving before surgery. Blood count, bleeding and clotting time, urinalysis, and semen analysis determinations may be useful. Semen analysis should be performed if the vasectomy candidate has never caused a conception.

Preoperative sedation is not advised if the procedure is being performed on an outpatient basis. The outpatient facility should have available emergency equipment, including oxygen, epinephrine, steroids, and other agents, consistent with local standards of ambulatory surgery and local statutory and health code requirements.

TECHNIQUE

Several general statements should be made about vasectomy techniques. Palpation and isolation of the vas from the spermatic cord are the first steps in the performance of vasectomy—usually the vas can be identified as a firm cord, approximately 1 to 2 cm in diameter, quite unlike other structures of the spermatic cord. Relaxation of the scrotal wall can assist in this maneuver. A warm room and a relaxed patient are essential. The patient is usually apprehensive and appreciates reassurances and a friendly relaxed attitude on the part of the surgeon. Downward displacement of the testicle assists the surgeon in localizing the vas. Occasionally, a thick, tough scrotum is encountered; vas isolation is difficult and may incur added pain.

Though reversibility should not be in the mind of the patient (it is requested approximately once in 10,000 cases), it should be in the mind of the surgeon. Vasocclusion by simple interruption of vas continuity, closure of the proximal (testicular) end by fulguration of the mucosal surface [33], or compression by tantalum clip or suture [25] followed by fascial interposition describes the technique considered most acceptable today. The danger of damaging the vital sympathetic innervation of the vas by removing a segment of the vas and accompanying nerves exists. An intact nerve supply may be vital to the transport of sperm from the epididymis at the time of ejaculation, should reanastomosis be performed [14].

Other technical considerations that may improve chances of restoration of fertility include sectioning of the vas as high as possible from the convoluted portion, careful preservation of the vas sheath, and preservation of the artery of the vas. Silber [34] has suggested that fulguration of the distal end of the cut vas be performed rather than of the proximal end, so as to allow sperm leakage to occur. He feels that this will promote sperm leakage and sperm granuloma formation, thereby reducing intravasal and epididymal tubular pressure so as to prevent epididymal rupture. This practice, however, has not been accepted by others, since recent unpublished communications suggest a higher failure rate with "open-ended" vasectomy. Although an increasing number of surgeons favor the Schmidt technique of mucosal fulguration described above, there is no evidence that external compression, particularly with inert tantalum clips with fascial interposition, is in any way less effective or more apt to result in sperm granuloma or failure.

Routine resection of the vas for pathologic study is not essential or recommended unless demanded by institutional rules. The presence of two vas specimens does not substitute for determining the end point of azoospermia. Since the same vas might have been sectioned twice or double vas may be present, the patient may still be fertile despite the fact that two separate specimens have been sent to the laboratory. Conversely, if the laboratory cannot confirm the presence of vasa on microscopic examination, the patient may still have had a successful procedure, since tissue can be distorted in removal or lost in transit to the laboratory. All patients must be followed carefully until complete healing has occurred and azoospermia has been demonstrated, regardless of the pathology report.

Moreover, removal of a segment is no assurance that spontaneous recanalization cannot occur. This unfortunate complication, though rare, is more apt to be prevented by interposition of fascia between the cut ends of the vas and avoidance of the use of catgut suture material. There is also evidence that removing portions of the vas may damage its sympathetic innervation, making subsequent efforts to reestablish fertility less successful, even though continuity of the end is achieved.

The vas is grasped and fixed between thumb and middle fingers while injecting approximately 3 to 5 cc of local anesthetic into the scrotal skin, scrotal layers, and perivasal tissues in the upper scrotal portion of the vas (Fig. 10-1). Anesthetic effect is almost immediate.

Fig. 10-1. The vas is injected with procaine.

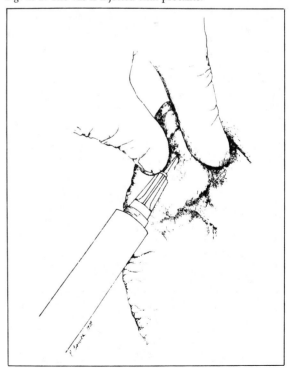

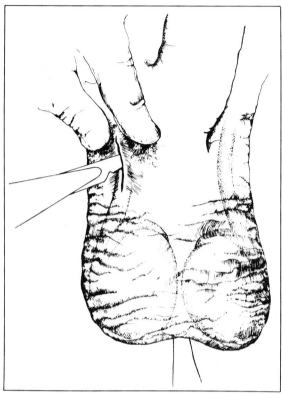

Fig. 10-2. The incision is made while the fingers are still grasping and fixing the vas.

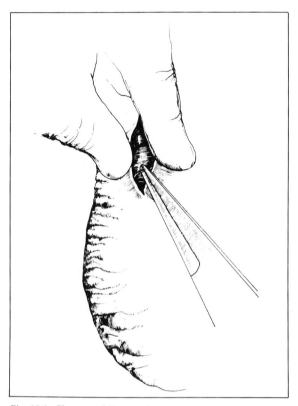

Fig. 10-3. Clamp and ligate subcutaneous bleeding points.

Fig. 10-4. The vas is grasped with an Allis clamp.

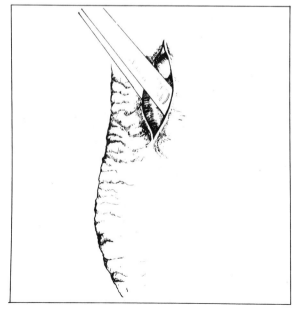

An incision is made with the fingers still grasping and fixing the vas (Fig. 10-2). A transverse incision is an acceptable alternative. The incision should be carried into the perivasal tissues.

It is important to clamp and ligate (or coagulate) subcutaneous bleeding points (Fig. 10-3). Attention to this operative detail will prevent hematomas, which can complicate the postoperative course.

The vas is grasped in its sheath (Fig. 10-4). With experience, the operator will learn how deep to make the initial incision, with the vas in a fixed position, so that the Allis or Babcock clamp can grasp the vas in its sheath with a minimal amount of overlying and surrounding tissues.

A vertical incision is made into the vas sheath (Fig. 10-5). Since the vas sheath will serve to provide tissue for a fascial barrier, care should be taken to define and separate the sheath from the vas itself. The definitive occluding procedure should not include the sheath but should be performed on the isolated vas. Once the sheath is opened, the vas can be readily immobilized by use of a second Allis clamp as illustrated in Figure 10-6.

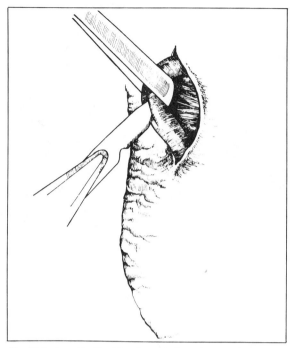

Fig. 10-5. A vertical incision is made into the vas sheath taking care to define and separate the sheath from the vas.

Fig. 10-6. The vas is immobilized using a second Allis clamp.

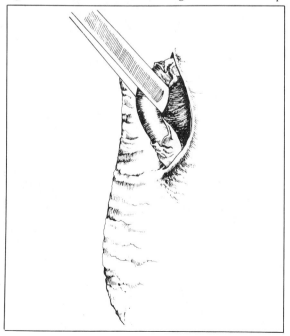

It may be advisable to place stay sutures in the vas sheath for future identification.

Two tantalum clips are applied to both the proximal and distal parts between which vas sectioning will be performed (Fig. 10-7A, B). The author prefers tantalum clips since they seem to cause less postoperative reaction and pain, and they are easy to apply.

Black silk or cotton sutures are a reasonable alternative but absorbable sutures should be avoided. Animal studies [21] suggest that clip migration can occur when a clip is applied to the vas in continuity. However, in over 1,000 reported vasectomies using this technique, there has been no evidence of this in the sectioned vas.

The vas sheath is then drawn over the distal end of the vas for fascial interposition (Fig. 10-7C). This maneuver is aided by the tendency of the distal vas (once clipped) to retract distally and is also assisted by drawing the proximal end forward, which further allows for ease in suturing over the distal end. A triple 0 chromic or triple 0 black silk suture is used for connective tissue interposition.

In the vas flush technique a blunt-tipped No. 23 gauge needle or attached polyethylene tubing can, with some practice, be inserted into the distal vas lumen (Fig. 10-8). One of several agents (the author has utilized 0.1% nitrofurazone solution) can be injected. Approximately 3 to 4 cc of the solution fills the vas to the ejaculatory duct. The patient usually feels a desire to void owing to stimulation of the ejaculatory duct at the level of the posterior urethra. The purpose of this technique is to shorten the end point of azoospermia. Albert [1] used the nitrofurazone solution to flush the distal vas at the time of vasectomy so that in the first ejaculation following the operation there were at most only a few immotile sperm. Following vas flushing, hematospermia has been observed in some cases. This may indicate irritation of the distal tract. Further evaluation of flushing techniques and use of appropriate agents are required as they hold the promise of further simplifying vasectomy procedures and reducing the time period to render the patient sterile [11, 27].

Schmidt [33] has described an excellent technique (Fig. 10-9). Utilizing coagulating current, fulguration of the proximal vas lumen for a distance of several millimeters is performed. This damages the vas mucosa and allows for the formation of scar, thereby "perfecting" vas occlusion by an intraluminal technique, rather than depending on external compression of the vas wall. It is Schmidt's observation that external compression, particularly with suture material, may result in pressure necrosis and gangrene of the devitalized tissue, allowing the proximal vas to open, followed by sperm leakage and sperm granuloma formation. In some instances the sperm granuloma may present postoperatively as a painful nodule, which may be so

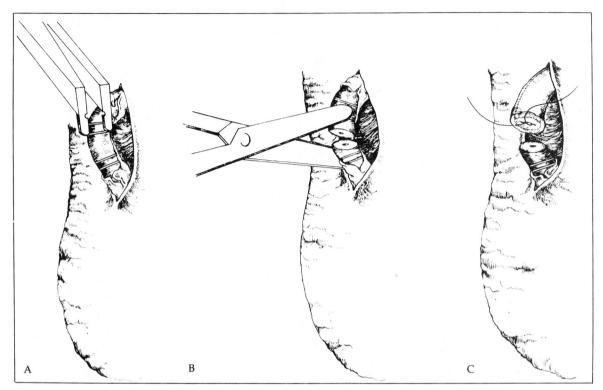

A   B   C

Fig. 10-7. (A and B) Two tantalum clips are applied to both the proximal and distal parts between which the vas sectioning will be performed. (C) The vas sheath is then drawn over the distal end of the vas for fascial interposition.

annoying to the patient as to require excision. Furthermore, recanalization between the proximal and distal ends may develop through the medium of the sperm granuloma. After mucosal fulguration, fascial interposition over the proximal end is usually performed (Fig. 10-9B).

The author utilizes an absorbable suture for skin closure (Fig. 10-10). The patient is told that these sutures will dissolve in 1 to 2 weeks, leaving a temporary gap in the skin which requires a daily dressing until healing is complete. Some surgeons prefer to use nonabsorbable sutures, which require removal after 1 week. This provides an opportunity to inspect the wound and observe signs of any possible complications.

A percutaneous injection technique for vasocclusion, utilizing a 4% formalin solution originally described by Coffey and Freeman [10], is currently under study by the author. A No. 25 gauge needle is used to inject 0.5 ml of the agent into the vas through the locally anesthetized scrotal skin. No attempt is made to find the vas lumen but simply to inject the agent into the vas wall. Very preliminary observations suggest that sperm transport can be affected by this technique, though several injections may be necessary to obtain azoospermia. Long-term follow-up of semen analysis is required.

EFFECTS AND SEQUELAE OF VASECTOMY

Disappearance of Sperm

Research into vasectomy and its sequelae has resulted in better understanding of the mechanism of sperm transport during ejaculation. Formerly, urologists had advised a period of from 6 weeks to several months of contraception following bilateral vasectomy, or until two semen specimens devoid of sperm had been produced. Freund and Davis [12] determined the exact end point in terms of the number of ejaculations postvasectomy required to render a patient's semen aspermic. Preoperative and consecutive postoperative semen specimens were studied. It was determined that approximately 60 to 70 percent of the sperm found in the normal ejaculate from an intact (i.e., unoperated) man come from that part of the vas proximal to the point of

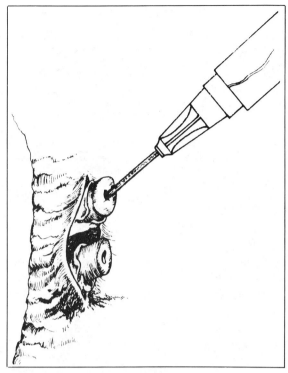

Fig. 10-8. The vas flush technique.

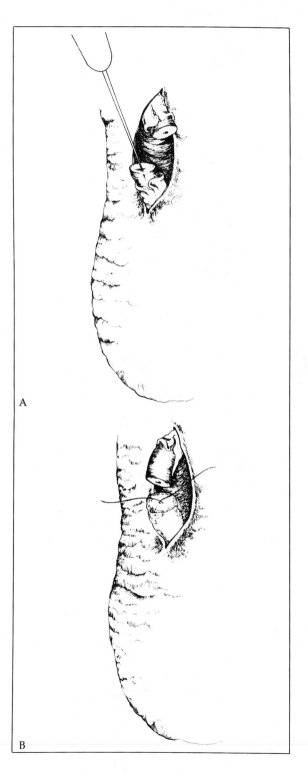

vasectomy and from the epididymis, since the first specimen after vasectomy consistently contained about 30 to 40 percent of sperm found in the preoperative specimen. A constant percentage decrease in sperm output with successive specimens after vasectomy suggested that ejaculation is a true biologic emptying phenomenon and that at ejaculation approximately 65 percent of the sperm distal to the point of vasectomy are expelled from the vasa. In more than 100 patients studied, absence of sperm was noted after 6 to 10 ejaculations following vasectomy. By virtue of this technique, the urologist and the patient, with the cooperation of the laboratory performing the sperm counts, can determine within a relatively short period of time after the operation that azoospermia has been produced and that the procedure has been successful.

Jouannet and David [22] repeated and confirmed these findings. They also observed that motile sperm were not observed in freshly ejaculated semen speci-

Fig. 10-9. (A) Utilizing coagulating current, fulguration of the proximal vas lumen for a distance of several millimeters is performed. (B) Fascial interposition over the proximal end is usually performed.

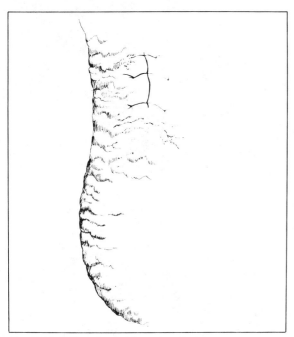

Fig. 10-10. Utilize absorbable suture for skin closure.

mens 15 days after successful vasectomy. The reappearance of any number of motile sperm 15 days postvasectomy strongly suggested failure or recanalization.

Effects of Vasocclusion

One prospective endocrine study suggests that there is an increase in mean plasma levels of testosterone, luteinizing hormone, and estradiol when compared with mean hormone levels measured before vasectomy. However, the changes were not found to be outside the normal range seen in adults [35]. An ongoing prospective study by the National Institutes of Health, studying many clinically significant parameters in vasectomized men matched with comparable non-vasectomized men, has failed to show any abnormality.

Morphologic effects of vasocclusion vary significantly from one species to another [3]. For example, sperm granulomas form rapidly in the rat vas and epididymis [24]. However, in biopsies of epididymal epithelium from the rhesus monkey [2], similarity of cellular organelles before and after vasectomy indicates that many functions of the epididymis, including secretion and resorption, continue and are probably not changed to any great extent. The epithelial cells appear to remain metabolically active.

To study the morphologic effects of vasectomy, testicular biopsy specimens from 3 to 7 years postvasec-tomy were fixed, embedded, and stained for light and electronmicroscopic examination. Sections of the seminiferous tubules demonstrated that (1) the blood supply to the tubules was intact; (2) the lumen of each tubule examined was patent; (3) the Sertoli cells appeared to be intact, with elongated cell outlines, radially oriented, dense cytoplasm, prominent endoplasmic reticulum, lipid droplets, subsurface cisternae adjacent to Sertoli cell junction, and nuclei with characteristic clefts and large tripartite nucleolus; however, a large number of lysosomes were present in the area between the nucleus and basement membrane as intact dense bodies and as membrane-coated electron-lucent formations; and (4) the germinal epithelium was present and showed normal stages of spermatogenesis, suggesting that vasectomy does not inhibit sperm formation. Spermatids were seen in the usual clusters of four to five. However, spermatozoa were not observed in their typical location close to the lumen, enwrapped by digitations of Sertoli cells, but rather were found to be abutting the vasal portion of Sertoli cells, often close to the basement membrane of the tubules. This peculiar location might indicate that these Sertoli cells were acting to absorb or eliminate the sperm. These ultrastructural findings suggest that the human testicle may do more than act passively toward those sperm that are not ejaculated and that do not pass through the vas deferens. Studies related to these findings are in progress and will be complemented by studies in animal models to determine ultrastructural and histochemical effects of vasectomy [19].

The question of immunologic consequences following vasectomy is of great interest today. Zappi et al. [43] and Ansbacher [5] have shown that in more than 50 percent of men in the first year following vasectomy, there are factors in the serum that cause agglutination of donor sperm. Normally, spermatozoa are sequestered from the vascular compartment by a barrier limiting both their potential to immunize the male and their vulnerability to immune damage. Disturbances of this barrier might occur after vasectomy when massive sperm absorption may take place somewhere in the genital tract or as a result of testicular biopsy through a transient release of an immunizing dose of spermatozoa. This immunity usually is not a high-titer response, and it may decline with time. Ansbacher [6] has shown that the titers of humoral antibodies decrease in 2 or 3 years following vasectomy. The mechanism of the humoral response is not yet known. It should be noted that the standard Kibrick test measures only IgG antibodies, while the sperm immobilization test measures both the IgG and IgA components. The origin of the immune response that may take place after vasectomy in man has not been demonstrated. Although antibodies have been reported in the blood of a certain percentage of men after vasectomy, the antigenic stimulus for antibody production has also not been localized.

Witkin et al. [42] have studied immune complexes postvasectomy in humans. Whether circulating immune complexes persist or are of medical consequence remains to be determined, but it would be reasonable to assume that in most cases they would be of sufficient size to be readily cleared from the circulation by the reticuloendothelial system. There are no substantial indications that vasectomy should induce significant levels of pathogenic circulating immune complexes.

Anderson et al. [4] have found that a large percentage of vasectomized men with sperm immunity were responsive to tumor-associated antigens in the leukocyte adherence assay and that antisperm antibodies or other serum factors played a role in this response. Further investigation of potentially adverse effects of vasectomy on the immune system is necessary, although to date no pathologic immunologic consequences of vasectomy have been reported in men.

Alexander and Clarkson [2] studied cynomolgus monkeys on high lipid diets and found a rapid development of arteriosclerosis in the vasectomized group. The arteries from the vasectomized monkeys contained significantly more total and esterified cholesterol than those from sham vasectomized rhesus monkeys maintained on a normal monkey diet. More severe arteriosclerosis was found in those animals than in age-matched nonvasectomized controls. Monkeys lacking circulating antisperm antibodies had more extensive arteriosclerosis than those with high levels of antibodies. It was postulated that those monkeys without detectable free antibodies are in a state of antigenemia and have higher levels of circulating immune complexes.

Human prospective epidemiologic studies up to ten years following vasectomy have indicated no increased instances of cardiovascular disease, including myocardial infarction [15, 16, 29, 38, 40]. No differences in the distribution of arteriosclerotic retinopathy evaluated by ophthalmoscopy and fundus photography were noted [26].

COMPLICATIONS

Surgical complications are technique-related, except where anomalous conditions or anatomic variations exist. The physician must pay particular attention to hemostasis and cannot hope for subcutaneous bleeding points to stop by themselves, since the complex scrotal fascial layers do not readily tamponade bleeding. Sterile technique is required. The occurrence of epididymitis, though rare, may be related to infection or may be a result of back pressure from the occluded vas. That this does not occur very often and that gross distention or pain from the epididymis is not noted clinically is indicative of some as yet unknown homeostatic mechanism in the human male not seen in other animals.

Sperm granuloma is an inflammatory response to the leakage of sperm from the vas or epididymis into surrounding tissues. Most granulomas are small and harmless, however, and would go unnoticed except in cases of later surgery. Thus, it is estimated that the true incidence may be as high as 20 percent in the vas and 15 percent in the epididymis. Some have been discovered only a few weeks after the procedure, others as long as 25 years later. Although generally asymptomatic, sperm granulomas can be troublesome if they become infected, create vasocutaneous fistulas, cause recanalization of the vas through ducts formed within the granuloma, or prevent later surgical reanastomosis. In theory at least, an immune response may result from absorption of sperm from the granuloma.

A diagnosis of sperm granuloma should be considered if the patient complains of pain and swelling at the site of vasectomy 1 or 2 weeks postoperatively. Specifically, if the patient has been asymptomatic for some time after the operation, a sudden onset of pain suggests a granuloma. On gross examination granulomas begin as an inflammatory response surrounding creamy-white, thick seminal fluids. The initial lesion is usually pea-sized. If the lesion becomes large and cystic, its contents may become tinged with blood. As the inflammation subsides, the lesion becomes yellowish-brown, and the walls become fibrous and sometimes calcified.

A sperm granuloma should be considered a complication of vasectomy. Sperm extravasation and resultant granuloma formation may be preventable by the fulguration technique of Schmidt [33] or by techniques of compression by inert instruments such as tantalum clips. Sutures that cause pressure necrosis, especially catgut, are more apt to be a setting for sperm leakage. Recanalization is more apt to occur in an area of sperm granuloma [33].

Although vasectomy is not completely foolproof, it is the most effective method of permanent male fertility control now available. It is becoming more effective as practitioners gain greater skill and experience. Nevertheless, a vasectomy candidate should understand that a small possibility of failure exists.

Failure may or may not result in pregnancy. Failure is usually discovered when semen examinations indicate the presence of sperm more than 4 to 6 weeks after the operation or after 10 to 12 ejaculations, when there are motile sperm in the semen after a period of azoospermia, or when pregnancy takes place. Pregnancy may occur as a result of even a few motile sperm in a patient's semen. The persistence of nonmotile sperm, assuming examination of a freshly ejaculated specimen, 4 to 6 weeks postoperatively probably relates to sperm retained in the distal tract, especially in the ampulla of the vas and seminal vesicle. Most investigators consider such a man to be sterile, whereas the presence of such number of motile sperm 4 to 6 weeks after vasectomy should raise suspicion of recanalization or failure. The emptying phenomenon is slower in older men.

The likelihood of recanalization may be influenced by the vasectomy technique employed. For example, crushing and tying the vas, particularly with absorbable sutures, a widely used procedure, can lead to recanalization. Members of the workshop on clinical aspects of male sterilization at the 1973 Geneva conference on voluntary sterilization agreed that separating the treated vas ends with a barrier of fascia is an effective means of preventing vasectomy failure.

The likelihood of operative failure is reduced if the surgeon has performed the procedure frequently. The importance of frequent practice was emphasized by Sobrero et al. [36] of the Margaret Sanger Research Bureau, New York. They reported six failures in 286 procedures performed during the first year of the vasectomy service at the bureau. Four of these procedures were performed by physicians-in-training and two by general surgeons with little experience in the operation. Failure also results from inadequate occlusion of the vas ends. If ligatures or clips are applied too loosely, sperm continue to pass through the vas; if they are applied too tightly, they may cut through the vas wall and permit the sperm to exit.

MORTALITY

The risk of death due to vasectomy is extremely low. Table 10-1 compares the mortality risks of reproductive alternatives for developed countries. Those data were derived from studies in the United States and the United Kingdom. After 1 year the mortality risks for vasectomies, IUD use, legal induced abortion, and female sterilization range from 0.1 to 4.0 per 100,000. The lowest rates are seen for IUD use and vasectomy and the highest rate (4 times that for female sterilization) is seen for pregnancy and delivery. After 5 and 10 years the mortality risks remain constant for the single-exposure events (vasectomy and tubal ligation) but increase with time for pregnancy and delivery and for those continuing oral contraceptive and IUD use [15, 23, 28, 31, 32].

Deaths related to vasectomy have been reported from India and Bangladesh as resulting from tetanus [17]. One study by Potts et al. [30] reported a mortality risk of 19.0 per 100,000 procedures. However, estimates

Table 10-1. Estimated cumulative death rates for different methods of fertility control in the United States and the United Kingdom*

Method of fertility control	Cumulative death rate		
	At 1 year	At 5 years	At 10 years
Female voluntary surgical contraception	4.0	4.0	4.0
Vasectomy	0.1	0.1	0.1
Intrauterine device	0.3	1.5	3.0
Abortion			
Before 12 weeks	1.1		
After 12 weeks	11.2		
Total	2.2		
Maternal mortality	18.7		

*Death rates expressed per 100,000 women per year for IUD users, per 100,000 procedures for abortion and female voluntary surgical contraception, and per 100,000 live births for maternal mortality.

of the risk of death from vasectomy in other developing countries have been reported as 0 to 1 deaths per 100,000 procedures.

SEMEN PRESERVATION AND VASECTOMY

That a man has fathered children is no guarantee that his sperm can be frozen, stored, and thawed years later for successful insemination. Since only semen from the best donors, with respect to recovery of motility, should be banked, there is little future in semen banking for purposes other than storage for an artificial insemination program or for men facing surgery for malignant testicular tumors [9]. The Association for Voluntary Sterilization has stated that it is inappropriate to consider semen banking for an individual considering vasectomy.

CONCLUSIONS

Vasectomy (vas sectioning and occlusion) is a short outpatient surgical procedure that has a demonstrable end point of azoospermia after 10 to 15 ejaculations (or shorter, using one of several vas flushing methods now available). As a contraceptive method, it is not coitally related, appears in prospective studies to cause no hormonal, biochemical, or other changes in the human male, and with appropriate screening and counseling should result in no psychologic problems. Refinements and improvements in technique, especially sectioning without resecting the vas to preserve blood and nerve supply, and emphasis on high sectioning of the vas away from the convoluted portion appear to result in even less postoperative discomfort and morbidity. As an added benefit, refinements may offer a better chance should a reversal be desired.

Appendix 10-1.
Conference on Vasectomy
Colombo, Sri Lanka
October 4 to 7, 1982
Plan of Action

The First International Conference on Vasectomy, held in Colombo, Sri Lanka, from October 4 to 7, 1982:

NOTES with approval the continuing efforts of international organizations, governments, and nongovernment organizations to provide safe and effective methods of fertility regulation as part of programs to improve the health and welfare of men, women, and families everywhere;

FURTHER NOTES the growing demand for permanent methods of contraception;

RECOGNIZES that men should share the responsibility for family planning and contraception;

CALLS the attention of policymakers and program administrators to evidence that men in every region of the world would use vasectomy services if they were available;

CONCLUDES that vasectomy is safe and should be offered as a choice in health and family planning programs; and therefore;

ADOPTS the following findings and recommendations for action:

FINDINGS

1. Vasectomy is one of the safest and most effective methods of contraception and is even safer and more widely deliverable than female methods of surgical contraception.
2. Men in every part of the world, and in every cultural, religious, or socioeconomic setting, have demonstrated interest in or acceptance of vasectomy, despite commonly held assumptions about male attitudes or societal prohibitions.
3. The greatest hindrance to increased acceptance of vasectomy appears to be lack of services in appropriate settings, reluctance of programs to initiate services, and lack of specific information about what vasectomy is and is not.
4. The most important factor in an individual's decision to request vasectomy appears to be having had personal contact and a conversation with a man who has had a vasectomy and is satisfied with the procedure.

RECOMMENDATIONS

Educating Health Providers and the Public

- Programs should be launched to increase the knowledge and awareness of vasectomy among all levels of health and family planning personnel. Greater clarification of health-provider attitudes and beliefs about vasectomy should be sought. Program administrators and health providers are too often convinced that men will not accept vasectomy for cultural, psychological, or religious reasons. It is recognized that an emotional inability to distinguish between masculinity and the ability to cause a pregnancy can be—and is—shared by providers as well as consumers; this belief can negatively influence the thinking of health providers.
- Special efforts must be made to inform and educate policymakers, health and family planning personnel, and the public about vasectomy, so that it can be an available choice for people who wish to control their fertility. The mass media should be used, in non directive and culturally appropriate ways, for public education, to make vasectomy an acceptable topic of conversation and to provide accurate information about it.
- More extensive information on vasectomy should be made available through commercial channels. Examples of commercial resources on which short messages about vasectomy can appear include soap wrappers, match boxes, bus tickets, postal envelopes, and pharmaceutical and personal hygiene products. To help desensitize the public about vasectomy, marketing techniques, such as advertising, can also be utilized. Information activities can be incorporated into daily or communitywide events, so that males will become better educated about the method and the local availability of services.

Counseling

- Since studies and experience show that the most important factor in a man's decision to accept vasectomy is contact with satisfied users, programs should make concerted and continuous efforts to include these users in education and counseling programs. Acceptor clubs for vasectomized men can be established, for example. Programs should continue to use interpersonal communication, primarily individual and group meetings, as the chief means of educating people about vasectomy.

Surveying the Needs of Consumers

- Establishing whether there is demand for vasectomy in a geographical area can best be accomplished by directly surveying the attitudes and wishes of men in that area. To guide planning for information activities, programs should undertake studies of men's attitudes toward vasectomy to determine specific barriers, if any, that exist.

Creative Quality Programming

- High-quality, prestigious service centers are essential in delivering vasectomy as a contraceptive choice. Quality is essential both to provide humanistic care and to increase the number of satisfied clients who are potentially important communicators about vasectomy. In all service-delivery centers preoperative screening and counseling and postoperative patient follow-up, in addition to expert surgical care, are essential.

- Male-oriented vasectomy centers that make men feel comfortable should be developed. These centers may offer other male health services in addition to vasectomy. Supportive services can be included, so that an atmosphere of fun and comfort is achieved.
- When a vasectomy program in a large rural area is initiated, mobile approaches should be used to help extend information and services. When acceptance in an area has increased, mobile services can be replaced by a reliable system for referring or transporting clients to a static center.

Surgical Personnel

- Planners should make every effort to use well-trained physicians for the delivery of services. Physicians should be motivated, encouraged, and reimbursed sufficiently so that they want to include vasectomy in their delivery systems, whether public or private.
- While it has been shown that paramedics have been trained in some settings to deliver safe, efficient vasectomy services, countries attempting to initiate national programs should do so through their network of trained physicians. In some instances, particularly in rural areas, where physicians are not in sufficient supply, paramedics can be trained to perform vasectomies according to high standards of competence and safety.

REFERENCES

1. Albert, P. S., Mininberg, D. T., and Davis, J. E. Nitrofurans: Sperm immobilizing agents. *Urology* 4:307, 1974.
2. Alexander, N. J., and Clarkson, Immunologic and morphologic effects of vasectomy in the rhesus monkey. *Fed. Proc.* 34:1692, 1975.
3. Alexander, N. J. Vasectomy: Morphological and Immunological Effects. In E. S. E. Hafez (ed.), *Human Semen and Fertility Regulation in Men*. St. Louis: Mosby, 1976.
4. Anderson, D. J., et al. Immunity to tumor-associated antigens in vasectomized men. *J. Natl. Cancer Institute* 69:551, 1982.
5. Ansbacher, R. Sperm agglutinating and sperm-immobilizing antibodies in vasectomized men. *Fertil. Steril.* 22:629, 1971.
6. Ansbacher, R. Vasectomy, sperm antibodies. *Fertil. Steril.* 24:788, 1973.
7. Batra, S. K., and Lardner, T. J. Sperm Transport in the Vas Deferens. In E. S. E. Hafez (ed.), *Human Semen and Fertility Regulation in Men*. St. Louis: Mosby, 1976.
8. Baumgarten, H. G., Owman, C., and Sjoberg, N. O. Neural Mechanisms in Male Fertility. In J. J. Sciarra, C.

Markland, and J. Spiedel (eds.), *Control of Male Fertility*. Hagerstown, Md.: Harper & Row, 1975.
9. Beck, W. W., Jr. Artificial insemination and preservation of semen. *Urol. Clin. North Am.* 5:593, 1978.
10. Coffey, D. S., and Freeman, C. Vas Injection: A New, Non-Surgical Procedure to Induce Sterility in Human Males. In J. J. Sciarra, C. Markland, and J. Spiedel (eds.), *Control of Male Fertility*. Hagerstown, Md.: Harper & Row, 1975.
11. Craft, I., and McQueen, J. Effect of irrigation of the vas on post-vasectomy semen counts. *Lancet* 1:515, 1972.
12. Freund, M., and Davis, J. E. Disappearance rate of spermatozoa from the ejaculate following vasectomy. *Fertil. Steril.* 20:163, 1969.
13. Freund, M., and Davis, J. E. A follow-up study of the efects of vasectomy on sexual behavior. *J. Sex Res.* 9:241, 1973.
14. Freund, M., and Ventura, W. Male Sterilization: Basic Science Aspects. In M. E. Schima, et al. (eds.), *Advances in Voluntary Sterilization (Proceedings of the 2nd International Conference, Geneva, Feb. 25–Mar. 1, 1973)*. Amsterdam: American Elsevier, 1974.
15. Goldacre, M. J., et al. Follow-up of vasectomy using medical record linkage. *Am. J. Epidemiol.* 108:176, 1978.
16. Goldacre, M. J., Holford, T. R., and Vessey, M. P. Cardiovascular disease and vasectomy: Findings from two epidemiologic studies. *N. Engl. J. Med.* 308:805, 1983.
17. Grimes, D. A., et al. Deaths from contraceptive sterilization in Bangladesh: Rates, causes, and prevention. *Obstet. Gynecol.* 1982.
18. Hackett, R. E., and Waterhouse, K. Vasectomy—reviewed. *Am. J. Obstet. Gynecol.* 116:438, 1973.
19. Hagedoorn, J. P., and Davis, J. E. Fine structure of the seminiferous tubules after vasectomy in man. *Physiologist* 17:236, 1974.
20. Hulka, J. F., and Davis, J. E. Sterilization of Men. In E. S. E. Hafez and T. Evans (eds.), *Human Reproduction: Conception and Contraception*. Hagerstown, Md.: Harper & Row, 1973.
21. Jhaver, P. S., et al. Reversibility of sterilization produced by vas occlusion clip. *Fertil. Steril.* 22:263, 1971.
22. Jouannet, P., and David, G. Evolution of the properties of semen immediately following vasectomy. *Fertil. Steril.* 29:435, 1978.
23. Kahn, H. S., and Tyler, C. W. Mortality associated with IUDs. *J.A.M.A.* 234:57, 1975.
24. Kwart, A. M., and Coffey, D. S. Sperm granulomas: Adverse effects of vasectomy. *J. Urol.* 110:416, 1973.
25. Leader, A. J., et al. Complications of 2,711 vasectomies. *J. Urol.* 111:365, 1974.
26. Linnet, L., et al. No increase in arteriosclerotic retinopathy or activity in tests for circulating immune complexes 5 years after vasectomy. *Fertil. Steril.* 27:798, 1982.
27. Mumford, S. D., and Davis, J. E. Flushing of distal vas during vasectomy. *Urology* 14:433, 1979.

28. Peterson, H. B., et al. Mortality risk associated with tubal sterilization in United States hospitals. *Am. J. Obstet. Gynecol.* 143:125, 1982.

29. Petitti, D. B., et al. Physiologic measures in men with and without vasectomies. *Fertil. Steril.* 37:438, 1982.

30. Potts, M., Spiedel, J. J., and Kessel, E. Relative Risks of Various Means of Fertility Control when Used in Less-Developed Countries. In J. J. Sciarra and G. I. Zatuchni (eds.), *Risks, Benefits, and Controversies in Fertility Control.* Hagerstown, Md.: Harper & Row, 1977.

31. Rochat, R. Maternal Mortality in the United States. In S. Aladjun (ed.), *Obstetrical Practice.* St. Louis: Mosby, 1980.

32. Rubin, G. L., et al. The risk of childbearing reevaluated. *Am. J. Public Health* 71:712, 1981.

33. Schmidt, S. S. Techniques and complications of elective vasectomy: The role of spermatic granuloma in spontaneous recanalization. *Fertil. Steril.* 17:467, 1966.

34. Silber, S. J. Microscopic vasectomy reversal. *Fertil. Steril.* 28:1191, 1977.

35. Smith, K. D., Chowdhury, M., and Teholakian, R. K. Endocrine Effects of Vasectomy in Humans. In J. J. Sciarra, C. Markland, and J. J. Spiedel (eds.), *Control of Male Fertility.* Hagerstown, Md.: Harper & Row, 1975.

36. Sobrero, A. J., et al. A vasectomy service in a free-standing family planning center: One year's experience. *Soc. Biol.* 20:303, 1973.

37. Ventura, W. P., Freund, M., and Davis, J. E. Influence of norepinephrine on the motility of human vas deferens. *Fertil. Steril.* 24:68, 1973.

38. Walker, A. M., et al. Hospitalization rates in vasectomized men. *J.A.M.A.* 245:2315, 1981.

39. Walker, A. M., et al. Vasectomy and non-fatal myocardial infarction. *Lancet* 1:13, 1981.

40. Wallace, R. B., et al. Vasectomy and coronary disease in men less than 50 years old: Absence of association. *J. Urol.* 126:182, 1981.

41. Westoff, C. R., and Jones, E. R. Contraception and sterilization in the U.S.: 1965–1975. *Fam. Plann. Perspect.* 9:4, 1977.

42. Witkin, S. S., Zelikovsky, G., and Bongiovanni, A. M. Sperm-related antigens, antibodies, and circulating immune complexes in sera of recently vasectomized men. *J. Clin. Invest.* 70:33, 1982.

43. Zappi, E., et al. Immunologic consequences of vasectomy. *Fed. Proc.* 29:728, 1970.

44. Zatuchni, G. Research in Fertility Regulation. In J. Sciarra (ed.), *Obstetrics and Gynecology* (vol. 6). Hagerstown, Md.: Harper & Row, 1982.

45. Ziegler, F. J. Vasectomy and adverse psychological reaction. *Ann. Intern. Med.* 73:853, 1970.

46. Ziegler, F. J., Rogers, D. A., and Prentiss, R. J. Psychosocial response to vasectomy. *Arch. Gen. Psychiatry* 21:46, 1969.

11. Male Sterilization Reversal

Stanley H. Greenberg

Approximately 500,000 men undergo vasectomy each year in the United States for the purpose of sterilization. If men seeking permanent contraception are properly evaluated and counseled before vasectomy, they should be physically and psychologically fit before and after the procedure. However, even if less than 1 percent of men who have had a vasectomy eventually request reversal of sterilization, this represents a considerable number of such operations. There have been significant developments in surgical techniques for vasectomy reversal (vasovasostomy) in recent years, and men considering such a step can be logically evaluated and often successfully treated.

CONSIDERATIONS IN PATIENT SELECTION

In the author's experience the majority of men seeking consultation for vasectomy reversal are 30 to 40 years old and have been divorced and remarried. If the option of donor insemination of the wife is not acceptable to the couple as primary treatment, then surgical vasectomy reversal will be the treatment of choice. Some men do request vasectomy reversal because they experienced adverse psychologic effects from sterilization but, as noted above, this is uncommon when proper prevasectomy consultation takes place. Finally, there certainly are individuals who simply change their minds about family size or who suffer the tragic loss of a child after vasectomy has been accomplished and request reversal for these reasons.

When the man is seen in consultation, a complete medical history and physical examination should be done. Marital history and the ages and physical status of the patient's children and wife are pertinent for proper consultation. Since sterilization reversal is truly an elective procedure in all cases, the patient's general medical status should be considered, and he should be fully advised as to the risks of surgery and anesthesia.

There are a number of pertinent points related to the history and physical findings that the clinician should particularly note. The length of elapsed time since the man's vasectomy was done is an important factor. Although successful vasovasostomy may be accomplished at any time after vasectomy and although varying results have been claimed by different investigators, nevertheless Silber [10] has found in an analysis of a large series of vasectomy reversals that the prognosis for both return of sperm to the semen and ultimate fertility is significantly reduced in men presenting for vasectomy reversal 10 years or more after the initial sterilization procedure. Whether this is due to impaired spermatogenesis, secondary epididymal obstruction, or patient age is not entirely clear. This time factor, however, must be seriously considered in patient selection.

149

Similarly, if the patient has had significant urologic infections, such as chronic prostatitis, severe epididymitis, or orchitis, the surgeon and patient must be prepared for more than a routine uncomplicated procedure.

When the patient is examined, testicular size and consistency, size and texture of the epididymis, presence or absence of cystic dilation, and position of the two ends of the vas should be particularly evaluated. If nothing abnormal is noted and the vas ends are easily palpable, it is rarely useful to consult the operative report or previous surgeon concerning the precise technique used for the original vasectomy. However, if the two ends of the vas are not readily palpable on each side or if the patient has already had one unsuccessful vasovasostomy, then operative findings, technique utilized in prior procedures, and any previous complications are of considerable significance. Determination of any extraordinary circumstances in a particular case, either social, emotional, or physical, may dictate that further consultation, additional considerations of informed consent, or preparation for variation of surgical techniques are needed.

Silber [10] has made an interesting observation regarding sperm granulomas with regard to the potential for reversal of vasectomy. He noted improved fertility rates in men undergoing vasovasostomy in a group of patients who had sperm granulomas. Such lesions result from sperm leakage from the testicular end of the severed vas with subsequent tissue reaction and granuloma formation in the scrotum. This event appears to be more likely when the vas end is ligated rather than cauterized, presumably because of more tissue necrosis caused by the ligation technique. Silber postulates that spontaneous release of intraductal pressure by sperm leakage at the vas end results in fewer epididymal obstructions than would otherwise occur secondary to rupture of that fragile structure and, hence, in those instances, better sperm counts and quality after vasectomy reversal. This observation has yet to be confirmed by other investigators, nor has the immunologic consequence of the presence or absence of sperm granulomas been adequately investigated. Therefore, Silber's recommendation of performing "open-ended" vasectomies has not gained popularity.

Although it has been repeatedly demonstrated that approximately 50 percent of vasectomized men have detectable serum levels of antisperm antibody, the significance of this phenomenon in terms of fertility potential after vasectomy reversal is not yet clear. There is a higher incidence of people with detectable titers of antisperm antibody in infertile populations compared with control groups; therefore, there is concern with regard to vasectomized men. However, the data available so far are contradictory. At present there is not enough evidence indicating serious compromise of success of vasectomy reversal by the presence of antisperm antibody to warrant routine testing of all men preoperatively. However, if a patient fails to father a child within 12 to 24 months after vasovasostomy, investigation into the cause or failure should be undertaken. If sperm counts are abnormally low, hormonal evaluation should be carried out. If normal, technical failure with persistent partial obstruction must be considered. Repeat surgery may be advised under these circumstances. If sperm counts are normal but motility parameters are poor, a significant effect of antisperm antibody should be considered. High-specificity radioimmunoassay determination of human antisperm antibody has been developed but is not widely available [1]. Cruder assay techniques dependent on sperm agglutinating or immobilizing phenomena are generally utilized in clinical practice. To a varying degree each technique presents problems of nonspecificity, false positive or false negative results, and lack of correlation with clinical response. Furthermore, the appropriateness of relying on serum or seminal assay results is unresolved. In practice the Kibrick macroagglutination test for assay of serum titers of antisperm antibody activity is probably reliable [4]. Treatment of men with normal sperm counts but chronic infertility apparently secondary to autoimmune factors generally yields a 30 percent pregnancy rate when high-dose steroid regimens are employed. No good data are available for men treated after vasovasostomy.

The ultimate success of sterilization reversal is measured in terms of pregnancy rates. However, there is a correlation between ultimate fertility and sperm count. It is helpful to do semen analyses at intervals after vasectomy reversal for the purpose of evaluating success or failure and for prognosis. Occasionally sperm will be seen initially with subsequent return to azoospermia, indicating stricture of anastomoses. No secondary surgery should be done, however, for at least 1 year after initial vasovasostomy, since temporary azoospermia from nonmechanical factors can occur. If a patient has persistent azoospermia or severe oligospermia, serum testosterone and gonadotropin determinations as well as testis biopsy may be necessary for full evaluation before exploration of the vas anastomoses. It is the author's opinion that preoperative sperm counts (i.e., before initial vasovasostomy) are generally not necessary, since the failure rate of vasectomy is not more than 1 in 300 and probably is more likely in the range of 1 in 10,000 with standard vasectomy techniques presently employed.

TECHNIQUES OF VASECTOMY REVERSAL

The historic development of vasectomy reversal techniques will not be outlined here in detail. However, it is relevant to note that from the time of O'Conor's [6] survey on vas reanastomoses done by urologists in the United States in 1948, suture material and operative techniques have been refined and results have improved. Questions concerning the use of splints or stents, absorbable versus nonabsorbable sutures, and other technical problems have been scientifically investigated. There presently is some controversy among urologists as to whether the use of intraoperative magnification is desirable or necessary. The debate about the appropriateness of macroscopic versus microscopic surgery of the vas as well as the significance and proper treatment of antisperm antibodies will probably continue for some time. In the following sections are described the presently accepted surgical techniques for vasectomy reversal, admittedly reflecting the author's bias.

Macroscopic Vasovasostomy

With the patient anesthetized with either general or spinal anesthesia, the scrotal area is thoroughly scrubbed. High scrotal incisions are necessary for adequate dissection of the upper end of the vas. The author prefers to deliver the entire scrotal contents into the operative field to allow examination of the testis and epididymis and to facilitate accurate and proper dissection. The ends of the vas are "freshened," and careful attention to hemostasis is crucial throughout. Any one of a number of commercially available vas approximating clamps with varying designs may be used to stabilize the vas ends during reanastomosis. The testicular end of the vas will normally leak fluid which, if examined microscopically, should contain sperm. Some authorities recommend such intraoperative microscopic examinations with debridement of the vas until fully formed sperm are found, even if this requires that epididymovasostomy be performed. In view of the generally low success rate of the latter procedure, however, others recommend making the anastomosis no more proximal than the tail of the epididymis at the initial procedure.

Even some proponents of the macroscopic technique recommend performing the anastomosis under $4\times$ loupe magnification. Fine nonabsorbable suture, such as 6-0 or 7-0 nylon or Prolene, is generally recommended with two to four full-thickness sutures placed symmetrically to realign the vas. Interrupted sutures of the same material are placed in the adventitial tissue to relieve tension on the anastomosis.

The scrotal contents are replaced and the incision closed in standard fashion, usually with absorbable sutures. Prophylactic antibiotics may be used at the surgeon's discretion. In the immediate postoperative period the patient's activity is limited only as comfort dictates, although strenuous physical activity is proscribed for at least 3 weeks. Considerable scrotal ecchymosis and edema are not unusual initially but should completely resolve.

Microscopic Vasovasostomy

In terms of initial patient preparation, surgical exposure, and postoperative care, macroscopic and microscopic techniques are similar. The anastomosis, however, is performed under at least $10\times$ magnification provided by an operating microscope that allows the operator and assistant to sit 180 degrees opposite each other. Standard microvascular instruments and technique are utilized. A complete description of the instrumentation and techniques is beyond the scope of this text. Any surgeon contemplating doing this surgery should be fully trained with initial practice under laboratory conditions.

Figure 11-1 illustrates the two-layer technique of Silber. This technique can be difficult and tedious, requiring four to six mucosal sutures of 9-0 or 10-0 nylon and eight to ten seromuscular sutures of 9-0 nylon. Figure 11-2 illustrates a modified microscopic anastomosis described by Howards [2] but additionally developed independently by others and utilized by many urologists. Four full-thickness sutures are placed to align the vas lumen. Four seromuscular sutures are placed between the initial sutures to make the anastomosis "sperm-tight." The author prefers to use 9-0 nylon throughout.

Macroscopic Epididymovasostomy

Epididymovasostomy may be required in some instances of failed vasovasostomies or initially when epididymal obstruction is discovered. Such obstruction is secondary to epididymitis or epididymal cysts or granulomas, which occur when the tubule ruptures from high intraductal pressures.

With macroscopic techniques a true anastomosis is not made, but rather an ellipse of scarred epididymal tissue is excised proximal to the point of obstruction and the epididymal fluid examined microscopically to confirm the presence of sperm. The vas is either incised or transected and spatulated and then sutured to the incised edge of the tunic covering the coiled epididymal tubule. When successful, this procedure results in a fistula formed between the epididymal tubule and the vas lumen.

Microscopic Epididymovasostomy

The technique for microscopic epididymovasostomy has been relatively recently developed and described by Silber [11]. The vas is transected, and the epididymis

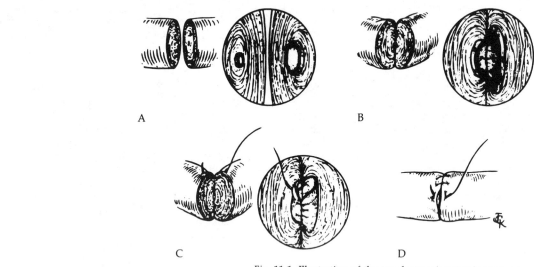

A   B

C   D

Fig. 11-1. Illustration of the two-layer microscopic vasovasostomy technique. Note discrepancy of the caliber of the vas lumen caused by higher pressure in the testicular end following vas occlusion. (After Silber, reproduced by permission of *Surgery, Gynecology & Obstetrics.*)

Fig. 11-2. Modified microscopic vasovasostomy technique. (After Howards, reproduced with permission.)

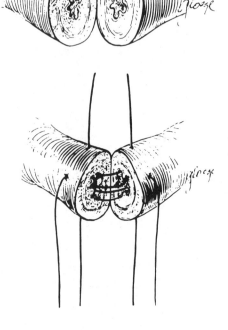

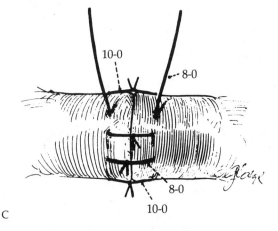

is sequentially sectioned transversely, beginning at the cauda and moving into the corpus and caput, if necessary, until the effluent fluid contains mature sperm. The cut edge is viewed with high power magnification, and the specific segment of tubule seen to be leaking fluid is identified. Using approximately three sutures of 9-0 or 10-0 nylon, the mucosa of the vas lumen is anastomosed end-to-end to the epididymal tubule itself, which has a diameter approximately equal to that of the

Table 11-1. Results of vasectomy reversal

Author	No. of patients	Patency (%)	Pregnancy (%)
Macroscopic			
O'Conor (1948) [6]*	420	35–40	
Phadke and Phadke (1967) [7]	76	83	55
Schmidt (1975) [8]	117	80	30
Middleton and Urry (1980) [5]	139		43
Microscopic			
Silber (1977) [9]	42	100	71

*Results of a survey taken of American urologists.

vas lumen. The muscularis of the vas is then sutured to the tunic covering the epididymis to relieve tension on the anastomosis.

RESULTS

Table 11-1 outlines results of vasovasostomy reported by a number of authors. Patency rates refer to the incidence of patients who have postoperative semen specimens with detectable mature sperm. Clearly, pregnancy rates are a more accurate reflection of the true success rate of sterilization reversal. Many recent reports of small series indicate that approximately 85 to 90 percent of men who undergo vasovasostomy by any technique will regain sperm in the semen. Pregnancy rates of 30 to 50 percent, however, have generally been the rule, except for the 70 percent rate reported by Silber. His claim that the two-layer microtechnique results in fewer anastomotic strictures and higher postoperative sperm counts with subsequently higher pregnancy rates is yet to be convincingly substantiated by other investigators. Experience and surgical facility with the procedure are indeed important factors and may account in part for Silber's results. It is probably desirable to include only patients who are at least 24 months postsurgery in the determination of pregnancy rates, which is not uniformly the case in all reported series.

When epididymovasostomy is performed by the macroscopic technique, patency rates and pregnancy rates are not expected to exceed 10 to 15 percent [3].

Silber has reported an 80 percent patency rate for his microscopic technique, but pregnancy rates have not yet been determined. Since the epididymal epithelium actually changes the physical and chemical characteristics of sperm cell membranes and is necessary for attainment of sperm motility and fertilizing capacity, it may be that this remarkable technical achievement in microsurgery will nevertheless be associated with disappointing pregnancy rates. Still, there has been a significant overall improvement in the technical aspects of surgical reversal of male sterilization with presently good expected results. The use of magnification as well as appreciation for the need for fine surgical technique have undoubtedly been major factors contributing to progress in this field. Further improvements in materials and instrumentation as well as the possibility of in vitro manipulation of sperm function and for in vitro fertilization may increase success rates further in the future.

REFERENCES

1. Haas, G. G., Cines, D. B., and Schreiber, A. D. Immunologic infertility: Identification of patients with anti-sperm antibody. *N. Engl. J. Med.* 303:722, 1980.
2. Howards, S. S. Vasovasostomy. *Urol. Clin. North Am.* 7(1):167, 1980.
3. Kar, J. K., and Phadke, A. M. Vaso-epididymal anastomosis. *Fertil. Steril.* 26:743, 1975.
4. Kibrick, S., Belding, D. L., and Merrill, B. Methods for detection of antibodies against mammalian spermatozoa. *Fertil. Steril.* 3:419, 1952.
5. Middleton, R. G., and Urry, R. L. Vasovasostomy and semen quality. *J. Urol.* 123:518, 1980.
6. O'Conor, V. J. Anastomosis of the vas deferens after purposeful division for sterility. *J. Urol.* 59:229, 1948.
7. Phadke, A. M., and Phadke, A. G. Experience in the reanastomosis of the vas deferens. *J. Urol.* 97:888, 1967.
8. Schmidt, S. S. Principles of vasovasostomy. *Contemp. Surg.* 7:13, 1975.
9. Silber, S. J. Microscopic vasectomy reversal. *Fertil. Steril.* 28:1191, 1977.
10. Silber, S. J. Vasectomy and vasectomy reversal. *Fertil. Steril.* 29:125, 1978.
11. Silber, S. J. Microscopic vasoepididymostomy: Specific microanastomosis to the epididymal tubule. *Fertil. Steril.* 30:565, 1978.

III. Hormonal Methods

12. Principles of Oral Contraception

William C. Andrews

Oral contraception provides reliable, reversible birth control for more than 50 million women around the world. "The pill" is one of the most thoroughly researched pharmacologic entities of the twentieth century and certainly the most closely monitored [86]. It has been the subject of numerous articles in the medical literature and even more in the lay press. The latter has produced confusion and uncertainty in the minds of many women. The protection from the risks of pregnancy outweighs the risks of potential untoward effects of the pill in the majority of women for whom the method is indicated. Additional benefits have been identified in recent years, suggesting that more lives may be saved as a result of the pill's protective effect against ovarian and endometrial cancer than may die as a result of cardiovascular accidents associated with oral contraceptive use [74].

The use of oral contraception involves a classic benefit versus risk equation. Thorough understanding of the risks as well as the benefits is essential for proper prescribing. Most of the serious complications are problems of the vascular system, often resulting from inappropriate coagulation. These concerns were initiated by individual case reports starting in 1961 [61], followed by case-control retrospective studies [39, 92, 97, 121]. These risks have been delineated by three prospective studies, whose findings have been published in ongoing fashion over the past 8 years [86, 93, 118].

The first of these studies, by the Royal College of General Practitioners in England, involved 46,000 women, half on oral contraceptives and half as controls [93]. The second study is that of the Oxford/Family Planning Association involving 17,000 women, 56 percent of them pill users and the others diaphragm or intrauterine device (IUD) users [118]. The third is the Walnut Creek Study from the Kaiser Permanente Foundation in Walnut Creek, California, involving 18,000 women in 107,000 woman-years of surveillance [86].

The first untoward complication of oral contraception to be statistically established was that of thrombophlebitis and thromboembolism [92]. Two retrospective case-control studies published in the *British Medical Journal* in April 1968 [39, 121] concluded that women taking oral contraceptives had a higher incidence of thrombophlebitis and pulmonary embolism. Although the incidence still remained low, the risk was estimated to be increased sevenfold by the use of oral contraceptives, and it increased with age for both users and nonusers, as it also does for pregnancy.

Another retrospective study, the Sartwell study from the United States [97], estimated the risk of vascular thrombosis to be increased 4.4 times for pill users. In 1974 the first of the prospective studies, that of the Royal College of General Practitioners [93], published its initial results, estimating an increased risk of 5.6 times for deep vein thrombosis. The Oxford/Family Planning Association in 1976 published its comparative study of the use of oral contraceptives, diaphragms, and IUDs and found a rate for new cases of venous thrombosis and pulmonary embolism of 0.86 per 1,000 woman-years for oral contraceptive users as compared to 0.38 for diaphragm users, a two- to threefold increased incidence [118].

The Walnut Creek Study [86] found no significant increase in thromboembolism in a comparison of current users, past users, and never-users. A number of objections have been raised to the Walnut Creek Study. Forty percent of the women in the study were over 40 years of age, only 19 percent were current users, and 19 percent were lost to follow-up. Thirty-two of the 170 deaths occurring in the study were excluded for a variety of reasons. Of those excluded, 26 percent were users whereas only 11 percent were nonusers. In spite of the acknowledged weaknesses, the study is valuable and suggests that at least in relatively healthy populations in the United States the risk, if present, is small.

The risk of thromboembolism is not related to length of use and disappears after stopping [58, 86, 110].

Two studies [33, 117] have shown an increased risk of postoperative thromboembolism in women using oral contraceptives immediately before major surgery. Increased risk declines rapidly after discontinuance of medication and is undetectable after 4 weeks. Women having elective surgery should cease oral contraceptive usage, when possible, at least 1 month in advance. If major surgery is necessary in a current user, prophylactic minidose heparin should be considered. Determination of antithrombin III levels has been suggested as a method to detect those patients at greatest risk of thrombophlebitis and aid in the decision regarding prophylactic heparin [78, 128].

Other factors influencing incidence rates of thrombophlebitis are obesity, genetics (3 times as common in mothers and sisters) [122], blood group (lower in group 0 patients, higher in group A) [43], chronic disease, and immobility.

Inman et al. [40] in 1970 reported finding a positive correlation between the dosage of estrogen and the risk of pulmonary embolism and deep vein thrombosis in the United Kingdom and in Sweden and Denmark. A discrepancy in this report is that a consistently lower incidence of thrombosis was noted in women using mestranol 100 μg norethynodrel 2.5 mg, which is one of the most estrogenic pills compared in the study. A 25 percent reduction in the incidence of venous thrombosis was noted with the use of 50-μg doses of estrogen, as compared with the higher doses in the Royal College of General Practitioners study [93]. In a follow-up report [48] these differences were found to be only

in superficial thrombophlebitis, and the incidence of deep vein thrombosis at the various doses was essentially the same. A lower incidence of thrombosis with oral contraceptives containing low doses of estrogen was also found by Stolley and associates [112].

A study from the Committee on Safety of Medicine in England [68] reported a small reduction in the incidence of pulmonary embolism with a 30-μg oral contraceptive as compared with a 50-μg variety but no reduction in incidence of thrombosis. They did find fewer venous and nonvenous deaths with the 30-μg than with the 50-μg oral contraceptive. More data are needed to confirm this trend.

No difference in the incidence of fatal myocardial infarction was noted between the users of 30-μg and 50-μg birth control pills in a study in England [2]. The authors concluded that a decrease may have been masked by the higher dosage of progestin in the 30-μg oral contraceptives.

CORONARY ARTERY DISEASE

No statistically significant association of oral contraceptive usage with coronary artery disease was shown in the initial case-control studies [39, 66, 97, 121], but in 1970 Inman et al. [40] reported finding such an association. Mann and Inman in 1975 [63] reported finding an increased risk of coronary thrombosis for oral contraceptive users, which was estimated to be 2.8 times for the age group 30 to 39 and 4.7 for the age group 40 to 44. They stress that this finding needs to be interpreted with caution as a number of assumptions necessarily had to be made in their calculation and the margin of error is likely to be fairly wide. In fact, in 1976 [64], following expansion of the study group, they reduced their estimate of risk for the age group 40 to 44 from 4.7 to 2.8.

In a companion study [65] of nonfatal coronary occlusion where it was possible to obtain a full history with regard to additional risk factors, only one case was found where the only risk factor was oral contraception. An increased incidence was found if pill use was combined with one or more of the following factors: hypertension, type II hyperlipoproteinemia, cigarette smoking, obesity, diabetes, or previous toxemias of pregnancy.

A reanalysis of the Mann et al. data was performed by Jain [42]. From this he calculated a relative risk of nonfatal myocardial infarction of 1.5 to 1 in women using oral contraception with no other risk factor, one-third of the overall risk estimated for all users. In comparison, the relative risk for obesity alone was 3.9 to 1, and for cigarette smoking alone 3.5 to 1. The estimated relative risk among those who use contraceptives as well as smoke was 11.7 to 1. Heavy smoking further increases the risk: The calculated risk is 5.4 for light smokers and 14.8 for heavy smokers. He concluded that "the use of oral contraception alone does not significantly increase the risk of nonfatal myocardial infarction but that smoking and oral contraceptive usage synergistically increase the risk." Mann [62], after further expansion of his series, has estimated that nonsmoking oral contraceptive users had a 1.8-fold increased risk of myocardial infarction as compared with an estimated 4.8-fold increased risk for oral contraceptive users who smoke. The number of nonusers was small, and the confidence limits for the risk estimate included one. He states "it is therefore possible that chance could explain an increased risk attributable to oral contraceptives in this group." He further found that the relative risk of myocardial infarction increased from 1.9 in smokers of 1 to 14 cigarettes daily to 19.1 for those who smoke 25 or more cigarettes a day.

Increased risk of smoking and the synergistic effect with oral contraception has been confirmed by the Boston Collaborative Drug Surveillance Program [89], the Johns Hopkins Cooperating Hospital Study [4], and other studies [44, 73, 99].

Jick et al. [44] concluded that "acute myocardial infarction in otherwise healthy, premenopausal women is almost exclusively an illness of cigarette smokers." The importance of hypercholesterolemia in predisposing to coronary occlusion in these women has been confirmed by several studies. In the report of Mann et al. [62] 41 percent of the patients with coronary occlusion before the age of 45 had type II hyperlipoproteinemia, while this was found in none of the group of matched controls. Shapiro et al. [99] reported a higher incidence of heavy smoking, diabetes, hyperlipoproteinemia, hypertension, and obesity in 234 cases of myocardial infarction in women aged 25 to 49, while Oliver [73], in a study of coronary occlusion in women under age 45, found that 48 percent had hypercholesterolemia, 39 percent were hypertensive, and 43 percent smoked 20 or more cigarettes a day. Eighty percent of his patients had one or more of these risk factors present.

The Walnut Creek Study [86] found an increased incidence of acute myocardial infarction with oral contraceptive usage only in smokers over the age of 40.

CEREBROVASCULAR DISEASE

An increased incidence of cerebrovascular disease has been reported in oral contraceptive users [11, 12, 98, 131]. The Collaborative Group for the Study of Stroke in Young Women [22, 23] has estimated the incidence of thrombotic stroke to be 3 to 4 times more common and

hemorrhagic stroke to be 2 times more common in oral contraceptive users than in nonusers. Hypertension was found to be a risk factor for stroke among women who use contraceptives as well as among those who do not. The degree of blood pressure elevation was highly correlated with increased relative risk in both thrombotic and hemorrhagic stroke. Migraine itself may be a risk factor for the occurrence of either thrombotic or hemorrhagic stroke but does not increase the risk of stroke in women using oral contraceptives. The risk of hemorrhagic stroke is increased by heavy smoking. The incidence of thrombotic stroke was estimated to be 1 per 10,000 woman-years of use. Nine percent of the strokes were fatal.

Data from the Walnut Creek Study in 1978 [80] indicated a risk of subarachnoid hemorrhage 6.5 times greater for users than nonusers. The risk for smokers was 5.7 times that for nonusers, and the risk for women who both smoked and used oral contraceptives was 21.9 times greater. The Walnut Creek Study [86] subsequently reported the incidence of thrombotic stroke as increased only for current users over age 40 and past users over age 50. Of a total of 31 cases of stroke included in the Royal College of General Practitioners and the Walnut Creek studies, only three of the 31 patients were under age 35.

HYPERTENSION

Hypertension has been reported to develop in 1 to 5 percent of oral contraceptive users [31, 53, 55, 56, 106, 107]. It is increased by age, parity, and obesity and is reversible after stopping the pills in the absence of intercurrent disease. Because of this, and the synergistic effect of hypertension in the development of other vascular complications, blood pressure should be monitored carefully in oral contraceptive users with discontinuance if hypertension develops. I would advise against the use of oral contraception in patients with established hypertension.

OVERALL EXCESS CIRCULATORY SYSTEM DISEASE MORTALITY

The excess circulatory system disease mortality is clearly concentrated in users over the age of 35 and primarily in smokers. Some increased risk in smokers can be shown above age 30. The Royal College of General Practitioners in 1981 published mortality rates for its study [58] and found a statistically significant excess mortality in oral contraceptive users only in smokers over age 35 and in all users over 45 (Table 12-1).

A number of studies have addressed national mortal-

Table 12-1. Circulatory disease mortality and risk by age, smoking status, and oral contraceptive use

Age and smoking status	Deaths per 100,000 woman-years (No. of deaths)		Relative risk	Excess risk per 100,000 woman-years
	Ever users	Never users		
15–24				
Nonsmokers	0.0(0)	0.0(0)		0.0
Smokers	10.5(1)	0.0(0)		10.5
25–34				
Nonsmokers	4.4(2)	2.7(1)	1.6	1.7
Smokers	14.2(6)	4.2(1)	3.4	10.0
35–44				
Nonsmokers	21.5(7)	6.4(2)	3.3	15.1
Smokers	63.4(18)	15.2(3)	4.2*	48.2*
45+				
Nonsmokers	52.4(4)	11.4(1)	4.6*	40.9*
Smokers	206.7(17)	27.9(2)	7.4*	178.8*

*Statistically significant differences in risk ($p < .05$).
Source: Royal College of General Practitioners. Further analyses of mortality in oral-contraceptive users. *Lancet* 1(8219):541, 1981. Reprinted in *Population Reports*, Series A, No. 6, Population Information Program, The Johns Hopkins University, Baltimore, Maryland.

ity trends [66, 94, 134], and most have shown no change that can be associated with the growth of pill usage. One study, that of Beral [10], concluded that there was a relationship between oral contraceptive usage and mortality trends in a study of 21 countries. A subsequent analysis of expanded data from the same 21 countries by Belsey [9] did not confirm such a relationship.

Tietze [116] analyzed United States mortality trends and concluded that an oral contraceptive effect could not be excluded but that the fourfold levels of relative risk found by the Royal College Study appeared to be exaggerated. No effect of oral contraceptive use can be seen in the mortality rates for the younger age groups.

A follow-up report of the Royal College of General Practitioners Oral Contraceptive Study [58] found no increase in cardiovascular mortality with the duration of oral contraceptive usage but reported that an increased risk may persist after discontinuance of the method. Most of the cases were women 35 years of age or older and most were smokers.

Slone et al. [103] have reported that former users of oral contraceptives aged 40 to 49 who used the pills for 5 to 10 years had a higher risk of myocardial infarction. Residual risk was not found in postmenopausal women. Persistence of risk after stopping oral contraceptive use has not been found by other investigators [63, 81, 90], and Slone et al. state that "the data in this report should be interpreted with caution." It should also be noted that pills used in the time frame of the former use in this study were of higher dosage than currently used.

The question of possible persistence of effect is, at the moment, unsettled [59]. If a lasting effect is present, the mechanism would be one of altered blood lipids accelerating atherosclerosis. Serum lipid levels, principally triglycerides, are increased in most women using oral contraceptives, as well as alterations in laboratory test values (Table 12-2) [105, 136]. Alteration in these levels is related to the estrogen and progestin content of the pills. Estrogen has been shown to raise high-density lipoproteins (HDL) while progestins lower these levels. The level of high-density lipoprotein is shown to be inversely related to the incidence of coronary occlusion. Bradley et al. [16] (Table 12-3) have shown higher levels of HDL protein with more estrogenic pills and significantly lower levels with progestin-dominant pills. The Royal College study has reported increased total arterial disease and a decrease in HDL cholesterol with increasing progestin levels in oral contraceptives [51]. Smoking may also have an adverse effect on HDL protein [29]. It appears to be preferable in any long-time usage of oral contraceptives to employ a formulation without a strong progestational component [130].

Cholesterol and triglycerides should be checked in all patients with a family history of coronary occlusion before age 50 and also should be checked in women over age 35 without risk factors who elect to continue oral contraception. Women over age 35 with any of the risk factors (hypertension, diabetes, obesity, hyperlipoproteinemia, cigarette smoking) should not be prescribed oral contraceptives.

Table 12-2. Altered clinical laboratory measurements with most clinical significance

Substances measured	Change in level
Albumin	Decreased
Glucose	Elevated glucose level at 1 hour
Triglycerides (S)	Elevated
Thyroid-binding globulin (S)	Elevated
Thyroxine (S)	Elevated (free thyroxine normal)
Triiodothyronine resin uptake	Decreased (FTI normal)
Cortisol-binding globulin (S)	Elevated
Cortisol (P)	Elevated
17-OH-Corticosteroids (U)	Decreased
17-Ketogenic steroids (U)	Decreased
Metyrapone test	Impaired responsiveness
Sulfobromophthalein test	Impaired excretion
Platelets (B)	Elevated, mild
Blood procoagulants (B)	Elevated*
Iron (S)	Elevated
Iron-binding capacity (S)	Elevated

S = serum; P = plasma; U = urine; B = blood; FTI = free thyroxine index.
*Not evident on routine testing.
Source: H. Weindling and J. B. Henry. Laboratory test results altered by "the pill." *J.A.M.A.* 229:1763, 1974. Copyright 1974, American Medical Association.

CARBOHYDRATE METABOLISM

Glucose tolerance is initially diminished in a significant number of women taking oral contraceptives. This is more pronounced in women predisposed to diabetes and with latent or overt diabetes. These changes return to pretreatment levels after stopping oral contraceptives [104].

The changes in carbohydrate metabolism appear to be related to the progestin content with little, if any, effect from the estrogen component. Spellacy has reported no adverse effect on carbohydrate metabolism with a low-dose pill containing norethindrone [109] but did find an adverse effect with oral contraceptives containing norgestrel [108].

Diabetes is not increased by the use of oral contraception [93, 118], but the lowering of glucose tolerance in predisposed patients could bring the prediabetic to insulin dependence sooner, thereby giving the individual a longer exposure to the atherogenic effect of diabetes. Patients with a family history of diabetes should be

Table 12-3. Serum high-density lipoprotein cholesterol concentration according to oral contraceptive or other hormone formulation

Compound dosage (μg)	Adjusted concentration (μg/dl)	Difference from nonuser level
Mestranol 0.05, norethindrone 1.0	60.1	+0.1
Mestranol 0.08, norethindrone 1.0	62.8	+2.8
Ethinyl estradiol 0.05, norgestrel 0.5	50.4	−9.6
Ethinyl estradiol 0.05, ethynodiol diacetate 1.0	66.2	+6.2
Mestranol 0.10, norethynodrel 2.5	73.1	+13

Source: Reprinted with permission from D. D. Bradley, et al. Serum high-density lipoprotein cholesterol in women using oral contraceptives, estrogens and progestins. *N. Engl. J. Med.* 299:17, 1978

screened with at least a 2-hour postprandial blood sugar followed by glucose tolerance if an abnormality is found in the postprandial glucose.

NEOPLASMS

Endometrium

A registry for endometrial carcinoma in young women taking oral contraceptives was started by Silverberg and Makowski [102]. By 1975 they had found 21 such cases. Eight of these patients had other significant factors that might contribute to the development of endometrial cancer. Of the remaining 13 patients, only two were employing the combined pills. Eleven of the 13 were using sequential pills, while 8 percent of users at that time were employing sequentials. It is of interest that ten of these 11 were using the sequential pill having only 5 days of progestin, while only one woman among those with endometrial carcinoma was found employing a sequential with 7 days of progestin. The combined pills, with their daily progestin component, appear to have a protective effect against endometrial cancer. Five case-control studies [38, 47, 60, 95, 132] have reported a lower incidence of endometrial cancer in ever or current users of oral contraceptives. Layde [60] has reported the negative relative risk of endometrial cancer in users to be 0.5 for the combination pills. The protective effect increases with use, and its protection persists for at least 5 years after use. The protection is greatest for nulliparas, who are at greater risk for endometrial cancer.

Cervix

Family planning clinics in New York in 1969 reported an increased incidence of carcinoma in situ of the cervix in women using the pill as compared with those using diaphragms [69]. Subsequent analysis of these data showed that the differences were attributable to differences in populations choosing and using the pill versus those choosing and using the diaphragm [27].

Stern et al. [111], studying a group of women with cervical dysplasia, reported that a greater number of patients using oral contraceptives progressed to carcinoma in situ as compared with a group using barrier methods. However, there was no increased incidence of dysplasia or carcinoma in women on the pill. Four other studies of cervical carcinoma, carcinoma in situ, and dysplasia have not shown a relationship of incidence with use of oral contraceptives [14, 15, 133, 135]. The Royal College of General Practitioners Study found the incidence of cancer of the cervix to be lower in users than nonusers, but the number was too small to be statistically significant [93], while Vessey [127] showed that the pill may have an adverse effect on the development of cervical neoplasia.

Sexual behavior influences the risk of developing dysplasia, and it is difficult to standardize accurately for this confounding factor. The Walnut Creek Study [86] reported a 6.8 relative risk for carcinoma and carcinoma in situ of the cervix for oral contraceptive users aged 20 to 39 and a relative risk of 1.8 for those aged 40 to 49. Swan and Brown [113] attempted to control for the variance in sexual behavior in analyzing the Walnut Creek data and concluded that the risk was significantly greater for women who have taken the pill for 4 to 6 years but not for shorter or longer periods. In the 4-to 6-year group of oral contraceptive users, relative risk ranged from 1.6 to 3.4, depending on the level of sexual activity. This issue is still unsettled, but it is my belief, after reviewing the literature, that there may be an attributable increase of dysplasia in oral contraceptive users; however, an increase in actual invasive malignancy has not been proven.

Ovarian Cancer

Five case-control studies have found a decreased incidence of ovarian cancer in oral contraceptive users [19, 60, 67, 71, 91]. A study by the Centers for Disease Control [60] reported a negative risk ratio for ovarian cancer in pill users of 0.6. The risk decreased with length of usage, and for those using the pills for more than 4

years, the risk ratio was 0.3. Protection was greater for nulliparas, with a 0.3 risk ratio as compared to parity greater than three, where the risk ratio was 0.7. The protection also persisted after cessation of usage.

The same overall relative risk of 0.6 was found by the Drug Epidemiology Unit of Boston University [91], which also reported a persistence of effect, with reduction of risk lasting as long as 10 years after cessation of use.

Breast Cancer

No increased incidence of breast cancer was found among users in the studies of Vessey, Doll, and Jones [123] or Arthes, Sartwell, and Lewisohn [5]. In the latter study the incidence was numerically less in users than nonusers, but the difference was not statistically significant. Thirteen percent of the patients with breast cancer in the reproductive age group in the Boston Collaborative Drug Surveillance Program [13] used birth control pills, while they had been employed by 20 percent of the controls. Fasal and Poffenbarger [30] estimated a relative risk of breast cancer among users of 1.1. The increased incidence was noted only in women who had used the pills for 2 to 4 years. It was not noted in those who had used the pills for a lesser or greater time. This is difficult to explain except as sampling error. If there were a cause and effect relationship, the incidence should have increased with duration of use.

A case-control study from California [83] reported an increased risk of breast cancer among women who used oral contraceptives before their first full-term pregnancy and were either long-term users or had had benign breast disease. An increased risk of breast cancer (risk ratio 2.4) among women having a first-trimester abortion before first full-term pregnancy was also found in this study. These conclusions have been questioned by Clifford Kay, Director of the Royal College of General Practitioners Study, because the study included only 163 out of a total of 293 eligible patients [49].

Follow-up studies published in 1981 of the two British prospective studies found no significant increase in breast cancer among ever or current users of oral contraceptives [49, 126]. The Royal College of General Practitioners Study [49] also reported no evidence of increased relative risk with duration of oral contraceptive use, estrogen dose, or history of benign breast disease, although the number of cases in the latter category was too small for firm conclusions. The Oxford/Family Planning Association Study [126] reported an overall relative risk of developing breast cancer in women who had used oral contraceptives of 0.96, as compared with never-users.

In a large-scale study by the Centers for Disease Control of 687 cases of breast cancer and 1,000 controls [76], the relative risk of breast cancer in oral contraceptive users was reported as 0.96 (95% confidence limits 0.8 to 1.1). They found no increased risk with duration of use or evidence of latency. No increased risk was noted in patients with a history of benign breast disease or with a family history of breast cancer in first- or second-degree relatives. Increased risk of breast cancer was noted in users as well as never-users with increasing age at first pregnancy. When standardized for this variable, no increased risk of breast cancer for oral contraception before the first pregnancy was noted. Ten percent less breast cancer was found in recent users of oral contraception as compared with controls. A report by Pike [84] stating that long-term use by young women of birth control pills containing "high-potency" progestins can cause breast cancer was rejected by the United States FDA's Fertility and Maternal Health Drugs Advisory Committee based on multiple methodologic problems with the study. Pill use and breast cancer require continuing research. At present there does not appear to be an association between pill use and development of breast cancer.

MELANOMA

The Walnut Creek Study [86] reported a standardized rate of 28 per 100,000 women for melanoma in oral contraceptive users as opposed to eight for never-users, for a relative risk of 3.5. It has been postulated that this apparent increased risk may be related to increased exposure to sunshine, which is a known factor in the development of melanoma. Neither of the prospective British studies [1, 50] showed any association between oral contraceptive usage and melanoma. In a United States case-control study [86] there was a small (risk ratio 1.8) but not statistically significant increased risk of melanoma with oral contraceptive use of 5 or more years. In the Oxford/Family Planning Association Study [62] there was a strong suggestion of a negative association between oral contraceptive usage and melanoma but the study involved only 12 women with the disease.

PITUITARY TUMORS

Pituitary tumors are rare, although they are being diagnosed with increasing frequency since the availability of prolactin determinations and more modern x-ray techniques. The number of cases reported in ever or current users of oral contraception is small and the data conflicting. No association has been established at this time [20, 24, 25, 101, 115].

LIVER TUMORS

Benign liver tumors have been shown to be increased in oral contraceptive users [21, 28, 52, 72, 119]. These reports involved women using higher dose pills than are presently prescribed. Liver tumors are rare, with an estimated incidence of 1.2 per 100,000 users [45], but may rupture with fatal consequences. The upper abdomen should always be palpated to search for any liver enlargement in follow-up examination of pill users. Tumors may regress with cessation of usage. There is no apparent increase in malignant tumors of the liver with oral contraceptive use.

SUBSEQUENT REPRODUCTIVE FUNCTION

Except for a delay in ovulation in the first cycle, there is usually prompt return of reproductive function after discontinuing oral contraceptives. Less than 1 percent of users have postpill amenorrhea, and most of these appear to be coincidental. The incidence is higher in patients with previous history of menstrual irregularities (approximately 40% having a history of previous oligomenorrhea), and it is not related to length of original pill usage [34, 57, 100]. Cumulative delivery rates for oral contraceptive users as compared with diaphragm users is the same by 30 months in parous women and by 42 months in nulliparous women [120]. There is no increase in spontaneous abortion rate or congenital anomalies in pregnancies occurring after discontinuance of oral contraception [8, 79, 87, 88, 93, 118]. There may be a small increase in congenital anomalies of the heart in infants exposed to oral contraceptives in utero during the first trimester [36]. These may be attributable to higher dose pills.

An increase in chromosomal anomalies, especially trisomies, which are uniformly lethal, has been reported in abortuses of women who became pregnant within 3 months after discontinuing the higher dose oral contraceptives used in the 1960s [18]. These abnormalities have not been found in two separate studies following the use of lower dose pills [52, 129]. The original report is difficult to explain in view of the absence of a rise in abortion rates. Because of the unpredictable time of ovulation in the first postpill cycle, patients are well advised to use barrier contraception during the first cycle off the pills to avoid confusion over the estimated date of confinement. If pregnancy does occur in the first cycle, patients should be reassured that there is no reason to expect any ill effects to the fetus.

SUBJECTIVE EFFECTS

Subjective symptoms such as depression, nervousness, headache, and alterations in libido have been reported in association with oral contraceptive usage. Depression has been reported to be increased [35, 37, 48], unchanged [7, 32, 54], or decreased [114] by the use of these compounds. A previous history of depression has been noted in most patients who have reported increase in this symptom.

A 30 percent increase in depression in takers was reported in the Royal College of General Practitioners Study [94], but they cautioned that "psychological effects of being a Pill user are at least as likely to cause emotional disorders as the pharmacological action of the sex steroids and reporting bias is likely to intrude." There was no evidence in that study that severe depression requiring hospitalization is more common in pill users. Depression occurring in women on oral contraception has been ascribed to a disturbance in tryptophan metabolism through a deficiency of pyridoxine, a coenzyme in its metabolism.

Mood scales of 5,151 never, past, and current oral contraceptive users were studied by Kutner and Brown [54]; 3,919 of these women also completed the Minnesota Multiphasic Personality Inventory (MMPI). No difference was found among the groups in the MMPI, and there was less premenstrual moodiness among users. This study reported no evidence of oral contraception aggravating preexisting depression.

Decreased libido has been reported in pill users by Grant and Pryse-Davies [32] and by the Royal College of General Practitioners Study [93]. The latter study noted that most of the reports of decreased libido were in first-year use, and the majority were postpartum. These investigators felt that the loss of libido may reflect the influence of recent birth rather than an effect of the pill. No change in libido was found by Bakker and Dightman [7], and improvement in sexual adjustment was noted by Zell and Crisp [137].

The difficulty of evaluating drug effects on subjective symptoms is demonstrated in the study of Aznar-Ramos et al. [6], who gave placebos in the guise of oral contraceptives to 147 women during 424 woman-months. Twenty-nine percent of the placebo patients reported decreased libido, 16 percent headaches, and 6 percent nervousness.

Similarly, headaches have been reported to be both more common [82] and less common [26] in women using oral contraceptives. Migraine can be precipitated or aggravated by these compounds. However, only a minority of migraine patients became worse, and some patients noted improvement of their migraine with oral contraception. In some women headaches do seem to be precipitated by oral contraceptives, and when significant, their use should be stopped. Since women having strokes while taking oral contraceptives often had a history of severe headaches before the stroke, it is important to take this precaution.

The effect of psychologic factors on the incidence of all these subjective symptoms is difficult to determine. Whether the effect is psychologic or pharmacologic, it seems best to discontinue the medication when these symptoms occur. The patient is thus allowed to be her own control.

BENEFICIAL RESULTS OF ORAL CONTRACEPTION

In addition to the prevention of pregnancy, other beneficial effects have been noted with the use of oral contraceptives. There is a significant decrease in menorrhagia, dysmenorrhea, and premenstrual tension with oral contraceptive usage [3, 93]. With the improvement in menstrual function, there is a concomitant decrease in iron deficiency anemia.

Benign cystic disease of the breast has been found to have a lower incidence in oral contraceptive users in six separate studies [13, 17, 77, 93, 97, 124]. In the Royal College Study [93] there was a progressive decrease in the incidence of benign cystic disease with duration of use up to 5 years. In the Oxford/Family Planning Association study [17] the risk ratio for fibroadenoma was 0.4, for chronic cystic disease 0.7, and for unbiopsied breast lumps 0.6.

A lower incidence of duodenal ulcer was found by both the Royal College Study [93] and the Oxford/Family Planning Association study [118]. The explanation for this is obscure.

Oral contraceptive users were found by the Centers for Disease Control [75] also to have a lower incidence of pelvic inflammatory disease, ectopic pregnancy, endometrial and ovarian cancer, and rheumatoid arthritis. Ory has summarized these findings and estimates that 50,000 hospitalizations are prevented annually in the United States by these benefits (Table 12-4). An ancillary benefit of the lower incidence of pelvic inflammatory disease is that a reduction in infertility owing to tubal occlusion should ensue.

Ory [74, 75] estimates that the reduction in ovarian cancer averts 850 deaths per year in the United States, and this benefit alone more than outweighs the near 500 cardiovascular deaths annually estimated to be related to pill use in the United States.

SUMMARY

The choice of contraception requires risk-benefit analysis into which individual wishes and concerns must be entered. For the healthy young woman, in my opinion, the benefits of oral contraception far outweigh the risk. For others, clinical judgment must be exercised, but I

Table 12-4. Rate of hospitalizations prevented annually by use of oral contraceptives per 100,000 pill users and estimated number of hospitalizations prevented annually, by specific disease, in the United States[a]

Disease	Rate	No.
Benign breast disease	235	20,000
Ovarian retention cysts	35	3,000
Iron deficiency anemia[b]	320	27,200
Pelvic inflammatory disease (first episodes)		
Total episodes[b]	600	51,000
Hospitalizations	156	13,300
Ectopic pregnancy	117	9,900
Rheumatoid arthritis[b]	32	2,700
Endometrial cancer[c]	5	2,000
Ovarian cancer[c]	4	1,700

[a]Except where noted, figures refer to hospitalizations prevented among the estimated 8.5 million current users of oral contraceptives in the United States.
[b]Episodes prevented regardless of whether hospitalizations occurred.
[c]Based on an estimated 39 million United States women who had ever used oral contraceptives.
Source: Reprinted with permission from H. W. Ory, The noncontraceptive health benefits from oral contraceptive use. *Fam. Plann. Perspect.* 14:183, 1982.

would strongly recommend against oral contraceptive usage in older women who smoke.

The most important benefit of oral contraception is reliable protection against pregnancy. The Oxford/ Family Planning Association study [125] found the failure rates for various forms of contraception shown in Table 12-5. It is seen that combination oral contraceptives provide much greater protection than any other method of contraception except sterilization. This tangible benefit coupled with the esthetic advantages of protection unassociated with coital activity may be of great importance to the individuals concerned.

REFERENCES

1. Adam, S. A., et al. A case-control study of the possible association between oral contraceptives and malignant melanoma. *Br. J. Cancer* 44:45, 1981.
2. Adam, S. A., Thorogood, M., and Mann, J. I. Oral contraceptives and myocardial infarction revisited: The effects of new preparations and prescribing patterns. *Br. J. Obstet. Gynaecol.* 88:838, 1981.
3. Andrews, W. C., and Andrews, M. C. The newer progestins in various gynecological disorders. *Va. Med. Monthly* 88:143, 1961.

Table 12-5. Failure rates per 100 woman-years for different contraceptive methods according to age of woman and duration of contraceptive use

Method	Aged 25–34: Duration of use			Aged 35+: Duration of use		
	24 Months	25–48 Months	49+ Months	24 Months	25–48 Months	49+ Months
Estrogen-progestogen OC						
50 µg	0.25	0.18	0.09	0.17	0.11	0.10
50 µg	0.38	0.40		0.23	0.00	
Progestogen only OC	2.5			0.5		
Diaphragm	5.5	4.0	2.3	2.8	1.7	0.8
Condom	6.0	4.0	3.6	2.9	1.3	0.7
Intrauterine devices						
Lippes loop C	2.4	3.0	2.0	1.1	1.0	0.6
Lippes loop D	2.3	2.4	2.3	1.8	0.0	0.4
Saf-T-Coil	2.3	1.8	1.4	1.6	1.2	0.5
Copper-7	3.1			0.6	1.1	
Sterilization						
Female	0.45	0.14	0.00	0.08	0.07	0.09
Male	0.08	0.00	0.00	0.00	0.00	0.03

OC = oral contraceptive.
Source: Reprinted with permission from M. Vessey, M. Lawless, and D. Yeates, Efficacy of different contraceptive methods. *Lancet* 1:841, 1982.

4. Arthes, F. G., and Masi, A. T. Myocardial infarction in younger women: Associated clinical features and relationship to use of oral contraceptive drugs. *Chest* 70:574, 1976.

5. Arthes, F. G., Sartwell, P. E., and Lewisohn, E. F. The pill, estrogens and the breast: Epidemiological aspects. *Cancer* 28:1391, 1971.

6. Aznar-Ramos, R., et al. Incidence of side effects with contraceptive placebo. *Am. J. Obstet. Gynecol.* 105:1144, 1969.

7. Bakker, C. B., and Dightman, C. R. Side effects of oral contraceptives. *Obstet. Gynecol.* 28:373, 1966.

8. Banks, A. L., Rutherford, R. N., and Colburn, W. A. Pregnancy and progeny after use of progestin-like substances for contraception. *Obstet. Gynecol.* 26:760, 1965.

9. Belsey, M., Russell, Y., and Kinnear, K. Cardiovascular disease and oral contraceptives: A reappraisal of vital statistic data. *Fam. Plann. Perspect.* 11:84, 1979.

10. Beral, V. Cardiovascular disease mortality trends and oral contraceptive use in young women. *Lancet* 2:1047, 1976.

11. Bickerstaff, E. R. *Neurological Complications of Oral Contraceptives.* Oxford: Clarendon, 1975.

12. Bickerstaff, E. R., and Holmes, J. M. Cerebral arterial insufficiency and oral contraceptives. *Br. Med. J.* 1:726, 1967.

13. Boston Collaborative Drug Surveillance Program. Oral contraceptives and venous thromboembolic disease, surgically confirmed gallbladder disease and breast tumors. *Lancet* 1:1379, 1973.

14. Boyce, J. G., et al. Cervical carcinoma and oral contraception. *Obstet. Gynecol.* 40:139, 1972.

15. Boyd, J. T., and Doll, R. A study of the aetiology of carcinoma of the cervix uteri. *Br. J. Cancer* 18:419, 1964.

16. Bradley, D. D., et al. Serum high-density lipoprotein cholesterol in women using oral contraceptives, estrogens and progestins. *N. Engl. J. Med.* 299:16, 1978.

17. Brinton, L. A., et al. Risk factors for benign breast disease. *Am. J. Epidemiol.* 113:203, 1981.

18. Carr, D. H. Chromosome studies in selected spontaneous abortions: l. Conception after oral contraception. *Can. Med. Assoc. J.* 103:343, 1970.

19. Casagrande, J. T., et al. "Incessant ovulation" and ovarian cancer. *Lancet* 2:170, 1979.

20. Chang, R. J., et al. Detection, evaluation, and treatment of pituitary microadenomas in patients with galactorrhea and amenorrhea. *Am. J. Obstet. Gynecol.* 128:356, 1977.

21. Christopherson, W. M., Mays, E. T., and Barrows, G. H. Liver tumors in women on contraceptive steroids. *Obstet. Gynecol.* 46:221, 1975.

22. Collaborative Group for the Study of Stroke in Young Women. Oral contraception and increased risk of cerebral ischemia or thrombosis. *N. Engl. J. Med.* 17: 871, 1973.

23. Collaborative Group for the Study of Stroke in Young Women. Oral contraceptives and stroke in young women. *J.A.M.A.* 231:718, 1975.

24. Coulam, C. B., et al. Pituitary adenoma and oral contraceptives: A case-control study. *Fertil. Steril.* 31:25, 1979.

25. Davajan, V., et al. The significance of galactorrhea in patients with normal menses, oligomenorrhea and secondary amenorrhea. *Am. J. Obstet. Gynecol.* 130:894, 1978.

26. Diddle, W. W., Gardner, W. H., and Williamson, P. J. Oral contraceptive medications and headaches. *Am. J. Obstet. Gynecol.* 105:507, 1969.

27. Dubrow, H., et al. A study of the factors affecting choice of contraceptive. *Obstet. Gynecol. Surv.* 24:1012, 1969.

28. Edmondson, H. A., Henderson, B., and Benton, B. Liver-cell adenomas associated with the use of oral contraceptives. *N. Engl. J. Med.* 294:470, 1976.

29. Enger, S. C., et al. High density lipoproteins (HDL) and physical activity: The influence of physical exercise, age and smoking on HDL-cholesterol and the HDL-/total cholesterol ratio. *Scand. J. Clin. Lab. Invest.* 37:251, 1977.

30. Fasal, E., and Poffenbarger, R. S. Oral contraceptives as related to cancer and benign lesions of the breast. *J. Natl. Cancer Inst.* 55:767, 1975.

31. Fisch, I. R., Freedman, S. H., and Myatt, A. V. Oral contraceptives, pregnancy and blood pressure. *J.A.M.A.* 222:1507, 1972.

32. Grant, E. C., and Pryse-Davies, J. Effects of oral contraceptives on depressive mood change and on endometrial monoamine oxidase and phosphatases. *Br. Med. J.* 3:777, 1968.

33. Green, G. R., and Sartwell, P. E. Oral contraceptive use in patients with thromboembolism following surgery, trauma or infection. *Am. J. Public Health* 62:680, 1972.

34. Golditch, R. P. Postcontraceptive amenorrhea. *Obstet. Gynecol.* 39:903, 1972.

35. Goldzieher, J. W., et al. A placebo-controlled double-blind crossover investigation of the side effects attributed to oral contraceptives. *Fertil. Steril.* 22:609, 1971.

36. Heinonen, O. P., et al. Cardiovascular birth defects and antenatal exposure to female sex hormones. *N. Engl. J. Med.* 296:67, 1977.

37. Herzberg, B. N., et al. Oral contraceptives, depression and libido. *Br. Med. J.* 3:495, 1971.

38. Herzberg, B. S., et al. Protection against endometrial carcinoma by combination-product oral contraceptives. *J.A.M.A.* 247:475, 1982.

39. Inman, W. H. W., and Vessey, M. P. Investigation of deaths from pulmonary, coronary and cerebral thrombosis and embolism in women of childbearing age. *Br. Med. J.* 2:193, 1968.

40. Inman, W. H. W., et al. Thromboembolic disease and steroidal content of oral contraceptives. A report to the Committee on Safety of Drugs. *Br. Med. J.* 2:203, 1970.

41. Jacobson, C. Cytogenetic study of immediate postcontraceptive abortion. Report of a study under Food and Drug Administration contract, 1974.

42. Jain, A. D. Mortality risk associated with the use of oral contraceptives. *Stud. Fam. Plann.* 8:50, 1977.

43. Jick, H. Venous thromboembolic disease and ABO blood type. *Lancet* 1:539, 1969.

44. Jick, H., Dinan, B., and Rothman, K. J. Oral contraceptives and non-fatal myocardial infarction. *J.A.M.A.* 239:1403, 1978.

45. Jick, H., and Herman, R. Oral contraceptive induced benign liver tumors: The magnitude of the problem (letter to the editor). *J.A.M.A.* 240:828, 1978.

46. Kane, F. J. Psychiatric reactions to oral contraceptives. *Am. J. Obstet. Gynecol.* 102:1053, 1968.

47. Kaufman, D. W., et al. Decreased risk of endometrial cancer among oral contraceptive users. *N. Engl. J. Med.* 303:1045, 1980.

48. Kay, C. R. Oral contraception, venous thrombosis and varicose veins. *J. R. Coll. Gen. Pract.* 28:393, 1978.

49. Kay, C. R. Breast cancer and oral contraceptives: Findings in Royal College of General Practitioners Study. *Br. Med. J.* 282:2089, 1981.

50. Kay, C. R. Malignant melanoma and oral contraceptives. *Br. J. Cancer* 44:479, 1981.

51. Kay, C. R. Progestogens and arterial disease: Evidence from the Royal College of General Practitioners Study. *Am. J. Obstet. Gynecol.* 142:763, 1982.

52. Kent, D. R., Nissen, E. D., and Nissen, S. E. Liver tumors and oral contraceptives. *Int. J. Gynaecol. Obstet.* 15:137, 1977.

53. Kunin, C. M., McCormack, R. C., and Abernathy, J. R. Oral contraceptives and blood pressure. *Arch. Intern. Med.* 123:362, 1969.

54. Kutner, S. J., and Brown, W. L. Types of Oral Contraceptives, Depression and Premenstrual Symptoms. In S. Ramcharon (ed.), *The Walnut Creek Study of the Side Effects of Oral Contraceptives* (Vol. I). Bethesda: U.S. Department of Health, Education, and Welfare, 1976.

55. Laragh, J. H. The pill, hypertension and the toxemias of pregnancy. *Am. J. Obstet. Gynecol.* 109:210, 1971.

56. Laragh, J. H., et al. Oral contraceptives, renin, aldosterone and high blood pressure. *J.A.M.A.* 201:918, 1967.

57. Larsson-Cohn, V. The length of the first three menstrual cycles after combined oral contraceptive treatment. *Acta Obstet. Gynecol. Scand.* 48:416, 1969.

58. Layde, P. M., Beral, V., and Kay, C. R. Further analyses of mortality in oral contraceptive users: Royal College of General Practitioners Study. *Lancet* 1:541, 1981.

59. Layde, P. M., Ory, H., and Schlesselman, J. The risk of myocardial infarction in former users of oral contraceptives. *Fam. Plann. Perspect.* 14:78, 1982.

60. Layde, P. M. Long-term oral contraceptive use and the risk of cancer. Presented at the First Annual Conference on Family Planning, Emory University, Atlanta, Georgia, Oct 4, 1982.

61. Loretz, I. T. Contraindications to oral contraception. *Br. Med. J.* 2:315, 1962.

62. Mann, J. I. Oral Contraception and Myocardial Infarction in Young Women: Data from Countries Other than the United States. In J. J. Sciarra, G. I. Zatuchni, and J. J. Speidel (eds.), *Risks, Benefits and Controversies in Fertility Control.* Hagerstown, Md.: Harper & Row, 1977.

63. Mann, J. I., and Inman, W. H. W. Oral contraceptives and death from myocardial infarction. *Br. Med. J.* 2:245, 1975.

64. Mann, J. I., Inman, W. H. W., and Thorogood, M. Oral contraceptive use in older women and fatal myocardial infarction. *Br. Med. J.* 2:245, 1976.

65. Mann, J. I., et al. Myocardial infarction in young women with special reference to oral contraceptive practice. *Br. Med. J.* 2:241, 1975.

66. Markush, R. E., and Seigel D. G. Oral contraceptives and mortality trends from thromboembolism in the United States. *Am. J. Public Health* 59:418, 1969.

67. McGowan, L., et al. The woman at risk for developing ovarian cancer. *Gynecol. Oncol.* 7:325, 1979.

68. Meade, T. W., Greenberg, G., and Thompson, S. G. Progestogens and cardiovascular reactions associated with oral contraceptives and a comparison of the safety of the 50 and 30 g. preparations. *Br. Med. J.* 280:1157, 1980.

69. Melamed, M. R., et al. Prevalence rates of uterine cervical carcinoma in-situ for women using the diaphragm or contraceptive oral steroids. *Br. Med. J.* 3:195, 1969.

70. Murawski, B. J., et al. An investigation of mood states in women taking oral contraceptives. *Fertil. Steril.* 19:50, 1968.

71. Newhouse, M. L., et al. A case control study of carcinoma of the ovary. *Br. J. Prev. Soc. Med.* 31:148, 1977.

72. Nissen, E. D., Kent, D. R., and Nissen, S. E. Liver tumors and the pill: Analyzing the data. *Contemp. Obstet. Gynecol.* 8:103, 1976.

73. Oliver, M. F. Ischaemic heart disease in young women. *Br. Med. J.* 4:253, 1974.

74. Ory, H. W. The non-contraceptive health benefits from oral contraceptive use. *Fam. Plann. Perspect.* 14:132, 1982.

75. Ory, H. W. Oral contraceptives and breast cancer. Presented to the National Medical Committee, Planned Parenthood Federation of America. Baltimore, Nov. 22, 1982.

76. Ory, H. W. Contraceptive safety: The need for epidemiologic research. Presented to the Symposium on the Regulation of Human Fertility: Needs of Developing Countries and Priorities for the Future. Stockholm, Feb. 7–9, 1983.

77. Ory, H., et al. Oral contraceptives and reduced risk of benign breast diseases. *N. Engl. J. Med.* 294:419, 1976.

78. Peterson, C., et al. Antithrombin III: Comparison of functional and immunologic assays. *Am. J. Clin. Pathol.* 69:500, 1978.

79. Peterson, W. F. Pregnancy following oral contraceptive therapy. *Obstet. Gynecol.* 34:363, 1969.

80. Petitti, D. B., and Wingerd, J. Use of oral contraceptives, cigarette smoking, and risk of subarachnoid hemorrhage. *Lancet* 2:234, 1978.

81. Petitti, D. B., et al. Risk of vascular disease in women: Smoking, oral contraceptives, noncontraceptive estrogens, and other factors. *J.A.M.A.* 242:1150, 1979.

82. Phillips, B. M. Oral contraceptive drugs and migraine. *Br. Med. J.* 2:99, 1968.

83. Pike, M. C., et al. Oral contraceptive use and early abortion as risk factors for breast cancer in young women. *Br. J. Cancer* 43:72, 1981.

84. Pike, M. C. Breast cancer in young women and use of oral contraceptives: Possible modifying effect of formulation and age at use. *Lancet* 2:296, 1983.

85. Public Information Program. Oral contraceptives. *Popul. Rep.* [A]. No. 6, May–June, 1982.

86. Ramcharan, S., et al. The Walnut Creek Contraceptive Drug Study: A comprehensive study of the side effects of oral contraceptives: Vol. III. An interim report: A comparison of disease occurrence leading to hospitalization or death in users and non-users of oral contraceptives. National Institutes of Health Publication No. 81-564, January, 1981.

87. Rice-Wray, E., et al. Pregnancy and progeny after hormonal contraceptives: Genetic studies. *J. Reprod. Med.* 6:101, 1971.

88. Robinson, S. C. Pregnancy outcome following oral contraceptives. *Am. J. Obstet. Gynecol.* 109:354, 1971.

89. Rosenberg, L., Armstrong, B., and Jick, H. Myocardial infarction and estrogen therapy in premenopausal women (Letter to the Editor) *N. Engl. J. Med.* 294:1290, 1976.

90. Rosenberg, L., et al. Oral contraceptive use in relation to nonfatal myocardial infarction. *Am. J. Epidemiol.* 111:59, 1980.

91. Rosenberg, L., et al. Epithelial ovarian cancer and combination oral contraceptives. *J.A.M.A.* 247:3210, 1982.

92. Royal College of General Practitioners. Oral contraceptives and thromboembolic disease. *J. R. Coll. Gen. Pract.* 13:267, 1967.

93. Royal College of General Practitioners. *Oral Contraceptives and Health: An Interim Report*. London: Pittman, 1974.

94. Sachs, B. P., et al. Reproductive mortality in the United States. *J.A.M.A.* 247:2789, 1982.

95. Salmi, T. Risk factors in endometrial carcinoma with special reference to the use of estrogens. *Acta Obstet. Gynecol. Scand.* 86:1, 1979.

96. Sartwell, P. E., Arthes, F. G., and Tonascia, J. A. Epidemiology of benign breast lesions: Lack of association with oral contraceptive use. *N. Engl. J. Med.* 288:551, 1973.

97. Sartwell, P. E., et al. Thromboembolism and oral contraceptives: An epidemiologic case-control study. *Am. J. Epidemiol.* 90:365, 1969.

98. Shafey, S., and Scheinberg, P. Neurological syndromes occurring in patients receiving synthetic steroids (oral contraceptives). *Neurology* 16:205, 1966.

99. Shapiro, S., et al. Oral contraceptive use in relation to myocardial infarction. *Lancet* 1:743, 1979.

100. Shearman, R. P. Secondary amenorrhea after oral contraceptives: Treatment and follow-up. *Contraception* 2:123, 1975.

101. Sherman, B. M., et al. Pathogenesis of prolactin-secreting pituitary adenomas. *Lancet* 2:1019, 1978.

102. Silverberg, S. G., and Makowski, E. L. Endometrial carcinoma in young women taking oral contraceptive agents. *Obstet. Gynecol.* 46:503, 1975.

103. Slone, D., et al. Risk of myocardial infarction in relation to current and discontinued use of oral contraceptives. *N. Engl. J. Med.* 305:420, 1981.

104. Spellacy, W. N. A review of carbohydrate metabolism and oral contraceptives. *Am. J. Obstet. Gynecol.* 104:448, 1969.

105. Spellacy, W. N., et al. The effects of estrogen, progestogen, oral contraceptives and intrauterine devices on fasting triglycerine and insulin levels. *Fertil. Steril.* 24:178, 1973.

106. Spellacy, W. N., and Birk, S. A. The effect of intrauterine devices, oral contraceptives, estrogens and progestogens on blood pressure. *Am. J. Obstet. Gynecol.* 112:912, 1972.

107. Spellacy, W. N., and Birk, S. A. The effects of mechanical and steroidal contraceptive methods on blood pressure in hypertensive women. *Fertil. Steril.* 25:467, 1974.

108. Spellacy, W. M. Carbohydrate metabolism during treatment with estrogen, progestogen and low dose oral contraceptives. *Am. J. Obstet. Gynecol.* 6:732, 1982.

109. Spellacy, W. M., et al. The effects of a "low estrogen" oral contraceptive on carbohydrate metabolism during six months treatment: A preliminary report of blood glucose and plasma insulin values. *Fertil. Steril.* 28:885, 1977.

110. Stadel, B. V. Oral contraceptives and cardiovascular disease. *N. Engl. J. Med.* 305:612, 1981.

111. Stern, E., Forsythe, A. B., and Coffelt, C. F. Steroid contraceptive use and cervical dysplasia, increased risk of progression. *Science* 196:1460, 1977.

112. Stolly, P. D., et al. Thrombosis with low estrogen oral contraceptives. *Am. J. Epidemiol.* 102:197, 1975.

113. Swan, S. H., and Brown, W. L. Oral contraceptive use, sexual activity, and cervical carcinoma. *Am. J. Obstet. Gynecol.* 139:52, 1981.

114. Swanson, D. W., et al. Use of norethynodrel in psychotic females. *Am. J. Psychiatry* 120:1101, 1964.

115. Teperman, L., et al. Oral contraceptive history as a risk indicator in patients with pituitary tumors with hyperprolactinemia: A case comparison study of twenty patients. *Neurosurgery* 7:571, 1980.

116. Tietze, C. The pill and cardiovascular disease. *Fam. Plann. Perspect.* 11:205, 1979.

117. Vessey, M. P., et al. Postoperative thromboembolism and the use of oral contraceptives. *Br. Med. J.* 3:123, 1970.

118. Vessey, M. P., et al. A long-term follow-up of women using different methods of contraception: An interim report. *J. Biosoc. Sci.* 8:373, 1976.

119. Vessey, M. P., et al. Oral contraceptives and benign liver tumors. *Br. Med. J.* 2:1064, 1977.

120. Vessey, M. P., et al. Fertility after stopping different methods of contraception. *Br. Med. J.* 1:265, 1978.

121. Vessey, M. P., and Doll, R. Investigation of relation between use of oral contraceptives and thromboembolic disease. *Br. Med. J.* 2:199, 1968.

122. Vessey, M. P., and Doll, R. Investigation of relation between use of oral contraceptives and thromboembolic disease: A further report. *Br. Med. J.* 2:651, 1969.

123. Vessey, M. P., Doll, R., and Jones, R. Oral contraceptives and breast cancer. *Lancet* 2:941, 1975.

124. Vessey, M. P., Doll, R., and Sutton, P. M. Investigation of the possible relationship between oral contraceptives and benign and malignant breast disease. *Cancer* 28:1395, 1971.

125. Vessey, M. P., Lawless, M., and Yeates, D. Efficacy of different contraceptive methods. *Lancet* 1:841, 1982.

126. Vessey, M. P., McPherson, K., and Doll, R. Breast cancer and oral contraceptives: Findings in Oxford Family Planning Association Contraceptive Study. *Br. Med. J.* 282:2093, 1981.

127. Vessey, M. P., et al. Neoplasia of the cervix uteri and contraception: A possible adverse effect of the pill. *Lancet* 2:930, 1983.

128. VonKaulla, E., et al. Antithrombin III depression and thrombin generation acceleration in women taking oral contraceptives. *Am. J. Obstet. Gynecol.* 109:868, 1971.

129. Vosbeck, E. Cytogenetic morphological and clinical aspects of 453 cases of human spontaneous abortions. Ph.D. Dissertation, George Washington University School of Graduate Studies, 1975.

130. Wahl, P., et al. Effect of estrogen/progestin potency on lipid/lipoprotein cholesterol. *N. Engl. J. Med.* 308:862, 1983.

131. Walsh, F. B., et al. Oral contraceptives and neuro-ophthalmologic interest. *Arch. Ophthalmol.* 74:628, 1965.

132. Weiss, N. S., and Sayvetz, T. A. Incidence of endometrial cancer in relation to the use of oral contraceptives. *N. Engl. J. Med.* 302:551, 1980.

133. Wied, G. L., et al. Statistical evaluation of the effect of hormonal contraceptives on the cytologic smear pattern. *Obstet. Gynecol.* 27:327, 1966.

134. Wiseman, R. A., and MacRae, K. D. Oral contraceptives and the decline in mortality from circulatory disease. *Fertil. Steril.* 35:277, 1981.

135. Worth, A. J., and Boyes, D. A. A case control study into the possible effects of birth control pills on pre-clinical carcinoma of the cervix. *J. Obstet. Gynaecol. Br. Comm.* 79:673, 1972.

136. Wynne, V., et al. Fasting serum triglyceride, cholesterol and lipoprotein levels during oral contraceptive therapy. *Lancet* 2:756, 1969.

137. Zell, J. R., and Crisp, W. E. A psychiatric evaluation of the use of oral contraceptives. *Obstet. Gynecol.* 23:657, 1964.

13. Oral Contraceptive Practice

Louise B. Tyrer

Provision of oral contraceptives ("the pill") has become one of the most widespread aspects of medical practice in the world [74]. Therefore, it is important for the physician to be knowledgeable about the essential and current elements of oral contraceptive practice.

INITIAL EVALUATION FOR ORAL CONTRACEPTIVE USERS

All women requesting oral contraceptives need to be educated and counseled as to the benefits and risks associated with all methods of fertility control so that they may make informed choices. A detailed personal and family history should be taken to identify women for whom the pill is contraindicated as well as those who may be at high risk for its use. Special attention needs to be given to the following aspects of the personal history: age; malignancies; breast disease; cardiovascular history including thrombophlebitis, heart disease, hypertension, stroke, and vascular headaches; diabetes or prediabetes; liver disease; menstrual history (oligomenorrhea); toxemia of pregnancy; obesity (30% or more over standard weight); and smoking (amount). With regard to family history the following elements should be ascertained for risk assessment: family history of diabetes (parents, siblings), and heart attack before age 50 in mother or father [84].

The physical assessment must include as a minimum the height (at initial visit only); weight; blood pressure; breast examination; abdominal palpation including the liver; pelvic examination including visual inspection of the cervix and vagina, bimanual examination, and, if indicated, rectal examination; inspection and examination of extremities for varicosities and signs of phlebitis; and further examination as indicated by history or laboratory findings.

The routine laboratory tests that need to be performed are hematocrit or hemoglobin and Pap smear. Other tests such as urinalysis and testing for sexually transmissible diseases should be performed as indicated.

Women who are identified as potentially at increased risk for oral contraceptive use related to certain risk factors should also have special laboratory tests to determine their blood lipid levels (e.g., triglycerides and cholesterol) and/or their diabetic potential (blood sugar) [18, 67]. These risk factors include but are not limited to the following: women aged 35 and older, especially if they smoke heavily (more than 15 cigarettes daily—highest risk group); obesity (30% or more above ideal weight); high blood pressure (140/90 or above or on antihypertensive drugs); history of elevated blood triglycerides or cholesterol; diabetes (both diet- and insulin-controlled); family history of diagnosed diabetes in parents or siblings; and parental history of death from heart attack under age 50. If laboratory testing reveals abnormal values, the woman needs to be counseled about her increased risk status and advised against the use of oral contraceptives. Women aged 35 or older who are heavy smokers should not be provided oral contraceptives in any event, because they are at highest risk for a serious cardiovascular complication related to pill use [47, 59].

CONTRAINDICATIONS

The Food and Drug Administration (FDA) [108] lists the following as contraindications to oral contraceptive use:

Thrombophlebitis or thromboembolic disorders
A past history of deep vein thrombophlebitis or thromboembolic disorders
Cerebrovascular or coronary artery disease
Known or suspected carcinoma of the breast
Known or suspected estrogen-dependent neoplasia
Undiagnosed abnormal genital bleeding
Known or suspected pregnancy
Benign or malignant liver tumor, which developed during the use of oral contraceptives or other estrogen-containing products

Other conditions that should be considered as contraindications are age 35 or older for smokers (most serious risk), 40 and older for nonsmokers; hypertension (140/90 and above); much-impaired liver functions; type II hyperlipidemia or hypercholesterolemia [64, 73, 90, 94].

Some important relative contraindications requiring individualized physician judgment are cardiac disease; renal disease; galactorrhea; hepatitis or mononucleosis (within past 6 months); history of cholestatic jaundice; gestational diabetes, prediabetes or either diet- or insulin-controlled diabetes; breast feeding; ulcerative colitis; sickle cell disease; use of drugs known to interact with oral contraceptives; family history of death from heart attack under age of 50; and family history of diabetes in parents or siblings [23].

COUNSELING AND INFORMED
REQUEST (CONSENT)

Once the initial evaluation has been completed and special blood test results evaluated (when appropriate), the patient needs to be counseled about all aspects of the findings. She should be provided with the patient pill package insert and additional information about pill use and have questions answered. A joint decision needs to be made between the physician and the pa-

tient as to pill use. In many clinics, as part of the patient's record, a written informed request for pill use, containing information about any special risk factors determined to be present, is signed by the patient and witnessed before oral contraception is provided. Such a form should be updated with any change in the patient's risk status.

Since cigarette smoking greatly increases the risk of serious cardiovascular side effects from oral contraceptive use, women electing to use the pill should be strongly advised not to smoke, particularly those aged 30 and older [108]. Women aged 35 and older who will not stop smoking should not be prescribed the pill. Additionally, patients must be warned to stop using the pill and consult their physician should any of the following symptoms occur: unilateral weakness, numbness, tingling in extremities, or slurring of speech (possible cause: stroke); loss of vision, diplopia, proptosis (possible cause: retinal artery thrombosis); severe leg pains, swelling, tenderness, warmth, palpable thrombosed vein (possible cause: thrombophlebitis); hemoptysis (possible cause: pulmonary embolism); severe chest pain that may radiate to the left arm or neck (possible cause: myocardial infarction); and pain or mass in the abdomen, particularly the right upper quadrant (possible cause: cholecystitis/lithiasis; mesenteric thrombosis; liver neoplasm). Some other symptoms to be reported to the physician that may require action are continuing breakthrough bleeding or spotting after the first 3 to 4 months of use or absence of menses for two or more cycles, particularly when associated with galactorrhea; initiation or exacerbation of severe headaches, particularly vascular in nature; breast mass or discomfort; jaundice; and depression.

PILL SELECTION; STARTING; MISSED PILLS

There are 28 combination estrogen-progestin and three progestin-only oral contraceptives on the market in the United States today, with no valid comparative studies on which to base selection. However, the failure rates have been well established: Combination oral contraceptives containing 30 μg of estrogen or more have a theoretic-effectiveness of 99.6 percent; those containing 20 μg of estrogen have a slightly lower theoretic-effectiveness (about 98%); and the progestin-only pill is about 97 percent. Use-effectiveness data on failures in the first year of use with the combination pill are higher, being about 2.5 percent, but considerably higher (8%) for women under age 22 who have annual family incomes of less than $10,000 [78]. Minipill failures may be 10 percent or more.

Since the data from the literature indicate that the incidence of serious cardiovascular complications has been reduced by lowering the level of both the estrogenic and progestational potency [66, 102, 118], initial selection should take these facts into consideration. The FDA recommends that the dosage for contraception not exceed 50 μg of estrogen except for specific indications (e.g., uncontrolled breakthrough bleeding or failure of withdrawal menses). In actual practice, use figures indicate that pills containing 30 to 35 μg of estrogen are now most commonly prescribed. Additionally, as data emerge suggesting an increased risk of heart attack and/or hypertension related to use of the more potent progestins, many physicians are prescribing pills that contain both low estrogen (50 μg or less) and a low dose of a less biologically active progestin [66]. For a listing of currently marketed oral contraceptives containing information about estrogens and progestins by type, dosage, and progestational effects, see Table 13-1.

When prescribing, it should be borne in mind that underweight women are more likely to experience immediate and unacceptable side effects related to hormone excess (e.g., nausea, vomiting, breast discomfort, and weight gain) than normal or overweight women and particularly need the lowest effective dosage of estrogen/progestin potency pills [104]. On the other hand, overweight women may have more breakthrough bleeding or spotting and require a pill of higher dosage or potency.

Younger women under age 18 have the lowest risk of serious complications related to pill use [78]. It is advisable to ensure that the onset of regular ovulation and menses have occurred before initiation of oral contraceptives. This age group is at greatest risk of unintended pregnancy with a mortality of 11.1 deaths per 100,000 live births as compared with an estimated risk of 1.5 deaths per 100,000 pill users [24, 77, 78]—a most positive benefit-risk ratio for pill use exists. Older women (age 35 and older) who smoke heavily and nonsmokers over age 40 have a negative benefit-risk ratio for mortality associated with pill use as compared with pregnancy [47, 48].

The pill is best initiated for the first time with either of the following schedules:

Start on the fifth day following the onset of menses
Start on the first Sunday following the onset of menses
 (if the woman wishes to avoid withdrawal menses occurring on weekends)

The choice of whether to prescribe the 21- or 28-day package is a matter of individual preference. Some hold that establishing the daily pill-taking habit provides less opportunity to forget. Concomitant use of a barrier method during the first months of pill use may be indicated for women likely to forget to take their pills regularly. After the first cycle the active pill should be started 7 days after taking the last active tablet from the previous cycle.

When starting the pill postpartum, it is advisable that only the "minipill" be used during full nursing [7, 13, 105]. It should not be started before 2 weeks postpartum, but preferably by 4 weeks. Non-nursing postpartum women should start the combination pill between the second and third week after delivery. Delaying initiation minimizes the risk of using the pill with a concomitant postpartum thrombophlebitis. For a patient undergoing late-midtrimester abortion (20 weeks from last menstrual period or more), applying the same principles for pill initiation as for non-nursing postpartum patients is appropriate. For patients having earlier abortion, the pill should be started at least within the first week following the procedure, as these patients may resume ovulation as early as 10 to 14 days following the abortion.

For oligomenorrheic women who wish to initiate oral contraception, once pregnancy and other pathology (e.g., pituitary adenoma) have been ruled out, the pill may be started on day 5 following a progesterone-induced withdrawal bleed. Such women must be counseled in advance of their increased risk of having post-pill amenorrhea [30, 60, 95].

If a patient reports that she has missed taking her pills, the following protocol [107] should be followed:

Regular pill use: If one pill is forgotten, take one as soon as remembered and the regular pill at the usual time. If the pill is forgotten 2 days in a row, take two pills daily for each of the next 2 days and use an additional method of protection (e.g., foam or condoms) for the rest of the month. If withdrawal bleeding does not occur, call the physician before restarting the pill. Continue to use another method until seen and evaluated.

Irregular pill use: If the patient has forgotten to take the pill for several days (3 or more), she may become pregnant. Discontinue the pill and use another method of protection (e.g., foam or condoms) for the rest of the month. If withdrawal bleeding does not occur, the patient must be evaluated. Advise the patient to continue to use another method of contraception until a determination can be made.

ONGOING EVALUATION OF ORAL CONTRACEPTIVE USERS

New pill users should be reevaluated within 6 months of initiation or sooner if problems develop. The patient needs to be queried as to symptoms suggestive of potential adverse effects or perceived problems. The weight and blood pressure should be checked and ex-

Table 13-1. Current oral contraceptives by name, dosage, and known effects on HDL-LDL cholesterol levels

Trade name	# per package	Manufacturer	Estrogen	Dose (μg)	Progestin	Dose (μg)	Adjusted serum HDL cholesterol concentration of certain OC formulations and difference from nonuser level[a]		Adjusted concentrations of lipids and lipoproteins in users and nonusers of certain OC formulations (mg/dl)[b,c]		
							Concentration (mg/dl)[c]	Difference from nonuser level	Cholesterol (median)		
									HDL nonusers	LDL	VLDL
Ovcon 35	21, 28	Mead Johnson	Ethinyl estradiol	35	Norethindrone	0.4			54	109	11
Ovcon 50	21, 28	Mead Johnson	Ethinyl estradiol	50	Norethindrone	1.0					
Ortho-Novum 7/7/7	21, 28	Ortho	Ethinyl estradiol	35	7-Norethindrone	0.5					
			Ethinyl estradiol	35	7-Norethindrone	0.75					
			Ethinyl estradiol	35	7-Norethindrone	1.0					
Ortho-Novum 10/11	21, 28	Ortho	10-Ethinyl estradiol	35	10-Norethindrone	0.5					
			11-Ethinyl estradiol	35	11-Norethindrone	1.0					
Modicon	21, 28	Ortho	Ethinyl estradiol	35	Norethindrone	0.5					
Ortho-Novum 1/35	21, 28	Ortho	Ethinyl estradiol	35	Norethindrone	1.0			Pooled data		
Ortho-Novum 1/50	21, 28	Ortho	Mestranol	50	Norethindrone	1.0	60.1	+0.1			
Ortho-Novum 1/80	21, 28	Ortho	Mestranol	80	Norethindrone	1.0	62.8	+2.8	58[d]	118	15[d]
Ortho-Novum-2	20, 21	Ortho	Mestranol	100	Norethindrone	2.0					
Loestrin 1/20	21, 28 Fe	Parke-Davis	Ethinyl estradiol	20	Norethindrone acetate	1.0					
Loestrin 1.5/30	21, 28 Fe	Parke-Davis	Ethinyl estradiol	30	Norethindrone acetate	1.5			Pooled data		
Norlestrin 1/50	21, 28, 28 Fe	Parke-Davis	Ethinyl estradiol	50	Norethindrone acetate	1.0					
Norlestrin 2.5/50	21, 28 Fe	Parke-Davis	Ethinyl estradiol	50	Norethindrone acetate	2.5			54	124[d]	14

Drug	Manufacturer	Days	Estrogen	Estrogen (μg)	Progestin	Progestin (mg)					
Demulen 1/35	Searle	21, 28	Ethinyl estradiol	35	Ethynodiol diacetate	1.0					
Demulen	Searle	21, 28	Ethinyl estradiol	50	Ethynodiol diacetate	1.0	66.2	+6.2	57	132[e]	20
Ovulen	Searle	21, 28	Mestranol	100	Ethynodiol diacetate	1.0			54	124[d] Pooled data	18[d]
Enovid-5	Searle	21	Mestranol	75	Norethynodrel	5.0					
Enovid-E	Searle	21	Mestranol	100	Norethynodrel	2.5	73.1	+13	73[d]	110	14
Enovid-10	Searle	21	Mestranol	150	Norethynodrel	9.85					
Brevicon	Syntex	21, 28	Ethinyl estradiol	35	Norethindrone	0.5					
Tri-Norinyl	Syntex	21, 28	Ethinyl estradiol	35	7-Norethindrone	0.5					
			Ethinyl estradiol	35	9-Norethindrone	1.0					
			Ethinyl estradiol	35	5-Norethindrone	0.5					
Norinyl 1 + 35	Syntex	21, 28	Ethinyl estradiol	35	Norethindrone	1.0					
Norinyl 1 + 50	Syntex	21, 28	Mestranol	50	Norethindrone	1.0	60.1	+0.1			
Norinyl 1 + 80	Syntex	21, 28	Mestranol	80	Norethindrone	1.0	62.8	+2.8			
Norinyl-2	Syntex	20	Mestranol	100	Norethindrone	2.0					
Nordette	Wyeth	21, 28	Ethinyl estradiol	30	Levonorgestrel	0.15					
Lo-Ovral	Wyeth	21, 28	Ethinyl estradiol	30	Norgestrel	0.3					
Ovral	Wyeth	21, 28	Ethinyl estradiol	50	Norgestrel	0.5	50.4	-9.6	43[d]	135[d]	15[d]
Progestin-only OCs											
Micronor	Ortho	28			Norethindrone	0.35					
Nor-Q.-D.	Syntex	42			Norethindrone	0.35					
Ovrette	Wyeth	28			d-1-Norgestrel	0.075					

[a] Adapted from D. D. Bradley et al. Serum high density lipoprotein cholesterol in women using oral contraceptives, estrogens and progestins. *N. Engl. J. Med.* 299:17, 1978.
[b] Adapted from P. Wahl et al. Effects of estrogen/progestin potency on lipid/lipoprotein cholesterol. *N. Engl. J. Med.* 308:865, 1983.
[c] To convert cholesterol values to millimoles per liter, multiply by 0.02586; to convert triglyceride values to millimoles per liter, multiply by 0.01129.
[d] Significantly different from nonusers at the 0.05 level.
[e] Not statistically significant related to small sample size.

aminations performed as indicated. For women who are at high risk for pill use related to elevated blood sugar and/or blood lipid determinations, these tests should be repeated to determine whether oral contraceptives should be continued. Thereafter, the special blood tests should be repeated every year or two as indicated as part of the decision on continued pill use.

Subsequent return visits should be individualized and occur at least annually. The history and physical assessment should be updated at that time and a repeat Pap smear taken. At each return visit a determination should be made as to the appropriateness of continuing oral contraceptives. Factors entering into this quantification are the occurrence of symptoms indicative of the development of potentially serious problems that may be associated with oral contraceptive use; minor side effects unacceptable to the patient; and patient desire to initiate pregnancy or patient request to discontinue or change contraceptive method.

There is no physiologic reason for patients to be "rested" periodically from the pill. Serious cardiovascular effects are not increased or related to duration of use at least until age 35 and older.

DRUG INTERACTIONS

A drug history should be taken on all oral contraceptive users and updated regularly. Additionally, pill users who are taking other drugs need to be advised about potential interactions and reduced effectiveness of both the pill and the other drug [2, 49, 56, 82]. This interaction may occur by altering drug absorption or by inhibiting or stimulating their metabolism by enzyme induction. Unexpected breakthrough bleeding or spotting may be an early warning sign of drug interaction and possibly lowered effectiveness. Absence of withdrawal bleeding may be indicative of pregnancy. Clinically important interactions occur between the pill and drugs such as rifampicin and anticonvulsants. There are three case reports of pregnancy in oral contraceptive users who were given ampicillin and one case with tetracycline. Diabetic control may also be affected. When the use of another drug is short term (e.g., 5 days of antibiotics), a backup barrier method may be prescribed. In the case of antidepressants and anticonvulsants, it may be necessary to increase the potency of the oral contraceptive to ensure efficacy and possibly increase the dose of the other drug to maintain control of the disease. However, if long-term therapy is required with potent enzyme-inducing drugs such as rifampicin or phenobarbital, pill users should employ a supplemental method or change to another method of contraception.

STOPPING PILL USE

Side Effects and Complications

Serious symptoms or potentially serious side effects require immediate discontinuation of oral contraception. In such instances further use is generally contraindicated. Such an assessment must be made by a physician. Other method(s) of contraception should be initiated. Minor side effects unacceptable to the patient, which do not diminish with continued use or switching pill dosage, may require discontinuation. In such situations the patient should be encouraged to continue at least through the tenth pill day to successfully suppress ovulation and ensure withdrawal menses.

Major Surgery/Hospitalization/Immobilization

Since major surgery, hospitalization, and immobilization increase the risk of thromboembolism, the pill should be stopped about 4 weeks in advance, when feasible. This recommendation need not apply to female sterilization by laparoscopy or minilaparotomy. When surgical emergencies occur to a pill user, some physicians recommend the use of minidose heparin as a precautionary measure along with cessation of use [33, 80, 116].

Pregnancy

When stopping oral contraceptives to initiate pregnancy, it is advisable but not essential to use a barrier method of birth control at least through one menstrual cycle, if for no other reason than to more accurately date gestation. The average delay in conceiving after stopping the pill is 2 months, with no increased risk of abortion, fetal anomalies in live births, or increase in subsequent infertility [9, 46, 81, 87, 88, 90, 111, 113, 117].

When pregnancy occurs with continuing use of the pill, there may be a slightly increased risk of congenital anomalies (heart) [37]. The pill must be stopped and the woman so counseled in order for her to make a decision as to whether she wishes to continue the pregnancy.

If a woman who is taking her pills regularly misses two menses, pregnancy should be ruled out through use of a highly sensitive pregnancy test before resumption of oral contraceptives. If the pregnancy test is negative and pelvic examination normal, in order to reestablish menses the dosage of the pill may have to be adjusted (e.g., decrease progestin potency or increase the estrogen from 35 µg to 50 µg).

MANAGEMENT OF SIDE EFFECTS AND COMPLICATIONS

Cardiovascular System Effects

MYOCARDIAL INFARCTION

Oral contraceptives exert a synergistic effect with other risk factors associated with an increased incidence of myocardial infarction. This synergism is greatly multiplied when the risk factor of heavy smoking is present [65, 115]; analysis of the risk of myocardial infarction with one of the risk factors being smoking reveals the following progression:

One factor—4 times increased risk
Two factors—10 times increased risk
Three factors—78 times increased risk

Good medical management calls for screening and eliminating from the pool of pill users women at high risk for heart attack, whether by history or physical or laboratory assessment; additionally, women at potentially increased risk found to have cholesterol values of 267 mg per 100 ml or above or triglycerides of 207 mg per 100 ml or more should not be given or continued on oral contraceptives. Occurrence of angina or a myocardial infarction mandates immediate cessation of oral contraceptives.

CARDIOVASCULAR ACCIDENT

Deaths from cardiovascular accidents associated with pill use are largely caused by subarachnoid hemorrhage. Thrombotic or nonhemorrhagic stroke is more rare and appears to be largely confined to women over age 35. Women who either develop persistent headache or note an exacerbation of headaches, especially migraine in type, or develop hemiparesis, even if transient, need to stop the pill and consult their physicians [42, 43, 90, 92, 109, 115].

HYPERTENSION

Hypertension, while rare, may have its onset at any time during pill use—hence the importance of checking the blood pressure at each visit [29, 54, 57, 58, 100, 101]. Usually such hypertension is mild to moderate with elevations of 10 to 20 mm Hg diastolic and 20 to 40 mm systolic. Both components of the pill are likely to contribute to the hypertension, but the progestin may have the greater effect. Mild elevations may subside when a pill with a lower dosage or level or progestational bioactivity is used. If this does not occur within 3 months, oral contraceptives should be discontinued, whereupon the blood pressure usually returns to pretreatment levels. A blood pressure of 140/90 should contraindicate pill use, as does the use of antihypertensive drugs.

THROMBOPHLEBITIS; DEEP VEIN THROMBOSIS

Suspicion of thrombophlebitis or deep vein thrombosis calls for immediate discontinuation of oral contraceptives [12, 42, 89–91, 93, 108]. Appropriate diagnostic techniques should be utilized to establish a diagnosis. Anticoagulant therapy is often indicated. If the diagnosis is confirmed, pills may not be resumed.

PULMONARY EMBOLISM

When symptoms of chest pain, shortness of breath, or hemoptysis occur, pulmonary embolism should be suspected and the pill immediately stopped [10, 42, 43, 89, 90, 92, 93, 109, 110, 115]. Once the diagnosis is confirmed, anticoagulant therapy is essential. If uncontrolled, ligation of the inferior vena cava may be necessary. Further pill use is contraindicated.

MESENTERIC ARTERY THROMBOSIS

Although rare, either venous or arterial thrombosis has been known to occur, but arterial thrombosis is the more serious, with a mortality approaching 50 percent related to delay in diagnosis. Abdominal pain, often of 2 or more weeks' duration, is characteristic. Later symptoms of vomiting, diarrhea, hematemesis, or bloody stools may occur. A series of upper gastrointestinal studies may show narrowing of a segment of small bowel. Although anticoagulant therapy may be tried in early cases, the therapy is usually surgical resection. Oral contraception should be discontinued if the diagnosis is suspected; if confirmed, pill use is contraindicated [40, 72].

RETINAL ARTERY THROMBOSIS

Retinal artery thrombosis is a rare condition heralded by the development of visual symptoms such as diplopia, blurred vision, or loss of vision [108]. Oral contraceptives should be immediately discontinued. The condition is treated with anticoagulants. Further oral contraceptive use is contraindicated.

Reproductive System Effects

BREAKTHROUGH BLEEDING/SPOTTING

Bleeding sufficient to require the use of a pad or tampon constitutes breakthrough bleeding. It is most common during the first 3 months of use of low-dose pills (50 μg of estrogen or less). It is cited as the most common reason why women discontinue pill use. Initiating pill use with a multiphasic pill may reduce breakthrough bleeding. Counseling and reassurance about early cycle breakthrough bleeding are often sufficient. Should it continue and be a problem after the first 3 to 4 months, adjustment of the formulation is indicated. However, other pathologic cause should first be ruled out, such as spontaneous abortion, neoplasia, ectopic pregnancy, and pelvic inflammatory disease (PID). It is advisable first to attempt to control the breakthrough bleeding by switching to a formulation with higher dosage or a biologically more active progestin, at least during a portion of the cycle. If not controlled and if the bleeding occurs during the first 10 days of the cycle, a higher dosage of estrogen is likely indicated. However, it is rarely necessary to exceed 50 µg of estrogen [21, 25, 31].

CHANGES IN MENSES
Primary dysmenorrhea usually improves with suppression of ovulation. Secondary dysmenorrhea related to adenomyosis or endometriosis also usually shows improvement. If dysmenorrhea occurs, prostaglandin antagonists produce effective relief. The number of days of menses and the amount of flow are also generally decreased.

Absence of withdrawal menses (exclusive of pregnancy) is usually related to insufficient endometrial proliferation. If pregnancy has been ruled out and withdrawal bleeding is important, a patient on a sub-50 µg pill may be switched to one containing 50 µg of ethinyl estradiol or mestranol (nearly equivalent). Another therapy is to continue the sub-50 µg pill but add 20 µg of ethinyl estradiol for 3 or more months [22].

UTERINE, CERVICAL, AND VAGINAL CHANGES
Pills containing higher doses of estrogen (100 µg) can stimulate growth of leiomyoma. However, the 50-µg estrogen pills have not been shown to either cause myomata or accelerate their growth.

All cases of persistent undiagnosed abnormal uterine bleeding require appropriate diagnostic procedures to rule out malignancy [68].

It is important to follow oral contraceptive users annually with Pap smears. Cervical dysplasias, more common among pill users, require colposcopic evaluation and treatment [61]. If cervical cancer is diagnosed, oral contraceptives should be permanently discontinued.

The vagina and cervix of diethylstilbestrol-exposed women may exhibit adenosis. Once malignancy has been ruled out, there is no contraindication to the use of oral contraceptives.

For treatment of cervical atrophy or hypertrophy, the estrogen dosage in the pill may be reduced with good results.

Moniliasis is common among oral contraceptive users. Five studies [14, 44, 98, 119, 124] reported an increased incidence of monilial infection among pill users, while five other investigators [20, 26, 62, 69, 106] found no difference in the incidence of this condition between users and nonusers. It requires treatment with an antifungal drug.

Pill use appears to significantly decrease a woman's risk of developing PID (by about 50%) and may offer some protective effect for her future fertility [3, 28, 90, 122].

POSTPILL AMENORRHEA/GALACTORRHEA
Postpill amenorrhea, occurring in about 1 percent of users, is usually defined as failure to resume menses by 6 months after discontinuation of oral contraceptives. It is more common in women who give a history of oligomenorrhea [4, 11, 15, 45, 106]. Such women need to be counseled in advance that they are at increased risk of having postpill amenorrhea. Associated galactorrhea occurs in about 20 percent of postpill amenorrhea. If galactorrhea is present, an evaluation should be started by 3 months. If a woman does not have galactorrhea but is anxious to achieve a pregnancy, an evaluation to include an endocrinologic workup should commence by the end of a 6-month period of amenorrhea. In the event pregnancy is not desired and galactorrhea is not present, one may wait up to a year for evaluation and possible therapy, as most women (about 99%) will resume menses within this time period [41]. Most women who have postpill amenorrhea/galactorrhea respond to therapy with daily bromocryptine (Parlodel, Sandoz) either alone or combined with chlomiphene citrate 50 to 100 mg daily for 5 days for up to 6 months. Care should be taken to rule out either dietary or exercise amenorrhea. Additionally, it is important to recall that pregnancy can occur before resumption of menses. Before initiation of sophisticated diagnostic tests or treatments, pregnancy must be ruled out.

BREAST PROBLEMS
Oral contraceptive use has not been found to cause breast cancer [5, 51, 61, 75, 76, 114] but may accelerate the growth of preexisting unnoticed neoplasm. Women who are at high risk for development of breast cancer according to the classification of the American Cancer Society require particularly careful monitoring while using oral contraceptives. If a woman develops a unilateral mass or pain while on oral contraceptives, the diagnosis of neoplasm should be considered and the pill discontinued while undergoing a diagnostic workup.

Women who experience bilateral breast pain, swelling, or masses are probably experiencing an estrogenic response. Reducing the dosage of estrogen and increasing the androgenic activity of the progestin (norgestrel/levonorgestrel) is often helpful. Reducing caffeine intake may also be helpful.

Breast feeding may be adversely affected by use of combination oral contraceptives, which may decrease the quantity and quality of breast milk and shorten the duration of lactation [35]. Small quantities of ingested oral contraceptives are excreted in breast milk, but no adverse effect has been demonstrated from this. It seems prudent at this time for breast-feeding women to avoid the use of the combination pills. However, progestin-only pills may be used, since they do not appear to adversely affect nursing [13].

Other Systemic Effects

METABOLIC AND CARBOHYDRATE METABOLISM; DIABETES
Although the pill does not cause diabetes, a significant deterioration in the glucose tolerance test (GTT) may occur in women on oral contraceptives [90, 96, 99, 111]. This effect is more likely to be marked with higher dose pills (above 50 μg of estrogen). Spellacy [97, 99] has found that this effect does not occur with pills containing 35 μg of ethinyl estradiol with norethindrone (0.4–0.5 μg norethindrone).

Women who are already insulin-dependent diabetics appear to be least affected; however, they are already at increased risk for atherosclerotic heart disease (ASHD), which the pill may worsen as does pregnancy. Ideally, a diabetic should use the pill only while she is young for the shortest possible time and elect permanent contraception upon completion of childbearing.

Other women who are at significantly increased risk for conversion to overt diabetes on oral contraceptives are those who experienced gestational diabetes and those with a strong family history of diabetes in parents or siblings. Such women should have a blood glucose determination to guide the decision as to whether to prescribe the pill. A fasting blood sugar (FBS) of 105 mg per 100 ml or greater or a 2-hour postprandial glucose of 120 mg per ml or above indicates possible diabetes. In these situations a diabetic workup is indicated before determining the contraceptive choice. If oral contraceptives are prescribed, the blood sugar (preferably the 2-hour postprandial test) should be repeated within 6 months of initiation of the lowest effective estrogen/progestin pill. If a marked increase in the blood sugar test has occurred, it is advisable to discontinue the pill and prescribe another method of contraception. After stopping the pill, glucose tolerance changes reverse in most patients.

ENDOCRINE-ADRENAL
Oral contraceptive use (estrogen effect) causes a reversible increase in corticosteroid-binding globulin but does not impair adrenal function [19, 121]. In addition, there is a rise in serum-free cortisol. As a result, conditions such as arthritis may improve during pill use and worsen when it is stopped.

ENDOCRINE-THYROID
Oral contraceptive use (estrogen effect) produces increased amounts of thyroid-binding globulin (TBG), al-

tering both T3 and T4 levels but not the thyroid function [19, 63, 121]. Thus it is not necessary to stop the pill during thyroid testing as the "T7 index" is unaffected.

The thyroid gland should be palpated at least annually for nodules and, if found, evaluated for malignancy.

Gastrointestinal System

Nausea, vomiting, epigastric distress, bloating, and loss of appetite are not uncommon upon initiation of oral contraceptives [90]. They can be minimized by prescribing a low-dose combination pill and recommending that it be taken at night with food. These undesirable effects, when they occur, usually subside within 3 months of continued use.

Duodenal ulcers are decreased by as much as 40 percent in oral contraceptive users. Gingivitis, mouth ulcers, and salivary calculi are increased and may require discontinuation of the pill.

Urinary System

Cystitis and urinary tract infection (UTI) occur slightly more often with pill use [53, 86, 90, 111]. The Royal College of General Practitioners Study found that 1.1 percent of users had kidney infections as compared with 0.7 percent of nonusers. Since estrogen can cause bladder hypersensitivity and progestin may decrease the tone of the ureters and bladder, decreasing the dosage and potency of both components may be helpful, along with therapeutic measures to clear up the UTI.

Hepatic and Biliary System

Hepatocellular adenoma of the liver is a rare benign tumor that may be associated with long-term pill use [16, 27, 71, 112]. It may produce a palpable mass or acute abdominal pain if rupture occurs. An intraabdominal hemorrhage is life-threatening. It is important to palpate the right upper quadrant for liver enlargement or tenderness at annual examinations. If suspected, the pill should be stopped. Selective hepatic angiography will usually demonstrate a lesion. Pill discontinuation results in regression of the tumor. Pregnancy must be avoided, as it may accelerate growth of the tumor. The pill is contraindicated for women with a previous history of severe liver disease or those who have abnormal liver function tests.

Cholestatic jaundice occurs in about 1 in 10,000 women on the pill [23, 36, 90]. Women who have either an inherited or acquired defect of hepatic excretory function may become jaundiced related to oral contraceptive use. Jaundice and pruritus are cardinal symptoms. Most cases occur within the first 6 months of pill use. Upon occurrence, the pill must be stopped.

If the jaundice appears to be unrelated to oral contraceptive use (e.g., hepatitis), the pill may be tried again about 3 months after a return to a normal state of health or normal liver function tests. Pregnancy, which can aggravate the condition, must also be avoided during this time.

Cholecystitis/Cholelithiasis

A small increased incidence of surgically confirmed gallbladder disease (1.2–twofold increased risk) in women prone to this disease appears to be limited to the first 6 to 12 months of use [12, 79, 86, 90]. One should be alert to this possibility during the first year of pill use.

Nervous System

While tension headaches are common and not likely related to pill use, migraine headaches may be caused by either component of the pill [26, 83, 90]. Patients who experience increasing severity of headaches, especially the vascular (migraine) type, should stop taking the pill and consult their physician. For headaches associated with fluid retention, reduction of the estrogen dosage may be helpful. If not, the pill should be discontinued.

Depression and Other Effects

Although there is a debate as to whether pill use causes depression, women with a history of psychic depression may be more prone to experience depressive effects with pill use [8, 32, 38, 50, 55, 70, 90, 103]. Treatment of depression in oral contraceptive users with pyridoxine (B_6) has been suggested, but there have been no well-controlled studies to demonstrate its therapeutic effectiveness [123]. However, should depression occur, and if daily supplementation with 25 mg of vitamin B_6 is not helpful, discontinuation of oral contraceptives should be tried.

Lowering the progestin activity or dosage may relieve symptoms of excessive fatigue. If not, other causes should be explored such as malnutrition related to dieting or hypothyroidism.

Emotional changes and dizziness may occur, which may or may not be related to pill use. Using a very low-dose estrogen pill combined with a high-protein diet may be helpful. Supplementation with vitamin B_6 may also be useful.

Epilepsy may increase in oral contraceptive users [90]. This may be related to drug interactions. Additionally, the efficacy of the oral contraceptives may be diminished. (See section on Drug Interactions.)

Changes in libido have been reported, which may or may not be pill related [6, 8, 90]. If decreased, prescribing a pill with low estrogen and higher androgenic activity (levonorgestrel) may be helpful.

Sensory System

Visual changes such as blurring of vision, scintillating scotoma, diplopia, proptosis, or suddenly diminished or lost vision require immediate cessation of pill use and evaluation [90]. If vascular spasm is identified on fundoscopic examination, appropriate diagnostic and therapeutic measures need to be initiated. Further oral contraceptive use is contraindicated. If related to edema and refraction problems (e.g., contact lenses), reduction of the estrogen dosage may be helpful.

Respiratory System

Upper respiratory symptoms, including asthma and nasal congestion, may be increased in oral contraceptive users [90]. Increased nasal congestion is known to occur during pregnancy and is likely related to an estrogen effect. Reducing the estrogen dosage may be helpful. If a problem develops and cannot be adequately controlled, it may be necessary to stop the pill.

Integumentary System

MELANOMA OF THE SKIN
Studies as to whether there is a pill-related increase in malignant melanoma of the skin are conflicting [1, 39, 52, 86]. However, oral contraceptive users would be well advised to limit exposure to the sun and use highly protective sun screens.

CHLOASMA
Since chloasma also commonly occurs in pregnancy when estrogen levels are highest, it may likely be estrogen related [90]. It has been noted in 3 to 5 percent of patients on oral contraceptives of higher dosage, but chloasma has decreased with a decrease in dosage. It is most common in women with dark complexions and is aggravated by exposure to sunlight. Once pigmentation has occurred, it may never disappear. Therefore, it is important to prescribe oral contraceptives with a low estrogen dosage and activity, advise users against exposure to the sun, and recommend highly protective sun screens.

ACNE AND HIRSUTISM
Estrogens decrease sebum production with improvement in acne and progestins have the reverse effect. Should acne worsen or hirsutism develop or worsen with pill use, decreasing androgenic activity through use of low-dose norethindrone may be helpful

[85, 90]. If further improvement is required, the estrogen dosage may be increased. The improvement may take several months to be noticeable.

HAIR LOSS

Androgens may cause loss of scalp and temporal hair [90]. Use of a pill with low androgenic activity (norethindrone) and more estrogenic activity may help. If symptoms persist, other medical conditions should be considered, such as hypothyroidism.

Nutritional Changes

Although oral contraceptive use may decrease levels of thiamine (B$_1$), riboflavin (B$_2$), pyridoxine (B$_6$), cobalamin (B$_{12}$), ascorbic acid (C), and folacin (folic acid), the evidence is conflicting as to whether these changes have any clinical significance [120, 123]. Therefore, in women who have an adequate diet, there is rarely a need for supplemental vitamins. Pyridoxine may occasionally be useful in counteracting symptoms of depression. However, in countries where nutrition is low or marginal, vitamin deficiencies may occur, and one should be alert to the symptoms of deficiency. Plasma levels of some nutrients such as copper and vitamin A may increase with pill use, but this is not clinically significant.

Weight Changes

The data show that as many women lose weight on the pill as gain [104]. Both hormones in the pill can contribute to weight gain, progestins mainly through an anabolic effect. The estrogen component may add weight by increasing subcutaneous fat, especially in the hips and breasts and/or through fluid retention.

Women who are distressed by weight gain should be placed on the lowest effective estrogen/progestin combination with a low potency progestin (norethindrone). They should also receive dietary counseling.

THERAPEUTIC USES AND
HEALTH BENEFITS

In addition to being the most highly effective reversible method of fertility control, the pill has the following therapeutic uses: suppression of fibrocystic disease of the breast; control of menses (regulation of cycle, diminished flow with less iron deficiency anemia and less dysmenorrhea); control of bleeding and size of uterine leiomyoma (low dosage of estrogen essential); control of bleeding with blood dyscrasias; control of endometriosis and adenomyosis; suppression of abnormal ovarian function in polycystic ovarian syndromes; hormonal replacement in ovarian dysgenesis; and treatment of acne [74]. Although these therapeutic claims are not identified as such in the labeling by the FDA, contraceptive use to treat such conditions has become a standard part of the physician's therapeutic armamentarium. Since the law does not prohibit the use of a drug by a physician for unapproved indications, one may do so. However, one is still subject to medicolegal challenge as is always the case in practice.

Oral contraceptive health benefits [74] are spelled out in Chapter 12, Principles of Oral Contraception.

CONCLUSION

Clearly oral contraceptive practice has become a complicated and sophisticated part of the physician's office services, requiring a continuous updating of our basic knowledge as the data base in this important area expands. By keeping current, we can offer our patients the best results through appropriate choices from the wide range available in oral contraception. Happily we can now assure our patients that from an overall perspective, the health benefits associated with pill use favorably outweigh their risks. But this positive benefit-risk ratio may not hold true for a particular individual patient; hence the continuing need for individualized assessment and follow-up of women who wish to utilize oral contraception for fertility control.

REFERENCES

1. Adam, S. A., et al. A case-control study of the possible association between oral contraceptives and malignant melanoma. *Br. J. Cancer* 44:45, 1981.
2. Altschuler, S. L., and Valenteen, J. W. Amenorrhea following rifampicin administration during oral contraceptive use. *Obstet. Gynecol.* 44:771, 1974.
3. Anonymous. Pill users protected against PID if they have used oral contraceptives for longer than one year. *Fam. Plann. Perspect.* 14(1):32, 1982.
4. Archer, D. F., and Thomas, F. L. The fallacy of the post-pill amenorrhea syndrome. *Clin. Obstet. Gynecol.* 24(3):943, 1981.
5. Arthes, F. G., Sartwell, P. E., and Lewisohn, E. F. The pill, estrogens and the breast: Epidemiological aspects. *Cancer* 28:1391, 1971.
6. Aznar-Romos, R., et al. Incidence of side effects with contraceptive placebo. *Am. J. Obstet. Gynecol.* 105:1144, 1969.
7. Badraoui, M. H. H., Fawzi, G., and Hefnawi, F. Effects of some progestational steroids on lactation. *J. Biosoc. Sci.* (Suppl. 4):135, 1977.

8. Bakker, C. B., and Dightman, C. R. Side effects of oral contraceptives. *Obstet. Gynecol.* 28:373, 1966.

9. Banks, A. L., Rutherford, R. N., and Colburn, W. A. Pregnancy and progeny after use of progestin-like substances for contraception. *Obstet. Gynecol.* 26:760, 1965.

10. Beral, V., and Kay, C. R. Mortality among oral contraceptive users. *Lancet* 2:727, 1977.

11. Berger, G. S., Taylor, R. N., Jr., and Treloar, A. E. The Risk of Post-Pill Amenorrhea. In L. G. Keith et al. (eds.), *The Safety of Fertility Control.* New York: Springer, 1980. Pp. 88–94.

12. Boston Collaborative Drug Surveillance Programme. Oral contraceptives and venous thromboembolic disease, surgically confirmed gallbladder disease and breast tumors. *Lancet* 1:1399, 1973.

13. Breast-feeding, fertility, and family planning. *Popul. Rep.* [J]. No. 24, Nov.–Dec. 1981.

14. Catteral, R. D. *Candida albicans* and the contraceptive pill. *Lancet* 2:830, 1966.

15. Chatterjee, R., et al. A study of postpill amenorrhea. *Int. J. Gynaecol. Obstet.* 18(2):113, 1980.

16. Christopherson, W. M., Mays, E. T., and Barrows, G. H. Liver tumors in women on contraceptive steroids. *Obstet. Gynecol.* 46:221, 1975.

17. Collected Letters of the International Correspondence Society of Obstetrics and Gynecology. Tests prior to prescribing oral contraceptives. Vol. 22, No. 9, May, 1981.

18. Collected Letters of the International Correspondence Society of Obstetrics and Gynecology. Oral contraceptives. Vol. 22, No. 23, Dec., 1981.

19. Corfman, P. A. Report of the task force on biologic effects: Second report on the oral contraceptives. Advisory Committee on Obstetrics and Gynecology, Food and Drug Administration. Washington, D.C., Aug. 1, 1969.

20. Davis, B. A. Vaginal moniliasis in private practice. *Obstet. Gynecol.* 34:40, 1969.

21. Dickey, R. P. The Pill: Physiology, Pharmacology and Clinical Use. In A. W. Isenman, E. G. Knox, and L. Tyrer, (eds.), *Seminar in Family Planning* (2nd ed.). Chicago: American College of Obstetricians and Gynecology, 1974.

22. Dickey, R. P. Diagnosis and management of patients with oral contraceptive side effects. *J. Contin. Educ. Obstet. Gynecol.* 20:19, 1978.

23. Dickey, R. P. *Managing Contraceptive Pill Patients* (3rd ed.). Durant, Okla.: D & B's Federal Printing, 1984.

24. Dickey, R. P. *Managing Contraceptive Pill Patients* (3rd ed.). Durant, Okla.: D & B's Federal Printing, 1984. Pp. 16, 17.

25. Dickey, R. P., and Dorr, C. H., III. Oral contraceptives: Selection of the proper pill. *Am. J. Obstet. Gynecol.* 33:273, 1969.

26. Diddle, W. W., Gardner, W. H., and Williamson, P. J. Oral contraceptive medications and headaches. *Am. J. Obstet. Gynecol.* 105:507, 1969.

27. Edmondson, H. A., Henderson, B., and Benton, B.

Liver-cell adenomas associated with the use of oral contraceptives. *N. Engl. J. Med.* 294:470, 1976.

28. Eschenbach, D. A., Harnisch, J. P., and Holmes, K. K. Pathogenesis of acute pelvic inflammatory disease: Role of contraception and other risk factors. *Am. J. Obstet. Gynecol.* 128:838, 1977.

29. Fisch, I. R., Freedman, S. H., and Myatt, A. V. Oral contraceptives, pregnancy and blood pressure. *J.A.M.A.* 222:1507, 1972.

30. Golditch, R. P. Postcontraceptive amenorrhea. *Obstet. Gynecol.* 39:903, 1972.

31. Grant, E. C. Hormone balance of oral contraceptives. *J. Obstet. Gynaecol. Br. Commonw.* 74:908, 1967.

32. Grant, E. C., and Pryse-Davies, J. Effects of oral contraceptives on depressive mood change and on endometrial monoamine oxidase and phosphatases. *Br. Med. J.* 3:777, 1968.

33. Green, G. R., and Sartwell, P. E. Oral contraceptive use in patients with thromboembolism following surgery, trauma or infection. *Am. J. Public Health* 62:680, 1972.

34. Gupta, K., et al. Coagulation studies in women on combination type of oral contraceptives. *J. Obstet. Gynaecol. India* 29:647, 1979.

35. Gupta, A. N., Mathur, V. S., and Garg, S. K. Effect of Oral Contraceptives on the Production and Composition of Human Milk. In A. S. Parkes et al. (eds.), *Fertility Regulation During Human Lactation: Proceedings of the 6th International Planned Parenthood Federation Biomedical Workshop. London, Nov. 23–24, 1976. J. Biosoc. Sci.* (Suppl. 4):123, 1977.

36. Haber, I., and Hubens, H. Cholestatic jaundice after triacetyloleandomycin and oral contraceptives. *Acta Gastroenterol. Belg.*, 43:475, 1980.

37. Heinonen, O. P., et al. Cardiovascular birth defects and antenatal exposure to female sex hormones. *N. Engl. J. Med.* 296:67, 1977.

38. Herzberg, B. N., et al. Oral contraceptives, depression and libido. *Br. Med. J.* 3:495, 1971.

39. Holly, E. A., et al. Cutaneous melanoma in relation to exogenous hormones and reproductive factors. *J. Natl. Cancer Inst.* 70:827, 1983.

40. Hoyle, M., et al. Small bowel ischaemia and infarction in young women taking oral contraceptives and progestational agents. *Br. Med. J.* 64:533, 1977.

41. Hull, M. G., et al. Normal fertility in women with postpill amenorrhea. *Lancet* 1:1329, 1981.

42. Inman, W. H. W., et al. Thromboembolic disease and the steroidal content of oral contraceptives. *Br. Med. J.* 2:203, 1970.

43. Inman, W. H. W., and Vessey, M. P. Investigation of deaths with pulmonary coronary and cerebral thrombosis and embolism in women of childbearing age. *Br. Med. J.* 2:193, 1968.

44. Jackson, J. L., III. Incidence of Moniliasis with Combined and Sequential Oral Contraceptives. In R. B. Greenblatt

(ed.), *Progress in Conception Control*. Philadelphia: Lippincott, 1966.

45. Jacobs, H. S., et al. Post-"pill" amenorrhea: Cause or coincidence? *Br. Med. J.* 2:940, 1977.

46. Jacobson, C. Cytogenetic study of immediate post-contraceptive abortion. Report of a study under Food and Drug Administration contract, 1974.

47. Jain, A. D. Mortality risk associated with the use of oral contraceptives. *Stud. Fam. Plann.* 8:50, 1977.

48. Jain, A. R. Cigarette smoking, use of oral contraceptives and myocardial infarction. *Am. J. Obstet. Gynecol.* 126:301, 1976.

49. Janz, D., and Schmidt, D. Antiepileptic drugs and failure of oral contraceptives. *Lancet* 1:1113, 1974.

50. Kane, F. J. Psychiatric reactions to oral contraceptives. *Am. J. Obstet. Gynecol.* 102:1053, 1968.

51. Kay, C. R. Breast cancer and oral contraceptives: Findings in Royal College of General Practitioners study. *Br. Med. J.* 282:2089, 1981.

52. Kay, C. R. Malignant melanoma and oral contraceptives. *Br. J. Cancer* 44:479, 1981.

53. Kunin, C. M. Urinary Tract Infections and Pyelonephritis. In P. B. Beeson, W. McDermott, and J. B. Wyngaarden (eds.), *Cecil's Textbook Of Medicine*, Vol. 2 (15th ed.). Philadelphia: Saunders, 1979.

54. Kunin, C. M., McCormack, R. C., and Abernathy, J. R. Oral contraceptives and blood pressure. *Arch. Intern. Med.* 123:362, 1969.

55. Kutner, S. J., and Brown, W. L. Types of Oral Contraceptives, Depression and Premenstrual Symptoms. In S. Ramcharon (ed.), *The Walnut Creek Study of The Side Effects of Oral Contraceptives* (Vol. I). Bethesda: United States Department of Health, Education, and Welfare, 1976.

56. Laenger, H., and Detering, K. Antiepileptic drugs and failure of oral contraceptives. *Lancet* 2:600, 1974.

57. Laragh, J. H., et al. Oral contraceptives, renin, aldosterone and high blood pressure. *J.A.M.A.* 201:918, 1967.

58. Laragh, J. H. The pill, hypertension and the toxemias of pregnancy. *Am. J. Obstet. Gynecol.* 109:210, 1971.

59. Layde, P. M., Beral, V., and Kay, C. R. Further analyses of mortality in oral contraceptive users: Royal College of General Practitioners study. *Lancet* 1:541, 1981.

60. Larsson-Cohn, V. The length of the first three menstrual cycles after combined oral contraceptive treatment. *Acta Obstet. Gynecol. Scand.* 48:416, 1969.

61. Lincoln, R. The pill, breast and cervical cancer, and the role of progestogens in arterial disease. *Perspectives* 16:55, 1984.

62. Logan, B. Is the "pill" a cause of vaginal candidiasis? Culture study. *N.Y. State J. Med.* 70:949, 1970.

63. Lowenstein, J. M. Thyroid function and oral contraceptives. *J. Reprod. Med.* 3:50, 1969.

64. Mann, J. I., et al. Myocardial infarction in young women with special reference to oral contraceptive practice. *Br. Med. J.* 2:241, 1975.

65. Mann, J. I., and Inman, W. H. W. Oral contraceptives and death from myocardial infarction. *Br. Med. J.* 2:245, 1975.

66. Meade, T. W., Greenberg, G., and Thompson, S. G. Progestogens and cardiovascular reactions associated with oral contraceptives and a comparison of the safety of the 50 and 30 mg. preparations. *Br. Med. J.* 280:1157, 1980.

67. Mishell, D. R., Jr. Oral Contraceptives Today: More Benefits Than Risks. *Mediguide Ob/Gyn*. West Haven, Conn.: Miles Pharmaceuticals, 1982. Vol. 1, #4.

68. Moghissi, K. S. Oral Contraceptives and Endometrial, Cervical and Breast Cancers. In E. S. E. Hafez (ed.), *Human Reproduction, Conception and Contraception* (2nd ed.). Hagerstown, Md.: Harper & Row, 1978.

69. Morris, C. A., and Morris, D. F. Normal vaginal microbiology of women of childbearing age in relation to the use of oral contraceptives and vaginal tampons. *J. Clin. Pathol.* 20:636, 1967.

70. Murawski, B. J., et al. An investigation of mood states in women taking oral contraceptives. *Fertil. Steril.* 19:50, 1968.

71. Nissen, E. D., Kent, D. R., and Nissen, S. E. Liver tumors and the pill: Analysing the data. *Contemp. Obstet. Gynecol.* 8:103, 1976.

72. Northmann, V. J., Chittinand, S., and Schuster, N. M. Reversible mesenteric vascular occlusion associated with oral contraceptives. *Am. J. Dig. Dis.* 18:361, 1973.

73. Oliver, M. F. Ischaemic heart disease in young women. *Br. Med. J.* 4:253, 1974.

74. Oral contraceptives. Public Information Program. *Popul. Rep.* [A]. No. 6, May–June, 1982.

75. Ory, H. W. Oral contraceptives and breast cancer. Presented to the National Medical Committee, Planned Parenthood Federation of America. Baltimore, Md., Nov. 22, 1982.

76. Ory, H. W. Contraceptive safety: The need for epidemiologic research. Presented to the Symposium on the Regulation of Human Fertility: Needs of Developing Countries and Priorities for the Future. Stockholm, Feb. 7–9, 1983.

77. Ory, H. W., et al. The pill at 20: An assessment. *Fam. Plann. Perspect.* 12:6, 1980.

78. Ory, H. W., Forrest, J. D., and Lincoln, R. *Making Choices: Evaluating the Health Risks and Benefits of Birth Control Methods*. Alan Guttmacher Institute, 1983.

79. Oxford Family Planning Association. New studies of malignant melanoma, gallbladder and heart disease help further define pill risk. *Fam. Plann. Perspect.* 14:95, 1982.

80. Peterson, C., et al. Antithrombin III: Comparison of functional and immunologic assays. *Am. J. Clin. Pathol.* 69:500, 1978.

81. Peterson, W. F. Pregnancy following oral contraceptive therapy. *Obstet. Gynecol.* 34:363, 1969.

82. Pettiti, D. Oral contraceptive drug interactions. *P. P. Med. Digest* 2:1, 1981.

83. Phillips, B. M. Oral contraceptive drugs and migraine. *Br. Med. J.* 2:99, 1968.

84. Planned Parenthood Federation of America. *Manual of Medical Standards and Guidelines*, Part I, section III.

85. Pye, R. J., et al. Effect of oral contraceptives on sebum excretion rate. *Br. Med. J.* 2:1581, 1977.

86. Ramcharan, S., et al. The Walnut Creek Contraceptive Drug Study: A comprehensive study of the side effects of oral contraceptives. Vol. III. An interim report: A comparison of disease occurrence leading to hospitalization or death in users and non-users of oral contraceptives. *National Institutes of Health Publication* No. 81-564, Jan. 1981.

87. Rice-Wray, E., et al. Pregnancy and progeny after hormonal contraceptives: Genetic studies. *J. Reprod. Med.* 6:101, 1971.

88. Robinson, S. C. Pregnancy outcome following oral contraceptives. *Am. J. Obstet. Gynecol.* 109:354, 1971.

89. Royal College of General Practitioners. Oral contraception and thromboembolic disease. *J. R. Coll. Gen. Pract.* 13:267, 1967.

90. Royal College of General Practitioners. *Oral Contraceptives and Health: An Interim Report from the Oral Contraception Study of the Royal College of General Practitioners.* New York: Pitman, 1974.

91. Royal College of General Practitioners. Oral contraceptives, venous thrombosis and varicose veins. *J. R. Coll. Gen. Pract.* 28:393, 1978.

92. Royal College of General Practitioners Oral Contraception Study. Further analysis of mortality in oral contraceptive users. *Lancet* 1:541, 1981.

93. Sartwell, P. E., et al. Thromboembolism and oral contraceptives: An epidemiological case-control study. *Am. J. Epidemiol.* 90:365, 1969.

94. Shapiro, S., et al. Oral contraceptive use in relation to myocardial infarction. *Lancet* 1:743, 1979.

95. Shearman, R. P. Secondary amenorrhea after oral contraceptives: Treatment and follow-up. *Contraception* 2:123, 1975.

96. Spellacy, W. N. A review of carbohydrate metabolism and oral contraceptives. *Am. J. Obstet. Gynecol.* 104:448, 1969.

97. Spellacy, W. N. Carbohydrate metabolism during treatment with estrogen, progestogen and low dose oral contraceptives. *Am. J. Obstet. Gynecol.* 6:732, 1982.

98. Spellacy, W. N., et al. Vaginal yeast growth and contraceptive practices. *Obstet. Gynecol.* 38:342, 1971.

99. Spellacy, W. N., et al. The effects of a "low estrogen" oral contraceptive on carbohydrate metabolism during six months treatment: A preliminary report of blood glucose and plasma insulin values. *Fertil. Steril.* 28:885, 1977.

100. Spellacy, W. N., and Birk, S. A. The effect of intrauterine devices, oral contraceptives, estrogens and progestogens on blood pressure. *Am. J. Obstet. Gynecol.* 112:912, 1972.

101. Spellacy, W. N., and Birk, S. A. The effects of mechanical and steroidal contraceptive methods on blood pressure in hypertensive women. *Fertil. Steril.* 25:467, 1974.

102. Stolly, P. D., et al. Thrombosis with low estrogen oral contraceptives. *Am. J. Epidemiol.* 102:197, 1975.

103. Swanson, D. W., et al. Use of norethynodrel in psychotic females. *Am. J. Psychiatry* 120:1101, 1964.

104. Talwar, P. P., and Berger, G. S. Side effects of drugs: The relation of body weight to side effects associated with oral contraceptives. *Br. Med. J.* 1:1637, 1977.

105. Toaff, R., et al. Effects of oestrogen and progestogen on the composition of human milk. *J. Reprod. Fertil.* 19:475, 1969.

106. Tolis, G., et al. Prolonged amenorrhea and oral contraceptives. *Fertil. Steril.* 32:265, 1979.

107. Tyrer, L. B. Suggested Patient Instruction Concerning Missed Pills. Planned Parenthood-World Population, Memorandum, Aug. 3, 1976.

108. United States Food and Drug Administration, Oral Contraceptive Labeling, 1980.

109. Vessey, M. P., and Doll, R. Investigation of relation between use of oral contraceptives and thromboembolic disease: A further report. *Br. Med. J.* 2:651, 1969.

110. Vessey, M. P., et al. Post-operative thromboembolism and the use of oral contraceptives. *Br. Med. J.* 3:123, 1970.

111. Vessey, M., et al. A long-term follow-up of women using different methods of contraception: An interim report. *J. Biosoc. Sci.* 8:373, 1976.

112. Vessey, M. P., et al. Oral contraceptives and benign liver tumors. *Br. Med. J.* 2:1064, 1977.

113. Vessey, M. P., et al. Fertility after stopping different methods of contraception. *Br. Med. J.* 1:265, 1978.

114. Vessey, M. P., McPherson, K., and Doll, R. Breast cancer and oral contraceptives: Findings in Oxford Family Planning Association Contraceptive Study. *Br. Med. J.* 282:2093, 1981.

115. Vessey, M. P., McPherson, K., and Yeates, D. Mortality in oral contraceptive users. *Lancet* 2:731, 1977.

116. VonKaulla, E., et al. Antithrombin III depression and thrombin generation acceleration in women taking oral contraceptives. *Am. J. Obstet. Gynecol.* 109:868, 1971.

117. Vosbeck, E. Cytogenetic morphological and clinical aspects of 453 cases of human spontaneous abortions. Ph.D. Dissertation, George Washington University School of Graduate Studies, 1975.

118. Wahl, P., et al. Effect of estrogen/progestin potency on lipid lipoprotein cholesterol. *N. Engl. J. Med.* 308:862, 1983.

119. Walsh, J., Hildebrandt, R. J., and Prystowsky, H. Candidal vaginitis associated with the use of oral progestational agents. *Am. J. Obstet. Gynecol.* 93:904, 1965.

120. Webb, J. L. Nutritional effects of oral contraceptive use: A review *J. Reprod. Med.* 25:150, 1980.

121. Weindling, H., and Henry, J. B. Laboratory test result altered by "the pill." *J.A.M.A.* 229:1762, 1974.

122. Westrom, L. Incidence, prevalence, and trends of acute pelvic inflammatory disease and its consequences in industrialized countries. *Am. J. Obstet. Gynecol.* 138:880, 1980.

123. Wynn, V. Vitamins and oral contraceptive use. *Lancet* 1:561, 1975.

124. Yaffee, H. S., and Grots, I. Moniliasis due to norethynodrel with mestranol. *N. Engl. J. Med.* 272:647, 1965.

14. Injectable Contraception

Allan Rosenfield

Interest in the provision of contraception by injection developed soon after oral hormonal contraception became available. In the late 1950s injectable depo medroxyprogesterone acetate (DMPA)* was introduced as an agent useful in the gynecologic treatment of endometriosis and endometrial cancer. Soon thereafter, its use as a contraceptive was explored. During the past 20 years extensive use in approximately 100 countries has resulted in the publication of a voluminous literature on DMPA and to a lesser extent on norethisterone enanthate (NET-EN),† including several review articles [21, 22, 47, 67, 68] and special reports from the World Health Organization [93], the American College of Obstetricians and Gynecologists [2], and an Ad Hoc Panel established for the United States Agency for International Development [66].

Use of DMPA as a contraceptive has generated an extraordinary amount of controversy, with some groups urging approval and others believing that the potential risks are so great that the drug should not be approved for general or even limited use [3, 52]. The reasons for this controversy relate in part to several potential adverse effects including carcinogenicity, teratogenicity, and interference with the return of fertility. Despite the controversy, it is estimated that over 2 million women throughout the world currently use DMPA for contraceptive purposes, with DMPA and/or NET-EN having been approved for contraceptive use in close to 100 developing and developed countries [47]. DMPA most recently has been approved, with some limitations, by the Swedish, British, and Canadian governments. In the United States, however, the U.S. Food and Drug Administration (FDA) has not yet approved DMPA for contraceptive use: in January 1983 it convened for only the second time in its history a Public Board of Inquiry to review the issues and make a recommendation to the commissioner of the FDA. This chapter will review the scientific and medical data and evidence concerning injectable contraception, with primary attention being given to DMPA.

HISTORY

In the mid-1950s long-acting progestin compounds were first used as a treatment for habitual abortion, endometriosis, and endometrial carcinoma [67]. Since the early 1960s several different compounds have been used for contraceptive purposes, although most of the literature and clinical experience relate to DMPA and only to a much lesser extent to NET-EN. Both provide protection from pregnancy for from 2 to 3 months.

*Depo-Provera, Upjohn Co.
†Norigest, Schering Co.

There also has been experience with the use of progestins (alone or in combination with estrogen) as a monthly injectable contraceptive [82]. This combination monthly approach has not been widely used in the United States.

Dosages of DMPA used for gynecologic indications such as treatment of uterine cancer usually were quite high, often in the range of 1,000 mg per week for several weeks with the reduction to maintenance levels thereafter [67]. Use of DMPA as a contraceptive was initiated in 1963. Based on experience, the most effective contraceptive dosage was found to be 150 mg given intramuscularly once every 3 months. Data have also been published on the use of 400 mg every 6 months [49]. In 1967 the manufacturer applied to the U.S. Food and Drug Administration to study the use of DMPA as a contraceptive in this country.

In 1974, after a positive review by the FDA Obstetrics and Gynecology Advisory Committee, notice was issued to doctors that the drug would be approved for limited use for those women who could not make use of other contraceptive methods [71]. However, several consumer groups felt that the drug should not be approved for this indication and brought the issue before a House of Representatives committee. After reviewing the evidence presented to it, the congressional committee concurred that approval was inappropriate and communicated this report to the secretary of the Department of Health, Education, and Welfare and, in turn, to the commissioner of the FDA. This sequence of events resulted in an apparent reversal at the FDA, and the expected approval was not issued. Instead the issue was referred to a combined committee of the Obstetrics and Gynecology Advisory Committee and the Epidemiology and Biometrics Advisory Committee [85]. After further review of the data, including new studies, their recommendation was the same as the earlier one, namely, that the drug should be approved for limited use.

For the next 3 years the commissioner did not act on this recommendation. Finally, in 1978 an official report was issued in which an agency denied approval of DMPA for use as a contraceptive [84]. Five reasons were given:

1. Safety questions raised by studies of beagle dogs in which an increased incidence of mammary carcinoma associated with DMPA was demonstrated
2. The availability of a number of safer contraceptive alternatives and the lack of clear evidence that a significant patient population in need of the drug existed in the United States
3. The possibility that vaginal bleeding might necessitate the administration of estrogen, imposing an added risk factor and decreasing the benefits of an estrogen-free hormonal contraceptive
4. The possibility of exposure of fetuses to DMPA if there is a contraceptive failure, producing a risk of congenital malformation, a risk potentially enhanced by the prolonged action of the drug
5. Serious reservations about the ability of a postmarketing study for carcinoma proposed by the Upjohn Company to yield meaningful data

The decision was appealed by the Upjohn Company and, after a delay of 2 years, the FDA appointed a Public Board of Inquiry which held hearings in January 1983. No final recommendation has yet been issued.

CHEMISTRY AND PHARMACOLOGY

DMPA is a microcrystalline suspension of 17-alpha-acetoxy-y-alpha-methol-tregn-4-ene-3,20-dione [14]. The drug is given by deep intramuscular injection and has a prolonged release as a result of its very low solubility in aqueous solution [19]. It is closely related chemically to natural progesterone. NET-EN is a long chain ester of norethisterone formulated in a castor oil–benzyl benzoate solution; it too is given by deep intramuscular injection.

After injection, there is an initial surge of steroid in the bloodstream [41]. The levels gradually fall during the period of activity, which for DMPA is 3 to 4 months; NET-EN is effective for a somewhat shorter period of time. DMPA circulates as an active progestin, while NET-EN circulates as both the ester and the active free steroid [69]. The prolonged activity is related to measurable levels of the drug continuing in the bloodstream, with serum levels of the two drugs varying from individual to individual.

These injectable contraceptives act primarily by inhibiting ovulation, probably through a hypothalamic effect [54, 63]. As a result, there is a reduction in the pituitary secretion of both follicle-stimulating hormone (FSH) and luteinizing hormone (LH), and the midcycle LH surge does not take place. Stimulation of the pituitary by gonadotropin-releasing hormone results in the secretion of FSH and LH, thus suggesting that the pituitary can react normally and that the site of action is at the level of the hypothalamus. As with oral contraceptives, there are also peripheral effects on luteal function, the endometrium, the cervix, and the fallopian tubes [21]. The drugs produce progestational changes in cervical mucus, making it relatively impermeable to spermatozoa. In addition, tubal motility is decreased. The endometrium becomes increasingly atrophic with use, a condition that may continue for 60 days or longer after cessation of the drug [44]. It has been shown that both DMPA and NET-EN bond strongly to progesterone receptors within the genital tract [75].

While the generally accepted dosage for DMPA is 150 mg intramuscularly every 3 months with the initial dose given during the menses, recent data have been published suggesting that dosages as low as 100 mg every 3 months are also effective in providing conception protection [19]. After injection of DMPA, blood levels as high as 7.8 nmol per liter are reached within 24 hours, then plateau to levels of 2.6 to 3.9 nmol per liter for about 3 months [59, 75]. Traceable amounts are still detectable 6 months later. There also has been experience with a 400-mg dosage given every 6 months [49, 65], but fewer data are available, and that dose currently is not in general use. Studies of NET-EN by the World Health Organization in which 200 mg were given intramuscularly every 3 months showed high pregnancy rates (3–4% per year) [89]. This resulted in a change in dosage schedule to 200 mg every 2 months for the first two to three injections with subsequent injections once every 3 months thereafter.

BENEFITS

There are a number of benefits attributable to injectable contraception, and, despite the controversies, it is because of these benefits that there has been continued interest in their use as contraceptive agents. DMPA has the highest use-effectiveness rates of any reversible method of contraception, with pregnancy rates of less than 0.5 per 100 women-years of use. One injection of DMPA provides contraceptive protection for 3 months; even if the woman is 2 to 3 weeks late for a repeat injection, the protective effect appears to continue for an extended duration. These extra weeks of protection are not found with NET-EN [89].

In addition, since injectables are progestins only, estrogen-related side effects and complications are absent. As with the pill and the intrauterine device (IUD), use is not related to coitus, a significant advantage for some women. DMPA is an attractive method for those women who prefer treatment by injection to other approaches. For example, there is freedom from daily contraceptive activities, such as pill taking. Its use produces no negative effects on the quantity or nutritive value of breast milk as may occur with oral contraceptive use [40]. Further, some data actually suggest that there may be an increase in breast milk [81]. It should be noted that there are still insufficient data on the effect of the drug on the breast-feeding infant. However, while DMPA is present in breast milk at almost the same concentration as in the mother's serum, the total exposure of the infant over the 3-month injection interval is about 0.2 percent of the maternal dose, a level unlikely to pose a risk [38, 73].

Because the amount of bleeding during menses is less while on DMPA, there is a positive impact on women who are slightly anemic [24]. Some studies suggest that progestins may prevent sickling, thus indicating that a progestin-only contraceptive like DMPA or NET-EN may be the contraceptive of choice for women with sickle cell disease [9, 32, 64]. There also appears to be a decreased incidence of vaginal candidiasis and probably of acute pelvic inflammatory disease (PID) in women with positive cervical cultures [74, 83]. Finally, despite widespread use worldwide for both gynecologic and contraceptive purposes, there has been only one death reported to date possibly related to the use of DMPA or of NET-EN [34].

MENSTRUAL SIDE EFFECTS

By far the most common side effect of present injectable contraceptives is disturbance of the normal menstrual pattern. The changes are unpredictable and initially appear predominantly as irregular spotting and staining [90, 93]. By the end of 1 year of use almost 50 percent of users become amenorrheic. A small percent of users will have one or more episodes of heavy vaginal bleeding, particularly when the drugs are used in the early postpartum period. Treatment is rarely required, but when necessary, the management is short-term estrogen therapy rather than dilatation and curettage. While amenorrhea is secondary to endometrial atrophy, the cause of the irregular bleeding pattern is less clear; abnormalities of lysosome function and prostaglandins as well as other vascular changes may contribute [24, 39].

When DMPA was first introduced, some recommended routine estrogen supplementation to lessen these symptoms as well as to ensure withdrawal bleeding [15, 62]. However, assessment of the effectiveness of estrogen showed it to be equivocal at best (except in producing withdrawal bleeding), and most clinicians currently do not recommend its use, particularly since it is preferable not to add potential estrogen-related problems [39, 90].

The various menstrual side effects are the most common cause of discontinuation of both DMPA and NET-EN, with significant variations in impact from culture to culture [80, 90]. In some areas of the world, for example, monthly bleeding is considered important, except during pregnancy, as a means of cleansing the body, and a nonpregnant state of amenorrhea is worrisome. If spotting, staining, or amenorrhea are unacceptable side effects, the appropriate course is to discontinue use rather than institute estrogen therapy.

Interestingly, one U.S. study found that approximately 60 percent of all women had possible indications for supplementary estrogens, but only 5 percent of these actually received even one course of estrogen therapy [28]. In only 0.2 percent of all cycles of DMPA use were estrogens actually used. Similarly, the World Health Organization, in a comparative trial of DMPA and NET-EN, reported that estrogens were used in 0.5 percent of the cases [24]. Thus, although estrogen use is uncommon, counseling about menstrual side effects is important before initiating use of injectable contraceptives. Studies to identify injectables that cause less disruption to the menstrual cycle are under way; long-term subdermal implants apparently have somewhat fewer problems in this regard [16].

OTHER SIDE EFFECTS

Other troublesome side effects include weight gain, headache, dizziness, abdominal bloating, mood changes, and a variety of other complaints, many of which may not be hormonally related [22, 91]. Perhaps the most common of these complaints is weight gain, which is probably a direct result of fat deposition [1]. The average weight gain reported is 0.5 to 2 kg after 1 year of use, although 20 to 40 percent of users note a decrease in weight [22].

Estrogen appears to be responsible for many of the cardiovascular complications in users, particularly those complications secondary to changes in the blood-clotting mechanism. However, progestins also may play a role in relation to some small-vessel disease [35]. Present data suggest that some progestins cause a decrease in high-density lipoproteins (HDL) with a possible acceleration of an atheromatous process [18, 42]. This appears to be particularly true of 19 nortestosterone progestins and less so with DMPA [36, 86, 87]. Estrogens, on the other hand, increase HDL levels, which appear to decrease the incidence of atherosclerosis. Further studies are needed concerning the possible role of progestins in relation to stroke and heart attacks. In the literature to date only one death has been reported resulting from a stroke in a woman using DMPA; the possible role of DMPA in this case has not been established [34].

Although a few studies suggest an elevation of blood pressure among DMPA users, most studies report no such increase [4, 45, 91].

A number of other metabolic effects have been described, but these, in general, have been reported as minor. There is a change in carbohydrate metabolism similar to that seen with oral contraceptives, the most common finding being an exaggerated insulin response to a glucose tolerance test but rarely frank diabetes [6, 79]. DMPA has a glucocorticoid effect and in high doses may suppress adrenal function [6], but at contraceptive dosages there is no evidence of clinical adrenal insufficiency, except for a possible weak suppressive effect on wound healing [46]. Most studies have shown no consistent changes in liver function [22, 23].

RETURN OF FERTILITY

Concern has arisen that DMPA may produce permanent sterility. The largest study to assess this problem was undertaken in Thailand, where 750 DMPA users who discontinued use of DMPA in order to get pregnant were compared with 437 oral contraceptive users who discontinued use for the same purpose [48]. The mean time for a pregnancy to ensue after discontinuation was 2.5 months for oral contraceptive users as compared with 5.1 months for DMPA users. Another study found a 5.5 month median delay after DMPA use as compared with 4.5 months after IUD use [61].

There is thus a significant delay in return of fertility, with substantial differences between oral contraceptive and DMPA users in pregnancy rates at both 6 and 12 months [48]. At 6 months 75 percent of oral contraceptive users had achieved a pregnancy as compared with 53 percent of DMPA users; at 12 months these rates increased to 85 percent and 75 percent respectively. However, by 20 to 24 months more than 90 percent of women in both groups had achieved a pregnancy. Thus, although permanent sterility does not appear to be a problem with DMPA use, potential users should be advised before initiation of this contraceptive method that there may well be a delay in return of fertility [48, 61].

CARCINOGENICITY

The most important issue concerning the use of DMPA is the finding of carcinogenicity in test animals. In some beagle dogs, one of the test animals required by the FDA to be used in steroid hormone testing, breast tumors developed on DMPA therapy, some of which were malignant [17, 20, 56]. Beagle dogs without treatment commonly develop benign breast adenomas, and there is evidence as well that they may have multiple microscopic foci of neoplasia [7, 55]. When treated with DMPA for long periods of time, these foci are apparently stimulated as they are by progesterone itself, although at a higher dosage than is the case with DMPA [7]. Mammary nodules developed in almost all the dogs who received treatment with DMPA over a long period of time, some becoming malignant and showing metastases. These findings are clear; the debate that has evolved concerns whether the beagle dog is a suitable model for safety studies of steroid hormones in humans.

The World Health Organization (WHO) and a number of drug regulatory agencies in other developed nations, after reviewing the evidence, have stated that the beagle dog is an inappropriate test animal for steroid hormones [21, 22, 93]. Much evidence suggests that the beagle dog reacts quite differently to progestins than does the human. For example, DMPA produces a hyperstimulation of the endometrium, resulting in mucometra and/or pyometra, often resulting in death of the animal [21]. Because of this particular complication, the FDA recommended that hysterectomies be performed on the dogs to permit survival of the animals and thus to allow other effects to be observed. In the human, on the other hand, after a brief period of stimulation, the endometrium becomes atrophic and remains so throughout therapy [53].

In addition, in response to DMPA, growth hormone levels increase in the beagle, often resulting in an acromegalic state [21]. A similar effect is not noted in the human. Finally, at the progesterone receptor site, progestins such as DMPA react much differently with increased binding capacity in the beagle breast than in the human [8]. The World Health Organization, in reviewing DMPA in 1978, concluded that "the beagle is an unsuitable model in which to observe potential adverse effects arising from the long-term use of progestins in women" [90].

It should be mentioned that in the hearings before the FDA Panel of Inquiry on Depo-Provera there were some pathologists who expressed different views, believing that the beagle dog data are indeed relevant despite these differences [11]. The Committee on the Safety of Medicines of the United Kingdom in reviewing the same issue, however, concluded "because of the differences between the beagle bitch and the human female in the sensitivity and the metabolism of progestogens, positive carcinogenicity studies in the beagle bitch can no longer be considered as indicative of significant hazard to women," and it therefore stopped requiring beagle dog studies of contraceptive steroids [10].

Although the time frame is still too short, a number of studies on humans have shown no increase in breast pathology [26, 95]. A preliminary report from the World Health Organization on a multicenter study supports the lack of any relationship in the human [94].

In late 1978, at the conclusion of a 10-year study of DMPA use in monkeys, it was reported that 2 of 10 monkeys receiving 50 times the human dose of DMPA

had developed endometrial cancer, while none of the 20 monkeys receiving other doses and none of the seven control monkeys showed any signs of endometrial diseases [84]. Interestingly, the two monkeys that did develop the disease were replacements for monkeys that had died, and although they had not received 10 years of continuous therapy, they had received more than 8 years of drugs. This finding was particularly surprising since DMPA is used in the palliative management of metastatic carcinoma of the endometrium and as treatment for those women with endometrial carcinoma in situ who do not wish a hysterectomy because of a desire for pregnancy. In addition, more recent epidemiologic studies with oral contraceptives have shown that the pill appears to protect women against the development of endometrial cancer and this protection is thought to be produced by the progestin component [60].

Nonetheless, the finding in monkeys obviously is of great concern, although no definitive conclusion can be drawn because the numbers are very small and may be of no statistical significance. In addition, there are reports from other studies of two monkeys developing precancerous conditions of the endometrium; in both these cases the monkeys were in control groups, one in a study of IUDs and the other in an oral contraceptive study conducted by a drug company [66]. Data have been presented to suggest that endometrial cancer is quite rare in the monkey species. However, it is not clear from the data presented how many of the monkeys mentioned were females of a sufficient age (over the age of 12) and whether there was adequate sectioning of the uterus to search for early endometrial carcinoma [76].

The Public Board of Inquiry was presented with data to suggest that the cancer noted in the monkeys may not be endometrial in origin but rather adenocarcinoma of the endocervix invading the endometrium [12]. This is an interesting but as yet unproven hypothesis; the implications if true are not clear. Review by a special group of pathologists for the Public Board of Inquiry stated the lesions were endometrial in origin.

The World Health Organization concluded that "endometrial carcinoma observed in women not receiving hormone treatment generally arises from hyperplastic endometrium, whereas the carcinomas in the two monkeys were in an otherwise atrophic endometrium. It appears that the tumors in the monkeys arose from a cell type not found in women. Furthermore, DMPA is used in relatively high doses with considerable success to treat some forms of endometrial carcinoma in women" [93]. While this issue cannot yet be put to rest, the accumulated human data are at least reassuring, and final answers will come from continued observations.

Clinical studies of DMPA are currently under way. In the northern province of Chiang Mai, Thailand, DMPA has been used extensively since the late 1960s, and currently the prevalence of DMPA use among women aged 15 to 44 is approximately 25 percent [50]. Records of hospitals in the area show no increase in the incidence of endometrial carcinoma in recent years; in those cases of endometrial cancer that could be traced, there was no evidence of the use of DMPA. While these data are not conclusive, it is reassuring that in an area where DMPA has now been in use for more than 15 years, where more than 100,000 women have accepted the use of the method, and where more than 1,000 women have used the method for more than 10 years, no increase in cancer has been noted.

The World Health Organization recently initiated a careful epidemiologic study of the relationship between DMPA and cancer of the breast, ovaries, cervix, and endometrium in nine countries, including three centers in Thailand. While the data are currently being analyzed and are not yet available, preliminary results appear to be promising; more definitive data will be available in the future [94].

TERATOGENICITY AND EFFECT ON BREAST-FEEDING INFANTS

A number of studies of steroid hormones have suggested that prenatal exposure may pose an increased risk of birth defects, although others have suggested that the results are equivocal [25, 27, 29, 33, 57]. Very little information is available on the specific effects of progestins alone, since most of the studies have been carried out on combined oral contraceptives. However, no evidence has been adduced to suggest that DMPA constitutes a greater risk than other steroid hormones. Further assessment suggests that even if there were a twofold increase, widespread use of the drug would actually result in a significant decrease in risk of birth defects because of a significantly decreased number of pregnancies [66].

Although animal data suggest that exposure in utero might produce masculinization of the female fetus, studies of DMPA in humans have not substantiated this finding. The effects of steroids in pregnancy require continued observation, but because the numbers of pregnant women exposed to these hormones are so small, the definitive data probably will not be forthcoming in the near future.

Some evidence suggests that DMPA and NET-EN produce a slight increase in the amount of breast milk, whereas oral contraceptives may produce a slight decrease [38, 81]. Further, there does not appear to be an adverse effect on milk composition. The amount of hormone actually ingested by the infant is so small that it is highly unlikely to have any deleterious effect, although this question requires further study.

CONCLUSION

After reviews of the evidence, a number of agencies, including the Drug Advisory Committee to the FDA, the World Health Organization, the International Planned Parenthood Federation, an Ad Hoc Consultative Panel for the U.S. Agency for International Development, and the drug regulatory agencies of more than 70 countries, have recommended approval of DMPA for contraceptive purposes. The World Health Organization concludes:

In summary, DMPA (and NET-EN) appear to be acceptable methods of fertility regulation. Clinical evidence of more than 15 years of use as contraceptive agents shows no additional, and possibly fewer adverse effects than are found with other hormonal methods of contraception. A particular advantage of DMPA and NET-EN as highly effective, long-lasting and reversible contraceptives makes them important as options for women desiring a method of fertility regulation [93].

However, the FDA and several consumer groups continue to strongly oppose the approval of DMPA. As a result a great deal of controversy has been generated over its use. The FDA Public Board of Inquiry currently is weighing the evidence presented by the FDA, the Upjohn Company, and a number of other interested parties, including the WHO, the International Planned Parenthood Federation, the Women's Health Network, a public interest health group, and other interested individuals. A decision on the use of DMPA as a contraceptive in the United States is expected in 1984.

REFERENCES

1. Amatayakul, K., Sivasomboon, B., and Thanangkul, O. A study of the mechanism of weight gain in medroxyprogesterone acetate users. *Contraception* 22:605, 1980.

2. American College of Obstetrics and Gynecology. Position paper: Depo medroxyprogesterone acetate use as a contraceptive, 1981.

3. Benagiano, G., and Fraser, I. The Depo-Provera debate: Commentary on the article *Depo-Provera: A critical analysis. Contraception* 24:493, 1981.

4. Black, H. R., Leppert, P., and Decherney, A. The effect of medroxyprogesterone acetate on blood pressure. *Int. J. Gynaecol. Obstet.* 17:83, 1979.

5. Bonte, J., et al. Hormono-prophylaxis and hormono-therapy in the treatment of endometrial adenocarcinoma

by means of medroxyprogesterone acetate. *Gynecol. Oncol.* 6:60, 1978.

6. Briggs, M. H., and Briggs, M. Glucocorticoid properties of progestogens. *Steroids* 22:555, 1973.

7. Cameron, A. M., and Faulkin, L. J. Hyperplastic and inflammatory nodules in the canine mammary gland. *J. Natl. Cancer Institute* 47:1277, 1971.

8. Capel-Edwards, K., et al., Long-term administration of progesterone to the female beagle dog. *Toxicol. Appl. Pharmacol.* 24:474, 1973.

9. Ceulaer, K., et al. Medroxyprogesterone acetate and homozygous sickle-cell disease. *Lancet* 2:229, 1982.

10. Committee on Safety of Medicines. Beagle bits: Carcinogenicity testing of progestogens. *Med. Act Inform. Lett.* 52:2, 1979.

11. Concannon, R. Testimony before the U.S. Food and Drug Administration, Public Board of Inquiry on Depo-Provera. January, 1983.

12. Dallenbach-Hellweg, G. Testimony before the U.S. Food and Drug Administration, Public Board of Inquiry on Depo-Provera. January, 1983.

13. Dodds, G. H. The use of sterile medroxyprogesterone acetate suspension as a contraceptive during a three-year period. *Contraception* 11:15, 1975.

14. Duax, W. L., Cody, V., and Griffin, J. Steroid structure and function: II. Conformational transformation and receptor binding of medroxyprogesterone acetate. *Steroid Biochem.* 9:901, 1978.

15. El-Habashy, M. A., Mishell, D. R., Jr., and Moyer, D. L. Effect of supplementary oral estrogen on long-acting injectable progestogen contraception. *Obstet. Gynecol.* 35:51, 1970.

16. Faundes, A., Sivin, I., and Stern, J. Long-acting contraceptive implants: An analysis of menstrual bleeding patterns. *Contraception* 18:355, 1978.

17. Finkel, M. J., and Berliner, V. R. The extrapolation of experimental findings (animal to man): The dilemma of the systemically administered contraceptives. *Lab. Invest.* 28:383, 1973.

18. Fotherby, K., et al. Effect of injectable norethisterone oenanthate (Norigest) on blood lipid levels. *Contraception* 25:435, 1982.

19. Fotherby, K., Koetsawang, S., and Mathrubutham, M. Pharmacokinetic study of different doses of Depo-Provera. *Contraception* 22:527, 1980.

20. Frank, D. W., et al. Mammary tumors and serum hormones in the bitch treated with medroxyprogesterone acetate or progesterone for four years. *Fertil. Steril.* 31:340, 1979.

21. Fraser, I. Long-acting injectable hormonal contraceptives. *Clin. Reprod. Fertil.* 1:67, 1982.

22. Fraser, I., and Weisberg, E. A comprehensive review of injectable contraception with special emphasis on Depo medroxyprogesterone acetate. *Med. J. Aust.* 1:1, 1981.

23. Garcia, C. R., and Wallach, E. E. Liver function studies and progestogen contraception: Review of an intramuscularly administered contraceptive. *Fertil. Steril.* 19:172, 1968.

24. Gray, R. H. Patterns of Bleeding Associated with the Use of Steroidal Contraceptives. In E. Diczfalusy, I. S. Fraser, and E. T. G. Webb (eds.), *Endometrial Bleeding and Steroidal Contraception: Proceedings of a Symposium on Steroid Contraception and Mechanisms of Endometrial Bleeding.* World Health Organization, 1980. P. 14.

25. Greenberg, G., et al. Maternal drug histories and congenital anomalies. *Br. Med. J.* 2:853, 1977.

26. Greenspan, A. R., et al. The association of depomedroxyprogesterone acetate and breast cancer. *Contraception* 21:563, 1980.

27. Harlap, S., Prywes, R., and Davies, A. M. Birth defects and estrogens and progesterones in pregnancy. *Lancet* 1:682, 1975.

28. Hatcher, R. A., et al. Depo-medroxyprogesterone acetate: Experience at the Grady Memorial Hospital Family Planning Program in Atlanta, Georgia: 1967–1979. Paper presented to the annual meeting of the Association of Planned Parenthood Physicians, Denver, Oct. 4, 1980.

29. Heinonen, O. P., et al. Cardiovascular birth defects and antenatal exposure to female sex hormones. *N. Engl. J. Med.* 296:67, 1977.

30. Howard, G., et al. The effect of norethisterone oenanthate on the full blood count. *Br. J. Fam. Plann.* 8:125, 1983.

31. Howard, G., Myatt, L., and Elder, M. G. The effects of intra-muscular norethisterone oenanthate used as a contraceptive on intravenous glucose tolerance and on blood coagulation factors 7 and 10. *Br. J. Obstet. Gynaecol.* 84:618, 1977.

32. Isaacs, W. A., Eltiong, C. E., and Ayerri, O. Steroid treatment in the prevention of painful episodes in sickle-cell disease. *Lancet* 1:570, 1972.

33. Janerich, D. T., et al. Congenital heart disease and prenatal exposure to exogenous sex hormones. *Br. Med. J.* 1:1058, 1977.

34. Jin, O. C., and Sun, L. Y. Medullary infarction: Was it Depo-Provera? *Singapore Med. J.* 21:717, 1980.

35. Kay, C. R. Progestogens and arterial disease: Evidence from the Royal College of General Practitioners' study. *Am. J. Obstet. Gynecol.* 142:762, 1982.

36. Keys, A. Alpha lipoprotein (HDL) cholesterol in the serum and the risk of coronary heart disease and death. *Lancet* 2:603, 1980.

37. Kistner, R. W. Histological effects of progestins on hyperplasia and carcinoma-in-situ of the endometrium. *Cancer* 12:1106, 1958.

38. Koetsawang, S. Injected long-acting medroxyprogesterone acetate: Effect on human lactation and concentrations in milk. *J. Med. Assoc. Thailand* 60:57, 1977.

39. Koetsawang, S. Present Management of Abnormal Bleeding Associated with Steroidal Contraceptives. In E. Diczfalusy, I. S. Fraser, and F. T. G. Webb (eds.), *Endometrial Bleeding and Steroid Contraception: Proceedings of a Symposium*

on Steroid Contraception and Mechanisms of Endometrial Bleeding. World Health Organization, 1980. P. 50.

40. Koetsawang, S., et al. Transfer of contraceptive steroids in milk of women using long-acting gestagens. *Contraception* 25:321, 1982.

41. Koetsawang, S., Shrimanker, K., and Fotherby, K. Blood levels of medroxyprogesterone acetate after multiple injections of Depo-Provera or Cyclo-Provera. *Contraception* 20:1, 1979.

42. Kremer, J., de Bruijn, H. W., and Hindriks, F. R. Serum high density lipoprotein cholesterol levels in women using a contraceptive injection of depot-medroxyprogesterone acetate. *Contraception* 22:359, 1980.

43. Laatikainen, T., Neiminen, U., and Adlercrentz, H. Plasma medroxyprogesterone acetate levels following intramuscular or oral administration in patients with endometrial carcinoma. *Acta Obstet. Gynecol. Scand.* 58:95, 1979.

44. Lees, R. A. Contraceptive and endometrial effects of medroxyprogesterone acetate. *Am. J. Obstet. Gynecol.* 104:130, 1969.

45. Leiman, G. Depo-medroxyprogesterone acetate as a contraceptive agent: Its effect on weight and blood pressure. *Am. J. Obstet. Gynecol.* 114:97. 1972.

46. Lenco, W., McNight, M., and McDonald, A. S. Effects of cortisone acetate, methylprednisolone and medroxyprogesterone on contraceptive and epithelialisation in rabbits. *Ann. Surg.* 181:67, 1975.

47. Liskin, L. S. Long-acting progestins: Promise and prospects. *Popul. Rep.* [K] 2:17, 1983.

48. McDaniel, E. B., and Pardthaisong, T. Depot-medroxyprogesterone acetate as a contraceptive agent: Return of fertility after discontinuation of use. *Contraception* 8:407, 1973.

49. McDaniel, E. B., and Pardthaisong, T. Use-effectiveness of six-month injections of DMPA as a contraceptive. *Am. J. Obstet. Gynecol.* 119:175, 1974.

50. McDaniel, E. B., and Potts, M. International forum update: Depomedroxyprogesterone acetate and endometrial carcinoma. *Int. J. Gynaecol. Obstet.* 17:297, 1979.

51. Mettler, L., Shirwani, D., and Brunnberg, F. J. Thrombocyte function in relation to the long-term application of medroxyprogesterone acetate as a female contraceptive agent. *J. Postgrad. Med.* 25:154, 1979.

52. Minkin, S. Depo-Provera: A critical analysis. *Women Health* 5:49, 1980.

53. Mishell, D. R., Jr., et al. Physiologic and morphologic alterations effected by the contraceptive use of depomedroxyprogesterone acetate. In *Proceedings of the Sixth World Congress on Fertility and Sterility*. 1970. P. 7.

54. Mishell, D. R., Jr., et al. The effect of contraceptive steroids on hypothalamic-pituitary function. *Am. J. Obstet. Gynecol.* 128:60, 1977.

55. Mulligan, R. M. Mammary cancer in the dog: A study of 120 cases. *Am. J. Vet. Res.* 36:1391, 1975.

56. Nelson, L. W., Carlton, W. W., and Weikel, J. H. J.

Canine mammary neoplasms and progestogens. *J.A.M.A.* 219:1601, 1972.

57. Nora, A. H., and Nora, J. J. Syndrome of multiple congenital anomalies associated with teratogenic exposure. *Arch. Environ. Health* 30:17, 1975.

58. Ojo, O. A. Depot medroxyprogesterone acetate for contraception: A continuing controversy. *Int. J. Gynaecol. Obstet.* 16:439, 1979.

59. Ortiz, A., et al. Serum medroxyprogesterone acetate (MPA) concentrations and ovarian function following intramuscular injection of Depo-MPA. *J. Clin. Endocrinol. Metab.* 44:32, 1977.

60. Ory, H. The noncontraceptive health benefits from oral contraceptive use. *Fam. Plann. Perspect.* 14:182, 1982.

61. Pardthaisong, T., Gray, R. H., and McDaniel, E. B. Return of fertility after discontinuation of depot medroxyprogesterone acetate and intra-uterine devices in northern Thailand. *Lancet* 1:509, 1980.

62. Parker, R. A., and McDaniel, E. B. The use of quinestrol for the control of vaginal bleeding irregularities caused by DMPA. *Contraception* 22:1, 1980.

63. Perez-Lopez, F. R., L'Hermite, M., and Robyn, C. Gonadotropin hormone releasing tests in women receiving hormonal contraception. *Clin. Endocrinol.* 4:447, 1974.

64. Perkins, R. S. Contraception for sicklers. *N. Engl. J. Med.* 285:290, 1971.

65. Rall, H. J. S., et al. Comparative contraceptive experience with three-month and six-month medroxyprogesterone acetate regimens. *J. Reprod. Med.* 18:55, 1977.

66. Report to USAID of the Ad Hoc Consultative Panel on Depot Medroxyprogesterone acetate. July, 1980.

67. Rosenfield, A. Injectable long-acting progestogen contraception: A neglected modality. *Am. J. Obstet. Gynecol.* 120:537, 1974.

68. Rosenfield, A., et al. The Food and Drug Administration and medroxyprogesterone acetate. *J.A.M.A.* 249:2922, 1983.

69. Sang, G. W., et al. Pharmacokinetics of norethisterone oenanthate in humans. *Contraception* 24:15, 1981.

70. Saxena, B. N., Shrimanker, K., and Grudzinskas, J. G. Levels of contraceptive steroids in breast milk and plasma of lactating women. *Contraception* 16:605, 1977.

71. Schmidt, A. M. Patient labeling of medroxyprogesterone acetate injectable contraceptive. *Federal Register* 39:32907, 1974.

72. Schrimanker, K., Saxena, B. N., and Fotherby, K. A radioimmunoassay for serum medroxyprogesterone acetate. *J. Steroid Biochem.* 9:359, 1978.

73. Schwallie, P. C. The effect of Depo-medroxyprogesterone acetate on the fetus and nursing infant: A review. *Contraception* 23:375, 1981.

74. Senanayake, P., and Kramer, D. G. Contraception and the etiology of pelvic inflammatory disease: New perspectives. *Am. J. Obstet. Gynecol.* 138:852, 1980.

75. Shapiro, S. S., Dyer, R. D., and Coles, A. E. Synthetic

progestins: In-vitro potency on human endometrium and specific binding to cytosol receptor. *Am. J. Obstet. Gynecol.* 132:549, 1978.

76. Sieber, S. M. Testimony before the U.S. Food and Drug Administration, Public Board of Inquiry on Depo-Provera. January, 1983.

77. Sodoff, L., and Lush, W. The effect of large doses of medroxyprogesterone acetate (MPA) on urinary estrogen levels and serum levels of cortisol, T_4, LH and testosterone in patients with advanced cancer. *Obstet. Gynecol.* 43:262, 1972.

78. Solash, J., et al. Hormonal steroids: Effects on the vascular system. *Gynecol. Invest.* 6:329, 1975.

79. Spellacy, W. M., et al. Medroxyprogesterone acetate and carbohydrate metabolism: Measurement of glucose, insulin and growth hormone during six months' time. *Fertil. Steril.* 21:457, 1970.

80. Swenson, I., Khan, A. R., and Jahan, F. A. A randomized single-blind comparative trial of norethindrone enanthate and depo-medroxyprogesterone acetate in Bangladesh. *Contraception* 21:207, 1980.

81. Toddywalla, V. S., Joshil, L., and Virkar, K. The effect of contraceptive steroids on human lactation. *Am. J. Obstet. Gynecol.* 127:245, 1977.

82. Toppazada, M. The clinical use of monthly injectable contraceptive preparations. *Obstet. Gynecol. Surv.* 32:335, 1977.

83. Toppazada, M., et al. The protective influence of progestogen only contraception against vaginal moniliasis. *Contraception* 20:99, 1979.

84. U.S. Food and Drug Administration. Approval of Depo-Provera for contraception denied. *FDA Drug Bull.* 8(2):10, 1978.

85. U.S. Food and Drug Administration (Bureau of Drugs). Obstetrics and Gynecology Advisory Committee and Biometric and Epidemiological Methodology Advisory Committee. Open Session: Depo-Provera, injectable, as a contraceptive: Report to the Committee, 1975.

86. Upjohn Company. Depo-Provera for contraception: Information for Public Board of Inquiry on Depo-Provera: Responses to the Board's question FDA Docket No. 78N-0124, 1982.

87. Wahl, P., et al. Effect of estrogen/progestin potency on lipid/lipoprotein cholesterol. *N. Engl. J. Med.* 308:864, 1983.

88. Whigham, K. A. E., et al. The effect of an injectable progestogen contraceptive on blood coagulation and fibrinolysis. *Br. J. Obstet. Gynaecol.* 86:806, 1979.

89. World Health Organization. Expanded Programme of Research, Development and Research Training in Human Reproduction. Task force on long-acting systemic agents for the regulation of fertility. Multinational comparative clinical evaluation of two long-acting injectable contraceptive steroids, norethisterone oenanthate and medroxyprogesterone acetate: 1. Use effectiveness. *Contraception* 15:153, 1977.

90. World Health Organization. Expanded Programme of Research, Development and Research Training in Human Reproduction. Task force on long-acting systemic agents for the regulation of fertility. Multinational comparative clinical evaluation of two long-acting injectable contraceptive steroids, norethisterone oenanthate and medroxyprogesterone acetate: 2. Bleeding patterns and side effects. *Contraception* 17: 395, 1978.

91. World Health Organization. Expanded Programme of Research, Development and Research Training in Human Reproduction. Task force on long-acting systemic agents for the regulation of fertility. Multinational comparative clinical evaluation of two long-acting injectable contraceptive steroids, norethisterone oenanthate and medroxyprogesterone acetate: A preliminary report. *Contraception* 25:1, 1982.

92. World Health Organization. The effect of female sex hormones on fetal development and infant health. *Technical Report Series* 657:1, 1981.

93. World Health Organization. Facts about injectable contraceptives. *Bull. W.H.O.*, 60:199, 1982.

94. World Health Organization. Testimony before the U.S. Food and Drug Administration, Public Board of Inquiry on Depo-Provera, 1983.

95. Zanartu, J., Onetto, E., and Dabancens, A. Mammary gland-nodules in women under continuous exposure to progestogens. *Contraception* 7:203, 1973.

15. Contraceptive Implants

Richard M. Soderstrom

With the exception of medicated intrauterine devices, no contraceptive implants have been approved for general use in the United States. Current research has, however, demonstrated several promising implant systems, some of which should reach the premarket trial stage in the near future. Much of the stimulus for this research stems from the continuing concern regarding the safety of conventionally employed steroidal contraceptives. One approach to the improvement of the effectiveness, safety, and acceptability of steroidal contraceptives is to develop long-acting preparations and methods of delivery that provide programmed medication.

If one considers oral contraceptives a pulselike delivery system, it is reasonable to assume there are periods following ingestion when serum steroid levels exceed the zone of therapeutic effectiveness. Overdosing can be obviated with implantable systems that meter the steroid into surrounding tissue and maintain the blood level in the desired range. This metered system over a prolonged period of time reduces the chance for human error associated with repetitive self-administration methods of contraception. This chapter will focus on nonbiodegradable subdermal implants as well as biodegradable systems.

NONBIODEGRADABLE SUBDERMAL IMPLANTS

In the mid-1960s silicone rubber was found to be an excellent carrier of contraceptive steroids for prolonged drug release [13, 22]. Early in clinical trials, subdermal Silastic implants impregnated with megestrol acetate (MA) were found to be effective as a contraceptive delivery system [9–12, 27]. However, multiple devices were needed to achieve the blood levels of progestin necessary to bring the failure rates into an acceptable range. By increasing the number of capsule implants, the duration of effectiveness also is increased.

A number of different steroids have been used with these Silastic implant systems. They include levonorgestrel, norgestrienone, norethindrone, gestrigone, 19 norsteroid ST-1435, and lynestrenol [5, 8, 14, 15, 19, 28]. Some of these compounds have higher rates of release than others with a correspondingly shorter duration of effect. With a slower release, an increased number of implants becomes necessary in order to achieve satisfactory serum levels. Because of this, levonorgestrel has become the most attractive compound for use with these Silastic implants.

A difference between capsules and rods of Silastic was noted in a clinical sense. Rods reduce the incidence of breakthrough bleeding but increase amenorrhea.

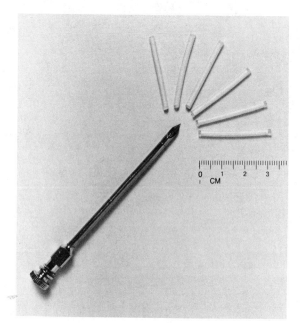

Fig. 15-1. The Norplant system consisting of six Silastic capsules and insertional trocar.

Mixing progestins with estradiol may achieve better control of bleeding problems [14].

Thus, Silastic implants can be considered advantageous in a number of ways. They can give better control of the therapeutic dose. The duration of use can be profound from 1 to 7 years. Repeat administration would be infrequent yet reliable. More importantly, upon removal ovulation should resume quickly. The disadvantages include (1) surgical insertion and removal; (2) the need for multiple capsules or rods; and (3) significant individual variation in steroidal blood levels.

Norplant

The contraceptive implant system that is currently undergoing clinical trials in the United States is named Norplant. This system, developed by the Population Council, consists of six Silastic capsules, each containing 36 ± 2 mg of levonorgestrel (Fig. 15-1). With a local anesthetic, a 5 to 6 mm incision is made in the skin of the upper arm or forearm. By means of a 10-gauge trocar, these capsules are deposited under the skin in a fanlike fashion. With experience, a clinician can complete the procedure in about 10 to 15 minutes (Fig. 15-2). After expiration the capsules must be surgically removed and, if desired, new capsules inserted.

The levonorgestrel diffuses from the Silastic, suppressing ovulation and causing a thickened cervical mucus, which inhibits sperm penetration. Though the blood levels of levonorgestrel are slightly higher shortly after implantation, a steady release of 30 µg per day is maintained throughout its use, with serum levels of about 0.4 µg/ml.

Clinical trials by Sivin et al. [25, 26] extending over 5 years showed an effectiveness rate of 7 pregnancies per 1,000 woman-years. A series of 492 acceptors was reported by Sivin et al. [25] in 1982. Of the five reported pregnancies, two occurred in the first month and may have been preexisting pregnancies. One pregnancy was reported but not confirmed. The remaining two pregnancies occurred in the third year, and one was an ectopic pregnancy.

Menstrual problems (~ 15%) are the leading reason for termination of the method. Infection in the implant site is unusual and does require removal, but permanent sequelae have not been reported. The medical reasons for removal are similar to those for oral contraceptives, but Sivin reports no difference in hypertension when compared with a matched series of patients using the Copper T.

Acceptance rates apparently are influenced by cultural differences. The combined average annual continuation rate is approximately 75 per 100. Reversibility as defined by a planned pregnancy following removal is 84 per 100 at 1 year.

BIODEGRADABLE SYSTEMS

The potential for a biodegradable system is just now being recognized. Though clinical trials are not as advanced as trials with implants like Norplant, a variety of systems are receiving intensive attention [1]. Such systems eliminate the need for removal.

An alternative to increasing the number of implants is to increase the surface-to-volume ratio, using multiple small particles or "mini-implants." Thus the therapeutic blood level can be more effectively controlled. Moreover, if the particle is 200 µm or less, a suspension of these particles can be administered by jet injection. However, once this suspension is injected, it cannot be removed as with Silastic implants.

Such miniparticles, to be effective, depend on the use of polymers that biodegrade without harm in living tissue. Polymers that are readily broken down by hydrolytic enzymes are potentially useful as drug carriers. As the degradation process continues, the carrier as well as the drug is delivered to the bloodstream. For this reason, toxicology investigation is a more important consideration.

One metabolite of carbohydrate metabolism, lactic

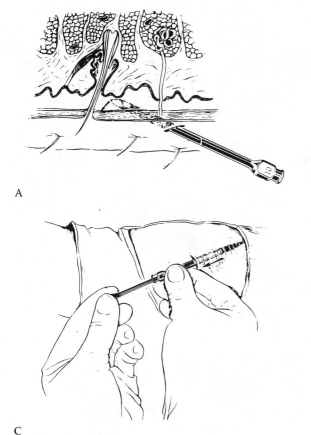

A

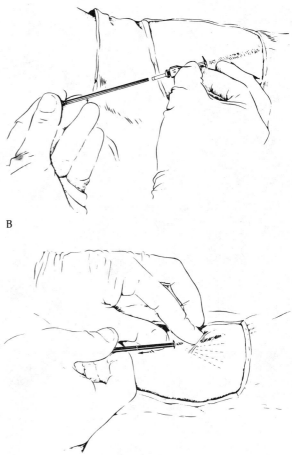

B

D

Fig. 15-2. (A) Under local anesthesia, the trocar is introduced into the subcutaneous tissues of the forearm. (B) A Silastic capsule is inserted into the trocar sleeve; an obturator is used to advance the Silastic capsule. (C) Once the Silastic capsule is in position, the trocar sleeve is slowly removed over the obturator, which holds the capsule in place. (D) The operator depresses the skin over the Silastic capsule to stabilize the capsule while the trocar and obturator are removed. The procedure is repeated in a fanlike position as shown.

acid, has two optional isomers. Polylactic acid (PLA) exists as a crystalline stereoregular polymer $L(-)$-PLA,$D(+)$-PLA or an amorphous racemic polymer D,L-PLA. Though similar to commercial polyesters such as Dacron, they decompose completely when exposed continuously to water and tissue fluids [20]. This aliphatic characteristic can be programmed for varying durations of effect by changing mixtures of these racemic particles and with other additives such as glycolic acid. The degradation by-product, therefore, is lactic acid, a nontoxic chemical.

Levonorgestrel and norethindrone (NET) are common progestins used in these biodegradable systems [3]. Micronized crystals of progestin can be homogeneously dispersed in microcapsules for intramuscular injection. One such study on baboons used a 6-month interval protocol with excellent suppression of ovulation. By increasing particle number, the desired blood level can be accurately reached [3].

It appears that there are no harmful effects at the site of injections. Also, the system can be sterilized without altering performance characteristics. By mixing particle size, number, and percentage of steroid present, the rate and duration of drug release can be predetermined [2].

The potential for the addition of other steroids such as estradiol is obvious. Concentric layers of hormone could be used to give sequential steroid therapy. Direct target organ injection is possible. Even microsphere inhalants could be programmed for accurate delivery. With many compounds now being administered via skin patch delivery systems, a transdermal contraceptive device employing the steroids now used orally is not a remote possibility.

Polycaprolactone, an aliphatic polyester similar to polylactic acid, can be extruded as a small bore tubing, which, when filled with steroid, can be implanted surgically yet would not require removal unless reversal is desired [7, 16, 18]. Toxicology studies of this polyester are under way.

Synthetic polypeptides as biodegradable polymeric carriers have been studied [6, 17, 23, 24]. Also, a new family of biodegradable polymers undergoes a time-predictable hydrolytic erosion in living tissue [4, 21]. These materials, called *chronomer*, are described as hydrophobic, biocompatible, and nontoxic. As the orthoester linkages on the surface of fabricated chronomer rods erode, the micronized progestin is released. Constant plasma levels can be maintained up to 6 months. As with the nonbiodegradable implants, these rods can be removed in order to restore fertility.

CONCLUSION

Subdermal implant systems are in various stages of investigation and development. Delivery systems include rods, capsules, and microparticles, all designed to meter a constant yet effective rate of contraceptive steroid. Some systems are nonbiodegradable and require minimal surgical training before they can be administered. Prolonged length of duration is a strong feature as is their rapid reversibility.

Biodegradable microparticles or microspheres can be readily injected without surgical trauma but in most instances are not readily reversible on demand. When impregnated with contraceptive steroids, a precise dosage schedule can be programmed.

With the development of more sophisticated systems, and with current technical capabilities, the future of nonbiodegradable and biodegradable systems for fertility control looks promising.

REFERENCES

1. Baker, R. W., and Lonsdale, H. K. Controlled Release— Mechanisms and Rates. In A. C. Tanquary and R. E. Lacey (eds.), *Controlled Release of Biologically Active Agents: Advances in Experimental Medicine and Biology.* New York: Plenum, 1974. Vol. 47, Pp. 15–72.

2. Beck, L. R., et al. A new long-acting injectable microcapsule contraceptive system. *Am. J. Obstet. Gynecol.* 135:419, 1979.

3. Beck, L. R., et al. Evaluation of a new three-month injectable contraceptive microsphere system in primates (baboon). *J. Contracept. Del. Systems* 1:79, 1980.

4. Benagiano, G., et al. Sustained release hormonal preparations for the delivery of fertility regulating agents. *J. Polymer Sci.* 66:129, 1979.

5. Bhatmagar, S., et al. Long-term contraception of steroid-releasing implants: II. A preliminary report on long-term contraception by a single Silastic implant containing norethindrone acetate (ENTA) in women. *Contraception* 11:505, 1975.

6. Choi, N. S., and Heller, J. Erodible agent releasing device comprising poly(orthoesters) and poly(orthocarbonates). United States Patent 4,138,344, Feb. 6, 1979. Assignee: Alza Corporation.

7. Cohen, M. R., Pandya, G. N., and Scommegna, A. The effects of an intracervical steroid-releasing device on the cervical mucus. *Fertil. Steril.* 21:715, 1970.

8. Coutinho, E. M., DaSilva, A. R., and Kraft, H. G. Fertility control with subdermal capsules containing a new progestin (ST-1435). *Int. J. Fertil.* 21:103, 1976.

9. Coutinho, E. M., et al. Long-term contraception by subcutaneous Silastic R capsules containing megestrol acetate. *Contraception* 2:313, 1970.

10. Croxatto, H., et al. Contraceptive action of megestrol acetate implants in women. *Contraception* 4:155, 1971.

11. Croxatto, H., et al. Adnexal complications in women under treatment with progestogen implants. *Contraception* 12:629, 1975.

12. Croxatto, H., et al. Fertility control in women with a progestogen released in microquantities from subcutaneous capsules. *Am. J. Obstet. Gynecol.* 105:1135, 1969.

13. Folkman, J., and Long, D. M. The rise of silicone rubber as a carrier for prolonged drug therapy. *J. Surg. Res* 4:139, 1964.

14. International Committee for Contraception Research of the Population Council. Contraception with long-acting subdermal implants: I. An effective and acceptable modality in international clinical trials. *Contraception* 18:315, 1978.

15. International Committee for Contraception Research of the Population Council. Contraception with long-acting subdermal implants. II. Measured and perceived effects in international clinical trials. *Contraception* 18:335, 1978.

16. Nuwayser, E. S., et al. A Microcapsule System for Drug Delivery. In H. L. Gabelnick (ed.), *Proceedings: Drug Delivery Systems.* DHEW Publication No. (NIH) 77-1238, 1977. Pp 193–251.

17. Peterson, R. V., et al. Controlled release of progestins from poly (alpha-amino acid) carrier. In Proceedings of the 6th International Symposium on Controlled Release of Bioactive Materials. New Orleans, La., August, 1979. Pp. I-21, I-27.

18. Pitt, C. G., et al. Biodegradable Polymers and Sustained Delivery of Contraceptive Drugs. In H. L. Gabelnick (ed.), *Proceedings: Drug Delivery Systems.* DHEW Publication No. (NIH) 77:1238, 1977. Pp 141–192.

19. Rahman, S. A., et al. Effect of norethindrone acetate–releasing single implant on hypothalamo-hypophyseal-gonadal axis in women. Symposium on General and Comparative Endocrinology. Abstract p. 77, 1976.

20. Schindler, A., et al. Biodegradable Polymers for Sustained Drug Delivery. In E. M. Pearce and J. R. Schaefgen (eds.), *Contemporary Topics in Polymer Science.* New York: Plenum, 1977. Vol. 2, pp. 251–289.

21. Schmitt, E. E. Pharmaceutical composition of poly(orthoester) co- and homopolymers and poly(orthocarbonate) co- and homopolymers having carbonyloxy functionality with drug. United States Patent 4,155,922, May 22, 1979. Assignee: Alza Corporation.

22. Segal, S. J., and Croxatto, H. B. Single administration of hormones for long-term control of reproductive function. Presented to the 23rd Meeting of the American Fertility Society. Washington, D.C., Apr. 14–16, 1967.

23. Sidman, K. R., et al. Use of synthetic polypeptides for biodegradable drug delivery systems. Polymer Preprints 20:27, 1979.

24. Sidman, K., Steber, W. D., and Burg, A. W. A Biodegradable Drug Delivery System. In H. L. Gabelnick (ed.), Proceedings: Drug Delivery Systems. DHEW Publication No. (NIH) 77-1238, 1977. P. 120.

25. Sivin I. The Norplant contraceptive method: A report on three years of use. *Stud. Fam. Plann.* 13:258, 1982.

26. Sivin, I., et al. Norplant: Reversible implant contraception. *Stud. Fam. Plann.* 11:227, 1980.

27. Tejuja, S. Use of subcutaneous Silastic capsules for long-term steroid contraception. *Am. J. Obstet. Gynecol.* 197:954, 1970.

28. Weiner, E., and Johansson, E. D. B. Effects on the ovarian function of subcutaneous implants containing lynestrenol. Presented to the 18th Nordiska Gynekologkongressen. Uppsala, June 4–8, 1974, Abstr. No. 92, *Acta Obstet. Gynecol. Scand.* [Suppl.] 47:50, 1976.

16. Vaginal Hormonal Devices

Subir Roy
Daniel R. Mishell, Jr.

It has been known for decades that many drugs, including steroids, when placed into the vagina, are absorbed through the vaginal epithelium into the general circulation. In 1965 Dzuik and Cook [7] demonstrated that steroids placed in Silastic tubes diffused out of the tubes into a saline solution at a constant rate. The rate of diffusion was related to the surface area of the Silastic as well as the thickness of the tubing. The amount of drug in the device determined its duration of action. Combining these two principles led to the development of contraceptive vaginal rings. A variety of contraceptive steroids have been placed into Silastic ring-shaped devices, which were then inserted into the vagina for various time periods. The steroids were absorbed through the vaginal epithelium at a relatively constant rate in amounts sufficient to inhibit ovulation. In this chapter the development of contraceptive vaginal rings (CVRs) will be reviewed. Initially, CVR development was undertaken by the pharmaceutical industry; however, since 1972 most development has been performed by the Population Council or the World Health Organization [21]. This chapter primarily reviews devices made and studied by the Population Council. The World Health Organization (WHO) has also developed and studied a CVR; however, very little information regarding this device has appeared in the scientific literature.

SIZE

Ascertainment of the optimal size of the toroidal-shaped CVRs has to take into account subject comfort as well as the possibility of spontaneous expulsion of the device with activities that increase intraabdominal pressure. The initial studies were performed with devices 70 to 80 mm in outer diameter and 10 mm thick [13]. Although no erosions or slippage occurred, because of concern about possible expulsions, devices 75 mm in diameter containing a flat spring much like a conventional diaphragm were fabricated and studied. Although none of the subjects complained of slippage, these spring rings were abandoned because vaginal erosions were produced in more than half the subjects [16]. A study of rings with an outer diameter of 65 mm and a 7-mm thickness demonstrated that the thinner rings produced more erosions than the thicker rings [18]. Subsequently rings with outside diameters of 61 mm [14, 15], 60 mm [17], 58 mm [17, 18], 55 mm [10], and 50 mm [24, 26] and 9 to 9.5 mm thickness have been shown to be well tolerated. The WHO Varlevo 20 ring has an outer diameter of 55.0 mm and a cross-sectional diameter of 9.5 mm [6].

From the results of these studies, it appears that CVRs with an outer diameter of about 50 to 58 mm and thickness from 7 to 9.5 mm are well tolerated by most acceptors. One size ring is suitable for all women. Unlike the diaphragm which acts locally, the device which acts systemically does not have to be fitted or placed in a certain position, although it generally assumes an orientation about the cervix. As long as the outer surface of the CVR is in contact with the vaginal epithelium, systemic distribution of the steroids will occur. Vaginal epithelial erosion occurs infrequently, and when it does, it heals spontaneously following simple removal of the CVR [15, 16, 18]. Spontaneous expulsion of the device can be easily corrected by having the user reinsert the device. No colposcopic changes of the vaginal epithelium adjacent to the CVR have been noted following 2 years of use [19].

FORMULATIONS

Homogeneous

The initial design of the CVR was a ring made of a homogeneous mixture of steroid and Silastic (Fig. 16-1A). This device was found to release high initial dosages of circulating steroid levels followed by a rapid reduction of steroid levels, which coincided with episodes of breakthrough bleeding or breakthrough spotting (BTB/BTS) [27].

Core

In order to eliminate the initial high steroid levels followed by the rapid decline associated with the homogeneous ring, the core ring (Fig. 16-1B) was developed. Rings that were 9 mm thick with steroids contained within a 3.5-mm central core were tested and found to produce fairly uniform serum levels while in situ except for an initial period, and they had sufficient steroid to allow use for several cycles [3]. The WHO Varlevo 20 ring is formulated as a core design containing about 6 mg of levonorgestrel [5].

Shell Design

In an effort to develop devices with more uniform release rates, rings with a so-called shell design were developed (Fig. 16-1C). These shell rings have a steroid and Silastic layer applied around an inner core of inert Silastic. The active layer is covered with another layer of inert Silastic tubing, thus providing an almost uniform distance through which the drug must travel in order to be absorbed [11]. The collagen band device (Fig. 16-1D) is another approach to stabilize release rates.

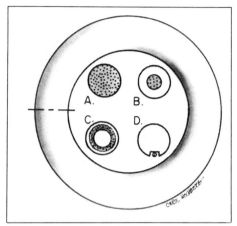

Fig. 16-1. A diagrammatic cross-sectional representation of the contraceptive vaginal ring. (A) The homogeneous vaginal ring is made of a homogeneous mixture of the contraceptive steroid and dimethylpolysiloxane [13]. (B) The core vaginal ring is comprised of a central core of 3.5 mm which is surrounded by 5.5 mm of dimethylpolysiloxane [3]. (C) The shell vaginal ring is fabricated around an inert core of dimethylpolysiloxane, which is surrounded by a layer of a homogeneous mixture of the contraceptive steroid and dimethylpolysiloxane, which is covered by a tube of dimethylpolysiloxane [15, 18, 28]. (D) The collagen band vaginal ring contains the contraceptive steroid in a band of collagen, which is kept in place by placement of the band in a groove in an inert dimethylpolysiloxane ring [30]. (From D. R. Mishell, Jr., et al. Clinical performance of endocrine profiles with contraceptive vaginal rings containing a combination of estradiol and d-norgestrel. Am. J. Obstet. Gynecol. 130:55, 1978.)

DRUGS TESTED

Studies have been performed utilizing the following various progestins alone or in combination with estrogens; medroxyprogesterone acetate (MPA), chlormadinone acetate (CMA), norethindrone (NET), R2323, dl-norgestrel (Ng), levonorgestrel (LNG), LNG + estradiol benzoate (EB), and LNG + estradiol (E_2). The 21-carbon compounds, MPA and CMA, produced similar blood levels as after oral administration, with suppressed ovulation; however, they were no longer studied following the reports of mammary tumors in beagle dogs [13, 16, 18]. Homogeneous NET rings releasing 850 to 1,529 µg per day produced unacceptable episodes of BTB/BTS associated with an offensive odor and were associated with ovulation in one-quarter of the cycles studied [16]. R2323 administered in a core device releasing 150 to 400 µg per day produced no

BTB/BTS, blocked ovulation, and upon removal was followed by prompt withdrawal bleeding [3]. Further tests with this promising agent were abandoned when it was reported that men ingesting 100 mg per week orally of this agent developed increased transaminase levels. In tests of rings releasing dl-Ng at rates of 120 to 350 μg per day the major problem was one of BTB/BTS, which occurred in 63 percent of cycles studied [28]. Ovulation also occurred in approximately 15 percent of cycles with this device in place. In an effort to reduce the incidence of BTB/BTS, a ring with LNG + EB was developed [30]. However, BTB/BTS was observed in 64 percent of cycles studied, suggesting that no benefit accrued from the addition of EB since such small amounts (50 to 100 μg) of estradiol benzoate were available for vaginal absorption. Shell rings releasing LNG alone demonstrated higher sustained circulating serum LNG levels (1.6—2.4 ng/ml) than those shell rings releasing dl-Ng (1.2–1.7 ng/ml), each over a 6-month period [23, 28]. These LNG shell rings were associated with BTB/BTS in 33 percent, lack of withdrawal bleeding in 5 percent, and ovulation in 3 percent of cycles studied. It was felt that the addition of E_2 to the LNG ring would produce better bleeding control and suppress ovulation.

In the first trial with rings releasing LNG + E_2, significantly improved bleeding control was observed: BTB/BTS occurred in only 7 percent of cycles studied. Withdrawal bleeding after ring removal occurred within 1 to 5 days with a mean of 2.6 days and lasted from 3 to 7 days with a mean of 4.5 days. There was no failure of withdrawal bleeding and no ovulation in any of the initial study cycles. These rings released an average of 289 μg of LNG per day and 212 μg of E_2 per day and produced fairly constant serum LNG levels of 1 to 3 ng per milliliter and an initial peak E_2 level of about 100 pg per milliliter, which rapidly declined but presumably stimulated the endometrium sufficiently to provide improved bleeding control.

USE SCHEDULE

The original use schedule was similar to that for oral contraceptives. The CVR was inserted on day 5 of the cycle and left in place for 21 days. In the first studies with rings containing medroxyprogesterone acetate a high incidence of BTB/BTS occurred with this schedule, suggesting that insufficient amounts of endogenous estrogen were being secreted during use of this progestin-only CVR [13, 16]. Therefore, a trial was performed in which this CVR was inserted on day 10, at which time more endogenous estradiol would be secreted by the ovary. Since the incidence of BTB/BTS was not re-

duced with the latter schedule, this approach was abandoned [18]. Another regimen, the bleeding signal, has been tested. In this novel approach, the subjects were instructed to leave the rings in place and only remove them for 5 days whenever they had BTB/BTS. In studies with this regimen the incidence of bleeding and spotting was usually lower than that expected during a comparable period of untreated cycles. The bleeding was also scantier than the subjects' ordinary menses and prolonged amenorrheic episodes occurred [29]. However, the fact that the patient does not have to remember when the ring has to be removed was thought to counterbalance the unpredictable occurrence of bleeding episodes with this schedule. In almost all instances, the ring was reinserted within 5 days after removal, and no ovulations were observed. Although no vaginal erosions occurred during this study, vaginal rugae were flattened. When questioned, most subjects preferred the fixed time schedule to the bleeding signal schedule.

Thus, the standard schedule for the use of the vaginal ring is to have the subject self-insert it on day 5 of the cycle for 3 weeks and then remove it for a 7-day period to allow withdrawal bleeding. The WHO Varlevo ring is designed to be worn continuously for 90 days [6].

Should the CVR interfere with coitus, it may be removed for up to 3 hours and then be reinserted without reducing the contraceptive effect [15]. In one study 25 percent of women sometimes or always removed the ring before coitus. Male discomfort during intercourse varied from 8 to 24 percent [8].

PHARMACODYNAMICS AND MECHANISMS OF ACTION

When the self-administered combination CVR releasing levonorgestrel and estradiol is placed in the vagina, the steroids are released from the surface and absorbed through the vaginal epithelium into the circulation at a fairly constant rate (Fig. 16-2). Patients using the rings containing estradiol and levonorgestrel had mean levonorgestrel levels of 2.5 ng per milliliter for the first cycle and 1.3 ng per milliliter during the sixth cycle [15]. These levels are sufficient to inhibit ovulation but several times less than the 4 to 8 ng per milliliter peak levels obtained with daily ingestion of tablets containing 500 μg norgestrel (250 μg levonorgestrel) [4]. Ovulation continues to be inhibited during the week that the rings are not in place. Although midcycle gonadotropin peaks are abolished, gonadotropin peaks have been observed during the 1-week interval when the ring was removed or soon after its reinsertion (Fig. 16-3).

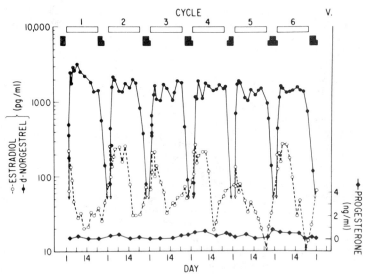

Fig. 16-2. Serum estradiol and d-norgestrel levels on a log-scale and progesterone levels during six treatment cycles with vaginal rings. Rings were inserted on day 1 and removed on day 21 during each cycle. Open bars represent 3-week treatment cycles with rings in place. Black bars represent bleeding days (full height for bleeding and half height for spotting) [21]. (From S. Roy and D. R. Mishell, Jr. Contraceptive Vaginal Rings: Mechanisms of Action and Historical Development. In E. S. E. Havez and W. A. A. van O [eds.], *Biodegradables and Delivery Systems for Contraception.* Lancaster, Eng.: MTP, 1980.)

In an earlier study with medroxyprogesterone acetate in which ovulation was also suppressed, the endometrial histology showed glands that were narrow, nontortuous, and widely separated, with the stroma having a pseudodecidual appearance [9].

Shell rings used for six or seven consecutive 21-day cycles with a 7-day nonuse interval between cycles have been analyzed for average steroid loss. In vivo, rings of 58-mm diameter were found to release levonorgestrel and estradiol at mean rates of 293 ± 54 μg per day and 183 ± 34 μg per day, respectively [11]. Rings of 50-mm diameter had mean levonorgestrel and estradiol release rates of 252 ± 34 μg per day and 152 ± 21 μg per day, respectively. Sufficient steroid was present in each of these rings so that they could be used for at least six treatment cycles before being replaced.

The WHO ring, releasing approximately 20 μg of levonorgestrel daily, has been found to suppress ovulation in 20 to 50 percent of cycles studied [6, 12, 31, 32]; postcoital tests found cervical mucus impenetrable to sperm in 11 of 12 cycles [31], providing an additional mechanism for contraceptive effectiveness.

Fig. 16-3. Three-times-a-week assay of serum LH (*solid line*) and FSH (*dotted line*) during six treatment cycles. Open bars represent the 3 weeks the rings were in place. These values for LH and FSH are for the same subject as in Figure 16-2 [21]. (From S. Roy and D. R. Mishell, Jr. Contraceptive Vaginal Rings: Mechanisms of Action and Historical Development. In E. S. E. Havez and W. A. A. van O [eds.], *Biodegradables and Delivery Systems for Contraception.* Lancaster, Eng.: MTP, 1980.)

d-Ng ESTRADIOL

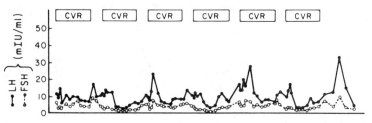

CLINICAL STUDIES

In order to assess the contraceptive effectiveness and acceptability of the shell CVR containing LNG and E_2, devices of two sizes—50 and 58 mm in outer diameter and 9.5 mm thick—were fabricated and compared with an oral contraceptive containing LNG (150 µg) with EE_2 (30 µg) (Nordette). These contraceptives were compared in a multicenter study from eight clinics in Brazil, Chile, Denmark, the Dominican Republic, Finland, the United States (Los Angeles), Nigeria, and Sweden [24–26]. A total of 547 50-mm CVR users, 556 58-mm CVR users, and 553 Nordette users were enrolled (Table 16-1). Both first and all segment 1-year net pregnancy rates among CVR users were less than 3 per 100, approximately the same as the pregnancy rates observed among users of Nordette. The continuation rate at 1 year was 50 per 100 users of the ring (all segments). This rate was significantly higher than or equal to the rate observed among the users of Nordette, 38.2 or

55.4, depending upon whether the lost-to-follow-up rates of these subjects were considered a termination or not, respectively. The profile of terminations was similar for the users of the two sizes of rings but differed significantly from that of the Nordette acceptors. Gross 1-year rates of termination for medical reasons ranged from 25 to 29 per 100 for the three regimens without a significant difference. However, ring users were more likely to terminate for vaginal problems and pill users for headaches, nausea, and other systemic symptoms. Problems relating to use of the regimen accounted for a significantly higher discontinuation rate among CVR than among Nordette users. Terminations for use-related reasons were coded into seven categories: frequent ring expulsion, interference with coitus, insertion or removal of ring unpleasant, ring odor, difficulties in storage of ring or pill, ring loss, and other problems associated with use of the pill. Lost rings, insertion and removal difficulties, or unpleasantness of insertion and removal accounted for the majority of use-related ter-

Table 16-1. All segments one-year termination and continuation rates per 100 acceptors by regimen and reason for termination

Rate	Net rates			Gross rates		
	CVR			CVR		
	50 mm	58 mm	Nordette	50 mm	58 mm	Nordette
Pregnancy	1.8	1.0	2.0	2.4	1.4	3.3
Medical termination	23.5	22.5	18.7	29.2	27.0	24.7
Use-related termination	6.6	4.4	2.0	8.4	5.4	3.6[a]
Personal termination	8.8	9.7	11.2	12.2	13.7	18.5
Moving	2.0	2.1	2.0	2.8	3.2	3.2
Loss-to-follow-up	8.5	9.9	25.9	9.5	11.3	31.0[b]
Continuation, LFU a termination	48.8	50.4	38.2	48.8	50.4	38.2[b]
Continuation, LFU not a termination	54.0	56.8	55.4	54.0	56.8	55.4
Type of termination	Events			Standard errors		
Pregnancy	9	5	10	0.8	0.7	1.1
Medical reasons	119	115	95	2.3	2.2	2.3
Use-related reasons	35	23	10	1.4	1.1	1.2
Personal reasons	45	47	55	1.8	1.9	2.4
Moving	10	10	10	0.9	1.0	1.1
Loss-to-follow-up	46	53	133	1.4	1.5	2.3
All	264	253	313	2.3	2.3	2.2
No. of women enrolled	547	556	553			
No. of women at risk, month 12	239	220	193			

[a]$P < .01$.
[b]$P < .001$.
Source: From I. Sivin et al. A multicenter study of levonorgestrel-estradiol contraceptive vaginal rings: I. Use effectiveness. An international comparative trial. *Contraception* 24:341, 1981.

minations. These trials indicate that CVRs of this design are as effective in use and have continuation rates equal to and possibly superior to Nordette under the same study conditions.

In addition, the side effects of the rings and Nordette were evaluated by noting spontaneous complaints, by recording additional medications taken, and by physical examination [25]. Inquiries about changes in the frequency of specific conditions were made at the end of the subjects' participation in the first year of the study (Table 16-2). The incidence of spontaneous complaints was similar among users of the two different-sized rings and of Nordette.

Vaginal complaints were significantly more frequent among ring users, while only users of the 50-mm ring had significantly greater menstrual complaints than users of either the 58-mm ring or Nordette. Headaches, dizziness, and nausea were reported significantly more frequently by users of Nordette. All three regimens were associated with weight gain of about 1 kg and increased hemoglobin levels of about 0.5 gm per deciliter. Nordette, but not the CVR, was associated with small but significant increases in both diastolic (0.9 mm Hg) and systolic (1.5 mm Hg) blood pressure.

A more detailed examination of the menstrual events based on diaries demonstrated that both the CVRs and Nordette produced approximately the same total number of bleeding and spotting days during six cycles of use [26], but the small (50-mm OD) ring was associated with somewhat more spotting (Table 16-3). This ring was also associated with somewhat more prolonged

bleeding and spotting runs and with more prolonged nonbleeding intervals than reported by users of the larger (58-mm OD) ring or Nordette. CVR users experienced a mean of about 1 day per month of bleeding or spotting with the ring in place. Evidence from menstrual diaries indicates that these CVRs, and in particular the 58-mm ring, provide control over the menstrual cycle comparable to that of Nordette.

With the use of the WHO Varlevo 20 ring, which is worn for 90 days continuously, only one method-related pregnancy has been reported in 554 woman-months of use, while breakthrough bleeding and spotting, although not completely eliminated with this ring, is reported to be slight on the average [6].

METABOLIC STUDIES

Carbohydrate and Liver Function

A prospective, long-term study was also undertaken to compare the metabolic effects of the contraceptive vaginal ring and Nordette in two groups of women consisting of 22 and 20 women, respectively. An intravenous glucose tolerance test (IVGTT), including determination of the insulin response to glucose, and liver function tests (bilirubin, alanine amino transferase [ACAT], asparagine amino transferase [ASAT], and alkaline phosphatase) were performed pretreatment after 3, 6, and 12 months of treatment and about 1 month after the treatment [2] (Table 16-4).

Table 16-2. First problems mentioned in response to question "How have you been feeling since last visit?" by regimen; all segments of use; incidence per 100 woman-years during first 12 months

Problem	50-mm ring	58-mm ring	Nordette	Significance (3 regimens)
Vaginal	34.1	37.8	9.6	—[a]
Lower abdominal pain	10.5	14.6	9.6	NS
Headache	7.7	7.1	19.4	—[a]
Nervousness	2.8	3.6	5.9	NS
Depression	1.7	2.1	0.7	NS
Menstrual	34.7	22.0	21.7	—[a]
Acne or other skin problems	7.7	8.0	5.3	NS
Mastalgia	0.3	0.9	1.6	NS
Other	21.0	21.4	31.6	—[b]
All first problems	120.5	117.6	105.4	NS
Woman-years	351.8	335.8	303.5	

NS = not significant.
[a] = $p < .001$; [b] = $p < .01$.
Source: From I. Sivin et al. A multicenter study of levonorgestrel-estradiol contraceptive vaginal rings: II. Subjective and objective measures of effects. An international comparative trial. *Contraception* 24:359, 1981.

Table 16-3. Bleeding and spotting days by regimen (data from menstrual diaries)

A. *Mean number of days of bleeding and spotting per 30-day reference periods*

Days from acceptance	CVR		Nordette
	50 mm	58 mm	
1–30	5.90	5.57	6.42
31–60	4.78	4.75	4.51
61–90	4.80	4.54	4.54
91–120	4.60	4.28	4.30
121–150	4.76	4.30	4.37
151–180	4.66	4.41	4.43
N, days 1–30	500	493	422
N, days 151–180	356	335	270

B. *Percentage distribution of bleeding and spotting days experienced in days 1–168 (6 × 28 day reference period)*

No. of days	50 mm	58 mm	Nordette
< 12	4.0	3.9	0.7
13–24	39.0	41.7	43.5
25–36	35.8	42.0	42.4
37–48	14.4	7.6	11.2
49–60	5.3	3.9	1.4
>60	1.3	0.8	0.7
Mean	28.67	26.80	27.29
Standard deviation	12.01	10.12	9.05
Number of women	374	357	278

C. *Mean number of bleeding and spotting days experienced in days 169–336*

	50 mm	58 mm	Nordette
Mean	25.30	24.55	24.42
Standard deviation	12.26	10.60	6.95
N	246	220	169

Source: From I. Sivin et al. A multicenter study of levonorgestrel-estradiol contraceptive vaginal rings: III. Menstrual patterns. An international comparative trial. *Contraception* 24:377, 1981.

Both the glucose tolerance and fasting values of glucose were unaltered. The early insulin response to glucose increased by 50 percent in the CVR group after 1 year of treatment, but not in the oral contraceptive group. All other insulin values were unchanged. The effect on the peak insulin is not related to or

Table 16-4. Mean increase of peak insulin in percent of pretreatment values (calculated on paired data)

Duration of use	CR	OC
3 months	26[a]	11
6 months	32[b]	17
12 months	50[b]	5

CR = contraceptive ring; OC = oral contraceptive.
[a]$p < .05$.
[b]$p < .01$.
Source: From T. Ahren et al. Comparison of the metabolic effects of two hormonal contraceptive methods: An oral formulation and a vaginal ring. *Contraception* 24:415, 1981.

indicative of any change of peripheral insulin sensitivity but rather of the sensitivity of the pancreas to the glucose stimulus. Since there is evidence of progesterone receptors in the beta cells, at least the initial insulin response to a glucose load might be directly influenced by progestins. The unchanged fasting and 60-minute insulin levels in this study, as well as the normal glucose tolerance, indicate that levonorgestrel by itself does not cause either impairment of glucose tolerance or peripheral insulin resistance.

Nordette produced no effect on the fasting glucose concentration or on glucose tolerance. The insulin concentrations, particularly in fasting states and at 60 minutes of the IVGTT, showed a tendency to higher values. This is in accordance with earlier findings of peripheral insulin resistance when estrogens of the synthetic type are used in combination with levonorgestrel [33].

All liver function values remained within the normal range in all subjects. There was a small significant decrease in alkaline phosphatase in both groups, which is in contrast to the elevation noted with a higher dosage of combined oral contraceptives.

It is concluded that neither of these two contraceptive methods, the effects of which are predominantly progestin dominant, seems to cause impairment of glucose tolerance or hepatic function.

GLOBULINS

A study comparing the combination CVR to various combination oral contraceptives has demonstrated that the CVR produces no changes in corticosteroid binding globulin-binding capacity (CBG-BC), angiotensinogen, or antithrombin III in contrast to oral contraceptives, which produce significant increases of the first two and a significant reduction in the last [22]. These globulins respond to estrogen-dominant preparations, which suggests that the combination CVR releasing levonorgestrel and estradiol is a relative progestin-dominant preparation. Indeed, the CVR produces a significant reduction of sex hormone binding globulin-binding capacity (SHBG-BC), no change in total serum norgestrel, but significantly greater non-SHBG-bound norgestrel (both percent and mass, μg/ml) when compared to an oral contraceptive containing norgestrel 0.3 μg and ethinyl estradiol 0.03 μg. The overall effect of such a preparation is to produce no estrogen-mediated effects while producing relative progestin dominance. Three factors account for the variation in estrogenic effect produced by the CVR as compared with the oral contraceptive steroids. First, a natural estrogen, estradiol, is released from the CVR instead of the more potent synthetic estrogen, ethinyl estradiol, found in the oral tablets. Second, a smaller amount of estrogen is absorbed from the CVR, and this absorption occurs only during the first few days of each treatment cycle because of the relatively lower solubility and diffusion of estradiol in comparison to levonorgestrel in dimethylpolysiloxane. Third, the CVR route of administration initially bypasses the liver, while the steroids absorbed orally pass directly to the liver after absorption in the gut. For these reasons the CVR has less of an effect on hepatic alterations than do combination oral contraceptives.

LIPIDS AND LIPOPROTEINS

Because of the concern that progestin-dominant contraceptive steroids may adversely affect lipids and lipoproteins, several studies investigating the effect of the CVR on lipids, lipoproteins, serum lipoproteins, and apolipoproteins have been undertaken. In a recent study lipids and lipoproteins as determined by analytic ultracentrifugation were studied in five controls and 10 women using 58-mm CVRs releasing 290 μg per day of LNG and 180 μg per day of E_2 [20]. The groups were comparable for race, age, parity, obesity indexes, alcohol ingestion, smoking, diet, and exercise. Fasting blood samples were obtained twice before CVR treatment, after 2 and 7 weeks of treatment, and 1 week thereafter (Table 16-5). The women using the CVR had a significant incremental reduction of cholesterol from baseline to treatment (15%), which was distributed among all the lipoprotein classes, especially HDL-C (27%). The cholesterol/HDL-C ratio was significantly increased with treatment. All mean changes were within the reference range. The reduction in HDL (21%) and especially in the subclasses HDL 2a (48%) and HDL 2b (71%) were significant and for the subclasses HDL 2a and HDL 2b outside the reference range. The LDL/HDL ratio increased significantly (44%), while the LDL/HDL 2a + 2b ratio increased significantly outside the reference range (131%) with treatment. Of the lipid and lipoprotein measurements that changed significantly with treatment, HDL-C, HDL, HDL 2a, LDL/HDL, and LDL/HDL 2a + 2b changed significantly toward baseline in the 1 week off treatment.

In a 1-year, prospective Swedish study the effects on lipoproteins, lipids, and apolipoproteins (apo) of a combined oral contraceptive (OC) (30 μg ethinylestradiol and 150 μg levonorgestrel) and a CVR releasing estradiol (about 180 μg per day) and levonorgestrel (about 290 μg per day) were compared (Table 16-6). The two treatments induced significantly different effects. In the OC group the lipoprotein-lipid concentrations showed only minor changes, but apolipoproteins (apo) B and A-I increased by about 15 percent. In contrast, during treatment with the CVR there was a 25 percent

Table 16-5. Average values of selected lipid and lipoprotein values (μg/dl)

Test	Reference range	Pretreatment	Treatment	Δ%[a]
Cholesterol	127–218	183	155	−15[c]
HDL-C	37–63	52	38	−27[c]
Chol/HDL-C	2.5–5.0	3.5	4.0	+14[c]
HDL	224–380	318	250	−21[c]
HDL 2a	79–165	115	60	−48[c]
HDL 2b	15–139	48	14[b]	−71[c]
LDL/HDL	0.5–1.4	0.9	1.3	+44[c]
LDL/HDL 2a + 2b	0.9–2.9	1.6	3.7[b]	+131

[a]Percentage change from pretreatment.
[b]Outside the reference range.
[c]Significant changes.
Source: Adapted from S. Roy et al. The effect on lipids and lipoproteins of a contraceptive vaginal ring containing levonorgestrel and estradiol. *Contraception* 24:429, 1981.

Table 16-6. Average values of selected lipids and lipoproteins

Test	Pretreatment	12 months	Δ%[a]
HDL-C	1.43	1.06	−24[b]
LDL-C	2.81	2.69	−10
LDL-C/HDL-C	2.00	2.7	+35[b,c]
Apo B[b]	88	103	+17[b]
Apo A-I[b]	97	98	NC

[a]Percentage change from pretreatment.
[b]Significant changes.
[c]Arbitrary unit.
Source: Adapted from T. Ahren et al. Comparison of the metabolic effects of two hormonal contraceptive methods: An oral formulation and a vaginal ring: II. Serum lipoproteins and apolipoproteins. *Contraception* 24:451, 1981.

decrement of cholesterol in high-density lipoprotein (HDL) and 10 percent in low-density lipoprotein (LDL) cholesterol, with only minor effects of apo B and A-I. The ratio of LDL and HDL cholesterol increased in the CVR group but not in the OC group. The results also indicate a change in the composition of the LDL and HDL particles, with an altered lipid-protein ratio, during both contraceptive treatments. Despite the impressive relative increase in the LDL/HDL ratio in the contraceptive ring group, the average absolute value of this ratio did not reach the mean for healthy men [1].

A possible potential reduction in the incidence of myocardial infarction with the use of the CVR suggested by a reduction in total cholesterol appears to be counterbalanced by a reduction in HDL-C and increases in the cholesterol/HDL-C and LDL/HDL ratios. The potential clinical implications of these findings, if any, remain to be determined.

VAGINAL FLORA

The CVR is a foreign body, which is placed into the vaginal vault for an extended period of time. Therefore, a concern has been expressed whether any changes in the flora of the vagina occur with CVR usage. A variety of studies with different agents (MPA, CMA, dl-NG, LNG E$_2$) have shown that although vaginal secretions, which in some instances were the result of pathogenic organisms such as *Candida*, are increased with CVR usage, the resulting vaginitis could be treated while continuing use of the CVR [10, 15, 18, 28].

To study this issue more carefully, a prospective study was undertaken in which premenopausal women seeking a steroid contraceptive method were allowed to choose between a CVR containing levonorgestrel and estradiol used in a 3-week-in, 1-

Table 16-7. Bacteriologic comparison of pretreatment with 6-month vaginal cultures

	CVR (N = 20)					
	↑	↓	=	+	−	0
Aerobes	10	2	8	0	0	0
Anaerobes	8	6	6	0	0	0
Lactobacilli	3	0	3	3	2	9
Candida	0	0	0	2	1	17
N. Gonorrhoeae	0	0	0	0	0	20
G. Vaginalis	0	0	1	2	5	11
	OC (N = 10)					
	↑	↓	=	+	−	0
Aerobes	3	2	5	0	0	0
Anaerobes	3	1	6	0	0	0
Lactobacilli	1	0	2	4	0	3
Candida	0	0	0	3	0	7
N. Gonorrhoeae	0	0	0	0	0	10
G. Vaginalis	0	0	0	0	2	8

CVR = contraceptive vaginal ring; OC = oral contraceptive; ↑ = increase; ↓ = decrease; = = no change in magnitude (> or < 10') of colony count from prestudy values; + = appearance of organism at 6 months when absent at prestudy; − = absence of organism at 6 months when present at prestudy; 0 = absence of organism at prestudy and at 6 months. Source: From S. Roy, J. Wilkins, and D. R. Mishell, Jr.: The effect of a contraceptive vaginal ring and oral contraceptives on the vaginal flora. *Contraception* 24:481, 1981.

week-out regimen (n = 20) and an oral contraceptive containing levonorgestrel (150 μg) and ethinyl estradiol (30 μg) in a 28-day regimen (n = 10) (Table 16-7) [23]. Cultures from the posterior vaginal fornix were obtained before therapy in both groups and monthly for 6 months for the CVR group and after 1, 3, and 6 months for the OC group. These cultures were streaked on specific media to provide quantitative aerobic and anaerobic, *Lactobacillus*, *Candida* sp., *Gardnerella vaginalis*, and *Neisseria gonorrhoeae* counts in microorganisms per milliliter. A comparison of the number of types of organisms isolated from vaginal cultures obtained initially and at 6 months demonstrated no statistically significant differences in colony counts between CVR and OC users. The results of this study suggest that the use of the CVR is not associated with a greater growth of pathogens than is oral administration of a progestin and estrogen combination.

In summary, the shell ring with an outer diameter of 58 mm and about 9 to 9.5 mm thick, releasing LNG (280 μg/dl) and estradiol (180 μg/d), which is self-administered and used for 3 continuous weeks and then removed for 1 week, is associated with acceptable rates of BTB/BTS, almost complete inhibition of ovulation, and acceptable rates of withdrawal bleeding upon ring removal and may be reused for at least 6 months. Upon discontinuation of the method, ovulation resumed promptly in all subjects studied.

These rings are as effective as and have continuation rates at least equal to those of oral contraceptives. Additionally, since headache and nausea are less common with ring use, this method of contraception may be preferred by women who complain of these or other symptoms while taking the oral steroid.

The ring produces few, if any, of the metabolic effects associated with oral estrogen administration, such as an increase in angiotensinogen and steroid-binding globulins as well as a decrease in antithrombin III. Thus, the side effects of hypertension and thrombosis, which can occasionally occur with oral contraceptives, would most likely not occur with CVR usage. Studies from some, but not all, centers indicate that women wearing vaginal rings have a decrease in total cholesterol, LDL cholesterol, and HDL cholesterol. The changes in the commonly used risk ratios (total cholesterol/HDL or LDL/HDL) are small in most women, and the values usually do not approach those found in normal men or male or female patients with cardiovascular disease. The relevance of these observations is undetermined and is currently being investigated.

The ring has proven to be acceptable in clinical trials in the United States as well as elsewhere. It is estimated that about 10 to 15 percent of women using contraception will choose this method. This method has been popular among women who have had problems with oral contraceptives or the IUD and is an effective alternative for women who cannot or will not use the other currently available methods.

REFERENCES

1. Ahren, T., et al. Comparison of the metabolic effects of two hormonal contraceptive methods: An oral formulation and a vaginal ring. II. Serum lipoproteins and apolipoproteins. *Contraception* 24:451, 1981.
2. Ahren, T., et al. Comparison of the metabolic effects of two hormonal contraceptive methods: An oral formulation and a vaginal ring. *Contraception* 24:415, 1981.
3. Akinla, O., Lahteenmaki, P., and Jackanicz T. Intravaginal contraception with a synthetic progestin R2323. *Contraception* 14:671, 1976.
4. Brenner, P. F., et al. Serum levels of d-norgestrel luteinizing hormone, follicle-stimulating hormone, estradiol and progesterone in women during and following ingestion of combination oral contraceptives containing dl-norgestrel. *Am. J. Obstet. Gynecol.* 129:133, 1977.
5. Burton, F. G., Skiens, W. E., and Duncan, G. W. Low-level, progestogen-releasing vaginal contraceptive devices. *Contraception* 19(5):507, 1979.
6. Diczfalusy, E., and Landgren, B. M. New Delivery Systems: Vaginal Devices. In C. F. Chang, D. Griffin, and A. Wolman (eds.), *Recent Advances in Fertility Regulation: Proceedings of a Symposium Organized by the Ministry of Public Health of the People's Republic of China and the World Health Organization's Special Programme of Research, Development and Research Training in Human Reproduction.* Beijing, Sept. 2–5, 1980. Geneva: Atarf, 1981. Pp. 43–69.
7. Dzuik, P. J., and Cook, B. Passage of steroids through silicone rubber. *Endocrinology* 78:208, 1966.
8. Faundes, A., et al. Acceptability of the contraceptive vaginal ring by rural and urban population in two Latin American countries. *Contraception* 24(4):393, 1981.
9. Granger L. R., Roy, S., and Mishell, D. R., Jr. Changes in unbound sex steroids and sex hormone binding globulins-binding capacity during oral and vaginal progestogen administration. *Am. J. Obstet. Gynecol.* 144:578, 1982.
10. Henzl, M. R., et al. Basic studies for prolonged progestogen administration by vaginal devices. *Am. J. Obstet. Gynecol.* 117:101, 1973.
11. Jackanicz, T. M. Levonorgestrel and estradiol release from an improved contraceptive vaginal ring. *Contraception* 24:323, 1981.
12. Landgren, B. M., et al. Pharmacokinetic and pharmacodynamic investigations with vaginal devices releasing levonorgestrel at a constant near zero order rate. *Contraception* 26(6): 567, 1982.
13. Mishell, D. R., Jr., et al. Contraception by means of a Silastic vaginal ring impregnated with medroxyprogesterone acetate. *Am. J. Obstet. Gynecol.* 107:100, 1970.
14. Mishell, D. R., Jr., et al. Clinical performances and endocrine profiles with contraceptive vaginal rings containing d-norgestrel. *Contraception* 16:625, 1977.
15. Mishell, D. R., Jr., et al. Clinical performance and endocrine profiles with contraceptive vaginal rings containing a combination of estradiol and d-norgestrel. *Am. J. Obstet. Gynecol.* 130:55, 1978.
16. Mishell, D. R., Jr., and Lumkin, M. E. Contraceptive effect of varying dosages of progestogen in Silastic vaginal rings. *Fertil. Steril.* 21:99, 1970.
17. Mishell, D. R., Jr., Lumkin, M., and Jackanicz, T. Initial clinical studies of intravaginal rings containing norethindrone and norgestrel. *Contraception* 12:253, 1975.
18. Mishell, D. R., Jr., Lumkin, M., and Stone S. Inhibition of ovulation with cyclic use of progestogen-impregnated intravaginal devices. *Am. J. Obstet. Gynecol.* 113:927, 1972.
19. Roy, S. Personal communication, 1983.
20. Roy, S., et al. The effect of lipids and lipoproteins of a contraceptive vaginal ring containing levonorgestrel and estradiol. *Contraception* 24:429, 1981.

21. Roy, S., and Mishell, D. R., Jr. Contraceptive Vaginal Rings: Mechanisms of Action and Historical Development. In E. S. E. Havez and W. A. A. van O (eds.), *Biodegradables and Delivery Systems for Contraception*. Lancaster, Engl.: MTP, 1980. Pp. 163–174.

22. Roy, S., et al. Comparison of metabolic and clinical effects of four oral contraceptive formulations and a contraceptive vaginal ring. *Am. J. Obstet. Gynecol.* 136:920, 1980.

23. Roy, S., Wilkins, J., and Mishell, D. R., Jr. The effects of a contraceptive vaginal ring and oral contraceptives on the vaginal flora. *Contraception* 24:481, 1981.

24. Sivin, I., et al. A multicenter study of levonorgestrel-estradiol contraceptive vaginal rings. I. Use effectiveness: An international comparative trial. *Contraception* 24:341, 1981.

25. Sivin, I., et al. A multicenter study of levonorgestrel-estradiol contraceptive vaginal rings. II. Subjective and objective measures of effects: An international comparative trial. *Contraception* 24:359, 1981.

26. Sivin, I., et al. A multicenter study of levonorgestrel-estradiol contraceptive vaginal rings. III. Menstrual patterns: An international comparative trial. *Contraception* 24:377, 1981.

27. Victor, A., et al. Peripheral plasma levels of d-norgestrel in women after oral administration of d-norgestrel and when using intravaginal rings impregnated with dl-norgestrel. *Contraception* 12:261, 1975.

28. Victor, A., and Johansson, E. D. B. Plasma levels of d-norgestrel and ovarian function in women using intravaginal rings impregnated with dl-norgestrel for several cycles. *Contraception* 14:215, 1976.

29. Victor, A., and Johansson, E. D. B. Contraceptive rings: Self-administered treatment governed by bleeding. *Contraception* 16:137, 1977.

30. Victor, A., et al. Collagen bands: A new vaginal delivery system for contraceptive steroids. *Contraception* 16:125, 1977.

31. World Health Organization (WHO) Special Programme of Research, Development and Research Training in Human Reproduction. *Seventh Annual Report*. Geneva, World Health Organization, Nov. 1978. (HRP/78.3) P. 167.

32. World Health Organization (WHO) Special Programme of Research, Development and Research Training in Human Reproduction. *Tenth Annual Report*. Geneva, World Health Organization, Nov. 1981.

33. Wynn, V., et al. Comparison of effects of different combined oral contraceptive formulations on carbohydrate and lipid metabolism. *Lancet* 1:1045, 1979.

17. Gonadotropin-Releasing Hormone (GnRH) Analogues as Contraceptive Agents

Sheldon Schlaff

The dramatic discovery of luteinizing hormone-releasing factor (LH-RH) structure in 1971 [20] after laborious purification of hypothalamic extracts was quickly followed by chemical synthesis [21]. The decapeptide (Fig. 17-1) was quickly shown to have intrinsic follicle-stimulating hormone (FSH) as well as luteinizing hormone (LH)-stimulating ability [4, 13], and in view of its dual function it was renamed *gonadotropin-releasing hormone* (GnRH). In the past few years many hundreds of analogues have been synthesized, with agonists up to 1,000-fold more potent than endogenous GnRH and antagonists 100- to 200-fold more active than the native compound [28]. As a result of new information in man and lower animals on the pulsatile nature of GnRH secretion [15], the control of pituitary GnRH receptors, and the direct involvement of GnRH in end-organ ovarian and testicular function [6], the agonist and antagonist derivatives are now being used in human studies in a wide variety of clinical states and disorders. These include ovulation induction, interruption and definitive treatment of precocious puberty, treatment of hormone-dependent cancers (breast and prostate), and of course evaluation as a contraceptive, luteolytic agent, and abortifacient. We shall discuss the physiology, pharmacology, and some clinical studies of GnRH and its derivatives predominantly as contraceptive agents.

GnRH PHYSIOLOGY

Gonadotropins (LH and FSH) in the adult are secreted by the pituitary in a periodic fashion, with peaks each 1.5 to 2 hours [36] presumably in response to periodic bursts of GnRH. The peak and nadir values generally are within 30 percent or so of the mean. The potentiation of the pituitary secretion of LH and to some extent FSH to exogenous bolus intravenous GnRH is greatest in normal females during the early luteal phase and can be reproduced with exogenous estrogen therapy. Progesterone can enhance the response even further during the luteal phase as well. Therefore, gonadal steroid secretion mediates the pituitary response to GnRH.

Why, however, is pulsatile secretion important or even necessary? The elegant primate experiments of Knobil [15] offer some explanation. Monkeys whose hypothalamus has been effectively disconnected from the pituitary by Halaz lesion experiments are hypogonadotropic, since GnRH activity is anatomically interrupted. When exogenous GnRH was pulsed intravenously every 1.5 hours for 28 days or more, a complete menstrual cycle was reproduced, including follicular development, steroid secretion, gonadotropin surges, and ovulation. When the pulsing was advanced to 60 minutes or 30 minutes, gonadotropin and steroid

Position Number	1		2	3	4	5	6	7	8	9	10
GnRH	(Pyro-Glu)	-	His	- Tryp -	Ser	- Tyr -	Gly -	Leu -	Arg -	Pro	- Gly - NH_2
Agonist (Buserilin)	(Pyro-Glu)	-	His	- Tryp -	Ser	- Tyr	-D-*Tryp*-	Leu -	Arg -	Pro	- NH
											C_2H_5

Substitution at position 6, deletion of residue 10, ethylamide terminus (Fujino modification)

Antagonist (Acetyl-Ala)			- D-CIF	-D-Tryp-	Ser	- Tyr	-D-Tryp-	Leu -	Arg -	Pro	- Gly - NH_2

Substitution at position 6 with major modifications at positions 1, 2, and 3

Fig. 17-1. Gonadotropin-releasing hormone (GnRH) and analogues.

secretion were blunted to increasing degrees. Therefore, a fixed rate of pulsatile GnRH secretion at a fixed dose with an intact pituitary and gonads can reproduce a completely normal menstrual cycle. Either a constant GnRH infusion or an increase in the frequency of GnRH pulses will significantly blunt or obliterate the normal cycle. This effect is caused by down-regulation of pituitary and gonadal receptors for GnRH [6], much as elevated insulin and growth hormone concentrations decrease their respective receptor concentrations. In addition, GnRH receptors at the level of the gonad are also uncoupled from the adenylate cyclase system [12], impugning still another means of physiologic down-regulation. These mechanisms provide levels of physiologic control to responses to peptide hormones. Thus, natural pulsatile GnRH secretion is a physiologic necessity.

GnRH is rapidly metabolized by hypothalamic peptidases with cleavage initially at the peptide bond between positions 6 and 7 [16, 19] (Fig. 17-1). Another subsidiary site of inactivation is the peptide bond between positions 9 and 10 by still another peptidase. The latter enzyme can also inactivate oxytocin and vasopressin. Synthesis of GnRH analogues is to a great degree based on this information. For example, insertion of d-amino acids at position 6 markedly decreases enzymatic degradation presumably by preventing peptidase cleavage. Glycine, the simplest amino acid, present in native GnRH at position 6, has no optical activity (d or l forms), inhibits the formation of peptide structural elements such as helixes and sheet forms, and is critically located at the center of the molecule. It is presumed to be a bridge holding the two pentapeptide ends in appropriate configuration for receptor binding. This native orientation is most likely preserved by a d-amino acid insertion. Insertion of a chemical "spacer" preventing metabolic degradation at position 6 is necessary for both agonist and antagonist activity.

Removal of the C-terminal glycine amide (position

10) and protection from proteolysis by a new amide bond attached to position 9 (Fujino modification) [10] markedly enhance GnRH potency. The combination of a d-amino acid insertion at position 6 and a Fujino modification which yields agonists 100 or more times as potent as the native compounds has been used in many of the clinical studies discussed below.

Antagonists are generally constructed by the substitution of d-amino acids and the N-terminal portion of the molecule, particularly the histidine in position 2. Newer derivatives modified at positions 1, 2, and 3 [27, 34] with d-amino acid substitution at position 6 to prevent enzymatic degradation have yielded inhibitors up to 1,000-fold more potent than native GnRH. One basic problem common to these derivatives is their route of administration. Some are so water insoluble that they can be administered only in oil bases by injection. Others are water soluble but must be taken intranasally, since rapid peptide cleavage occurs through the oral route.

The clinical rationale for the use of agonist and antagonist GnRH cogeners was initially straightforward: Antagonists could be used as reversible, safe, and effective contraceptive agents, while agonists would be suitable for treatment of hypothalamic hypogonadism. This rationale has been abandoned or significantly modified, since all agonists tested exhibit a paradoxical antagonist effect evident both in vivo and in vitro at the pituitary and gonadal level. The pituitary, testes, and ovary contain receptors for GnRH [6]. Not only does LH and FSH stimulation result from pituitary stimulation, but Leydig cells in the testes are stimulated to produce testosterone, and luteal cells in the ovary are induced to produce progesterone by GnRH. Both agonists and antagonists bind to these nonpituitary receptors in a manner proportional to their agonist or antagonist potency in stimulation or prevention of LH stimulation. Both classes of derivatives then cause significant down-regulation of GnRH receptors in all these structures. The loss of ovarian GnRH receptors is a direct gonadal effect not necessarily mediated through increased LH levels, since hypophysectomized animals also have blunted luteal cell stimulation of progesterone under these conditions. In addition, luteal cells in tissue culture show a marked decrease in progesterone stimulation. Since dibutyl cyclic AMP (an adenylcyclase analogue) can stimulate progesterone production directly from luteal cells [12] and is unaffected by GnRH analogue, it is felt that the decapeptide may interfere with the mechanism of hormonal stimulation of cyclic AMP in addition to receptor down-regulation.

These observations have led to clinical studies testing both agonist and antagonist derivatives to GnRH as contraceptive agents. None of these agents, however, is available as an oral preparation.

CLINICAL STUDIES

Theoretically, if an agonist and an antagonist exert comparable biologic effects, it should make little difference pharmacologically which is used. In practice, however, the much greater availability and the water solubility of GnRH agonists have led to intranasal administration. The bulk of clinical information has been obtained with these agents.

GnRH agonists in rodent and in man inhibit ovulation and cause luteolysis [8] and in rodents may interrupt pregnancy. Thus, they seem to be active at many different points in the reproductive cycle and have pharmacologic characteristics of a potent contraceptive. The major agonist compound used in clinical studies is Buserilin (shown in Fig. 17-1). This compound has 140-fold potency relative to native GnRH.

Initial reports [2, 23] demonstrate that either the subcutaneous or intranasal administration of Buserilin for 1 month in 39 normally menstruating women inhibited ovulation and menses. The same group expanded their study to include 27 normally menstruating women for 89 cycles of 3 to 6 months of administration of 400 to 600 micrograms of intranasal Buserilin [1]. Eighty-seven of the 89 cycles were anovulatory, and the two failure cases were seemingly related to a technical problem with the nasal spray, since subsequent cycles in the latter two patients were anovulatory. While 21 women experienced one or more small bleeds resembling menstruation, no dysfunctional uterine bleeding occurred. Biopsy specimens from three of these women showed weak proliferative endometrial activity. The six amenorrheic women had significantly lower serum estradiols than those 21 patients with some evidence of

bleeding. Menses resumed within 34 days after drug discontinuation. Other than bleeding, no major side effects occurred.

Other reports, however, are not as glowing. With the same continuous regimen (400 μg/day nasal spray of Buserilin) morphologic alterations of the endometrium indicated that unopposed estrogen effect in 156 treatment-months was much more extensive [29]. This study was expanded, covering 411 treatment-months in 70 women with three different dosage levels of GnRH agonist [31] (Buserilin) consisting of 400 μg, 200 μg, and 100 μg per day; endometrial biopsy showed significant endometrial stimulation in 77 percent of the group, with no great differences noted between endometrial stimulation at the various dosage levels. This degree of presumptive unopposed estrogen effect (i.e., endometrial hyperplasia) is extremely disturbing. Clearly, the contraceptive effects at 400 and 200 μg per day were excellent. The dosage level of 100 μg was not sufficient in many cases to inhibit normal corpus luteum function, however.

Thus, at the dosage level used with daily intranasal spray evidence of unopposed estrogen effect was evident in the majority of cases that were carefully studied, although the contraceptive effect was clearly maintained. The drug seemed to be efficacious, but its safety is in question with this regimen.

Other studies in primate and man have examined [17, 18, 26, 32] the use of intermittent doses on specific cycle days to cause luteolysis. The mechanism of action consisted of GnRH receptor down-regulation as well as uncoupling those receptors from the cyclase leading to decreased progesterone secretion. The action is distinct and separate from $PGF_{2\alpha}$-induced luteolysis. Thus, intermittent postovulatory therapy should be able to induce a marked drop in progesterone production. However, vulnerability in man is limited to 5 to 10 days after the LH peak with the early corpus luteum (1–4 days) refractory to GnRH [17, 18, 32]. All these studies used 50 to 250 μg subcutaneous Buserilin injections one or more times per day. These studies were small, with approximately 15 subjects or less. The failure of luteolysis before day 5 was more than 75 percent compared with less than 5 percent if the lowest dose (50 μg/day) was given on days 5 to 8. The end point consisted of menses and decreased progesterone level. Luteolysis has also been reproduced in primates using intramuscular injections [26].

Thus, if drug use for luteolysis is dependent on basal body temperature chart timing, a cumbersome and possibly inaccurate method for the general population, problems of drug efficacy would be legion. The explanation for the corpus luteum refractory period is unclear. Rodent luteal cells respond in tissue culture to GnRH agonists within hours [12] with significant drops in progesterone secretion. There may be, however, a species difference. Yen [36] suggests that the delivery of GnRH agonist to its appropriate receptor site may play a role in luteolysis. The human corpus luteum apparently has a significant increase in blood supply 5 to 8 days after ovulation [24], coinciding with the drug sensitivity at that time. It may also relate to the level of GnRH receptors at various cycle times.

These studies suggest that GnRH agonists may be used as postcoital contraceptives. However, since hCG (endogenous or exogenous) in humans can overcome the luteolytic effect of GnRH agonists [3], the rationale is tenuous at best. The major objection to these hCG injection studies is the large daily dose (1,500 and 5,000 IU/day) administered to several patients for 7 to 10 days, which is certainly unphysiologic for early pregnancy. Subcutaneous administration of GnRH agonist for 2 days, however, was not effective as an abortifacient on menstrual days 37 to 54 in pregnant women with serum levels of hCG of 2,000 to 5,000 mIU per milliliter [5]. Since hCG is secreted early after implantation with a logarithmic increase in serum levels, GnRH agonists may thus exhibit a significant failure of luteolysis if pregnancy ensues. Certainly, use as an early abortifacient, at least in the dosages studied, was a failure.

These studies utilized a simple GnRH agonist of high potency. Do antagonists offer a more appropriate choice? To date, no major clinical studies are available in humans with antagonists because of their relatively low solubility and limited availability. Studies carried out in rodents and primates indicate quantitative differences in the suppression of gonadotropins, with primates requiring larger doses, further confusing the situation [35].

What began as high hopes regarding the unlimited promise of the contraceptive effect of GnRH analogues has yielded to a cautious optimism at best. Intranasal doses of agonist derivatives either yield good contraception with a chemical castration or a high incidence of unopposed estrogen effect. Although luteolysis is achieved, it is only in the midluteal phase, and it is unclear whether early pregnancy would obliterate this response. Its use as an abortifacient is improbable. Unless more potent analogues that can be easily administered become available and until the physiology of luteolysis and its relation to early pregnancy is understood, the future for GnRH analogues as female contraceptives is clouded.

The use of GnRH analogues seems to be uncertain in the area of male contraception as well. Normal males receiving agonist (Buserilin) in subcutaneous doses of 50 μg daily [25] showed a significant decrease in sperm count and testosterone over a 10-week period with, however, an associated decline in libido and potency and, surprisingly, occasional hot flashes. These effects were all reversible over a 10- to 14-week period, with testosterone and gonadotropin returning to normal in several weeks, even at the highest dosage used. Little effect on these parameters was seen with 50 μg every 4 days [25]. Therefore, at present, daily injections and use of testosterone as an adjunctive agent are necessary to achieve contraception without unwanted clinical effects. Intranasal Buserilin at doses of 200 μg daily also can almost completely inhibit testosterone production in normal males in 7 to 10 days [9].

There are areas, however, where the use of GnRH analogues has been strikingly effective: It is now the treatment of choice in precocious puberty [7], it is being used experimentally as a treatment for hormonally responsive cancers (prostate [33] and breast [14]), and in significant dosages it achieves a chemical castration with decreased gonadotropins and sterility. It also holds some theoretical possibilities for the treatment of endometriosis [22]. Its role as a contraceptive agent, however, must await further studies.

REFERENCES

1. Bergquist, C., Nillius, S. J., and Wide, L. Intranasal GnRH agonist as a contraceptive agent. *Lancet* 2:215, 1979.
2. Bergquist, C., Nillius, S. J., and Wide, L. Inhibition of ovulation in women by intranasal treatment with an LH-RH agonist. *Contraception* 19:497, 1979.
3. Bergquist, C., Nillius, S. J., and Wide, L. Luteolysis induced by an LH-RH agonist is prevented by hCG. *Contraception* 22:341, 1980.
4. Besser, G. M. Hormonal responses to synthetic LH-RH and FSH-RH in man. *Br. Med. J.* 3:267, 1972.
5. Casper, R. F., Sheehan, K., and Erickson, G. Neuropeptides and Fertility Control in the Female. In G. I. Zatuchni, M. H. Labbock, and J. J. Sciarra (eds.), *Research Frontiers in Fertility Regulation.* New York: Harper & Row, 1980. P. 409.
6. Clayton, R. N., and Catt, K. J. GnRH receptors: Characterization, physiological regulation and relationship to reproductive function. *Endocr. Rev.* 2:186, 1981.
7. Comite, F., et al. Short-term treatment of idiopathic precocious puberty with a long acting analogue of LH-RH. *N. Engl. J. Med.* 305:1546, 1981.
8. Corbin, A., et al. The anti-reproductive pharmacology of LH-RH and its agonist analysis. *Int. J. Fertil.* 23:81, 1978.
9. Faure, N., et al. Inhibition of Androgen Biosynthesis in the Human Male by Chronic Administration of Buserilin. In G. I. Zatuchni, J. D. Shelton, and J. J. Sciarra (eds.), *LH-RH Peptides as Female and Male Contraceptives.* Hagerstown, Md.: Harper & Row, 1983. P. 307.
10. Fujino, M., Kobayashi, S., and Obayashi, M. Structure activity relationships in the C-terminal part of LH-RH. *Biochem. Biophys. Res. Commun.,* 49:863, 1973.

11. Harwood, J. P., et al. Ovarian GnRH receptors. II. Regulation and effects on ovarian development. *Endocrinology* 107:414, 1980.

12. Harwood, J. P., Clayton, R. N., and Catt, K. J. Ovarian GnRH receptors. I. Properties and inhibition of luteal cell function. *Endocrinology,* 107:407, 1980.

13. Kastin, A. J., Gual, C., and Schally, A. V. Clinical experience with hypothalamic releasing hormones. Part A. LH-RH and other hypophysiotropic releasing hormones. *Recent Prog. Horm. Res.* 28:201, 1972.

14. Klijn, J. G. M., and DeJung, F. H. Treatment with an LH-RH analogue (Buserilin) in premenopausal patients with metastatic breast cancer. *Lancet* 1:1213, 1982.

15. Knobil, E. The neuroendocrine control of the menstrual cycle. *Recent Prog. Horm. Res.* 36:53, 1980.

16. Koch, Y., Baram, T., and Chobsieng, P. Enzymatic degradation of LH-RH by hypothalamic tissue. *Biochem. Biophys. Res. Commun.* 61:95, 1974.

17. Koyama, T., Ohkura, T., and Kumasaka, T. Effect of postovulatory treatment with LH-RH on the level of plasma progesterone in women. *Fertil. Steril.* 10:549, 1978.

18. LeMay, A., Labrie, F., and Farland, L. Possible luteolytic effects of LH-RH in normal women. *Fertil. Steril.* 31:29, 1979.

19. Marles, N., and Stern, F. Enzymatic mechanisms of inactivation of LH-RH. *Biochem. Biophys. Res. Commun.* 61:1458, 1974.

20. Matsuo, H., et al. Structure of the porcine LH and FSH releasing hormone: The proposed amino acid sequence. *Biochem. Biophys. Res. Commun.* 43:1334, 1971.

21. Matsuo, H., et al. Synthesis of porcine LH and FSH releasing hormone by the solid phase method. *Biochem. Biophys. Res. Commun.* 45:822, 1971.

22. Meldrum, D. R., et al. "Medical oophorectomy" using a long acting GnRH agonist: A possible new approach to the treatment of endometriosis. *J. Clin. Endocrinol. Metabol.* 54:1081, 1982.

23. Nillius, S. S., Bergquist, C., and Wide, L. Inhibition of ovulation in women by chronic treatment with a stimulatory LH-RH analogue, a new approach to birth control. *Contraception* 17:537, 1978.

24. Novak, E. R., and Woodruff, J. D. *Gynecologic and Obstetric Pathology.* Philadelphia: Saunders, 1974. Pp. 335–337.

25. Rabin, D., et al. Experience with a Potent GnRH Agonist in Normal Men: An Approach to the Development of a Male Contraceptive. In G. I. Zatuchni, J. D. Shelton, and J. J. Sciarra (eds.), *LH-RH Peptides as Female and Male Contraceptives.* Hagerstown, Md.: Harper & Row, 1983. P. 296.

26. Raymond, J. P., and Moguilensky, M. I. Inhibition of progesterone secretion during the luteal phase by two LH-RH segments in Macca Fasicullaris. *Fertil. Steril.* 34:593, 1980.

27. Rees, R. W., Foell, T. J., and Chai, S. Y. Synthesis and biological activities of analogues of LH-RH modified in position 2. *J. Med. Chem.* 17:1016, 1974.

28. Rivier, C., Rivier, J., and Vale, W. Chronic effects of (D-tryp^6-Pro^9-Ne) LH-RH on reproductive processes in the female rat. *Endocrinology* 103:2299, 1978.

29. Schally, A. W., Arimura, A., and Coy, D. H. Recent approaches to fertility control based on derivatives of LH-RH. *Vitam. Horm.* 38:257, 1981.

30. Schmidt-Gollwitzer, M., Hardt, W., and Schmidt-Gollwitzer, K. Influence of the LH-RH analogue Buserilin on cyclic ovarian function and on endometrium; A new approach to fertility control? *Contraception* 23:187, 1981.

31. Schmidt-Gollwitzer, M., et al. In G. T. Zatuchni, J. D. Shelton, and J. J. Sciarra (eds.), *LH-RH Peptides as Female and Male Contraceptives.* Hagerstown, Md.: Harper & Row, 1983.

32. Sheehan, K. L., and Yen, S. S. C. Clinical Studies with LH-RH Agonists. In G. T. Zatuchni, J. D. Shelton, and J. J. Sciarra (eds.), *LH-RH Peptides as Female and Male Contraceptives.* Hagerstown, Md.: Harper & Row, 1983.

33. Tolis, G., et al. Tumor growth inhibition in patients with prostate cancer treated with LH-RH agonists. *Proc. Natl. Acad. Sci. U.S.A.* 79:1658, 1982.

34. Vale, W., Grant, G., and Rivier, J. Synthesis of polypeptide antagonists of the hypothalamus LH-RH. *Science* 176:933, 1972.

35. Wilks, J. W., Folkers, K., and Bowers, C. Y. Inhibition of preovulatory secretion in the Rhesus monkey by ((Glu-Pro)^{1}D-Phe^2,D-tryp^{3,6}) LH-RH. *Contraception* 22:313, 1980.

36. Yen, S. S. C., et al. The operating characteristics of the hypothalamic pituitary system during the menstrual cycle and observation of the biological action of somatostatin. *Recent Prog. Horm. Res.,* 31:321, 1975.

IV. Barriers and Vaginal Chemical Agents

18. The Diaphragm

Andrew T. Wiley

HISTORY

Although use of mechanical barriers for contraceptive purposes dates back to antiquity, it was not until the development of vulcanization of rubber in the 1840s that commercial manufacture of such devices became feasible. The contraceptive industry began with the manufacture of condoms and a prototype of the cervical cap in the 1850s and 1860s.

The diaphragm came somewhat later: In 1882 Dr. C. Hasse, professor of anatomy at Breslau, Germany, writing under the pseudonym of Wilhelm Mensinga to protect his reputation, described a rubber vaginal contraceptive diaphragm, which became known as the Mensinga diaphragm. Later during that same decade articles describing this device appeared in Holland and England, explaining its use and referring to it as the Dutch cap or the Mensinga pessary. By the end of the nineteenth century diaphragms in several sizes could be obtained in both Holland and England.

Margaret Sanger, the American birth control pioneer, became acquainted with the devices while in Holland and England during the early part of the twentieth century, but her importation of them into the United States was blocked by the Comstock laws. Undaunted, she managed to smuggle enough of them to open a clinic in New York City in 1923.

In 1924 Dr. W. A. Püsey, President of the American Medical Association, wrote an editorial [24] endorsing contraception as an effective health measure, thus helping to establish its credibility. By the mid-1920s the Holland-Rantos Company had been formed for U.S. manufacture of diaphragms. In 1929 Dr. James Cooper published an extensive report on contraception [3], which fully described the diaphragm and promoted its use in the United States. The development and improvement of clinical spermicides during the 1920s and 1930s [13] by the pharmaceutical industry completed the cycle, and the U.S. contraceptive revolution was under way.

The 30 years between 1930 and 1960 witnessed increasing acceptance and use of the diaphragm, but the advent of the pill and the intrauterine device (IUD) in the early 1960s caused use of the diaphragm to decrease markedly. With the realization during the early 1970s that modern contraceptive methods could be associated with health problems, a steady revival of interest in and use of the diaphragm began in the United States and in several other developed countries.

MECHANISM OF ACTION

The diaphragm acts as a barrier to cervical entry by spermatazoa. This occurs because the diaphragm fits snugly between the inferior rim of the symphysis pubis

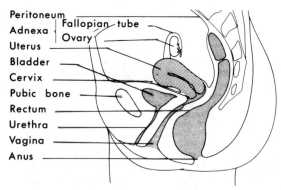

Fig. 18-1. Section of female pelvis. (From R. H. Gray. *Manual for the Provision of Intrauterine Devices [IUDs].* Geneva: World Health Organization, 1980.)

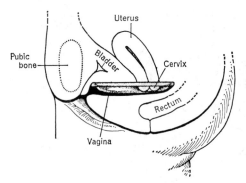

Fig. 18-2. A properly fitted diaphragm. (From *Population Reports*, Population Information Program, Series H, No. 4, The Johns Hopkins University, January 1976.)

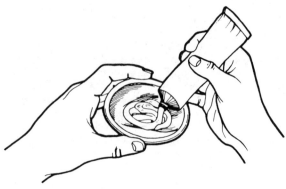

Fig. 18-3. Applying spermicide to the diaphragm. (Reprinted with permission from R. A. Hatcher et al. *Contraceptive Technology: 1982–1983* [11th rev. ed.]. New York: Irvington Publishers, 1982.)

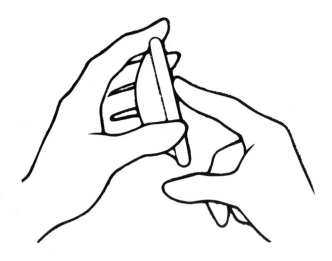

Fig. 18-4. Applying jelly to diaphragm rim. (From *Ortho Diaphragms.* Raritan, N.J.: Ortho Pharmaceutical Corp., 1981.)

proximally and the posterior vaginal fornix distally and because it is in firm contact with both lateral and vaginal walls, thus completely separating the cervix from the vaginal space (Figs. 18-1, 18-2). A well-fitted diaphragm tends to remain firmly in place and usually can be dislodged only by the woman or her partner using the fingertips.

Application of a cream or jelly to the side of the diaphragm that will contact the cervix before insertion is the recommended method of diaphragm use in this country. The composition of these creams and jellies has been greatly modified over the years, but many people believe that the viscosity of the jelly or cream is as important to its contraceptive effectiveness as its spermicidal qualities. The original creams and jellies were composed of ingredients such as glycerin, starch, boric acid, and acetic acid; later, mercurials were used for their more specific spermicidal action. In recent years the principal active ingredient has been nonoxynol-9, a potent spermicide.

Most health care providers recommend that, in addition to cream or jelly applied to the concave surface of the diaphragm, a thin layer should also be applied to the rim of the diaphragm so that, after placement, the uterus is sealed off chemically as well as mechanically (Figs. 18-3, 18-4).

Craig and Hepburn [5] recently challenged the need for a spermicide with diaphragm use. They cite the inconvenience involved and point out that Johnson et al. [15] demonstrated that spermicide around the rim of the diaphragm can contribute to excessive lubrication causing diaphragm displacement during coitus.

Routine use of spermicide with the diaphragm, however, dates back to the 1920s when Boucher [2] reported a lower failure rate with diaphragm plus spermicide than with diaphragm alone.

CONTRACEPTIVE EFFECTIVENESS

A variety of studies in the United States and Great Britain [4, 11, 13, 16, 20, 25–28, 32] have shown diaphragm failure rates ranging from a low of 2 to a high of 23 pregnancies per 100 women per year. The fact that a large study [28] involving more than 70,000 months of diaphragm use reported a pregnancy rate of 2 per 100 women per year illustrates the high theoretical effectiveness of a properly fitted diaphragm when used regularly with a spermicide by a conscientious woman. On the other hand, a pregnancy rate of 12 to 19 per 100 women per year [11, 25] illustrates the wide discrepancy possible between theoretic- and use-effectiveness of the diaphragm. Some [13, 32] feel that a failure rate of 2 or 3 per 100 women per year is a sound reflection of the overall effectiveness for married women who are long-term users of a properly used diaphragm. Tietze calculates 10 percent among married women.

Several factors have been shown to affect diaphragm effectiveness: Failure rates are higher for new users than for women who have used the diaphragm for some time; failure rates are higher for younger women than for older women; and failure rates are higher for women seeking to delay pregnancy than they are for women seeking to prevent pregnancy [20, 22, 27].

Although motivation is a critical factor, in addition to patient carelessness, diaphragm failure can result because the patient (1) was inadequately trained in its use, (2) was incompletely instructed in insertion technique, (3) was improperly fitted, (4) used a device that was defective, or (5) had the device displaced during coitus. That such diaphragm displacement can occur in certain coital positions (e.g., female superior) has been shown by Johnson, Masters, and Lewis [15].

PREVALENCE OF USE

Diaphragm use slowly but steadily increased during the 40 years between its introduction in the United States and the advent of the pill and the IUD in the early 1960s. In 1934 Kopp [17] and Pearl [22] found that the diaphragm was used by only 3 to 4 percent of the contracepting couples they questioned. A 1955 U.S. National Fertility Survey, reported by Westoff and Ryder [29], found that 25 percent of 1,900 white married

women of reproductive age questioned were using the diaphragm. The only method reported more widely used in this survey was the condom, which was reported used by 27 percent of the couples. The 1960 survey showed no substantial changes, but by the time of the 1965 survey only 10 percent of the 2,500 women questioned reported using the diaphragm. U.S. service statistics on contraceptive acceptance in a large number of clinics between 1972 and 1974 revealed that only 2.7 percent of patients chose the diaphragm.

More recently, however, diaphragm use in the United States began to increase. For example, the California State Health Department reported that diaphragm use among its clientele had increased from 7 percent in 1976 to 13 percent in 1979 [1]. Similarly, a report from Albany, New York, indicated that the 13 percent of student contraceptors choosing the diaphragm in 1973 had increased to 49 percent in 1976 [8]. By 1977 approximately 12 percent of Planned Parenthood's clients across the country were choosing the diaphragm. According to a 1979 report from the University of Oregon, 41 percent of contracepting medical and nursing students at that institution were using diaphragms [16].

Just how far this trend will go or whether it has already peaked is not clear, but it is now evident that the diaphragm, after 10 years of relative unpopularity, is once again considered an acceptable and important contraceptive method.

TYPES OF DIAPHRAGMS

The three basic types of diaphragms in general use are the arcing spring, the coil spring, and the flat spring.

The arcing spring diaphragm has two types of springs in the rim. These springs are designed in such a way that when the rim is compressed, the diaphragm assumes the shape of an arc (Fig. 18-5).

The coil spring diaphragm, which folds in one plane, has a round spiral coiled in the rim, which is encircled with rubber (Fig. 18-6).

The flat spring or Mensinga diaphragm has not changed much over the years. It has a flat metal band or spring embedded in the rubber rim, which makes it quite firm (Fig. 18-7).

All these three types of diaphragms come in a wide range of sizes between 50 and 105 mm in diameter, the sizes varying by 5 mm. The sizes in most frequent use are 70 mm, 75 mm, and 80 mm.

The flat spring diaphragm has a thin rim and, therefore, is often well suited for use by the woman who has a shallow arch behind the symphysis pubis. This diaphragm can generally be easily worn by women who have not yet had children.

The coil spring diaphragm is generally very satisfac-

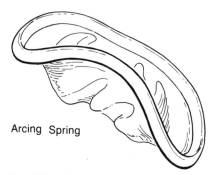

Fig. 18-5. Arcing spring diaphragm. (Reprinted with permission from R. A. Hatcher et al. *Contraceptive Technology: 1980–1981* [10th rev. ed.]. New York: Irvington Publishers, 1980.)

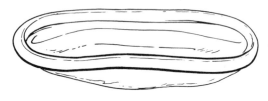

Fig. 18-6. Coil spring diaphragm. (Reprinted with permission from R. A. Hatcher et al. *Contraceptive Technology: 1980–1981* [10th rev. ed.]. New York: Irvington Publishers, 1980.)

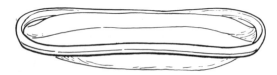

Fig. 18-7. Flat spring diaphragm. (Reprinted with permission from R. A. Hatcher et al. *Contraceptive Technology: 1980–1981* [10th rev. ed.]. New York: Irvington Publishers, 1980.)

tory for a parous woman whose vaginal muscle tone is good, whose pubic arch is reasonably deep, and whose uterus is neither markedly anteflexed nor retroverted.

The arcing spring diaphragm, because of its double spring component, tends to provide firm pressure on the lateral vaginal walls and is often quite effective in women whose vaginal muscle tone is poor. The arcing form it takes when compressed makes it relatively simple to insert. The arcing shape it assumes also makes it useful for women with a mild uterine prolapse as well as for women with marked uterine anteflexion or retroversion. The arcing spring diaphragm in proper

size can be satisfactorily worn by most women and therefore is increasingly popular with patients and providers.

SOURCES AND COMPOSITION

Diaphragms are marketed in the United States by Ortho Pharmaceutical Company, Holland-Rantos, Schmid Laboratories, and Milex Products and in England by London Rubber. The brand names of the various types are listed by manufacturer in Table 18-1. All are made of vulcanized rubber with steel springs, but the coil spring is cadmium plated to prevent erosion. Diaphragms made of synthetic plastic instead of rubber are also available for the occasional woman found to be allergic to rubber. The prices of diaphragms vary, but in general each one costs between $10 and $15 (U.S.) when purchased at a pharmacy.

FITTING OF THE DIAPHRAGM

In addition to strong and sustained patient motivation, proper fitting of the diaphragm by a clinician is essential to its effective use. For that reason, adequate time must be allowed for the fitting. Because paramedicals often have more time to spend with their patients than do some physicians, there is a growing tendency for paramedicals to do the fitting and provide the detailed instruction, an important aspect of effective use.

A pelvic examination is necessary to rule out obvious gynecologic abnormalities, to estimate the size and position of the uterus, and to allow the examiner to determine what size diaphragm is needed. This determination is made by inserting the index and middle finger until the middle finger reaches the end of the vaginal canal behind the cervix. With the middle finger in this

Table 18-1. Various types of diaphragms

Brand name	Type	Manufacturer
Koromex	Coil spring	Holland-Rantos
Koroflex	Arcing spring	Holland-Rantos
Durex	Flat spring	London Rubber
Ortho White	Flat spring	Ortho Pharmaceutical
Ortho	Coil spring	Ortho Pharmaceutical
All-Flex	Arcing spring	Ortho Pharmaceutical
Ramses	Coil spring	Schmid Laboratories
Ramses Bendex	Arcing spring	Schmid Laboratories
Omni-Flex	Coil spring	Milex Products
Wide Seal	Arcing spring	Milex Products

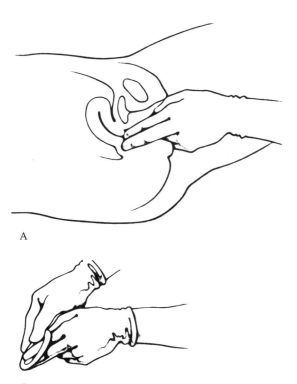

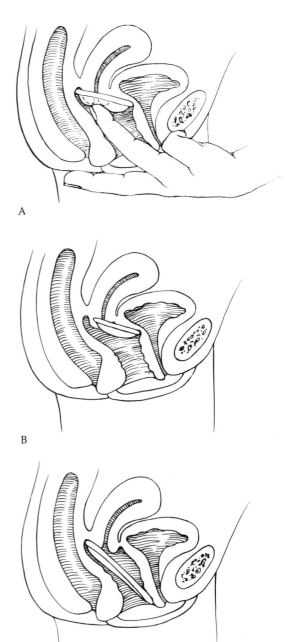

Fig. 18-8. (A and B) Determining diaphragm size. (From *Ortho Diaphragms.* Raritan, N.J.: Ortho Pharmaceutical Corp., 1981.)

position, the examiner then notes where the index finger comes in contact with the symphysis pubis and marks this point with the thumb of the same hand before withdrawing the fingers. A diaphragm is then selected by placing the tip of the middle finger against the rim and choosing that diaphragm whose opposite rim is exactly at the spot on the index finger previously marked by the thumb (Fig. 18-8).

As noted, diaphragms are graded by diameter in millimeters and range between 50 and 105 mm, with most patients needing diaphragms measuring between 65 and 85 mm.

The diaphragm chosen should touch the lateral vaginal walls and should fit snugly but comfortably between the posterior vaginal fornix and the symphysis pubis. The cervix, of course, should be completely covered. With too loose a fit the diaphragm will not stay in place with coital activity. Too tight a fit is uncomfortable and might unduly compress the urethra and result in difficulty in voiding. The three sagittal drawings in Figure 18-9 illustrate a proper diaphragm fit (A), too small a fit (B), and too large a fit (C).

Fig. 18-9. (A) To check proper placement, the cervix is felt through the dome of the diaphragm by the index finger. (B) A diaphragm that is too small. (C) A diaphragm that is too large. (From *Population Reports,* Population Information Program, Series H, No. 4, The Johns Hopkins University, January 1976.)

Teaching the patient to properly place and remove the diaphragm requires time. The patient is generally advised to stand with one foot propped up on the toilet seat or on a chair. However, she can also be advised to insert it while lying on her back with her knees propped up or while squatting. After placing the spermicide on the side of the diaphragm to be placed against the cervix, she is advised to use one hand to separate the labia and the other to squeeze the two sides of the diaphragm together and insert it along the posterior wall of the vagina until the posterior rim of the diaphragm is far enough into the vagina that she is able to press the anterior rim up behind the symphysis and have it comfortably remain there. She is taught to remove the diaphragm by using the index finger to pull down on the anterior rim and dislodge it. In this maneuver, it should be pointed out to the patient that care should be taken that a fingernail does not perforate the diaphragm surface. Patient insertion technique is shown in Figure 18-10.

INSTRUCTIONS FOR USE

The patient is advised always to use the diaphragm with contraceptive cream or jelly; approximately one teaspoonful is placed on the cervical side of the diaphragm where it will come into direct contact with the cervix.* Most clinicians also advise the patient to smear a thin film of the contraceptive cream or jelly around the rim of the diaphragm before insertion to ensure immobilization of any spermatozoa able to penetrate between the diaphragm rim and the vaginal walls. Whether or not this is essential is unknown, but it seems a reasonable precaution.

The diaphragm with contraceptive cream or jelly applied to it can be inserted any time before intercourse, but if more than 6 hours have elapsed between insertion and first intercourse, the patient should remove the diaphragm and reapply the contraceptive cream or jelly or insert an extra applicator full in the vagina.

After the initial exposure, if one or more subsequent acts occur with the diaphragm in place, it is advisable for the patient to insert additional spermicide into the vaginal canal before each subsequent coital act. The diaphragm should remain in place at least 6 hours after the last act of intercourse, but care should be exercised to ensure that the diaphragm does not remain in place beyond 24 hours.

It is quite feasible for the patient to utilize the diaphragm during menstruation, but it should be used

*Because some women have a tendency to invert the diaphragm during insertion, application of the spermicide to both sides of the diaphragm may be appropriate.

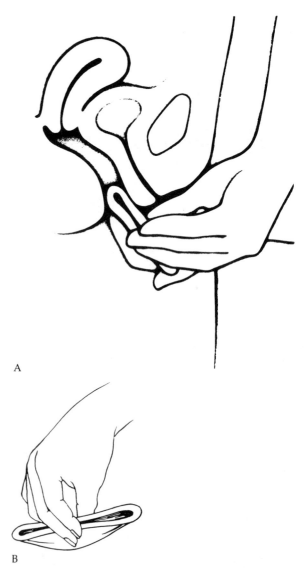

A

B

Fig. 18-10. (A and B) For insertion, the rim of the diaphragm is pinched between the fingers and the thumb. (Figure 18-10A from *Population Reports,* Population Information Program, Series H, No. 4, The Johns Hopkins University, January 1976.)

with the spermicidal cream or jelly and the patient should be assiduous about changing and cleaning it at least every 24 hours. Removal technique is illustrated in Figure 18-11.

It is important that the woman learn to correctly place and easily remove the diaphragm by doing it sev-

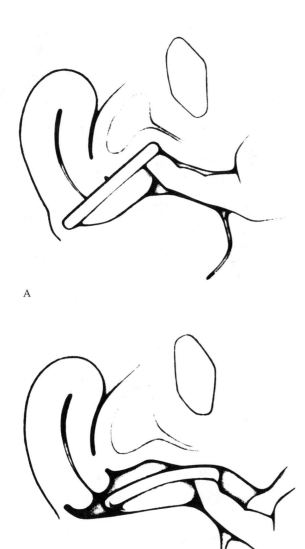

A

B

Fig. 18-11. (A and B) Technique for removal of the diaphragm. (From *Ortho Diaphragms.* Raritan, N.J.: Ortho Pharmaceutical Corp., 1981.)

eral times under supervision before her initial fitting is over. It is also important that she learn to recognize the knoblike feel of the cervix so that she can assure herself that the cervix is completely covered when the diaphragm is correctly placed. It is also generally thought

important for the patient to be rechecked in about 2 weeks to ensure that she is placing and using the diaphragm correctly (see Fig. 18-9A).

Although no longer much in use, it is possible for the patient to obtain a diaphragm inserter by which the diaphragm is pushed into the vagina stretched over a Y-shaped piece of plastic, which is notched to accommodate various diaphragm sizes. After the diaphragm is all the way in, the patient disengages the inserter by giving it a quarter turn as it is withdrawn, and then she secures the diaphragm by manually pressing the anterior rim up behind the symphysis pubis.

Diaphragm fitting rings were once widely used, but most clinicians now prefer to use a real diaphragm when fitting a patient.

Refitting of a diaphragm is generally advisable after a weight gain or loss in excess of 15 pounds and is necessary after pregnancies and pelvic surgery. When refitting after a full-term pregnancy or a miscarriage or abortion occurring beyond 12 weeks of gestation, it is advisable to wait 4 to 6 weeks until uterine involution is complete, being sure to advise the use of some other means of protection if coitus takes place before that time.

It is important before use to periodically inspect the diaphragm for holes or tears, especially near the rim where a fingernail might have perforated it. After use the diaphragm should be rinsed and then cleaned thoroughly with mild soap in warm water. It should then be dried and stored in a protected place. The diaphragm container generally serves well for this purpose. It is important to avoid the use of any strong agents such as harsh detergents and antiseptics when cleaning the diaphragm. The use of talc should also be avoided because of the potential for upward migration into the abdominal cavity. The diaphragm should never be boiled or subjected to extremely hot water. If properly used and cared for, a diaphragm should be able to serve the woman for several years.

CONTRAINDICATIONS

There are a number of contraindications to diaphragm use. These fall into several categories:

Anatomic
Allergic
Situational
Personal

The anatomic reasons are by far the most important. Included in these are such complete contraindications as uterine prolapse and rectovaginal or vesicovaginal fistulas and such possible contraindications as severe cystocele or rectocele, severe uterine anteflexion or retroversion, short anterior vaginal wall, scarring from perineal or vaginal tears or surgery, and very poor vaginal muscle tone. Another contraindication in this category is a history of recurrent cystitis associated with diaphragm use. This could indicate an undesirable degree of diaphragm pressure on the urethra.

The allergic reasons include allergic reactions to the rubber in the diaphragm or to some ingredient in the spermicide. Generally, these allergic reactions can be dealt with by use of a diaphragm made of synthetic plastic or by switching to a different spermicidal preparation.

Situational contraindications would include the immediate postpartum period when the diaphragm cannot be properly put in place and those situations where there are no personnel available to fit the patient with a diaphragm or to demonstrate its use. Unfortunately, such situations are the rule in much of the developing world.

Personal contraindications would include patients who are averse to handling their own genitalia, who object to the "messiness" of the method, and who are either too careless to use it regularly or seemingly unable to learn to use it properly.

HEALTH BENEFITS OF THE DIAPHRAGM

The contraceptive health benefits of using the diaphragm and spermicide are basically the same as those obtained using other contraceptive methods and, of course, are considerable. In addition, however, diaphragm use provides at least two other significant noncontraceptive health benefits.

One of these is the prophylactic effect against sexually transmitted diseases (STD) and vaginal infections. For example, Jackson et al. [13] report a lower incidence of cervical gonorrhea among diaphragm users than among women using nonbarrier methods.

The other significant health benefit was shown in studies conducted in England [7]: A decrease in cervical abnormalities in diaphragm users was demonstrated. After adjusting for the effects of other variables, the risk of cervical neoplasia in diaphragm users was found to be only one-quarter that of users of other methods. Reduced incidence of STD and of precancerous lesions of the cervix, therefore, are important potential health benefits of diaphragm use.

COMPLICATIONS OF THE DIAPHRAGM

Several complications are known to be associated with diaphragm use. One, of course, is the possibility of a local allergic reaction owing either to the rubber in the diaphragm or to an ingredient in the spermicide. Such complications are relatively easy to recognize and treat. Another possible complication is pressure ulceration or tissue necrosis caused by excessive pressure of the diaphragm rim against the vaginal wall [30]. This is unusual and represents an improper fitting of the diaphragm. Still another is cystitis resulting from partial urethral blockage by the diaphragm, which should be suspected when cystitis recurs in a diaphragm user.

The complication most likely to cause concern for diaphragm users at present is toxic shock syndrome, because its association with tampons has received wide publicity. A few nonfatal cases of toxic shock syndrome have been reported in diaphragm users [14, 18, 19]. In all cases patients had left the diaphragm in place for 36 hours or longer. *Staphylococcus aureus* was cultured from the cervix in most of these reported cases. The occurrence of this complication points out the importance of carefully instructing diaphragm users never to leave the diaphragm in longer than 24 hours in order to prevent its action as a culture medium receptacle for staphylococci and streptococci.

Other possible complications associated with diaphragm use that warrant further study include:

1. The potentially harmful effect of dusting the diaphragm with talcum powder after washing it. In a recent study Dr. Daniel Cramer of Harvard [6] found that women with epithelial ovarian cancer were almost twice as likely as controls to have used talcum powder on the perineum or on sanitary napkins. Although no definite link with diaphragm use was found, it would seem prudent to avoid the use of talc in the genital area altogether.
2. The possibility of congenital malformation in a child conceived as a result of diaphragm failure. Although a recent study by Huggins of the University of Pennsylvania [12] reported no increase in the total rates of malformations in offspring of diaphragm users, he did find several times the expected incidence of neural tube defects. This finding points out the importance of providing full counseling to diaphragm and spermicide users, so that any choice they make will be a fully informed one.
3. The possibility that reduced exposure to human seminal fluid factors is associated with an increase in the risk of developing breast cancer. This hypothesis, postulated by Gjorgov in a recent publication [10], would implicate a couple's use of condoms, abstinence, withdrawal, and the diaphragm all as likely to increase the risk of developing breast cancer. Whether or not all the many possible variables involved have been fully taken into account in this study remains to be seen.

EXPERIMENTAL DIAPHRAGM USE

Recently several new and experimental diaphragms have been or are being produced in the United States. The Searle company recently introduced a disposable 60-mm spring diaphragm intended for one-time use; it is enclosed in a small packet, which the potential user can easily carry in a handbag. The Battelle Memorial Institute [9] is currently testing a nonfitted spermicide-releasing diaphragm designed for one-time use. The simplicity of such a medicated diaphragm could well make it appealing to many users.

PRESENT PERSPECTIVE

From the time of its introduction over 100 years ago in Germany and Holland, the vaginal diaphragm has been increasing in use and popularity in many of the developed countries of the world. This gradually increasing popularity, soundly based on the reproductive freedom it confers on women, was interrupted for approximately 15 years beginning in the early 1960s with the advent of the oral contraceptive and the IUD. Since about 1975, however, with the realization that the newer contraceptive methods also had drawbacks, a steady increase in diaphragm use and popularity is once again under way.

It is now fully realized that a diaphragm should never be left in the vagina for longer than 24 hours, and it is also recognized that it is important to clean the diaphragm well and dry it after removal. These precautions are necessary because of cases of toxic shock syndrome associated with diaphragms left in place more than 24 hours.

A patient who becomes pregnant in spite of using a diaphragm and spermicide should be advised that at least one study indicates that the risk of a neural tube defect in the fetus is likely to be increased. The patient can then decide whether she wants her clinician to test for this possibility.

In general, therefore, while not entirely free of drawbacks and possible complications, the diaphragm is an acceptable, effective contraceptive used by an increasing proportion of women of reproductive age in the United States and a number of other developed countries.

REFERENCES

1. Aved, B. M. Trends in contraceptive method of use by California family planning clinic clients, age 10–55, 1976–1979. *Am. J. Public Health* 71:1162, 1981.
2. Boucher, D. Birth control methods. American Birth Control League, 1924. Cited by E. M. Stim in The non-spermi-cide fit-free diaphragm: A new contraceptive method. *Adv. Plan. Parent.* 15:88, 1980.
3. Cooper, J. F. *Techniques of Contraception*. Day-Nichols, 1929.
4. Corderoy, E. C. Condom effectiveness. (Letter to the Editor) *Fam. Plann. Perspect.* 11:271, 1979.
5. Craig, S., and Hepburn, S. The effectiveness of barrier methods of contraception with and without spermicide. *Contraception* 26:347, 1982.
6. Cramer, D. W., et al. Presented to the 10th World Congress of Obstetrics and Gynecology. Reported in *Ob-Gyn News* 18:33, 1983.
7. Derman, R. An agenda for vaginal contraceptive development. In Proceedings of the International Workshop on New Developments in Vaginal Contraception, Guatemala City, 1979.
8. Dotterer, W. H., Berlin, L. E., and Henriques, E. S. Increase in diaphragm use in a university population. *J. Obstet. Gynecol. Nurs.* 8:280, 1979.
9. Edelman, D. A., and Thompson, S. Vaginal contraception: An update. *Contraceptive Delivery Systems* 3:75, 1982.
10. Gjorgov, A. N. Barrier contraception and breast cancer. *Contrib. Gynecol. Obstet.* 8:162, 1980.
11. Hagen, I. M., and Beach, R. K. The diaphragm: Its effective use among college women. *J. Am. Coll. Health Assoc.* 28:263, 1980.
12. Huggins, G. R., et al. Vaginal spermicides and outcome of pregnancy: Finding in large cohort study. Presented to the 10th World Congress of Obstetrics and Gynecology (Reported in *Ob-Gyn News* 18:24, 1983.) *Contraception* 25:219, 1982.
13. Jackson, M., Berger, G. S., and Keith, L. G. *Vaginal Contraception*. Boston: G. K. Hall, 1981. Pp. 136–161.
14. Jaffe, R. Toxic shock syndrome associated with diaphragm use (Letter to the Editor). *N. Engl. J. Med.* 305:1585, 1981.
15. Johnson, V., Masters, W., and Lewis, K. C. The Physiology of Intravaginal Contraceptive Failure. In M. S. Calderone (ed.), *Manual of Family Planning and Contraceptive Practice*. Baltimore: Williams & Wilkins, 1970.
16. Keith, L. G., Berger, G. S., and Jackson, M. A. Effective use of vaginal contraception: A method for the 1980s. *Contemp. Obstet. Gynecol.* 19:64, 1982.
17. Kopp, M. I. *Birth Control in Practice (A Statistical Analysis of 10,000 Cases at the Clinical Research Bureau in New York)*. New York: McBride, 1933.
18. Lee, R., Dillon, M. P., and Bashler, E. Barrier contraceptives and toxic shock syndrome. (Letter to the Editor). *Lancet* 1:221, 1982.
19. Loomis, L., and Feder, H. M. Toxic shock syndrome associated with diaphragm use (Letter to the Editor). *N. Engl. J. Med.* 305:1585, 1981.
20. McLure, Z. Failure rate of contraceptive methods. *Fam. Plann. Inform. Serv.* 1:59, 1981.
21. Mishell, D. R. *Current Therapy in Obstetrics and Gynecology*. Philadelphia: Saunders, 1980. Pp. 167–172.

22. Pearl, R. Contraception and fertility in 4945 married women: A second report on a study in family limitation. *Hum. Biol.* 6:355, 1934.

23. Penfield, A. J. Contraception and female sterilization. *N. Y. State J. Med.* 81:255, 1981.

24. Püsey, W. A. The prevention of conception. *J.A.M.A.* 83:2020, 1924.

25. Schirm, A. L., et al. Contraceptive failure in the United States. *Fam. Plann. Perspect.* 14:68, 1982.

26. Tatum, H. J., and Connell, E. B. Barrier contraception: A comprehensive overview. *Fertil. Steril.* 36:1, 1981.

27. Vaughn, B., et al. Contraceptive efficacy among married women 1970–1973. National Center for Health Statistics. *Fam. Plann. Perspect.* 9:251, 1977.

28. Vessey, M., Lawless, M., and Yeates, D. Efficacy of different contraceptive methods. *Lancet* 1:841, 1982.

29. Westoff, C. F., and Ryder, N. B. United States' methods of fertility control: 1955, 1960 and 1965. *Stud. Fam. Plann.* 17:1, 1967.

30. Widhalm, M. V. Vaginal lesion: Etiology—a malfitting diaphragm? *J. Nurse Midwif.* 24:39, 1979.

31. Wortman, J., et al. The diaphragm and other intravaginal barriers: A review. *Popul. Rep.* [H]. No. 4, 1976.

32. Zatuchni, G. I., et al. *Vaginal Contraception: New Developments.* New York: Harper & Row, 1979. Pp. 2–12.

19. The Cervical Cap

Richard J. Derman

Almost 150 years have elapsed since the availability of the first cervical cap. Throughout this period the cap's popularity has fluctuated widely, generally in relation to the availability of other contraceptive modalities. This chapter will review some of the factors that have permitted present advocates of the cervical cap to "breathe new life" and at the same time explore historic factors leading to present-day cervical cap technology.

Actually the use of cervical/vaginal pessaries, the category still employed for the cervical cap by the United States Food and Drug Administration, predates modern medicine by almost 4,000 years. Probably by trial and error, women in Asia and the Middle East selected natural herbs, plants, and food products to occlude the cervix and to develop a vaginal environment hostile for sperm viability. Most of the ingredients used were either highly acid or alkaline, thus incorporating two principles used in modern contraceptives—a barrier plus a spermicide. Perhaps most often cited is the description in the Petrie papyrus (1850 B.C.) of three vaginal pessaries, all of which possessed a consistency that would harden and most probably occlude the cervix. The base of one was crocodile dung, the second was composed of honey and sodium carbonate, and the third utilized a gum resin [8].

Less esoteric ingredients used in other neighboring countries included pessaries woven from the opium plant containing significant amounts of tannic acid [9], linen rags, beeswax, natural sponges, algae, a hollowed-out half lemon, and collections of feathers—a common practice in ancient India.

In modern times Friedrich Wilde's [40] text on infertility, published in Germany in 1838, is the first reference cited in the medical literature to a cervical cap. These were custom-made rubber devices not dissimilar in appearance to those still marketed in England today. In his writings Wilde also noted the postpartum use of contraceptive cervical covers inserted by midwives at the time of delivery.

Recognizing the different shapes and sizes of cervices, Wilde advocated that a special mold be made for each patient by first taking a wax impression of the cervix [8]. It is interesting that the newest of the cervical caps (still in testing) employs this same technique.

Even in the mid-1800s consumer demand for barrier contraception was evident, as Wilde's cervical caps gained widespread popularity throughout Europe, with many references being made in the medical literature [8] to the personalized "cautchuk pessarium."

Approximately 25 years later a New York physician named E. B. Foote developed his own cervical cap. It is still unclear whether his original design predated that of Wilde or simply built upon the German gynecologist's earlier work. In any event, Foote did not attempt to gain widespread use of the cap, and it was never

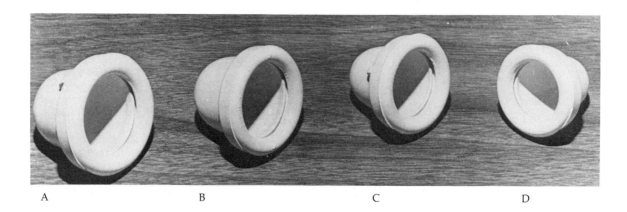

Fig. 19-1. Prentif Cavity Rim Cervical Caps. (A) 31 mm. (B) 28 mm. (C) 25 mm. (D) 22 mm.

commercialized [8, 10], probably because of the restrictive Comstock laws in effect in the 1870s.

Shortly thereafter, the cervical cap appeal became somewhat fragmented owing primarily to the work of another German gynecologist, Mensinga, whose cap design more closely approximated the present-day diaphragm. The "Dutch cap" as it was often referred to, because of its great popularity in that country, was known in England, Germany, and the United States as the Mensinga diaphragm. It was to become the prototype of modern diaphragms.

However, modifications of cervical caps continued to be introduced, and in 1908 Kafka, a Viennese gynecologist, developed a firm variety of the pliable cervical cap. There are indications that in this period cervical caps were the most frequently physician-prescribed contraception method in Europe [41].

With these early breakthroughs in contraceptive technology, the family planning movement was rapidly beginning to emerge in both Europe and the United States, pioneered by the leadership of Marie Stopes and Margaret Sanger. Interestingly, each of these two remarkable women selected a different method with which to prevent conception and limit family size. Dr. Stopes developed her own cervical cap, and the Prorace cap was used almost exclusively in her English clinics with recommendations that it need be removed only during the menses. Margaret Sanger preferred the Mensinga diaphragm and introduced it in the United States; even in this early period of contraceptive knowledge, she suggested its use with a spermicide to improve efficacy.

Despite the cap-diaphragm controversy, new varieties of cervical caps continued to proliferate, often incorporating such materials as silver, gold, aluminum, stainless steel, ivory, and even platinum. Most important to the evolution of the cervical cap was the use of a

celluloid-like material as modified by Pust, another German physician. Metal and celluloid caps almost replaced those made with rubber, and the Pust-designed cap is still manufactured and widely used in Germany today [31].

Other recently developed caps have employed lucite and polyethylene. However, it is of interest that the most widely used caps today use the original rubber material. These are primarily manufactured by the Lamberts Company of London, England. However, both soft as well as firm caps continue to be manufactured in Denmark, Germany, and Israel. Cervical caps are routinely measured in millimeters of the inner diameter. Unfortunately, the gradations of cap size are limited, perhaps owing to the low profit margin associated with sales of these devices. For example, the Prentif Cavity Rim Cap (Fig. 19-1), which is most commonly used, is available in only four sizes: 22, 25, 28, and 31 mm.

Of great importance is the fact that the early bias in favor of diaphragms in the United States and the pessary designation given to the cap have to the present precluded its approval as a contraceptive device. Cervical caps may be obtained and fitted in this country only under a research-status exemption granted by the Food and Drug Administration with the requirements of reporting and informed consent, despite a 150-year history of a relatively inert device often used without an accompanying spermicide.

Research in this country with cervical caps occurred long before restrictive United States government device legislation. Reports by Gräfenberg [12] and Dickinson [7], as well as those by Stone [34], Greenhill [13], Moses [29], Lehfeldt [25], and Tietze [35], appeared in the 1930 to 1965 period. Most of the work reported was with the rigid cervical cap and utilized a spermicide in conjunction with the device [35]. It is of interest that there were at least three U.S. companies manufacturing devices during the period 1920 to 1950. Despite the routine use of the cap plus spermicide, Lehfeldt et al. [28] questioned the ability of the spermicide to be effective beyond the initial 7-day period. This was particularly important in that most caps were fitted for use over the entire intermenstrual period. His studies indicated that creams as opposed to gels were somewhat more effective in prolonging the duration of spermicidal activity [28], but in almost all cases such activity was absent after 7 days, despite the cream and jelly being retained within the cap. Lehfeldt concluded that "the cap affords protection without a spermicidal supplement" [28].

In 1953 Tietze et al. reported in the *American Journal of Obstetrics and Gynecology* on perhaps the first significant use-effectiveness study with the cervical cap. He pointed out that most United States gynecologists were still unfamiliar with the cervical cap and its mode of action [35] and noted that this device had not gained widespread popularity as it had in Europe. The collective data of Tietze et al. reported 7.6 pregnancies per 100 woman-years of experience with 143 lucite-cap-wearing patients who also used a spermicide. These data incorporated women who may have used the device incorrectly, without spermicide, or not at all [35]. In comparison, a parallel group of their diaphragm patients yielded a rate of 13.7 per 100 woman-years of use. In fact, until the 1980s the Tietze data comprised the only statistically valid cervical cap study in the United States and only one of three studies comprising more than 100 patients [21, 23, 42]. The authors also pointed out that of the 28 unplanned pregnancies in their study, 21 were related to faulty technique or omission of spermicide and 10 were instances of admittedly irregular use. Omitting these patients yielded a theoretical (or method) effectiveness of 98 percent.

The paper also noted the contraindications to cervical cap use that prevailed at that time. They included:

Deep cervical laceration extending to the vaginal vault
Cervical erosion or nabothian cysts
Extreme shortness or elongation of the cervix
Acute or subacute salpingitis [35]

Recent investigators include herpetic lesions and condyloma accuminata as additional contraindications, while questioning some of the earlier ones.

The original authors specifically prescribed the cap for some women who could not utilize the diaphragm for anatomic or functional reasons such as short anterior vaginal wall, cystocele, lacerated or relaxed pelvic floor, third-degree retroversion, acute anteflexion of the uterus, or allergy to rubber by either partner [35]. The authors even suggested that small caps could be inserted into virgins who apparently could not be adequately fitted for a diaphragm [35].

The popularity of the diaphragm and condoms and the approval of oral contraceptives in 1962 temporarily led to a situation where use of the cap in the United States was minimal. All United States manufacturing ceased, and few devices were imported from Europe.

Why then has there emerged a recent interest in the cervical cap, particularly in the United States? No single answer will suffice. Clearly, the emergence of the feminist movement and the establishment of a feminist health network are important factors. Many women view the cap as a noncoitally dependent method, having minimal risks and affording the opportunity for additional familiarity with one's pelvic organs. The potential risks associated with both oral contraceptives and intrauterine devices (IUDs) have also served to reinforce the impact of the cap. Published data showing a reduced incidence of cervical dysplasia with the use of all barriers coupled with a near epidemic of pelvic inflammatory disease particularly associated with IUD use represent additional stimuli to use.

However, as is often the case, particularly when the supply of available devices does not approach the demand, perceived attributes often outweigh scientific reality. Under the best conditions the cervical cap data rarely appear to produce effectiveness in excess of that associated with the diaphragm. In addition, some unpleasant features have been reported as being associated, or theoretically associated, with cervical cap use. They include:

1. Increase in vaginal odor, particularly when the device remains in place more than 48 hours
2. Significant time necessary for proper initial fitting of the cap
3. Recognition that at least 25 to 30 percent of women cannot be properly fitted with those caps presently available either because of cervical size, configuration, or acute cervicovaginal angulation, or, with equal frequency, because of factors related to discomfort or displeasure with self-insertion and removal
4. Difficulty with removal and reinsertion of the device
5. Dislodgment during coitus
6. Reports of cervical fissures and crater ulcers secondary to suction (extremely rare with Prentif caps)
7. Recent reports of vaginal laceration particularly attributable to one type of cervical cap—the Vimule [1].
8. Theoretical increased risk of toxic shock syndrome or anaerobic bacterial proliferation because of lack

of egress of cervical secretions (although no cases of TSS have ever been reported)

9. Potential increase in urinary tract infection rates
10. Possible contraindication to use in women with erosion of the cervix (although evidence shows "erosions" improve)
11. Theoretical consideration of retrograde menstruation with subsequent development of endometriosis
12. The continuing controversy regarding disposition of large amounts of nonoxynol-9 in the vagina, its rate of systemic absorption, and its potential for toxicity and teratogenicity

The importance of these factors in terms of both ultimate FDA approval and widespread consumer acceptance warrants a closer look at the data.

Perhaps the most significant recent data collected on cervical cap use come from Koch at the Brigham and Women's Hospital [22]. He surveyed 413 acceptors of the Prentif contraceptive cervical cap* and received 371 responses. In relation to the broad area of acceptability, two categories of reporting were perhaps most important: questions on those features most disliked about the cap and questions as to why cap use was stopped. An overall 37.7 percent odor rate was reported; it was one of the prime reasons for cessation of cap use. This confirms earlier anecdotal reports in the literature but is in conflict with the paper of Tietze et al. [35] where no dropouts were attributable to odor. Koch felt that perhaps the unique oil/water base present in the particular vaginal cream employed in the study may have, to some degree, effected the high reported rate of odor.

The Tietze data [35] with the rigid cap list difficulty with self-insertion as a prime cause for discontinuation. While 20 percent of respondents in the Koch survey indicated difficulty with insertion, only 10 percent saw this as a major problem and less than 5 percent as the prime reason for discontinuation [22].

While dislodgment was not listed as a reporting category in the Tietze paper, it is most important to recognize that of the 69 respondents in the Boston study who reported stopping cap use, dislodgment and pregnancy each accounted for 18.8 percent, ranking first in order of frequency. These data, reported from a center where careful cervical cap fitting by a committed clinician was obviously undertaken, suggest that modifications in future cap design may be important if the utility of cervical cap contraception is to improve.

Perhaps the most comprehensive data, albeit anecdotal, on the time requirements for cervical cap fitting emerged from a cervical cap symposium sponsored by

the Feminist Women's Health Center in Atlanta (May, 1983). This meeting was significant in that it probably represented the first international symposium ever held on the subject of cervical caps. Participants in this meeting indicated that not only did the initial fitting require one-half to 1 hour per recipient, but additional time in self-help groups was suggested as being the best vehicle for ensuring both adequate fit and consumer well-being with the cap [37]. Inability to fit a very short or flat cervix (less than 1.5 cms) was reported by Cappiello et al. [3]. Tietze [35] and Koch [22] report a similar difficulty and noted as well that proper fitting can also be impossible with extreme elongation of the cervix.

Clearly, the paucity of meaningful data substantiating safety and efficacy is probably the single most important reason for the present lack of FDA approval. Few of the questions raised regarding relative risk factors have been addressed in the literature. The Koch data [22] has helped to dispel some concerns previously thought to either specifically contraindicate cap use or increase the potential for serious local or systemic illness.

The early reports of Gräfenberg, Tietze, and Lehfeldt listed cervical erosion as a contraindication to cap use, although no references for this conclusion are cited. Most recent data seem to agree with the earlier observations of Kafka [18, 19] and Pust [32] indicating a lessening or disappearance of the erosion, or at very least no deterioration of the condition [22]. It is therefore not surprising that alterations in Pap smears in this study were infrequent and less than those found in the general population. Koch suggests that by promoting normal squamous metaplasia, the cap and diaphragm [15, 38] may prove to reduce the risk of both dysphasia and cervical carcinoma.

Other health issues associated with cap use remain arcane. Urinary tract infections were a significant problem in 6 percent of the Boston group and one reason for discontinuation of use. The relatively large numbers of symptomatic patients suggest that future controlled studies should include routine urine cultures as part of the protocol.

The toxic shock issue in relation to the cap needs to be addressed. While there are inadequate numbers of cap users in the United States to deny a possible causal relationship, no TSS cases have to date been reported in any cap user.

A recent publication by the National Academy of Sciences [30] indicates that fewer than 10 of 10,000 menstruating women per year may develop symptoms suggestive of toxic shock syndrome. It would therefore require many thousand patient-years of cervical cap use to determine if an increased risk for TSS truly exists. Koch [21], however, points out that 28 percent of

*In this study the cap was used in conjunction with a spermicidal cream.

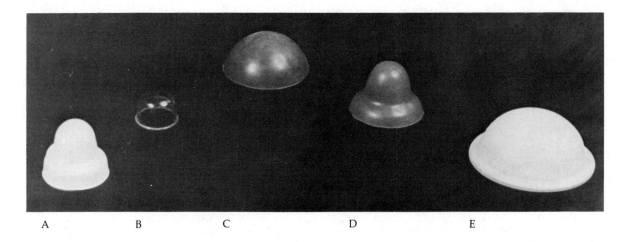

A   B   C   D   E

Fig. 19-2. Five types of barriers: (A) Prentif 22 mm. (B) Celluloid Cervical Cap. (C) Dumas Cap. (D) Vimule Cap. (E) Ortho Diaphragm.

women surveyed could not determine menses with the Prentif cap, and egress of menstrual fluid may be prevented. The concomitant use of spermicides with the cervical cap should theoretically reduce risk because of a lowering of the vaginal pH. The reports of Cutler [5] and Singh [33] note the bacteriocidal effects of nonoxynol-9, which may be a deterrent to the development of this *S. aureus*–related condition.

Toxicity issues surrounding all vaginal methods that employ the standard nonoxynol-9 spermicide appear to be waning. Despite long-term usage by millions of consumers, no major systemic effects have been reported other than contact irritation. A consensus on the Jick [16] data, which suggested teratogenicity, has not developed, and moreover the study design and conclusions of that report have been challenged. Animal absorption studies employing nonoxynol-9 reported by Chvapil [4] are covered more extensively in this text in the chapter dealing with vaginal spermicides.

Koch may have been the first investigator to report on menstrual changes with cap use, with about 20 percent of respondents indicating menstrual irregularities. A heavier flow with increased cramping was noted by two-thirds of this subgroup [22]. Because menstrual flow patterns may vary and reported differences were of a diverse nature, a true association with cap use is still speculative. However, Koch theorizes that one possibility for an increase in dysmenorrhea symptoms may be the development of endometriosis secondary to tubal outflow of menstrual fluid. Resistance to such outflow caused by a cap worn during intervals of bleeding may theoretically promote endometriotic im-

plants. The author rightly points out, however, that no evidence now exists linking the cervical cap to endometriosis.

Investigators of cervical caps have long been familiar with a "suction ring" appearance on the cervix when the cap is removed. This is particularly prevalent with the Prentif Cavity Rim Cap (CRC). Most of these findings are transient, however, and rarely, if ever, does one see actual laceration of the mucosa [11]. It was therefore significant that Bernstein et al. [1], working through a NICHD grant, reported that two-thirds of users of a particular cap, the Vimule, had traumatic lesions on the portio vaginalis ranging from erythematous impressions to abrasion and frank laceration. The two caps studied had different edge configurations, with the CRC being more rounded than the sharperedged, more rigid Vimule cap. Despite its rather infrequent usage in this country, restricted primarily to women with short cervices, Bernstein has discontinued the use of the Vimule cap and has urged all investigators to carefully inspect the cervix and vaginal mucosa in all cap users. Recently the FDA curtailed research on the Vimule cap [1]. Figure 19-2 shows some of the more commonly used devices.

Effectiveness data on all barrier contraceptives are confusing at best. The diaphragm has been the subject of a number of efficacy studies. Often such study results inappropriately compare use- and method-effectiveness or Pearl index rates with life-table analyses. Most biostatisticians concur that these data are not comparable among studies because of major differences in reporting practices and protocol design. Despite two diaphragm studies that suggest an effectiveness of 98 percent [24], other studies cite pregnancy rates in the magnitude of almost 20 percent [37, 39].

Perhaps because there are not as many studies available with the cap, the range of effectiveness data should be viewed with caution. If all reported studies of more than 100 woman-users are considered, reported failure rates in more than 3,000 women have ranged from 3.5 [42] to 16 per 100 woman-years of use [6, 14].

Examples of such data (primarily expressed in the Pearl formula) include reports from the following clinics:

1. Fink (Germany), 1931
   99 women: Clinic insertion (50%)—4 pregnancies
   Self insertion (50%)—8 pregnancies
2. Kabanova (U.S.S.R.), 1936 [17]
   300 women: 100 ivory caps—8% failure rate
   100 aluminum caps—8% failure rate
   100 rubber caps—11–15% failure rate
3. Lehfeldt (U.S.), 1949 [27]
   156 women (6–22 months of use)—14 failures
*4. Tietze (U.S.), 1953 [35]
   143 women (greater than 90% used method more than 1 year)—7.6 pregnancies per 100 woman-years of use
5. Childbearing-Childrearing Center (U.S.), 1980 [2]
   76 women (397 months of cap use)—19.6% failure rate
6. Denniston (U.S.), 1980 [15]
   110 women (based on 6 months' data, est. 1 yr)—16% failure rate
*7. Koch (U.S.), 1981 [21]
   413 women (372 respondents to questionnaire)—8.4 pregnancies per 100 woman-years of use

Perhaps more divergent than the efficacy data are dropout rates, which even among the most enthusiastic proponents of cervical caps are rather high. Denniston [6] reported a dropout rate of 38.5 per 100 woman-years of use, Boehm [2] noted a 49.5% dropout after 1 year, and Koch [21], in perhaps the largest series, reports a 32.6 percent rate of dropout.

When one critically reviews all the data, it becomes apparent that in highly motivated women with proper fitting and follow-up, reasonable continuation rates exist with pregnancies reported in an acceptable range.

Figure 19-3 depicts appropriate insertion and removal techniques. Many instruction guides have been written on the proper techniques for cap insertion. Capiello's recommendations [3] are as follows:

1. Fill cap one-third to two-thirds full of spermicide and apply around rim. Oil-based spermicides may be more likely to cause an odor when used with a cap.
2. The cap may be inserted any time† before intercourse and must remain in place for at least 8 hours after last act of intercourse.
3. To insert the cap assume a squatting or half-squatting position with one leg raised on a stool. Hold cap together and insert tab end of cap first. Slid the cap into the vagina and push it along the floor of the vagina as far as it will go. Use your finger to press cap onto cervix. Now sweep the finger around cap to see if cervix is covered by cap. Also try depressing the dome of the cap to feel cervix through the rubber.
4. To remove, place finger on top of lateral rim, pull down on cap to break suction, then hook finger into cap and pull out of vagina.
5. Check to ensure cap is on cervix before and after intercourse during the first month of use. During this month, also check cap fit after using various positions of intercourse. Check fit after intercourse if with a new partner. It might also be possible for cap to be dislodged with a bowel movement.
6. Douching is not recommended when the cap is in place.
7. The cap should not be used as a contraceptive during your period. Another method of contraception is recommended at this time.
8. There are varying opinions as to length of time cap may be left in place and still be effective. In our area, most cap providers recommend 2 to 3 days.
9. Wash cap with mild soap and water and dry thoroughly. Sometimes when the cap is removed you may notice an unpleasant odor. This can be alleviated by (a) soaking the cap in 1 cup of water mixed with 1 tablespoon of vinegar or lemon juice for 20 minutes; or (b) placing one drop of liquid chlorophyll on top of the spermicide before inserting the cap. Chlorophyll is available at pharmacies and some natural food stores.
10. Childbirth and abortion may affect the size of the cap needed.

The cap appears to have survived a tumultuous 150-year history and is being eagerly welcomed by some segments of the health and consumer community. There is little question that a safe, efficacious, noncoitally dependent device that requires minimal physician interaction would be most welcome. Unfortunately,

---

*Utilized life-table analysis.

†Note that the efficacy of spermicidal cream is vastly diminished after 7 days.

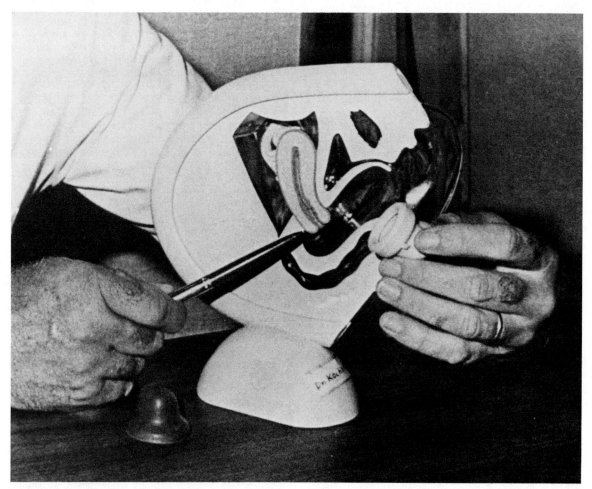

Fig. 19-3. Demonstration of cervical cap placement.

present-day caps do not entirely fulfill those criteria. Goepp and associates are taking plaster impressions of the cervix in order to generate a form-fitting cap. Unfortunately, the first round of clinical trials with the Contra-Cap led to disappointing rates of pregnancy with abandonment of the trial. New technology has apparently been developed in the impression and molding process, and clinical studies are likely to resume. Modifications of this cap now include the use of an outlet valve to allow for continued in vivo use over long periods of time. Although promising, no published clinical data have as yet appeared.

Koch [21] suggests that another modification could entail a small, thin, noncontact cap produced in a variety of assorted sizes and shapes. Ideally it would contain a timed-release spermicide and most importantly have those features that would allow for ease of insertion and removal. In his view, suction is not maintained constantly within the cap but occurs only at onset of withdrawal of the cap from the cervix and ceases when the seal at the rim is broken.

REFERENCES

1. Bernstein, G. S., et al. Studies of cervical caps: I. Vaginal lesions associated with use of the Vimule cap. *Contraception* 26:443, 1982.
2. Boehm, D. The cervical cap: Effectiveness as a contraceptive. *J. Nurse Midwif.* 28:3, 1983.
3. Cappiello, J. D., and Grainger-Harrison, M. The rebirth of the cervical cap. *J. Nurse Midwif.* 26:13, 1981.

4. Chvapil, M., et al. Studies on nonoxynol-9: Intravaginal absorption, distribution, metabolism and excretion. *Contraception* 22:3, 1980.

5. Cutler, J. C., et al. Vaginal contraceptives as prophylaxis against gonorrhea and other sexually transmissible diseases. *Adv. Plann. Parent.* 12:1, 1977.

6. Denniston, G. C. Presented to meeting of Planned Parenthood Physicians. Denver, Oct. 1980.

7. Dickinson, R. L. *J. Contraception* 2:103, 1937.

8. Fairbanks, B., and Scharfman, B. The cervical cap: Past and current experience. *Women Health*, p. 60, July 16, 1980.

9. Finch, B. E. Balls, Feathers and Caps. In B. E. Finche and H. Green (eds.), *Contraception Through the Ages*. Springfield, Ill.: Thomas, 1962. Pp. 38–45.

10. Gentile, G., and Helbig, D. Barrier contraceptives and spermicide: Revealed wisdom reconsidered. Presented to the annual meeting of the Association of Planned Parenthood Physicians. Denver, Oct. 4, 1980.

11. Goepp, R. Presented to meeting of Planned Parenthood Physicians. Denver, Oct. 1980.

12. Gräfenberg, E., and Dickinson, R. L. *West. J. Surg.* 52:335, 1944.

13. Greenhill, J. P. *The 1949 Year Book of Obstetrics and Gynecology*. Chicago: Year Book, 1949. P. 384.

14. High rates of pregnancy and dissatisfaction mark first cervical cap trial. *Fam. Plann. Perspect.*, 13:48, 1981.

15. Jackson, M., Berger, G. S., and Keith, L. G. *Vaginal Contraception*. Boston: G. K. Hall, 1981.

16. Jick, J., et al. Vaginal spermicides and congenital disorders. *J.A.M.A.* 245:13, 1981.

17. Kabanova, A. Mechanical methods of contraception. *J. Contraception* 1:111, 1936.

18. Kafka, K. Uber den Neuen Kappenverschluss des Muttermundes und sein Indikationen. *Klin. Therapeutische Wochenschr.* 50:1390, 1908.

19. Kafka, K. Uber Kappenbehandlung. *Wien. Med. Wochenschr.* 41:2272, 1908.

20. Kelashan, J., et al. Barrier-method contraceptives and pelvic inflammatory disease. *J.A.M.A.* 248:184, 1982.

21. Koch, J. The experience of 372 women using the Prentif contraceptive cervical cap. Distributed to the International Cervical Cap Symposium. Atlanta, May 1983.

22. Koch, J. The Prentif contraceptive cervical cap: A contemporary study of its clinical safety and effectiveness. *Contraception* 25:135, 1982.

23. Konikow. Report on experience with the French pessary. Proceedings of the 1st American Birth Control Conference, 1921.

24. Lane, M. E., Arceo, R., and Sobrero, A. Successful use of the diaphragm and jelly by a young population: Report of a clinical study. *Fam. Plann. Perspect.* 8:81, 1976.

25. Lehfeldt, H. *J. Contraception* 2:106, 1937.

26. Lehfeldt, H. *J. Sex. Educ.* 1:132, 1949.

27. Lehfeldt, H. Cervical Cap. In M. E. Calderone (ed.), *Manual of Family Planning and Contraceptive Practice* (2nd ed.). Baltimore: Williams & Wilkins, 1970. P. 373.

28. Lehfeldt, H., Sobrero, A. J., and Inglis, W. Spermicidal effectiveness of chemical contraceptives used with the firm cervical cap. *Am. J. Obstet. Gynecol.* 82:446, 1961.

29. Moses, B. L. *Hum. Fertil.* 6:138, 1944.

30. The National Academy of Sciences, Institute of Medicine. Toxic shock syndrome, an assessment of current information and future research needs, 1982.

31. Pust, W. Ein Brauchbarer Frauenschutz. *Dtsch. Med. Wochenschr.* 29, 1923.

32. Pust, W. Discussion of Mechanical Occlusive Methods. In M. Sanger and H. M. Stone, (eds.), *The Practice of Contraception*. Baltimore: Williams & Wilkins, 1931. P. 24.

33. Singh, B., and Cutler, J. C. Vaginal Contraceptives for Prophylaxis Against Gonorrhea and Other Sexually Transmissible Diseases. In G. I. Zatuchni (ed.), *Vaginal Contraceptives*. Hagerstown, Md.: Harper & Row, 1979. Pp. 175–185.

34. Stone, H. M. *J. Contraception* 2:102, 1937.

35. Tietze, C., Lehfeldt, H., and Liebmann, H. The effectiveness of the cervical cap as a contraceptive method. *Am. J. Obstet. Gynecol.* 66:904, 1953.

36. Unpublished data from International Cervical Cap Symposium, Atlanta, May 1983.

37. Vaughn, B., et al. Contraceptive efficacy among married women 1970–1973. National Center for Health Statistics 62:26, 1979.

38. Vessey, M., et al. A long-term follow-up study of women using different methods of contraception: An interim report. *J. Biosoc. Sci.* 8:373, 1976.

39. Vessey, M., Lawless, M., and Yeates, D. Efficacy of different contraceptive methods. *Lancet* 1:841, 1982.

40. Wilde, F. A. Das Weibliche Gebar-Unvermogen, Friedrich-Wilhelms Universitat, Berlin 1938.

41. Wortman, J. Barrier methods. *Popul. Rep.* [H]. No. 4, Jan. 1976.

42. Yarros, R. S. Report of the Illinois Birth Control League, Chicago, 1927.

20. The Contraceptive Sponge

Richard M. Soderstrom

With the renewed interest in barrier methods, it was only a matter of time before one of history's oldest methods of contraception would be rediscovered. Historians tell us of the use of natural sea sponges for vaginal contraception dating back to the ancient Egyptians. A variety of solutions and oils were used to enhance its effectiveness, but, of course, statistics are lacking.

During the mid-1970s a collagen sponge shaped like a thick round wafer was studied seriously but never in a large-scale fashion. Early in 1982 research on this product was abandoned [1].

A cylindrical device made out of resilient polyurethane was tested by Jost in the late 1970s. It contained the commonly used spermicide nonoxynol-9. During coitus, compression of the device by coital thrusting released the spermicide. In vitro studies indicated that the device contained enough spermicide to be effective for 72 hours before disposal and subsequent insertion of a new sponge tampon [5]. At the time of this writing, development and research of this product have been discontinued.

At this time, there is only one contraceptive vaginal sponge that has been developed, clinically tested, and reviewed by the Food and Drug Administration (FDA). Approval for marketing was delivered to the manufacturer, the VLI Corporation, in March 1983. Eight months earlier, the device was approved and is currently marketed in the United Kingdom. These approvals followed a 7-year development and research program initiated by its inventor and president of the VLI Corporation, Bruce Vorhauer, Ph.D., a biomedical engineer.

A confusing historic event is worth mentioning at this point. On October 28, 1982, a formal presentation was made by the VLI Corporation to a medical advisory panel of the FDA [7]. The request for marketing and the claims presented were approved by these medical professionals. However, at the time of this writing, the FDA has chosen to alter the panel's recommendation. Because of this divergence of opinion, the claims for this product will be described as presented to the medical advisory panel. These claims are currently approved in the United Kingdom and several other European countries.

PRODUCT DESCRIPTION

The vaginal contraceptive sponge consists of a resilient, hydrophilic, polyurethane foam sponge impregnated during manufacture with an aqueous solution of preservative compounds plus nonoxynol-9. Because of its properties as a nonionic surfactant, this common sper-

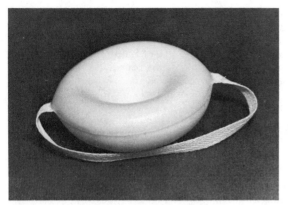

Fig. 20-1. The vaginal contraceptive sponge.

micide facilitates the formation of the open-celled sponge.

The sponge is placed in the vagina by the user any time up to 24 hours before contemplated coitus. In its position in the upper vault of the vagina, the sponge works as a contraceptive in three ways:

1. It releases the spermicide to kill the sperm.
2. It blocks the path of the sperm.
3. It absorbs the male ejaculate, thereby reducing the number of sperm available for fertilization.

The sponge (Fig. 20-1) is a cup-shaped device about 6 cm in diameter and 3 cm thick, incorporating a woven polyester retrieval loop, 1 gm of nonoxynol-9, and minimal amounts of inactive preservatives.

Nonoxynol-9 has been recommended for classification as "Category I" by the FDA's advisory panel on over-the-counter (OTC) vaginal contraceptives and considered safe and effective for OTC use as a vaginal contraceptive (*Federal Register*, December 12, 1980, pp. 82014–82049). This spermicide has had worldwide use for more than 20 years. Since the quantity of spermicide delivered from the sponge in situ averages that of currently marketed OTC spermicidal products, there is no reason to suspect pharmacologic activity at variance with the established historic behavior of nonoxynol-9.

The sponge itself is a specifically formulated new biomaterial, a water-reactive polyurethane polymer. This material has been fully tested and adjudged safe.

During their development sponges were studied for nonoxynol-9 content after coital activity. Even following multiple acts of intercourse over a 2-day period, the residual content of the spermicide found in the sponge was in the range of 900 mg. Because of the continuous availability of the spermicide while the sponge is being worn, coitus can occur multiple times during the recommended wearing time.

This barrier contraceptive is a nonsystemic, reversible barrier method of birth control; it is not an occlusive device and does not function like the cervical cap or diaphragm. The following features set it apart from other available contraceptives:

1. There is an absence of the potential adverse side effects that are associated with oral contraceptives and intrauterine devices.
2. There is one universal size, eliminating the need for professional fitting.
3. It is easily inserted and removed by the user.
4. It is marketed over the counter.
5. Unlike the condom and other spermicidal methods, the user may engage in multiple acts of coitus without additional preparation.
6. It combines spermicidal activity with a barrier method of contraception.
7. There is no need to wait after insertion.
8. It can be inserted hours in advance of intercourse to avoid interruption of sexual gratification.
9. It is disposable, unlike the diaphragm.
10. Excess medication does not extrude from the vagina during coitus.

EFFECTIVENESS

Comparative studies of the sponge are ongoing and have involved about 2,000 women worldwide in 1,000 woman-years of sponge use as of late 1982. To date, the effectiveness of the sponge is in the range of other vaginal contraceptives, essentially equivalent to that of the diaphragm and greater than that of the Neo-Sampoon foaming tablet suppository.

Because the effectiveness of barrier methods improves with use, a new method is at a disadvantage when compared with another method with which women have experience [6]. Also, it should be remembered that the effectiveness of these methods appears to depend on certain user characteristics that influence the user's ability and motivation to use the method consistently and correctly. To some extent, this ability and motivation may depend on the degree of instruction and counseling that users receive from family planning providers. For example, one landmark study documented a failure rate of only 2 per 100 users per year among diaphragm-using women who were, for the most part, young and unmarried but who received thorough education [4].

The most sophisticated study of this contraceptive sponge was conducted by the International Fertility Research Program, Research Triangle Park, North Carolina, under the direction of David A. Edelman, Ph.D (biostatistics) [3]. This recently published pro-

Table 20-1. Twelve-month cumulative life-table rates (per 100 women)

Event	Contraceptive method mainly used prior to admission			
	Vaginal contraceptive		Nonvaginal contraceptive	
	Contraceptive sponge (n = 264)	Diaphragm (n = 249)	Contraceptive sponge (n = 452)	Diaphragm (n = 470)
Pregnancy	13.2*	5.9	16.1	12.0
Medical reasons	7.0*	2.4	7.5	3.9
Discomfort	1.8	2.2	7.0*	3.5
Planned pregnancy	3.1	3.8	5.5	8.8
Other personal reasons	18.3	22.7	24.1	28.5
Continuation rate	62.7	66.9	51.7	53.2

*$p < 0.05$.
Source: From D. A. Edelman, S. C. Smith, and S. McIntyre. Comparative trial of the contraceptive sponge and diaphragm: A preliminary report. *J. Reprod. Med.* 28:781, 1983.

spective study involved a nationwide collaboration of 13 different institutions. Patients were randomly assigned either the contraceptive sponge or a diaphragm with jelly.

A total of 729 sponge users and 723 diaphragm users were studied. Comparisons were made between these two groups according to whether the patient had previously used a vaginal contraceptive agent or not. As shown in Table 20-1, the pregnancy rate per 100 women as a cumulative life-table event was 13.2 for contraceptive sponge users who previously used a vaginal contraceptive approach; the rate was 16.1 for those sponge users who were unfamiliar with vaginal contraceptive means. Similar figures for the diaphragm users were 5.9 for those experienced with the diaphragm, and 12.0 for those using the diaphragm for the first time. Statistical significance was reached only when comparing the contraceptive sponge with the diaphragm in those patients familiar with vaginal contraception. The continuation rates were similar within both groups, with those experienced in vaginal contraception showing a greater continuation rate, as expected.

NONCONTRACEPTIVE RISKS AND BENEFITS

With more widespread use the noncontraceptive benefits of the sponge may become more apparent. For the most part, use of the sponge is associated with no significant side effects. Since there are no foaming or effervescent agents in the sponge, irritation has been quite low in clinical trials (less than 2 percent of users).

Persons sensitive to spermicides, however, may experience an allergic response.

At least one study suggests that nonoxynol-9 as a vaginal contraceptive offers some prophylaxis against gonorrhea and other sexually transmitted diseases [2].

Because tampon use has been associated with toxic shock syndrome (TSS) and since prolonged diaphragm retention has led to anecdotal events of the same, studies have been conducted to discover whether the use of the sponge may lead to the same risk. In vitro testing (USP Antimicrobial Test) has shown that the contraceptive sponge has a bacteriostatic effect on the growth of several microorganisms, including *Staphylococcus aureus* associated with TSS [7]. Further, the presence of acidic agents in the sponges lowers the vaginal pH. Additionally, the sponge is a nonabrasive material as opposed to tampons. These facts tend to support the view that the sponge will not encourage growth of *S. aureus*. Seven cases of TSS associated with use of the vaginal sponge have been reported to the FDA. Some have been disputed diagnoses, and in all cases the user did not follow the instructions for use supplied by the manufacturer.

THE SPONGE AND THE FDA

As previously mentioned, the administration of the FDA and its medical advisory panel presently disagree in the area of appropriate claims by which the contraceptive sponge may be marketed. As of this printing, approval for marketing would restrict the duration of use of this sponge for 24 hours rather than 48 hours as initially approved by the advisory panel. It is expected, however, that continued studies in support of the 2-day use of the sponge will surface over ensuing years.

SUMMARY

A new sponge for vaginal contraception as a barrier method is now available in the United States. This method combines a barrier with a known spermicide and is available over the counter. Its universal size obviates the need for prescription fitting by a medical professional, and it is divorced from a critical timetable for peak effectiveness, unlike other spermicidal methods. Its convenience with multiple acts of coitus sets it apart from all other barrier methods of family planning.

With the increasing public awareness of body functions and the potential risks associated with various contraceptive techniques, safety and effectiveness become a prime concern of contraceptive users. The demonstrated high level of safety and competitive effectiveness of this intravaginal sponge barrier contraceptive makes it a desirable entry in the "cafeteria" of available birth control methods.

REFERENCES

1. Chvapil, M., et al. Preliminary testing of the contraceptive collagen sponge. *Obstet. Gynecol.* 56:503, 1980.
2. Cutler, J. C., et al. Vaginal contraceptives as prophylaxis against gonorrhea and other sexually transmissible diseases. *Adv. Plan. Parenthood* 12:45, 1977.
3. Edelman, D. A., Smith, S. C., and McIntyre, S. Comparative trial of the contraceptive sponge and diaphragm: A preliminary report. *J. Reprod. Med.* 28:781, 1983.
4. Lane, M. E. Contraception in adolescence. *Fam. Plann. Perspect.* 5:19, 1973.
5. Tyrer, L. B., and Bradshaw, L. E. Jost Intravaginal Device: A Spermicidal Sponge (IUD). In G. I. Zatuchni et al. (eds.), *Vaginal Contraception: New Developments* (PARFR Series on Fertility Regulation). Hagerstown, Md.: Harper & Row, 1979.
6. Vessey, M. P., et al. Efficacy of different contraceptive methods. *Lancet* 1:841, 1982.
7. Vorhauer, B. Presentation to the Food and Drug Administration Fertility and Maternal Health Drug Products Advisory Committee. Washington, D.C., Oct. 28, 1982.

21. Foams, Creams, and Suppositories

Louis G. Keith
Gary S. Berger
Marianne A. Jackson

The popularity of vaginal spermicides has fluctuated since pharmaceutical companies first introduced them in the 1930s. The market for vaginal spermicides in the United States peaked during the 1950s, only to drop precipitously with the introduction of hormonal contraception and the intrauterine device (IUD) in the 1960s. Now, in the 1980s, there is renewed interest in vaginal spermicides as an effective method of contraception [12].

Two factors have led to the widening acceptance that spermicides are beginning to enjoy. First, the women's health movement has generated increased awareness among women of their bodies and sexuality. Second, two decades of experience with both the pill and the IUD have revealed potential health risks for women who use them. Among the medical complications reported for pill users are blood clotting disorders and various cardiovascular, neurologic, hepatic, and dermatologic problems.

As an alternative to the pill or IUD, spermicides offer the advantages of showing few, if any, systemic interactions or toxic effects and of being the most accessible method of birth control. The couple who chooses spermicide-containing products for these advantages, however, must make some compromises with regard to effectiveness, convenience, and aesthetic issues.

In this chapter, after an analysis of the available products and their modes of action, we intend to discuss spermicides on the basis of the three issues that most influence the consideration of any contraceptive method: safety, effectiveness, and acceptability. We hope that our discussion will help show that the ideal contraceptive has not yet been developed and that the selection of any method over another always requires some compromise.

AVAILABLE PRODUCTS

Among the chemical preparations available as vaginal contraceptives are foams, creams, jellies, suppositories (also called *pessaries* or *vagatories*), and effervescent suppositories and tablets. Table 21-1 lists some of the products available in the United States. All these preparations contain a spermicide, a chemical agent that interferes with the functional activity of spermatozoa, and a vehicle, usually an inert ingredient, that carries the spermicide and holds it against the cervix. Foams and creams also rely on their ability to block the cervical os to achieve their maximum effectiveness, while jellies and some types of vaginal suppositories derive almost

The authors gratefully acknowledge the able editorial assistance of Vito Maiorano.

Table 21-1. Commercial spermicides currently available

Product	Manufacturer	Active ingredient	Concentration
Creams			
Conceptrol	Ortho	Nonoxynol-9	5%
Delfen	Ortho	Nonoxynol-9	5%
Koromex II Contraceptive Cream*	Holland-Rantos	Octoxynol	3%
Ortho-Creme*	Ortho	Nonoxynol-9	2%
Jellies			
Conceptrol Gel	Ortho	Nonoxynol-9	4%
Gynol II Jelly	Ortho	Nonoxynol-9	2%
Koromex II Contraceptive Jelly*	Holland-Rantos	Octoxynol	1%
Koromex II-A Contraceptive Jelly	Holland-Rantos	Nonoxynol-9	2%
Koromex Crystal Clear Gel	Holland-Rantos	Nonoxynol-9	2%
Ortho-Gynol Jelly*	Ortho	Nonoxynol-9	2%
Ramses Vaginal Jelly	Schmid Products	Nonoxynol-9	5%
Foams (without diaphragm)			
Because	Schering	Nonoxynol-9	8%
Delfen	Ortho	Nonoxynol-9	12.5%
Emko	Schering	Nonoxynol-9	8%
Emko Pre-Fill	Schering	Nonoxynol-9	8%
Koromex	Holland-Rantos	Nonoxynol-9	12.5%
Suppositories			
Encare	Thompson Medical Corp.	Nonoxynol-9	6.9%
Intercept	Ortho	Nonoxynol-9	5.6%
Prevetts	Fox Pharmacal	Nonoxynol-9	6.9%
Semicid	Whitehall Labs	Nonoxynol-9	6.3%
Vaginal sponge			
Today	VLI Corp.	Nonoxynol-9	125 mg

*For use with diaphragm only.

all their effectiveness from the chemical nature of their active ingredient.

Chemical Nature of Active Ingredients

A partial list of chemicals used as active ingredients in vaginal contraceptives is provided in Table 21-2. Although there may be considerable overlap, the mode of action of most spermicides falls into one of five general categories: (1) electrolytes, (2) sulphydryl-binding agents, (3) bactericides, (4) surfactants, and (5) enzyme inhibitors [22].

ELECTROLYTES
Electrolytes rely on the decreased spermatozoal activity and metabolism that has been associated with hypertonicity. Some preparations of high-salt jellies have been shown to be highly spermicidal in vitro [11], although none have made their way into commercial products. Boric acid and tartaric acid, which are used in some effervescent commercial products to generate the foam-

ing action, also exert some spermicidal effect through their electrolytic activity.

SULPHYDRYL-BINDING AGENTS
The category of sulphydryl-binding agents includes compounds that disrupt cellular function by oxidation, alkylation, or the formation of mercaptides. Oxidizing substances, such as hydrogen peroxide, o-iodobenzoate, and several hydroquinones, destroy the tertiary protein structure by converting the thiol group of cysteine residues into disulfide linkages. Some hydroquinones were incorporated into commercial products until the late 1950s, when they were banned because of potentially carcinogenic effects. Alkylating agents exert a similar effect, although through an entirely different mechanism. Mercaptide-forming agents, which include many different organometallic compounds, have been successfully incorporated into several commercial products. The most notable of these is phenylmercuric acetate, which was widely used as the active ingredient in such products as Koromex until a potential association

Table 21-2. Partial list of spermicidal agents

Surfactants
  Dodecaethylene glycol monolaurate
  Methoxypolyoxyethylene glycol 550 laurate
  Nonoxynol-9*
  p-diisobutylphenoxypolyethoxyethanol (Octoxynol)*
  p-methanylphenylpolyoxyethylene (8.8) ether (Menfegol)

Sulphydryl-binding agents
  Hydrogen peroxide
  Phenylmercuric acetate (PMA)
  Ricinoleic acid
  Sodium borate
  Zinc phenosulfonate

Bactericides
  Benzetonium chloride
  Chloramine
  8-Hydroxyquinoline sulfate (Chinosol)

Electrolytes
  Boric acid
  Tartaric acid
  Lactic acid

*Most commonly used in commercial preparations today.
Source: Adapted from J. L. McGuire and F. C. Greenslade.
Research in Vaginal Contraception: An Overview. In G. I.
Zatuchni et al. (eds.), *Vaginal Contraception: New Developments.*
Hagerstown, Md.: Harper & Row, 1979.

with chronically absorbed mercury (Minamata disease) was suggested.

BACTERICIDES

Bactericides constitute a very large group of agents that work through various mechanisms to immobilize sperm. Some, such as phenylmercuric acetate, overlap into other categories, but all have microbicidal activity and also provide protection against venereal diseases. Chloramine, benzethonium chloride, and Chinosol have had significant roles in modern contraceptive preparations, but most agents in this category have been subjected to governmental banning [22].

SURFACTANTS

Surface-active agents constitute the most widely used active ingredients of currently available spermicidal products. They are characterized by long-chain alkyl groups that can penetrate the lipoproteic membrane of spermatozoa with high affinity. Through this interaction with the cell membrane, surfactants increase the cell's permeability, leading to the leakage of cell components and the irreversible loss of sperm motility. Surfactant activity, however, is not entirely limited to sperm cells; the membranes of bacteria or any parasite that might be present in the vagina, as well as (unfortu-

nately) the cells forming the vaginal mucosa itself, all show some susceptibility to the potent effects of these agents. It is for this reason that a lower incidence of sexually transmitted diseases (STDs) is associated with the use of spermicidal products containing certain surfactants. And it is also for this reason that vaginal irritation is occasionally reported by women using these products. The issues of potential side effects and benefits of spermicides will be discussed more fully later.

Among the many long-chain surfactants that possess spermicidal activity, nonoxynol-9 (nonylphenoxypolyethoxyethanol) represents a special case: It is the single most widely used spermicide, worldwide. Its structure is given below.

$$C_9H_{19}-\!\!\!\!\bigcirc\!\!\!\!-(OCH_2CH_2)_9OH$$

Despite the fact that nonoxynol-9 is one of only six spermicidal agents to receive a safe rating from the FDA, some controversy has recently surfaced regarding the possible systemic effects of this compound. Questions have been raised based on a series of recent findings on the pharmacokinetics of nonoxynol-9. In tests on rats, Chvapil and coworkers [8] showed that continued intravaginal administration of large doses (5mg/100gm/day) of nonoxynol-9 resulted in significant elevation of serum glutamic oxaloacetic transaminase (SGOT), a marker of tissue injury, after 5 days and a significant increase of collagen accumulation in liver cells, as determined by total hydroxyproline content, after 15 days. Another study by the same group showed that nonoxynol-9 is rapidly transported from the vagina to the blood in rabbits in which a collagen sponge containing 110 mg of the agent had been inserted intravaginally. The surfactant (a small portion of which had been ^{14}C-labeled) was detected in the blood within a few minutes of its intravaginal application, and almost 100 percent of it was found to be reabsorbed from the sponge within 6 days. Table 21-3, which shows the distribution of the labeled material after 6 days, also raises questions about the ability of animal tissue to metabolize surface-active agents. Only half the dose was detected in the fecal and urinary excretions, and the muscle tissue retained a far greater percentage than did adipose tissue. The labeled material noted in exhaled carbon dioxide cannot be construed as evidence that nonoxynol-9 was being metabolized, because the purity of the sample was no better than 70 to 80 percent, as determined by thin layer chromatography [8].

Almost no information is available on the metabolic effects of nonoxynol-9 in humans. One preliminary study found significant reductions in serum cholesterol levels in women using nonoxynol-9, but the study was

Table 21-3. Distribution of ^{14}C-labeled nonoxynol-9 in the rabbit after 6 days*

Body tissue or excretion	% of dose
Muscle (estimated, assuming 40% of total body mass)	28.7
Fat (estimated, assuming 18.8% of total body mass)	2.2
Body tissues other than skin, bone, and bone marrow	1.0
Feces (collected up to 144 hr)	9.8
Urine (collected up to 144 hr)	39.9
CO_2 (estimated from 6-hr rat study)	3.0
Retained in sponge	0.4
Total recovered	85.0
Amount not accounted for	15.0

*Single intravaginal dose of 111 mg administered by collagen sponge.
Source: Reprinted with permission from M. Chvapil et al. New Data on the Pharmacokinetics of Nonoxynol-9. In G. I. Zatuchni et al. (eds.), *Vaginal Contraception: New Developments.* Hagerstown, Md.: Harper & Row, 1979.

based on a very small sample, and no conclusions were reached [8]. Further research must be conducted in this area.

ENZYME INHIBITORS

The utilization of enzyme inhibitors, agents that neutralize the acrosomal enzymes needed by the spermatozoon to penetrate the egg, as vaginal contraceptives is a relatively recent innovation [28]. Although these substances hold much promise for the future, none has as yet found their way into commercially available preparations.

The most recent evidence indicates that at least three acrosomal enzymes are active on the sperm cell: hyaluronidase, which allows the spermatozoon to pass through the cumulus oophorus; corona-penetrating enzyme (CPE), which facilitates penetration between corona cells; and acrosin, a proteolytic enzyme that permits the spermatozoon to transverse the zona pellucida (Fig. 21-1). Several researchers [7, 17, 24] have reported on the use of hyaluronidase inhibitors as contraceptive agents in animal studies. Chang and Pincus [7] found up to 80 percent inhibition of fertility with oral and intraperitoneal administration of phosphorylated hesperidin. Joyce et al. [15] used two hyaluronidase inhibitors, phosphorylated hesperidin and hydroquinone sulfonic acid (53 D/k), and two acrosin inhibitors, TLCK (N-a-p-tosyl-L-lysine chloromethyl ketone HCl) and

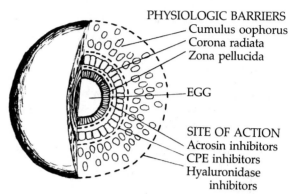

PHYSIOLOGIC BARRIERS
Cumulus oophorus
Corona radiata
Zona pellucida

EGG

SITE OF ACTION
Acrosin inhibitors
CPE inhibitors
Hyaluronidase inhibitors

Fig. 21-1. The physiologic barriers that the spermatozoa must traverse to fertilize the egg. The broken lines indicate the site of inhibition for each of the acrosomal enzyme inhibitors.

NPGB (p-nitrophenyl-p-guanidinobenzoate), as intravaginal contraceptives in studies on the rabbit. Using a dosage of 200 μg per milliliter, they found 100 percent fertility inhibition with 53 D/k, 100 percent with TLCK, 98 percent with NPGB, and 79 percent with phosphorylated hesperidin. The high specificity of acrosomal enzyme inhibitors, both in their area of activity within the body and in their ability to differentiate among species, suggests that these agents may become the ideal topical contraceptive, once testing has established their safety and effectiveness in humans.

Vehicles

Several pharmaceutical modalities possess the properties necessary for effectively transporting the active ingredient into the vagina: jellies, creams, pastes, nonfoaming suppositories, effervescent suppositories, plastic films, and the sponge.

Although the vehicle is usually an inert ingredient, it does provide some additional contraceptive activity of its own because it prevents the spermatozoa from coming into direct contact with the cervical mucus. Nonfoaming suppositories, creams, and jellies rely on the body temperature to melt them, allowing them to achieve the dispersion necessary for their effectiveness. Creams and jellies need only a few minutes to complete this process, but suppositories should be inserted 15 to 30 minutes before intercourse. Foams, creams, jellies, and suppositories must be placed high up in the vagina in order to cover the cervical os.

Effervescent suppositories were developed in an attempt to increase the vehicle's ability to disperse the active ingredient throughout the vagina. This vehicle uses sodium carbonate and an organic acid to interact with acidic vaginal secretions and create the carbon dioxide foam that disperses the active ingredient throughout the vagina within 3 to 10 minutes. Some women, however, have reported that the heat generated by this process can be uncomfortable.

Johnson, Masters, and Lewit [14] studied the dynamics of using vaginal contraceptives, taking into account such variables as changes in vaginal shape and in the quantity of secretions during sexual arousal and after orgasm. They found that vaginal creams and aerosol foams were dispersed immediately during sexual arousal to cover the mucosa of the vaginal vault and the cervical os. In contrast, jellies and suppositories dispersed unevenly, and foaming tablets showed inconsistent foaming capacity. This research group also reported on the ability of single doses of various preparations to prevent conception after multiple ejaculations. They found that, of the seven products tested, the most effective performers were a cream, a foam, and a gel—in that order—and concluded that the vehicle had little if any impact on long-term effectiveness [14].

Plastic films represent a recent innovation in vehicle technology. These devices are water soluble and rapidly dissolve upon insertion into the vagina. Preliminary findings show that they may find acceptance among couples who have rejected the latex condom on the grounds that it reduces sensation and among those women who consider foams and suppositories too messy or who experience a burning sensation with foaming tablets. Soluble film as a vehicle for spermicide also has the advantage of introducing less material into the vagina [2].

SAFETY CONSIDERATIONS

In the United States six commonly used spermicides have been deemed safe by the FDA: menfegol, nonoxynol-9, octoxynol-9, dodecaethyleneglycol monolaurate, laureth 10S, and methoxypolyoxyethyleneglycol 550 laurate. (The mode of action of these agents, as well as some recently raised concerns regarding nonoxynol-9, have been discussed in the section on Available Products.) On the other hand, phenylmercuric acetate, which had been successfully utilized in several commercial products, was recently classified as unsafe [9]. Although no dangers have been directly linked to the use of this compound, the general neurogenic toxicity of other mercury-containing agents is well established. Two bits of specific evidence sealed the fate of phenylmercuric acetate: (1) Toxic effects have been linked to it in animal embryos; and (2) in humans it has been detected in the maternal circulation, in breast milk, and in fetal tissue after vaginal administration. Quaternary ammonium compounds and boron-containing compounds, both of which have been used in contraceptive preparations as preservatives, have also been classified as unsafe [9].

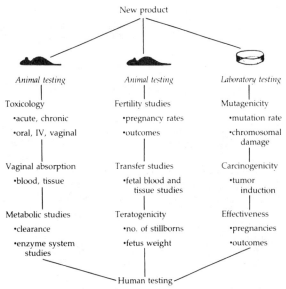

Fig. 21-2. Screening process for vaginal contraceptive development. (Modified from E. B. Connell. Vaginal Contraception: Current FDA Status. In G. I. Zatuchni et al. [eds.]. *Vaginal Contraception: New Developments.* Hagerstown, Md.: Harper & Row, 1979.)

The FDA's classification method is based primarily on animal studies in which the agents are administered intravaginally and on laboratory testing. The December 1980 report of the FDA Panel on Vaginal Contraceptives recommended that an extensive series of studies be conducted on all new products. These tests, which are designed to ensure an adequate level of safety before testing proceeds to studies on humans, cover such safety issues as toxicology and teratogenicity in animals, mutagenicity and carcinogenicity in cell cultures, and transfer and metabolic rates in animal tissues [9]. The schema presented in Figure 21-2 illustrates the extensiveness of the screening process.

Despite the careful and comprehensive testing that each of the approved spermicidal agents has been subjected to, a couple of safety issues remain. One such issue is the vaginal irritation that has occasionally been reported with the use of topic contraceptives. In this case the concern centers on the mechanism by which this minor skin irritation develops. As epithelial membrane disruption occurs after use of surface-active spermicides, the vaginal epithelium becomes increasingly thin, and vaginal intolerance and irritation develop [22]. As the epithelium wears down, the risk that surface-active ingredients may penetrate into the submucosa and be absorbed there increases. The tissue is well vascularized and has a high resorption capacity, and it is possible that spermicidal agents readily pass into the systemic circulation and exert effects that have not yet been recognized.

Another area of concern has been raised by a study by Jick et al. [13], in which it was reported that the risk of some specific congenital birth defects may be 2 times greater among women using vaginal spermicide. In a review of computerized records, they found an excess of limb-reduction abnormalities, neoplasms, chromosomal abnormalities, and hypospadias in infants born to women who *presumably* had been exposed to spermicides. *The report did not establish when the spermicide was used in relation to pregnancy—or even that it was used at all—because exposure was simply defined as having filled at least one prescription for a spermicide-containing product within 600 days of the termination of pregnancy.*

A more recent study by Mills et al. [19] was designed to further explore some of the concerns raised by Jick's report; these workers were unable to find any association between maternal spermicide exposure before or after the last menstrual period and congenital malformations. This study design identified the type of spermicide and the time it was used in relation to pregnancy. These features and the large sample size employed make it a far more accurate representation of the possible teratogenic effects of spermicide use. The investigators conclude by observing that the data indicate that even accidental exposure to spermicides after conception is probably not teratogenic.

Other studies have suggested that spermicides may damage the newly fertilized ovum [23, 26]. The abortuses of women who had been exposed to spermicidal agents around the time of conception were found to have higher risks of chromosomal abnormalities than abortuses from unexposed women. These observations do not agree with the findings of Mills et al. [19] or a large study in Japan on abortus material.

HEALTH BENEFITS OF SPERMICIDES

Changes in sexual mores have led to an increase in the incidence of sexually transmitted diseases (STDs). The toll of these infections is great, not only in terms of death, disease, and disability, but also in terms of loss of work, frequent outpatient visits, and expensive therapies. Therefore, the emergence of data suggesting that widespread and consistent use of vaginal contraceptive products could dramatically reduce the incidence of STDs contributed greatly to the resurgence of interest in vaginal methods [12].

Gonorrhea

A lowered incidence of cervical gonorrhea is associated with the use of chemical vaginal contraception [3]. The only difference observed among gonorrhea cultures from cervical, rectal, and oropharyngeal sites, in a study comparing contraceptive methods, was the significantly lower rate of cervical gonorrhea in women using any form of barrier contraception. Since incidences of oral and rectal infection showed no variations, the chemical barrier contraceptives probably determined the reduction.

Studies in vitro have demonstrated that many of the surface-active ingredients commonly used in modern spermicidal preparations also inhibit the growth of gonococci [5, 10, 21]. Moreover, in the only available clinical study [10], contraceptive foam appeared to reduce the recurrence rate for infections of *Neisseria gonorrhoeae* among high-risk women. The protection afforded by foam may stem from its ability to lower vaginal pH and thereby create an environment that is either bactericidal or bacteriostatic for *N. gonorrhoeae*.

Candidiasis and Trichomoniasis

Laboratory studies suggest that most spermicides inhibit the growth of *Candida albicans* and *Trichomonas vaginalis*. Although more clinical studies are needed to establish the effectiveness of these compounds as antifungal and antiparasitic agents, the one published clinical report that we are aware of suggests that they are potent indeed. In that study Lazar [16] compared the incidence of *T. vaginalis* infection among women using the pill, IUDs, diaphragms, condoms, foams, and no contraceptive method at all. Examining the cytologic smears of 11,197 women, he diagnosed trichomoniasis in nearly 6 percent of pill users and IUD users compared with only 3 percent of diaphragm users and less than 1 percent of women using foam.

Herpesvirus Infections

Genital infection with herpes simplex virus types 1 and 2 (herpes hominus 1 and 2) has reached epidemic proportions in the United States. The relatively mild physiologic effects of the infection have, in many cases, become a secondary concern to the severe depression that commonly is seen among patients with this disease, for which there is no known cure. Only methods that prevent primary infection are likely to be successful in decreasing its incidence. Two recently published reports provide evidence that the use of vaginal contraceptives may prevent the spread of herpes.

Postic et al. [20] studied two spermicidal compounds

in terms of their ability to inactivate herpesvirus. They examined Preceptin Gel, whose active ingredient is a surfactant similar to nonoxynol-9, and a spermicide-germicide compound (SGCA) that is currently under development. Each strain of virus tested was inactivated by a 5% emulsion of Preceptin Gel. The potency of SGCA even exceeded that of the Preceptin Gel.

Asculai and coworkers [1] conducted a similar study to determine the virucidal effects of surface-active ingredients in commercially available spermicidal preparations. They exposed herpesvirus strains to various dilutions of nonoxynol-9 and triton X-100 and to unaltered samples of six other available products (Delfen cream, Preceptin Gel, Emko foam, Koromex jelly, Lorophyn gel, and Ramses gel). All the products were found to inactivate the viruses. Electron microscopy studies revealed that the viruses were quickly denuded of their outer, lipid-containing envelopes and that degradation of the inner core began shortly thereafter. In this state the virus apparently loses its infectivity [1].

EFFECTIVENESS REVIEW

In general, all contraceptive failures can be placed into one of two categories: failure of the method itself, often called *biologic failure*, and failure of the contraceptive user to apply the method properly. In reporting efficacy rates, many researchers do not attempt to distinguish between these two types of failures because, in a very real sense, the frequency with which a method induces user errors can be plausibly thought of as a flaw in the method itself.

As is the case with other barrier methods, most instances of spermicide failure can be traced to problems in patient compliance. User-related problems include acts of intercourse when the method is not used, failure to use the recommended amount of spermicide, failure to use additional spermicide when intercourse is repeated, insertion of spermicide too long before intercourse, and failure to leave diaphragm or cap in place long enough after intercourse (if spermicide is used as part of a combined method) or premature douching (if spermicide is used alone). The specific issue regarding the acceptability of spermicide methods and the reasons behind user-initiated failures will be discussed in the next section. Here, we will review efficacy rates as determined by tests in humans under controlled conditions and in clinical field trials.

Controlled Conditions Testing in Vivo

Although no one would dispute the value of compiling substantial data on in vivo human testing under various controlled conditions, relatively few researchers have tested spermicides in this way. The problems associated with in vivo testing include (1) the time and cost required for such testing, (2) the lack of established test standards that would allow results to be compared and that would determine which tests most accurately reflect clinical effectiveness, and (3) the limitations imposed by medicolegal and ethical requirements for protection of subjects.

Despite these formidable problems, in vivo human testing has established itself as an important intermediate step in the screening of new spermicide products—subsequent to in vitro and animal studies similar to the ones recommended by the FDA and before the initiation of field trials. In vivo tests have been conducted both after coitus and after artificial insemination under a variety of conditions. The method generally involves the microscopic examination of cervical and endocervical mucus for motile sperm; unfortunately, these tests have frequently given inconclusive results, largely because of inconsistencies in the study methods.

In testimony to the FDA Over-the-Counter Panel on Vaginal Contraceptives, Masters emphasized the need for further study in the area of in vivo human testing and the importance of developing standardized guidelines for such testing [18]. If progress is made in these areas, such methods may assume a greater role in efficacy testing; but for now, controlled in vivo testing serves in the screening process for new products, while actual efficacy can only be determined from clinical field studies.

Clinical Field Trials

Researchers have attempted to determine the effectiveness of spermicides through clinical field trials since 1937 and have documented failure rates ranging from less than 1 to nearly 30 per 100 woman-years of use (Table 21-4). The wide variation among failure rates reflects differences in study designs as well as differences in the actual effectiveness of various spermicides themselves. The lack of standardization of study protocols makes it very difficult to compare results. Some of the features of Table 21-4 demonstrate just how widely the study methods differed: The number of women included in the studies ranged from 130 to more than 10,000; the duration ranged from 12 months to 5 years; some studies excluded the first month, two months, or even 12 months of method exposure in calculating results; and different statistical procedures were used to calculate failure rates.

Perhaps the most significant factor contributing to the wide variation in documented failures among these

Table 21-4. Clinical field tests of spermicides, 1955–1977

Authors	Date of study	Product	Active ingredient	No. of women	No. of months	Duration of observation	Use failure	Method failure
Jellies								
Dingle & Tietze	1958–1961	Lactikol	Glyceryl monoricinoleic acid; nonoxynol-9	170	1,789	1–36	23.5	
Margolis et al.	1958–1960	Lanesta Gel	Ricinoleic acid	259	3,250	1–24	7.7	3.6
Kasabach	1958–1960	Koromex	PMA 0.02%; polyoxyethylene nonylphenol 0.5%	195	2,058	2–24	20.9	7.5
Frank	1959–1961	Koromex	PMA 0.02%; polyoxyethylene nonylphenol 0.5%	684	6,594	1–26	23.1	
Finkelstein & Goldberg	1955–1958	Immolin	Methoxypolyethylene glycol 550 laurate 5%	176	3,354	12–36	5.7	3.2
Foam Tablets								
Dingle & Tietze	1958–1961	Durofoam	Nonoxynol-9, 5%	240	1,749	1–36	22.0	
Ishihama & Inoue	1967–1969	Neosampoon	p-Methanylphenylpolyoxyethylene 8.8 ether	475	8,955	1–14	3.2	
Creams								
Rovinsky	1956–1962	Delfen	Nonoxynol-9, 5%	251	2,915	1–67	9.1	3.7
Aerosol foams								
Kleppinger	1962–1965	Delfen	Nonoxynol-9, 5%	138	1,116	1–19	7.6	2.2
Tietze & Lewit	1961–1963	Emko	Nonoxynol-9, 8%	779	4,590	1–57	28.3[a]	
Bushnell	1961–1965	Emko	Nonoxynol-9, 8%	130	2,737	1–57	1.75	
Bernstein	1968–1970	Emko	Nonoxynol-9, 8%	2,932	28,322	1–22	4.0	3.0
Foam suppository								
Brehm & Haase[b]	1970	Encare Oval	Nonoxynol-9	10,017	67,759	6.2 avg.	0.8	
Suppository								
Squire et al.	1972–1977	Semicid	Nonoxynol-9	326		1–49	0.6[a]	

PMA = phenylmercuric acetate.

[a]These rates are given as gross cumulative failure, the 28.3 figure after 1 year and the 0.6 after 2 years.

[b]This study is based on a questionnaire sent to 287 practitioners.

studies is the motivation of the patient population. For example, the exceptionally high efficacy (1.75 failures per 100 woman-years) reported by Bushnell [6] in his prospective clinical study of Emko contraceptive foam reflects the fact that he insisted that patients selected for his study demonstrate adequate motivation to adopt a contraceptive method and adhere to it. The study was conducted in a private practice setting, where the investigator had more of an opportunity to develop the kind of rapport with his patients that could foster the continued motivation necessary to achieve the results. The fact that none of the women in the study were lost to follow-up supports this contention.

The other criteria that Bushnell applied to his patient population included a reasonably regular menses, the absence of any disease that might interfere with conception, prior pregnancy (which was taken as evidence of fertility), and the ability of the subject to accurately report the medical history and any observations that might be relevant to the study. Bushnell's patient population showed a wide range in the duration of involvement in the study (1–57 months) and accrued 2,737 woman-months of exposure. Four pregnancies occurred; although all were linked to lapses in user compliance, there was not one clear-cut method failure.

Although this study speaks eloquently for the effectiveness of spermicide contraception, it may not provide the most representative picture. A small single-center study such as Bushnell's, in which the patient population is selected against stringent criteria, may reflect the influences of the researcher and experiment design. To get a more realistic view of the motivation for contraception in the general population, we would have to look at the larger multicenter studies.

The early 1960s report of Tietze and Lewit [25] and the late 1960s report of Bernstein [4] merit attention in this regard. These two studies, which utilized the same product and which were conducted according to similar guidelines, show vastly different results. Tietze and Lewit, calculating results according to the life-table method, reported a gross cumulative failure rate of 28.3 per 100 women. In contrast, Bernstein found an overall Pearl rate of only 4 per 100 woman-years and 3.0 method failures per 100 woman-years. Again, motivation provides the clue that explains this great discrepancy. Tietze and Lewit studied several contraceptive methods concurrently, and all of them showed method failures far in excess of theoretical rates. This makes one suspect a predominance of patient rather than method failures. In contrast, the difference between method failures and overall failures in Bernstein's study is small, indicating that the selected population was probably more motivated and diligent.

It is clear to see that the vagaries and errors of various study methods have led to wildly disparate efficacy rates being reported throughout the literature, but we still have not established which rate gives the most accurate picture. From the point of view of a woman selecting a contraceptive method, perhaps the most accurate estimates are the failure rates obtained in prospectively designed studies of highly motivated, intelligent women who have been adequately instructed in the proper application of the method and who have received some follow-up. Under these conditions, modern foams, creams, and jellies have a biologic failure rate of about 2 to 5 per 100 woman-years [12].

ACCEPTABILITY

In his review of an article on the possible adverse effects of vaginal spermicides, Williamson [27] noted that this method of contraception has an actual failure rate considerably in excess of the theoretical failure rate, which raises some questions about usage patterns. Usage patterns are a reflection of the acceptability of a method; they include all those characteristics of a particular method—things like cost, convenience, comfort, aesthetics, and availability—that induce a woman to use it. Thus, acceptability has a great deal to do with the ultimate effectiveness of a contraceptive method. Cultural aspects often play an important role in the selection of a method, but no single acceptability issue will determine whether a particular choice is more acceptable than another; rather, all these issues, along with safety and effectiveness, must be weighed together.

Accessibility and Cost

Of all the contraceptive methods available, spermicidal preparations are the most accessible. Sold over the counter in pharmacies, retail stores, and outlets and distributed by family planning clinics and even physicians, they require no prescription, little, if any, counseling, and no fitting examination. The easy access of spermicidal products enhances their appeal for women who do not wish to be examined genitally, who do not wish to reveal their sexual relations, and who do not have access to appropriate medical care facilities. The same basic reasons make them attractive to adolescents.

Another factor that increases the appeal of spermicides is their low cost. Spermicides have a long shelf life and represent an excellent way to keep an inexpensive method of contraception in constant reach for women who need occasional use.

Table 21-5. Essential instructions for the use of spermicides

- Foams can be inserted within a minute or two before intercourse. Creams and jellies need a few minutes more to reach body temperature, melt, and achieve even distribution. Suppositories should be inserted 15 to 30 minutes before intercourse.

- The patient should make sure that foams, creams, jellies, and suppositories are applied high up in the vagina in order to cover the cervical os.

- The patient should wait at least 6 hours before douching. If the combination of spermicide and semen becomes too messy, she should let the excess drain into the toilet and wash the external genitalia with a damp cloth. Additional acts of coitus require repeated applications of spermicide.

- In the event that minor burning or irritation develops, the user should try switching to another brand or, if irritation is experienced with many different products, consider using an alternative method.

- The cervical cap minimizes the amount of spermicide exposed to the vagina or penis. The use of condoms will also protect the male from exposure to spermicidal agents and thus help him to avoid undesired side effects associated with spermicidal preparations.

Source: Adapted from M. Jackson, G. S. Berger, and L. G. Keith. *Vaginal Contraception.* Boston: G. K. Hall, 1981.

Convenience and Comfort

Spermicides are convenient in the sense that infrequent users are not tied to the method. On the other hand, if spontaneity is an important concern in the selection of a contraceptive method, spermicides cannot be the method of choice; Table 21-5, which lists the essential instructions for the use of spermicides, shows what an important element time is in the effective use of spermicidal preparations.

Among comfort issues, burning and irritation are the most frequently mentioned by spermicide users; this is especially the case for users of foaming suppositories, with which a burning sensation has been reported by both partners. Aesthetic issues, such as the excessive leakage or odor that is perceived by some women, may also play an important role in a woman's selection of one method over another.

In addition to these general acceptability issues, special considerations sometimes exist in certain circumstances. For example, spermicides have appeal as a backup method in cases where a woman misses a pill or has reason to suspect the reliability of her IUD. Spermicides can also serve as an interim measure between other methods or before a regimen of oral contraceptives is initiated or an IUD is inserted.

REFERENCES

1. Asculai, S., et al. Inactivation of herpes simplex viruses by nonionic surfactants. *Antimicrob. Agents Chemother.* 13:10, 1975.

2. Belsky, R. Water-Soluble Condom and Vaginal Contraceptive Film Insert. In G. I. Zatuchni et al. (eds.), *Vaginal Contraception: New Developments.* Hagerstown, Md.: Harper & Row, 1979.

3. Berger, G. S., Keith, L. G., and Moss, W. Prevalence of gonorrhea among women using various methods of contraception. *Br. J. Vener. Dis.* 51:307, 1975.

4. Bernstein, G. S. Clinical effectiveness of an aerosol contraceptive foam. *Contraception* 3:37, 1971.

5. Bolch, O. H., Jr., and Warren, J. C. In vitro effects of Emko on *Neisseria gonorrhoeae* and *Trichomonas vaginalis. Am. J. Obstet. Gynecol.* 115:1145, 1973.

6. Bushnell, L. F. Aerosol foam: A practical and effective method of contraception. *Pacific Med. Surg.* 73:353, 1965.

7. Chang, M. C., and Pincus, G. Does phosphorylated hesperidin affect fertility? *Science* 117:274, 1953.

8. Chvapil, M., et al. New Data on the Pharmokinetics of Nonoxynol 9. In G. I. Zatuchni et al. (eds.), *Vaginal Contraception: New Developments.* Hagerstown, Md.: Harper & Row, 1979.

9. Connell, E. B. Vaginal Contraception: Current FDA Status. In G. I. Zatuchni et al. (eds.), *Vaginal Contraception: New Developments.* Hagerstown, Md.: Harper & Row, 1979.

10. Cutler, J. C., et al. Vaginal contraceptives as prophylaxis against gonorrhea and other sexually transmissible disease. *Adv. Plann. Parenthood* 12:45, 1977.

11. Gamble, C. J. An improved test of spermicidal activity without dilution or mixing. *J.A.M.A.* 152:1037, 1953.

12. Jackson, M., Berger, G. S., and Keith, L. G. *Vaginal Contraception.* Boston: G. K. Hall, 1981.

13. Jick, H., et al. Vaginal spermicides and congenital disorders. *J.A.M.A.* 245:1329, 1981.

14. Johnson, V. E., Masters, W. H., and Lewit, K. C. The Physiology of Intravaginal Contraceptive Failure. In M. S. Calderone (ed.), *Manual of Contraceptive Practice.* Baltimore: Williams & Wilkins, 1964.

15. Joyce, C., Freund, M., and Peterson, R. N. Contraceptive effect of intravaginal application of acrosin and hyaluronidase inhibitors in the rabbit. *Contraception* 19:95, 1979.

16. Lazar, A. *Trichomonas vaginalis* infection: Incidence with use of various contraceptive methods. *J. Med. Soc. N.J.* 67:225, 1970.

17. Martin, G. L., and Beiler, J. M. Effect of phosphorylated hesperidin and other flavonoids on fertility in mice. *Science* 115:402, 1952.

18. Masters, W. Testimony before the Food and Drug Administration. Panel on Vaginal Contraceptives, May 20, 1978.

19. Mills, J. L., et al. Are spermicides teratogenic? *J.A.M.A.* 248:2148, 1982.

20. Postic, B., et al. Inactivation of clinical isolates of herpesvirus hominis, types 1 and 2, by chemical contraceptives. *Sex. Transm. Dis.* 5:22, 1978.

21. Singh, B., Cutler, J. C., and Utidjian, H. M. D. Studies on the development of a vaginal preparation providing both prophylaxis against venereal disease and other genital infections and contraception. II. Effect in vitro of vaginal contraceptive and noncontraceptive preparations on *Treponema pallidum* and *Neisseria gonorrhoeae*. *Br. J. Vener. Dis.* 48:57, 1972.

22. Sobrero, A. J. Spermicidal Agents: Effectiveness, Use and Testing. In G. I. Zatuchni et al. (eds.), *Vaginal Contraception: New Developments*. Hagerstown, Md.: Harper & Row, 1979.

23. Strobino, B., et al. Exposure to contraceptive creams, jellies, and douches and their effect on the zygote. *Am. J. Epidemiol.* 112:434, 1980.

24. Thompson, R. Q., Sturtevant, B., and Bird, O. D. Effect of phosphorylated hesperidin, a hyaluronidase inhibitor, on fertility in rats. *Science* 118:657, 1953.

25. Tietze, C., and Lewit, S. Comparison of three contraceptive methods: Diaphragm with jelly or cream, vaginal foam, and jelly/cream alone. *J. Sex. Res.* 3:392, 1967.

26. Warburton, D., et al. Environmental influences on rates of chromosomal anomalies in spontaneous abortions, abstracted. *Am. J. Hum. Genet.* 32:92, 1980.

27. Williamson, R. A. Commentary. In R. M. Pitkin and F. J. Zlatnik (eds.), *Year Book of Obstetrics and Gynecology*. Chicago: Year Book, 1982. P. 207.

28. Zanefeld, L. J. D., Robertson, R. T., and Williams, W. L. Synthetic enzymes as antifertility agents. *FEBS Lett.* 11:345, 1970.

22. Condoms: The Rubber Remedy

Michael J. Free

The condom is the only reversible method of contraception available to the male at the present time. Since no other promising contraceptive methods are emerging from current clinical trials, it is safe to assume that the condom will remain the predominant and perhaps the only reversible male method for at least the next 10 years. Although the condom has a long history of use in human sexual practice, present-day condoms are thoroughly up-to-date devices. They remain the only method that is effective both as a contraceptive and as a prophylactic against diseases transmitted by genital contact. Furthermore, even in combination with backup postcoital steroid regimens or abortion in the event of disuse, misuse, or method failure, they provide the lowest health risk of any method of contraception.

There is a growing need for male involvement in the practice of contraception as well as a need for solutions to reproductive health and social problems such as unwanted pregnancy in teenagers, and aversion to or rejection of side effects attendant upon systemic or uterine contraceptive methods. The condom can address all these problems in a remarkably effective way. It is time for health professionals to come to terms with the condom.

The condom is usually categorized as a "traditional" method; thus, it is often viewed as a historic artifact. Since it was the only effective method available during an age of sexual repression, it retains the stigma of association with promiscuity and venereal disease and may offend sensibilities with its obvious penile shape and size. As a nonprescription item, it is often forgotten during discussions within the doctor's office or clinic. Too many physicians erroneously assume that their patients who are seeking birth control advice have already rejected the over-the-counter options. This withholding of professional emphasis on the condom as a serious option conveys to the patient an impression that the method is less worthy of consideration than the prescription methods, even when his or her lifestyle, sexual behavior patterns, age, or risk factors indicate condoms as a method of choice. The failure of physicians to consider this method can have far-reaching implications, even for people who for one reason or another do not seek medical advice on contraception. The emphasis that is placed or withheld by physicians generates opinions in the community that ultimately affect laws, institutional sanctions, and attitudes. The editorial pleas issued by the *Journal of the American Medical Association* in 1979 for organized medicine and public health to take the lead in influencing public attitudes toward the condom have gone relatively unheeded [33]. The problems that can be effectively ameliorated by widespread condom use are continuing to mount.

Why did an instantly reversible contraceptive with 98

percent method effectiveness, no negative side effects, wide availability, and relatively low cost, which offers good protection against sexually transmitted diseases (STD), become so neglected in the United States? What are the flaws inherent in this method such that it should be rejected in favor of methods with similar or only slightly better protection, tangible and disruptive side effects, and little or no protection against sexually transmitted diseases, and which require a doctor's office visit? How can these flaws be neutralized or minimized so that the potential of this method can be brought to bear upon the problems of teenage pregnancy, sexually transmitted diseases, and aversion to or rejection of side effects attendant upon the use of other methods?

CONDOMS REVISITED

The idea of a physical barrier against venereal disease must have become obvious quite early in the history of civilization. Use by the male of barriers for the prevention of pregnancy came later [20, 36]. A variety of materials and contrivances for these purposes have been recorded in the literature and include linen, plant pods, animal skin, and animal intestines. A refined version of the last material, a product prepared from the caecum of lambs, has survived to the present day and is now a luxury product costing $1 to $2 per condom. Although the vast majority of condoms produced in the past 130 years have been rubber, the tough, porous, relatively thick caecal ("skin") condom is considered an optimum barrier device by many condom users, suggesting that:

Thinness is not the ultimate criterion for sensitivity in a condom.
Elasticity is not an absolute necessity for condom function; in fact, the movement of the penis inside the lubricated condom may be an enhancing attribute (however, size is more important with nonelastic condoms).
Pinholes and porosity are not directly related to condom effectiveness.

The development of vulcanization in the mid–nineteenth century and the introduction of the latex dipping process in the 1930s made possible the mass production of rubber condoms at a much lower cost in comparison with animal caecum condoms [20]. Rubber condoms were, by nature, highly elastic, relatively impermeable, and less conductive of heat than the animal products. While early reusable intestine and rubber condoms were offered in different sizes for proper fit, the modern, thin, dipped latex membranes with 600 to 900 percent stretchability permitted a one-size-fits-all

approach to condom marketing. This approach became standard for the industry until recent times when different sizes were again introduced to provide maximum comfort and sensitivity. The changes in condom technology since the introduction of the rubber condom have brought about a progressive improvement in the average effectiveness, reliability, sensitivity, and attractiveness of the method.

The original rubber condoms were made of crepe rubber, ground up and dissolved in organic solvents. The solvent rendered the product "smelly" and sometimes irritating to the tissues. These condoms were thick and frequently defective. The change to a process of dip molding in latex concentrate, the centrifuged and ammonia-stabilized aqueous exudate of the rubber tree, brought about a substantial improvement in the product by eliminating solvent residues and permitting the manufacture of thinner products with increased resistance to aging. Automation of the latex dipping process increased the uniformity of the product. The development of a hot curing process further increased the durability of condoms, resulting in a shelf life of 5 or more years under temperate conditions. The United States Food and Drug Administration (USFDA) introduced a formal regulatory program for condoms in 1949, which became progressively more stringent until 1968 [3]. The British Standards Institute also published quality standards in 1964 and began to award their seal of approval to products that complied.

Although these standards and regulations were based on pinholes which, in themselves, have questionable relevance to the failure of condoms as a contraceptive or even as a disease prophylactic, they nevertheless provided an easily measurable and apparently effective test for monitoring good manufacturing practices in the condom industry. Under this climate of regulation, changes in all phases of production brought about substantial improvement in the reliability of the product. In the 1960s the practice of electronic screening became widespread in the condom industry. This process, in which every condom is tested for electric conductance, ensured that condoms would meet the increasingly stringent standards for pinholes. It is still not clear whether electronic screening did indeed weed out the weak condoms, and with the present high state of the dipping art and proposed changes in U.S. and international test procedures for pinholes, the cost-benefit ratio of electronic screening is in question.

Special finishing processes, including "dry" silicone lubrication introduced in the 1960s, have given condoms some of the "feel" of the natural membrane product. About 80 percent of the condoms sold in the United States are lubricated with silicone or water-based lubricants. Lubrication reduces the frictional stress and therefore the chance of breakage in a localized area of the condom wall. This process also makes the condom more comfortable and pleasurable for both partners when natural secretions are inadequate. Thinness of the rubber membrane in the modern condom compensates for the lower heat-transmitting properties of rubber when compared with the collagenous natural "skin" membrane. New untextured condoms vary in thickness from 0.03 to 0.07 mm, compared with those of 0.06 to 0.09 mm of only a decade ago. By flaring the glans area of the thin-walled condoms and lubricating both inside and out, a quality similar to that of the animal caecum condom has been achieved in some models, whereby the penis is free to move to some extent inside the condom.

The shape of the condom is determined by the shape of the condom molds (forms or formers). The incorporation of reservoirs into the tip of the condom was a very useful early modification of the basic shape, providing space for the ejaculate and a more obvious tactile and visual means whereby the user can verify that the method was effective. The production of other shape changes required refinements in the stripping of the dipped product from the mold. In the past few years improved stripping techniques have led to the production of various shapes, most of which may have no more than aesthetic or novel appeal. However, some shapes like the flared-glans condom mentioned earlier may have sensory significance, and others may be better adapted to the circumcised penis.

Changes in condom packaging have ensured durability in temperate climates and provided some additional protection against "pocket" damage. While the early individual foil and plastic laminated packages were difficult to open, the introduction of serrated package edges makes opening easy, even in the dark.

The most evident changes in condoms over the past years have been aesthetic. Introduction of color and texture, attractive packaging, and marketing appeal to women were common more than 15 years ago in Japan but are relatively recent innovations in the U.S. market. Much of the impetus for innovation and creative merchandising of condoms comes from Japan, where 75 percent of contraceptors use condoms [42]. The extensive experience with ultrathin products in Japan has led to enormous improvements in strength and incidence of pinholes in these condoms, so that they are now able to pass the regulatory requirements of the United States and are in the American marketplace. However, the thinnest U.S. product (Nuda; Ansell Inc., Dothan, Ala.) is now quite similar to the ultrathin Japanese products when thickness over the important glans area is compared (Table 22-1).

The latest innovation in condom design arose from the condom industry in the Western world and involves the incorporation of spermicide in the condom

Table 22-1. Typical thickness of condoms

Brand	Thickness (mm)		
	Open end	Middle	Closed end
Japanese, U.S., or U.K. standard brands	0.05	0.06	0.07
Japanese "ultrathin" brands	0.03	0.04	0.045
Thinnest U.S. brand	0.04	0.04	0.045
Animal caecum "skin" brand	0.07	0.06	0.08

lubricant. This product (Ramses Extra; Schmid Laboratories, Inc., Little Falls, N.J.), recently approved conditionally by the USFDA [42], may provide an additional measure of protection in those cases where the condom slips off due to postejaculatory detumescence while the penis is still in the vagina or in the rare instance of breakage. Spermicide-lubricated condoms now account for 40 percent of all condom sales in the United Kingdom.

These developments in condom production technology over the past 40 years have brought about a remarkable improvement in the quality of the product. The USFDA estimated that 75 percent of the condoms produced in the United States in 1939 were defective; between 1942 and 1960 this proportion declined to 4 percent and in 1961 fell to between 0.4 and 0.7 percent [3].

Even with the new, more stringent standards that permitted the USFDA to seize condom shipments containing more than 0.24 percent of defective units, the proportion of questionable shipments between 1969 and 1972 was only one-third of that for the previous 3-year period [42].

Obviously, the much-quoted estimate of condom breakage of 1 in 150 to 1 in 300 [44], based on studies carried out in the 1940s, is unlikely to have much meaning for condom users today. Since old-style condom dipping machinery is still operating in some parts of the world, it is possible to gain an impression of the difference in condom strength of old-style products compared with that of the modern product (Fig. 22-1). The crucial difference is in the uniformity of strength in the modern product, making for greatly improved reliability. If properly stored and handled, the modern product can be expected to be uniformly strong, whereas 20 to 40 years ago up to 30 percent of condoms might be so weak that they would stand a high chance of being broken during use. Some indication of the relationship between this strength of condoms and breakage during use was obtained from a clinical study, using condoms

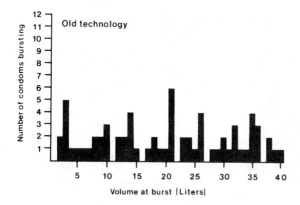

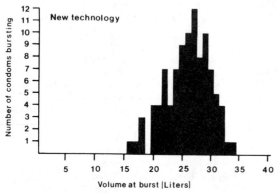

Fig. 22-1. Uniformity in strength of condoms: Old versus new technology.

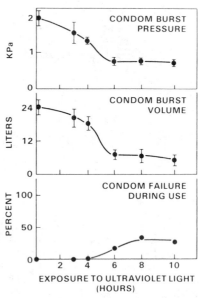

Fig. 22-2. Relationship between condom strength and breakage during use.

that had been artificially deteriorated to different levels of strength (Fig. 22-2) [11]. These data demonstrate the considerable reserve of strength that exists in the modern condom and also show that the strength of the condom, as determined by air burst tests, can relate to actual use conditions. The study also demonstrates the importance of keeping condoms out of the light and, if possible, of avoiding transparent packaging, since ultraviolet light destroys condoms in a matter of just a few hours.

Progress in Marketing and Promotion

The number of condom users throughout the world is estimated to be about 40 million, including 3 million in the United States and Canada, more than 10 million in Japan, and nearly 7 million in northern and western Europe, including the United Kingdom. In Japan condoms are used by 75 percent of contracepting couples; in Scandinavian countries 20 to 40 percent of contraceptors rely on the condom.

The United Kingdom, Trinidad, Tobago, and Singapore all had a prevalence of condom use of more than 20 percent of contracepting couples in recent years [42]. These countries reflect a wide range of sexual attitudes, cultural practices, and traditions of contraception. While there are often special factors that enhance condom use, such as the absence of other legal modern methods in Japan, these high use rates point to the possibilities for condom use in the United States. It is clear that condoms can be integrated successfully into diverse patterns of sexual behavior and practice. Freed of its cultural stigmata and promoted by the powerful media and advertising techniques of our day, condom use could probably become a more widespread practice in the United States.

Many new condom users are emerging from the ranks of couples who had previously relied upon oral contraceptives, as indicated by nearly 70 percent of respondents to a consumer survey on condom use, who switched from the use of the pill because of fear of the side effects [38]. The important population of condom users reflected in this report were mostly married and using condoms for contraception rather than for prevention of a sexually transmitted disease. From the promotional and public health points of view, this group must be viewed in an entirely different light than young, single, sexually active people. This latter group is more likely to have more than one sexual partner, is more at risk of sexually transmitted disease, and is less

Table 22-2. Effectiveness of the condom

	Couple-years of use	Total failures	Method failure	Total failure rate per 100 years	Method failure rate per 100 years	Reference
Group of highly fertile urban couples	127	4	1	3.1	0.8	34
Urban couples beginning at marriage	308	12	5	3.9	1.6	35
National Health Service patients in a small town practice	248	12	1	4.8	0.4	21
Married patients of family planning clinic who used oral contraceptives, diaphragm, or IUD before study	1,543	62	Unknown	4.0	Unknown	14
Aggregate of above studies	2,226	90	7	4.0	1.0	

predictable in its behavior, but it can be influenced by certain segments of the media using specific types of advertising and motivational messages. Therefore, the promotion of condoms for contraception alone must be kept distinctly separate from promotions targeted at groups with a high risk of sexually transmitted disease.

Condom marketing in the United States has improved enormously over the past 10 years, but it is still a long way behind that of other countries and even farther behind the state of American advertising art as reflected, for example, in advertising for cigarettes, blue jeans, and soft drinks. Although the restrictive National Association of Broadcasters Radio and Television Codes fell by the wayside in 1982, most television and radio stations have been reluctant to air commercials for contraceptives. Indeed, most polls show that people respond unfavorably to questions about contraceptive advertising on the broadcast media. They also have responded unfavorably to the broadcasting of advertisements on feminine hygiene products, hemorrhoid medication, and numerous other personal products. Interestingly, most respondents to surveys recognized the possible advantages and benefits of airing contraceptive commercials [8].

Despite these impediments to condom merchandising in the United States, condoms are now available and on open display in drug stores throughout the country, and the appeal of the product through colorful packaging and promotional display racks undoubtedly has some impact on the use of the product. There are, however, a variety of anachronistic practices in the commercial distribution of condoms and in birth control clinics. These will be discussed in the section on Strategies for Reintroduction.

THE CONDOM AS CONTRACEPTIVE

The contraceptive effectiveness of the modern condom is probably best represented by the result of a few British studies carried out in the past 10 years. These British studies have used diverse approaches:

A longitudinal study of highly fertile couples (4 pregnancies in the previous 6 years) who used condoms exclusively [34]

A 5-year follow-up study of contraceptive use by urban couples beginning at marriage [35]

A study of contraceptive use by patients in a small town medical practice [21]

A large study of married patients of family planning clinics who had substituted the condom for the pill, diaphragm, or intrauterine device [14]

The results of these studies (Table 22-2) suggest combined use plus method failure rates of 3.1 to 4.8 per 100 woman-years and rates based on method alone of only 0.4 to 1.6 per 100 woman-years. In contrast, for even the more successful intrauterine devices, pregnancy rates of 1.5 to 3.0 per 100 women are common in the first year of use [28], and among women using combined oral contraceptives the failure rate from pills missed during the dosage cycle can approach one pregnancy per 100 woman-years [23].

These figures on contraceptive effectiveness, which reflect the experience of well-motivated people, compare well with the figures on the method effectiveness of the condom (Table 22-2). For poorly motivated or otherwise ineffective users of contraception, the failure rate with either the pill or the condom can soar to levels on the order of 11 to 28 failures per 100 woman-years

[19, 23]. In the United Kingdom the condom has always maintained a level of respectability and was available through barbershops and surgical goods stores even before the pill made contraception a household word [36]. Presumably the good results obtained in the British studies cited in Table 22-2 reflect this attitude of familiarity and acceptance of condoms as well as the absence of negative associations, which impede condom use in the United States. In a 1970-1971 U.S. national fertility study, pregnancy rates of nearly 10 percent were reportedly in the first year of condom use [40]. Later U.S. surveys yielded first-year pregnancy rates of 7.1 per 100 women trying to prevent pregnancy and 12.3 per 100 women trying to delay pregnancy [15]. However, recent studies show pregnancy rates as low as 0.9 percent in highly motivated U.S. women intending to prevent pregnancy who are older than 29 years and with a family income greater than $15,000 [41].

Condoms fail as contraceptives primarily because of disuse. Wallets, overnight bags, and nightstand drawers are full of good intentions. Somehow the good intentions must be translated into action at a time when other pressing concerns and insecurities are operating. For new or casual sexual partners, disuse of the condom may carry disease as a risk in addition to pregnancy. This group will be discussed in the next section. For familiar sexual partners, even those who are consistent condom users, there are the occasional times, unfortunately often coinciding with fertility peaks, when the experience transcends all earthly routines and the condom goes unused. Since these couples are likely to be highly motivated to take action to prevent pregnancy, the doctor could provide an effective form of postcoital contraception for such situations [18].

Counseling for Effective Condom Contraception

In addition to disuse, condoms also fail because of misuse. Instructions are not always included with condoms, and clinical counseling practice is often out-of-date, stressing the need to use spermicide in combination with the condom and the need to place the condom on the penis before sexual contact because of sperm in the preejaculatory fluid; and mingling information about contraception and venereal disease so that the two reasons for using the condoms are associated in the mind of the user.

While the last two of these instructions are vital for the user at risk of sexually transmitted diseases, none are appropriate for the monogamous contracepting couple. For these stable sexual partners using the condom only for contraception, the condom need be placed on the penis only before ejaculation. The possibility that enough sperm to cause conception are present in the lubricative fluid before ejaculation is very slight to nonexistent [4, 12]. The user can introduce the condom during foreplay or late in extended intercourse without fear of interrupting coitus if the sexual partners learn to make these procedures a natural, even playful, part of the sexual exchange. For such contracepting couples, the disease prophylactic qualities of the condom are irrelevant and should not enter into the discussion. Furthermore, the use of adjunct foam or cream is a major inconvenience with marginal benefits unless the user desires to avoid pregnancy at all costs and cannot accept postcoital methods in case of method failure.

Condoms lubricated with spermicide have been available for several years in the United Kingdom and are now available in the United States. Although the extra effectiveness of these condoms is difficult to demonstrate [37] since condom failure is already a rare event, the spermicide offers theoretical protection against failure resulting from slow leakage, as through a hole or small tear, or where the condom slips off during withdrawal.

Instructions for the use of condoms that are to be used only for contraceptive purposes might be as follows:

Use a condom every time.

Use an appropriate size of condom, preferably lubricated and with a reservoir tip. Handle the condom with reasonable care (watch out for fingernails and jewelry).

Roll the rim of the condom all the way to the base of the penis.

After intercourse and before the loss of erection, hold onto the condom when withdrawing the penis, taking care not to spill any semen in the vagina.

Check the condom before putting it aside. If the semen cannot be seen or felt in the reservoir tip, take prescribed postcoital precaution or insert contraceptive foam or jelly in the vagina. If none of these are available, the female partner should contact her clinician.

In any case, if menstruation is delayed, the woman should contact her clinician.

THE CONDOM AND SEXUALLY TRANSMITTED DISEASE

Clinical Effectiveness

In the history of the condom venereal disease prevention and contraception have become inextricably interwoven; in previous centuries use of the condom was undoubtedly a prerogative of rich men who cared less about what they might leave behind than what they might bring home. Moreover, in recent times U.S. law has permitted the condom no other image than that of

Table 22-3. Number of Australian soldiers with and without venereal disease by number of exposures and condom used

Number	Group 1: No condom or wash		Group 2: Condom or wash sometimes		Group 3: Condom always	Group 4: Wash always	
	V.D.	No V.D.	V.D.	No V.D.	No V.D.	V.D.	No V.D.
1–5	14	53	10	24	48	8	16
6–10	7	9	9	14	5	4	1
11–20	3	6	4	0	1	0	0
More than 20	2	2	5	0	1	0	0
Total	26	70	28	38	55	12	17
Percent of group	27	73	42	58	100*	41	59

*Note that this is "No V.D." column.
Source: Adapted from S. D. Clark, Jr. An examination of the sperm content of human pre-ejaculatory fluid. Unpublished data, 1982.

a prophylactic against disease, causing this perception to persist in the minds of all but the highly sexually active who, according to social studies of venereal disease, are more inclined to rely on serendipity or the pill for contraception [7]. The dearth of personal concern by this subgroup appears to stem not from ignorance but from certain attitudes that characterize their lifestyle [17]. This fact, along with the high incidence of asymptomatic infections, has unfortunately limited the effectiveness of the condom as a public health adjunct.

Nevertheless, the preponderance of evidence seems to suggest that when used properly the condom is an effective barrier against gonorrhea and other venereal infections [6, 17, 29]. Its effectiveness is reflected in the data on Australian soldiers in Vietnam, whose consistent use of the condom appears to have afforded them adequate protection against venereal disease (Table 22-3) [17]. The results of studies of the general population in Scandinavian countries, where the public is better informed about the condom and its proper use than in the United States, also show the prophylactic effectiveness of this device: The frequency of condom use by infected Danish teenagers was only 25 percent of that of uninfected controls [9].

Laboratory studies have also demonstrated the effectiveness of latex and caecum condoms as barriers against Neisseria gonorrhoeae and herpes simplex vaginalis type 2 organisms [5, 43]. The herpesvirus (0.1μ diameter) was unable to penetrate the condom membrane even after the condom was subjected to pressure and stretch while in contact with the contaminated media. Although additional and larger scale studies along these lines would be useful in building a strong case for condoms against herpes infection, the present results are reassuring and should be used to encourage the use of condoms for people at risk of this disease. Although the potential exists for the transfer of some disease entities (e.g., herpes or syphilis from genitals to some other parts of the sexual partner's body), this risk is considered to be relatively low compared with genital-to-genital transmission [42].

The vigorous promotion of the condom in Sweden coincided with an arrest of the rapidly increasing incidence of gonorrhea followed by its dramatic fall in that country [1]. The United States has experienced a similar rapid increase in the reported cases of gonorrhea over the past 15 years, which could be curtailed by even a modest improvement in the frequency of effective condom use [25].

Counseling for Condom Use in Prophylaxis

It is possible to state with some degree of confidence that most people would be protected against sexually transmitted diseases if condoms were used throughout the entire period of genital contact. However, even among those who have not rejected the condom outright, conflicts may arise when contemplating condom use "in the clinch." These conflicts may be due to fear that the condom, with its cultural baggage of bad associations, may prove disagreeable or insulting to a new partner, especially if the partner is already taking contraceptive precautions (oral contraceptives, intrauterine devices, or surgical sterilization). Clinical counselors and other health professionals in contact with teenagers and other single people can suggest to their clients some culturally appropriate words of reassurance that deal with this conflict. For example:

Condoms keep me going longer (male).

I've gotten used to condoms and feel more at ease when I use them (male or female).

I like to be reassured that contraception is successful (female, male).

I want you to tell me if you like this new texture (male).

My doctor told me not to let semen come in contact with my cervix (female).

Some additional strategies for encouraging and promoting condom use in high-risk populations will be discussed in the section on Strategies for Reintroduction.

THE CONDOM IN CLINICAL PRACTICE

Quite apart from contraception and protection from common sexually transmitted diseases, the condom has other indications for general and reproductive health:

Protection against other diseases of the reproductive tract:
    Cervical cancer
    Pelvic inflammatory disease
    Amniotic fluid infection
Treatment of reproductive dysfunction:
    Premature ejaculation
    Infertility due to sperm antibodies
Other uses:
    Collection of semen specimens
    Collection device for urinary incontinence or diversion
    Emergency urinal

Protection from Diseases of the Reproductive Tract

Dysplastic changes of the cervix have often been linked statistically to the frequency of intercourse, multiple sexual partners, and sexually transmitted diseases (especially herpes and condyloma) [42]. If these aspects of an individual's sexual history are linked in a cause and effect relationship to the risk of cervical cancer, it follows that condom use would reduce the risk of this disease. Recent studies have tested this hypothesis, and the results suggest that condom use not only reduced the risk of cervical dysplasia or carcinoma [2, 10, 25] but also appeared to have a therapeutic effect on cervical cell abnormalities [39].

Organisms implicated in the etiology of pelvic inflammatory disease might be carried through the cervix by sperm [46]. Some of these organisms are involved in common sexually transmitted diseases. Condoms can

therefore prevent some of the organisms associated with pelvic inflammatory disease (PID) from entering the reproductive tract [24]. This protective effect of condoms is reflected in the results of case-control studies in the United States, where users of barrier methods were only 60 percent as likely to be hospitalized for PID as those using all other methods or no method at all [23]. Similarly, condoms can offer valuable indemnity against amniotic fluid infections, especially during late pregnancy when the cervix offers less of a barrier to transmission of the disease organisms [31].

The Condom in Treatment of Reproductive Dysfunction

The condom has long been used in the management of premature ejaculation, and while it is not a substitute for treatment of the underlying psychologic problems, it has been effective for some patients [22]. From the neurophysiologic standpoint, some aspects of sensation in the penis are probably transduced into sensory nerve signals by special vibration-sensing receptors found in areas of transition between skin and mucous membrane (mucocutaneous corpuscles; genital corpuscles). These receptors are stimulated by motion and, unlike pressure and other tactile receptors, generally do not attenuate with overstimulation. The loss of sensation that often occurs with prolonged penile stimulation is more probably due to fatigue occurring at a more central point in the sensory nervous pathways. The presence of a latex barrier between the receptors and the source of stimulus might be expected to reduce the level of stimulation. However, if the penis moves against the barrier, as in a flared or nonelastic condom, the stimulus level could be restored, at least in part. Addition of a texture to the barrier material may enhance this stimulus even further. In the absence of reliable sensory neurophysiologic information on the human penis and vagina, we may speculate that shape and texture can be significant in the sensory quality of condoms and should be considered in prescribing for the premature ejaculator or the understimulated.

Infertility related to antisperm antibodies in women has been treated by use of the condom for 3 to 6 months between unprotected intercourse, carefully timed to coincide with ovulation [27]. Although the success of this method is mixed, the therapy is simple and cheap and has been judged to increase the chance of pregnancy in these patients by 20 to 30 percent [42].

Other Uses for Condoms

The use of condoms for the collection of semen specimens presents problems owing to the lubricant or powder, which can distort or clutter the microscopic field of view during examination. Moreover, rubber itself may be injurious to sperm. Special plastic condoms may be used for the collection of semen for analysis and insemination.

Condoms have been used as collective devices for urinary incontinence or diversion in patients with senility or neurogenic bladder disease or following a cerebrovascular accident. The condom is cemented onto the skin of the penis with skin cement [24]. Usually the condom is connected to a catheter and a collection bottle, although the modern condom can safely hold several liters of fluid without bursting. This high elasticity has also rendered the condom useful in situations such as during flight in small aircraft where no facilities for urination were available.

STRATEGIES FOR REINTRODUCTION

The present-day condom is a thoroughly up-to-date device, having little in common with its ancient or recent progenitors. It deserves a more prominent place in the little black bag of choices offered to the sexually active person at risk of pregnancy or sexually transmitted disease. In order for it to attain this well-deserved status in the United States, old myths surrounding the condom must be dispelled and the method reintroduced to meet the needs of today's society.

Condom Mythologies

Several widely held and published opinions on condom use do not hold true for modern condoms or today's condom user. Some of these opinions had relevance 20 or 30 years ago, while some merely reflect the past taboos of U.S. culture, which still prevail in some quarters. Some comments on the most prevalent of these anachronistic opinions are as follows:

Condoms must be tested by the user before use. Some present-day texts on contraceptive practice still advocate blowing into the condom to test for leaks before use. Pinholes will occur on the average in less than four condoms per thousand for all the reputable brands manufactured in the United States, the United Kingdom, and Japan. These rare leaky products will in most cases contain microscopic holes that cannot be detected without sensitive laboratory equipment. Only a fraction of these pores will be in the functionally important closed end of the condom. In any case, pinholes are extremely unlikely to permit egress of sufficient sperm to bring about a failure of

contraceptive effectiveness. Passage of low numbers of disease organisms is not likely to be consistent with the initiation of infection either. The low probability of pinholes, the risk of physical damage attendant upon the user's efforts to test the condom, as well as the need to avoid impediments to condom use *dictate that self-testing should not be advocated.* Rather, the user should purchase products of high reputation, store them in a dry, dark place away from excess heat, and avoid carrying the same condom around in a wallet for more than a few weeks.

Preejaculatory fluid contains viable sperm and can therefore cause pregnancy. This has not been found to be true except in cases where a previous ejaculation occurred a short while before with no intervening urination [4, 12]. Even then, the probability of conception is small enough to be insignificant. In some men ejaculation can occur in part or entirely without orgasmic sensation. For these individuals, early placement of the condom is necessary. However, for monogamous couples with good control and motivation, the condom need not be placed on the penis before genital contact, only before ejaculation.

Condoms break frequently. A modern condom will characteristically burst at 25 to 40 liters of air or 2 to 6 kg of water. The reserve strength, as seen in Figure 22-2, is enormous, and condoms from established and reputable manufacturers are remarkably uniform (see Fig. 22-1). The probability of breakage is very low and in most cases will not be experienced in a reproductive lifetime. The few individuals who, for reasons that are uncertain, tend to experience a higher than average incidence of breakage should be advised to use a larger size of condom or to use a flared latex or skin condom (Table 22-4).

Contraceptive foam or jelly should be used with condoms. Instructing the use of adjunct spermicides with condoms can be seriously counterproductive in many instances. This is especially true for the sexually active adolescent population. Young people often are already burdened by uncertainties and insecurities, which make the use of condoms alone a logistic, psychologic, and functional problem, without the additional complication of spermicides. Proper use of the condom alone would be quite enough to dramatically improve the prognosis for teenage unwanted pregnancy and venereal disease. Use of adjunct spermicides should only be advocated for couples who must avoid pregnancy at all costs and cannot accept backup postcoital methods of fertility control.

Condoms are too disruptive during coitus. In today's less self-conscious, more creative approach to lovemaking, the male or female partner can introduce condoms during foreplay or late in extended intercourse

Table 22-4. Regional or racial differences in erect penis size

Present U.S. condom sizes		Penis size	Percent of sample		
Class A	Class B		White/U.S.[a]	Black/U.S.[a]	Thailand[b]
Length (mm)					
		75–100	1	0	3
		100–125	7	3	27
	150	126–150	30	23	51
160					
	170	151–175	46	39	17
200		176–200	14	21	2
Circumference (mm)					
	94				
100		76–100	3	2	16
	102				
108		101–112	13	9	37
	Flare[c]				
	124	113–127	29	34	30
		128–137	34	29	14
Flare[c]					
140		138–150	15	15	3

[a]Measured at point of maximum circumference [13].
[b]Measured at base [30].
[c]Applies to a few styles of condoms with a shaped (flared) profile about the glans portion.

without interruption. Most modern condoms lend themselves to placement as a natural and even playful part of the sexual exchange. In Europe sexually active adolescent boys are counseled to place a lubricated condom onto the penis before going out on a date. The lubrication will usually hold the condom in place on the flaccid penis, and if it is not needed, nothing is lost. If it is needed, it is already in place and requires no fumbling or explanation. This approach works and should be introduced into clinic counseling practice.

American condoms are the thickest in the world. Condoms manufactured in the United States offer a range of functional thickness similar to Japanese products (see Table 22-1). Japanese ultrathin products are also available in the U.S. market and differ from the thinnest U.S. manufactured condoms only with respect to their different finish and smaller amount of lubricant (approximately 50–100 mg versus 150–300 mg for U.S. products). These very thin products have proved popular and are just as elastic as the thicker models. However, they will break at lower stress forces than thicker condoms.

Strategies

Although condoms have come out from under the counter in most drugstores in the United States, the act of selection from an open shelf and presentation of the condoms at the cashier's counter still constitutes a public proclamation of sexuality, which, for many adolescents and some adults, presents a difficult obstacle. Mail order condoms are available but are not a useful option for most adolescents, since small parcels in plain brown wrappers arouse undesirable curiosity in the family home. The family planning clinic is still predominantly a female environment and therefore not a comfortable place for males. Slot machine condoms are available in many places but often contribute negatively to the condom image because of their location and in some cases their substandard merchandise. In general, the emphasis on the drugstore and clinic as a source of condoms contributes an air of authenticity and respectability to the method. In the present U.S. cultural climate of negative associations surrounding condoms, extending condom marketing to other commercial outlets may not be useful. However, some creative schemes for improving availability in a reinforcing and an image-enhancing way could be devised. For example:

Many more doctors' offices can stock and sell condoms to their patients together with advice on use of the method and the means of postcoital indemnification in the event of disuse, misuse, or failure.

Family planning clinics can provide male environments or discrete service counters for over-the-counter supply of condoms and other supplies.

Arrangements between clinics (or schools, colleges, clubs, or other youth-oriented institutions) and local drugstores could provide for phone-in orders to be plain-wrapped for pickup at the drug counter or checkout area. The purchaser need only request a package for the named person; the transaction would not be distinctly different from phone-in and pickup of prescriptions.

Some progress has been made over the past 5 years in the commercial promotion of condoms. Magazines and professional journals are being used for tasteful and attractive advertisements by the industry. One U.S. company (Young Rubber Corp., Trenton, N.J.), together with the American Public Health Association, Planned Parenthood, and other interested organizations are doing battle in the Supreme Court to remove the last of the Comstock barriers in order to permit the mailing of commercial promotional and informational literature about condoms [32]. Although the U.S. National Association of Broadcasters Radio and Television Code, which prohibited contraceptive advertising among its members (75% of all radio and television stations), was canceled in March 1983, most individual stations remain opposed or at least unwilling to encourage such advertisements. The canceling of the code opened up a significant opportunity for selective use of the media for informing people about products for reproductive health. The few stations that have aired such advertisements have experienced little opposition or negative reaction to them [8]. Other promotional measures might include more attractive posters for clinics, doctors' offices, and public places where young people gather; more articles in popular magazines and newspapers; and informative advertisements in clinical journals.

The *American Journal of Public Health* and the *Journal of the American Medical Association* have published editorials to urge the medical profession to consider the condom as a serious and important health tool for the sexually active teenager as well as for many adults. Publicity on the side effects of the pill and the IUD, although often ill-considered and out of perspective from a risk-benefit point of view, has nevertheless brought about widespread movement toward barrier methods. This movement can be encouraged if health providers counsel their clients on the proper use and high method effectiveness of condoms and offer postcoital indemnities and backup routines to be used in the event of failure.

The concerted efforts of clinicians and other health providers, youth counselors, public health officials, pharmacists, public-spirited media, and the condom industry in facilitating, promoting, and desensitizing condom use could have a dramatic effect upon the epidemic of venereal disease, the tragedy of unwanted teenage pregnancies, and the family planning failures and unsettling compromises that arise when individuals decide to forego chemical and intrauterine contraceptive methods.

REFERENCES

1. Ajax, L. How to Market a Non-Medical Contraceptive. In M. H. Redford, G. W. Duncan, and D. J. Prager (eds.), *The Condom: Increasing Utilization in the United States.* San Francisco: San Francisco Press, 1974. Pp. 5–21.
2. Beral, V. Cancer of the cervix: A sexually transmitted infection? *Lancet* 1:1037, 1974.
3. Butts, H. E. Legal Requirements for Condoms Under the Federal Food, Drug, and Cosmetic Act. In M. H. Redford, G. W. Duncan, and D. J. Prager (eds.), *The Condom: Increasing Utilization in the United States.* San Francisco: San Francisco Press, 1974. Pp. 202–209.
4. Clark, S. D., Jr. An examination of the sperm content of human pre-ejaculatory fluid. Unpublished data, 1982.
5. Conant, M. Problems with sexual activity. Presented to the Herpes Simplex Clinical Practice and Research Symposium. San Francisco, Jan., 1982.
6. Darrow, W. W. Contraceptives as venereal disease prophylactics. Presented to the 101st annual meeting of the American Public Health Association. San Francisco, Nov. 5, 1973.
7. Darrow, W. W., and Weisner, P. J. Personal prophylaxis for venereal disease. *J.A.M.A.* 233:444, 1975.
8. Donovan, P. Airing contraceptive commercials. *F. Plann. Perspect.* 14:321, 1982. 11. Peel, J. A male oriented fertility control experiment. *Practitioner* 202:677, 1972.
9. Ekstrom, K. Patterns of sexual behavior in relation to venereal disease. *Br. J. Vener. Dis.* 46:93, 1970.
10. Fish, E. N., et al. Update on the relation of herpesvirus hominis type 2 to carcinoma of the cervix. *Obstet. Gynecol.* 59:220, 1982.
11. Free, M. J., and Alexander, N. J. Male contraception without prescription. *Public Health Rep.* 91:437, 1976.
12. Free, M. J., Skiens, W. E., and Morrow, M. M. Relationship between condom strength and failure during use. *Contraception* 22:31, 1980.

13. Gebhard, P. H., and Johnson, A. B. *The Kinsey Data: Marginal Tabulations of the 1938–1963 Interviews Conducted by the Institute for Sex Research.* Philadelphia: Saunders, 1979.

14. Glass, R., Vessey, M., and Wiggins, P. Use-effectiveness of the condom in a selected family planning clinic population in the United Kingdom. *Contraception* 10:591, 1974.

15. Grady, W. R., et al. Contraceptive Failure and Continuation Among Married Women in the United States, 1970–76 (Working paper No. 6). Hyattsville, Md.: National Center for Health Statistics, 1981.

16. Harris, R. C. W., et al. Characteristics of women with dysplasia or carcinoma in situ of the cervix uteri. *Br. J. Cancer* 42:359, 1980.

17. Hart, G. Factors influencing venereal infection in a war environment. *Br. J. Vener. Dis.* 50:68, 1974.

18. Hatcher, R. A., et al. Contraceptive technology 1973–1974. Emory University Family Planning Program, Atlanta, Ga., 1973.

19. Hatcher, R. A., et al. *Contraceptive Technology 1982–1983.* (11th ed.). New York: Irvington, 1982.

20. Himes, N. E. History of the Condom or Sheath. In *Medical History of Contraception.* New York: Shocken, 1970. Pp. 186–206.

21. John, A. P. K. Contraception in a practice community. *J. R. Coll. Gen. Prac.* 23:665, 1973.

22. Karafin, L., and Kendall, A. R. Advantages and disadvantages of the condom. *Medical Aspects of Sexuality* 3:73, 1969.

23. Kols, A., et al. Oral contraceptives in the 1980s. *Popul. Rep.* [A]. No. 6, 1982.

24. Kelagan, J., et al. Barrier-method contraceptives and pelvic inflammatory disease. *J.A.M.A.* 248:184, 1982.

25. Ledger, W. J. Relationship of pelvic infection to various types of contraception. *Clin. Obstet. Gynecol.* 17:79, 1974.

26. Lee, T. Y., et al. Potential impact of chemical prophylaxis on the incidence of gonorrhoea. *Br. J. Vener. Dis.* 48:376, 1972.

27. Li, T. S. Sperm immunology, infertility, and fertility control. *Obstet. Gynecol.* 44:607. 1974.

28. Liskin, L., and Fox, G. IUDs: An appropriate contraceptive for many women. *Popul. Rep.* [B]. No. 4, 1982.

29. McCormack, W. W., Lee, Y., and Zinner, S. H. Sexual experience and urethral colonization with genital microplasma. *Ann. Intern. Med.* 78:696, 1973.

30. Muangman, D. Report on measurement of Thai male genital sizes and recommendation for appropriate condom usage. Unpublished data, 1978.

31. Naeye, R. L., and Ross, S. Coitus and chorioamnionitis: A prospective study. *Early Hum. Dev.* 6:91, 1982.

32. *The Nation's Health.* American Public Health Association, December, 1982.

33. Nonmedical birth control: A neglected and promising field (Editorial). *Am. J. Public Health* 63:473, 1973.

34. Peel, J. A male oriented fertility control experiment. *Practitioner* 202:677, 1972.

35. Peel, J. The Hull Family Survey: II. Family planning in the first 5 years of marriage. *J. Biosoc. Sci.* 4:333, 1972. United Kingdom. *Contraception* 10:591, 1974.

36. Peel, J., and Potts, M. *Textbook of Contraceptive Practice.* London: Cambridge University Press, 1969.

37. Potts, M., and McDevitt, J. A use-effectiveness trial of spermicidally lubricated condoms. *Contraception* 11:701, 1975.

38. Report to Consumers: Condoms. *Consumer Reports*, October, 1979. Pp. 583–589. (See also the corrections and revised ratings, *Consumer Reports*, March, 1980, p. 183).

39. Richards, A. C., and Lyon, J. B. The effect of condom use on squamous cell cervical intraepithelial neoplasia. *Am. J. Obstet. Gynecol.* 140:909, 1981.

40. Ryder, N. B. Contraceptive failure in the United States. *Fam. Plann. Perspect.* 5:133, 1973.

41. Schirm, A. L., et al. Contraceptive failure in the United States: The impact of social, economic and demographic factors. *Fam. Plann. Perspect.* 14:68, 1982.

42. Sherris, J. D., Lewison, D., and Fox, G. Update on condoms: Products, protection, promotion. *Popul. Rep.* [H]. No. 6, 1982.

43. Smith, L., Jr., et al. Efficacy of condoms as barriers to HSV-2 and gonorrhea: An in vitro model (Abstract). Presented to the 1st STDs World Congress. San Juan, Puerto Rico, Nov. 15–21, 1981.

44. Tietze, C. *The Condom As Contraceptive* (Publication No. 5). New York: National Committee on Maternal Health, 1966.

45. Tietze, C. The Condom. In M. S. Calderone (ed.), *Manual of Family Planning and Contraceptive Practice.* Baltimore: Williams & Wilkins, 1970. P. 424.

46. Toth, A., O'Leary, W. M., and Ledger, W. Evidence for microbial transfer of spermatozoa. *Obstet. Gynecol.* 59:556, 1982.

V. Intrauterine Contraception

23. Intrauterine Contraception

Michael S. Burnhill

Most physicians know that the use of intrauterine contraceptive devices (IUDs) has been gradually declining since the early 1970s. The reasons for this are basically:

1. Fear of inflammatory disease related to the use of the IUD.
2. Fear of ectopic pregnancies related to the use of the IUD.
3. Intrauterine pregnancies related to the use of the IUD.
4. Most important of all, malpractice actions resulting from the first three reasons or other IUD-related problems.

This has not been an unexpected phenomenon. As with most medical and other innovations, there is always a rapid period of acceptance and enthusiasm, followed by a long plateau in which the negative aspects of the innovation begin to be recognized, and then decline, as disenchantment spreads throughout the profession.

Modern intrauterine contraceptives were first described in 1908 by Richter [95], who used a coil of silkworm gut tied with a small piece of nickel bronze wire that protruded through the cervix. His device was very rapidly modified by Püst [93], who took off the nickel bronze wire because it had a tendency to irritate the penis and replaced it with a catgut tail to which a small collar button had been tied so that it could be felt with a finger pressed up against the cervical os. The Püst devices were associated with a number of pelvic infections, and in the early 1920s Gräfenberg [49, 50] decided that removing the tail would alleviate some of the infections. His idea proved to be correct, and over the next two decades all intrauterine devices in use were tailless ones. The Gräfenberg silkworm gut was promptly followed by a silver and then stainless steel coil manufactured in four sizes. It was adopted and modified in Japan by Ota [86], who added a hub and spokes to the device, a modification that reduced the expulsion rate and the possible dangers of intestinal obstruction should the device perforate. However, this second wave of IUDs was also doomed to failure [33], as a worldwide pandemic of gonorrhea, which took place during the depression of the 1930s, discredited the use of the IUD. The entire field lay quiet until the Population Council in the late 1950s, in searching for possible means of reducing rapid population increases in the Third World, invited Dr. Ishihama [61] from Japan and Dr. Oppenheimer [82] from Israel to report on the use of the Ota ring and Gräfenberg ring, respectively. Their publications stirred the start of the modern IUD revolution. Within a short period of time, the loop [69–71], the spiral [75], and the bow [9] appeared in the United States and were widely tested. They were followed by a plethora of other inert plastic devices, and Hall revived interest in the Gräfenberg ring [51–53]. During the 1960s these devices were studied in great detail by the Population Council [119–121], the Pathfinder Fund [7, 8], and many other researchers. A number of problems began to be noted, such as expulsions, perforations, bleeding, and higher than expected pregnancy rates. It was with great interest that the contraceptive community noted that the addition of copper wire, as developed by Zipper [132], was shown to improve the contraceptive effect of IUDs. Dr. Howard Tatum at the Population Council adapted this concept and produced the currently marketed TCu 200.

Independently, Dr. Harry Rudel developed a copper device now being marketed as Cu-7 [43]. These were the first of the bioactive devices of which a number of other copper-coated models are in use outside of the United States. By the mid-1970s the Alza Corporation [88, 89] developed a hormonal delivery system built into the skeleton of the T device, and this is now marketed as the Progestasert. However encouraging these developments were, there were ominous signs developing on the horizon, as the Dalkon shield [29, 30, 68, 85], one of the earlier entirely plastic devices, was found to be associated with a number of midtrimester pregnancy infections, shock, and deaths. This started a period of intense reporting of IUD-associated infections [11, 21, 24, 32, 34–38, 40, 41, 44, 45, 57, 63, 65, 67, 74, 77, 81, 83, 84, 92, 99, 105, 109, 111, 115, 117, 124]. In addition, increasing numbers of papers reporting on complications, difficult removals, embeddings, perforations [5, 22, 26, 36, 39, 42, 66, 94, 96, 102, 106, 110, 129–131], etc., worked their way into the literature and were reported with much distortion by the popular press. This resulted in a steady eroding of confidence in the use of IUDs, particularly with respect to nulligravid women. The focus of this chapter, however, is to point out to family planners that when properly used, when carefully inserted, and when patients are properly selected and counseled, IUDs remain one of the most effective coitus-independent forms of contraception available [73, 90, 102, 123].

SELECTING THE APPROPRIATE PATIENT

The most important general characteristic for determining whether a patient is a suitable candidate for wearing an IUD is the overall health of the genital tract [40]. While a list of contraindications can be easily printed [36, 56, 73, 86, 90, 102, 123], it is important to remember that the guiding principle is that *the reproductive tract should be healthy and nonpregnant.* This one sentence embodies all the general principles that are important in determining whether an IUD should be inserted. It

seems almost superfluous to have to remind people that

1. The uterus should be nonpregnant at the time of insertion.
2. No unexplained genital bleeding should be noted in the patient's history.
3. The cervix, uterus, and tubes should be uninfected and there should be no recent history of cervicitis or salpingitis.
4. No genital tract cancer should be present.
5. The uterus should be large enough and the canal straight and large enough for an IUD to be inserted.
6. There should be no condition in the body that would be seriously jeopardized by an IUD-related infection, such as subacute bacterial endocarditis, chronic glomerulonephritis, renal failure, etc.
7. There should be a single cavity of the uterus (noted on sweeping the canal during the insertion)—i.e., no severe congenital anomalies that would limit the IUD to one side of the uterus.
8. The patient should be mentally capable of noting and reporting any IUD-associated infection signs, the expulsion of the IUD, the possibility of pregnancy, or the occurrence of extremely heavy periods.

The patient must understand the limitations of an IUD and its possible effect on the uterus and that there should be no gynecologic disease present that would interfere with the efficacy of the IUD or predispose her to infection.

TYPES OF IUDS

At the present time in the United States there are four IUDs being marketed. Average results for pregnancy, expulsion, and removal are given in Table 23-1.

The Lippes Loop (Ortho Pharmaceutical Corporation)

The Lippes loop [7, 8, 36, 70–72, 102, 120, 121, 126, 127] as currently marketed is a polyethylene device with barium powder mixed into the polyethylene to provide radiopacity. It is shaped like a double S and comes in four sizes. Sizes A and B were the original ones designed by Dr. Lippes and are basically unsuited for use because of the unacceptably high pregnancy rate associated with them. They are both the same size, more or less, as loops C and D, but because they are thinner, they are more likely to be expelled or associated with pregnancy. Loop D is about the same size as loop C, but it is stiffer and is only recommended in those cases where a multiparous woman has expelled loop C. The

Table 23-1. One-year net cumulative life-table rates per 100 women for IUDs commercially available in the United States

	Number of insertions	Pregnancy	Expulsion	Medical removal
Lippes loop[a]				
Size A	1,015	5.3	23.9	12.2
B	1,305	3.4	18.9	15.1
C	3,489	3.0	19.1	14.3
D	7,553	2.7	12.7	15.2
Copper TCu 200[b]	4,127	2.2	8.3	13.3
Cu-7 (Gravigard[b])				
Nulliparas	N.S.[d]	1.6	8.0	13.7
Multiparas	N.S.	1.9	5.7	10.7
Progestasert[c]				
Nulliparas		2.6	7.4	15.1
Multiparas	7,614	1.8	3.1	11.2

[a]Ortho Pharmaceutical Corporation, Raritan, N.J. [43].
[b]Searle Laboratories, Chicago, Ill. [48].
[c]Alza Pharmaceuticals, Palo Alto, Calif. [1].
[d]Not stated; 11,852 women completed 12 months of IUD use.
Source: Adapted from D. A. Edelman, G. S. Berger, and L. Keith. *Intrauterine Devices and Their Complications.* Boston: Hall, 1979.

device is extremely useful, with low complication rates, particularly in those women who have had children, and whose uterus is large enough to hold them comfortably. Loop C is generally recommended. Unlike medicated devices, the loop may remain in place indefinitely.

The Cu-7 (Searle Laboratories)

The Cu-7 was the first bioactive device marketed in the United States [36, 43, 58, 62]. It consists of a slender, 7-shaped device with pure copper wire wound around the stem. This device is relatively easy to insert and is not associated with a great deal of dysmenorrhea, but it does have problems owing to the slender, pointlike end of the long arm. This has resulted in embedding of the device in the lower uterine segment or cervix and in either partial or complete perforation of the long arm of the device into the peritoneal cavity. This kind of embedding and partial perforation can make the removal of the device difficult if not almost impossible. From my point of view, there is no real advantage of the 7 that would suggest its preferential use over the TCu 200.

The TCu 200 (Searle Laboratories)

Though the TCu 200 is the older of the copper IUDs, various marketing and licensing problems led to its being adopted for United States use only in the past sev-

eral years. The straight arm of the device is well adapted in the uterine cavity, and the bulbous lower end has a tendency to limit and reduce the number of embeddings and perforations [22, 36, 87, 96] (though these are not completely eliminated). The device is relatively easily tolerated, even in nulligravida uteri, provided the uterine cavity is long enough to accept the device, which, unfortunately, may be a little too long for the average uterus. It is, however, in this country, my choice for a copper IUD.

Progestasert (Alza Pharmaceuticals)

The Progestasert is structurally similar to the TCu 200 except that the long arm [88, 89], instead of being wound with copper wire, consists of a hollow cylinder comprised of a special plastic designed to exude a tiny amount of progesterone directly onto the endometrial surface over a period of a year (and probably in the future 2 years). The device's contraceptive action is related not only to its foreign body presence in the uterus but also to the effect of micro doses of progestin on implantation. The device is particularly well suited for those women who have painful or heavy periods, as the progestin contributes to the quieting of the uterus and thus seems to be beneficial. However, the use of the device is associated with a fair amount of spotting, which can be troublesome, and with the necessity of relatively frequent reinsertions, which is both expensive and uncomfortable for the woman. Except as indicated in women with dysmenorrhea and possibly premenstrual distress syndromes, there seem to be few indications for the use of this device.

INSERTION OF THE IUD

The insertion of the IUD [14, 36, 56, 58, 73, 86, 90, 102, 123] is carried out only after

1. The patient has read about the advantages, disadvantages, and limitations of IUD use.
2. The woman has signed an informed consent indicating that she understands the nature and limitations of the IUD.
3. A very careful history has been taken, indicating that there is nothing in her medical history that might contraindicate the use of an IUD.
4. A careful physical examination has been performed, including evaluation of the cardiovascular system so that no unsuspected valvular heart disease or major arrhythmia is overlooked.

After a complete physical examination has been done, the operator must determine in his or her own mind whether an insertion can be carried out. This decision will be based on the health of the genital tract as indicated by

1. Lack of tenderness or pain on movement of the cervix or compression of the uterus
2. The absence of a purulent discharge
3. The absence of an acute cervicitis
4. The absence of any undiagnosed uterine or adnexal masses
5. The estimation that the uterus is large enough to hold an IUD without the device being compressed or forced downward

If after this evaluation all the criteria are met, the operator may then select the appropriate IUD, as determined by examination, conversations with the patient, and physician preference.

Equipment for inserting an IUD [56, 58, 102] includes:

1. Speculi, in a range of sizes and shapes.
2. Medicine cup, for antiseptic solution, cotton balls, and a sponge stick for applying them. Alternatively, large-size cotton swabs or folded sponges may be used to clean the cervix.
3. A cervical grasping instrument, preferably a Bierer forcep (available from Rocket Instruments), a White's tonsil seizing forcep (available from most instrument companies), a long, heavy Allis clamp, or failing any of these, a square-ended, single-toothed tenaculum.
4. A uterine sound marked in centimeters or inches.
5. A sterile IUD in its package.
6. A 10- or 20-cc syringe, either disposable or Luer-lok pressure control type, with either a 22-gauge spinal needle or a tonsil needle.
7. Povidone-iodine solution.
8. 1% Carbocaine, Nesacaine, or Xylocaine.

The insertion technique [14, 20, 56, 58, 73, 90, 102], proceeds as follows. First, a bimanual examination defines the uterine position within the pelvis. The speculum is inserted and the cervix prepped with an antiseptic solution such as povidone-iodine. One may choose to anesthetize the cervix using a paracervical block to diminish the cramping and pain of insertion and to lessen the chances of a hypotensive reaction [1, 25, 56, 102] (which may occur from discomfort during insertion). The cervix is visualized, and 1 or 2 ml of anesthetic placed submucosally at 12 o'clock about 1 cm from the tip of the cervix. The cervix is then grasped and pulled laterally to the right where submucosal infiltration takes place at 3 o'clock and then

again at 5 o'clock. The mucosa should blanch. This is repeated at 7 and 9 o'clock so that a total of about 8 to 10 ml of 1% local anesthetic is placed underneath the mucosa. The blanching is very important, as it lets the operator know that the local anesthetic has not been injected directly into a descending branch of the cervical artery or vein.

The anesthetic is allowed to diffuse for 2 to 5 minutes (depending on the parity of the patient, firmness of the cervix, and the operator's perception as to the patient's anxieties and/or pain threshold). As soon as the block appears effective, the IUD is loaded into the inserter, and the cervix grasped at 12 o'clock and pulled downward. The uterus is then sounded, and the depth at which the sound reaches the fundus is noted. If the sounding is less than 6 cm [14, 17, 20, 43, 66, 118], it is highly unlikely that any current intrauterine device can be placed without serious side effects. This is particularly a problem with the long T- or 7-shaped devices, as placement across the cervical os may produce bleeding and cramping, expulsion, and/or embedding or perforation of the cervix.

The sound is also moved from side to side to determine whether a single cavity is present or whether there is a septum extending for a substantial distance into the uterine cavity. While one can insert two IUDs if necessary in a bicornuate uterus, this is frequently impossible unless the gravidity of the patient is high, because there is usually not enough room to place both IUDs. Placing an IUD in one cavity provides some contraceptive protection, but it is associated with a higher pregnancy rate than one would like.

If the uterus is deemed to be large enough and access to the fundus is clear and easy, the contraceptive device is then loaded into its inserter as indicated on the manufacturer's instructions. These should be read carefully *before inserting an IUD for the first time.* Moreover, the first several IUD insertions should be supervised by an appropriately trained individual.

After the IUD is loaded, the insertion into the uterine cavity should be performed slowly and gently, either by push or pull on the plunger (depending on which type device is being inserted). Following the removal of the inserter, it is extremely important that the sound be used to make sure that the device is entirely placed within the uterine cavity and that no part of it protrudes downward through the cervix. This single maneuver, *seating the device* [14, 20], is extraordinarily important in reducing IUD-related problems. With the sound in place to prevent downward displacement, the tail of the IUD is pulled reasonably taut so as not to leave any redundant tail in the uterine cavity. The thread is then cut, leaving a half to three-quarters of an inch protruding through the cervical canal. If one is absolutely sure (by feel with the sound in the uterus) that the device is well placed in the fundus, the shorter length of protruding tail is preferable. After cutting the tail, the instruments are removed.

If the block has been successful or if the patient was of sufficient gravidity and composure to do without one, she should be experiencing only some minor cramping. One may wish to send her home with a prescription for some mild analgesic for the first day or two. Of particular value for perhaps the first two cycles is the use of a prostaglandin inhibitor such as Anaprox, Motrin, or Ponstel. These prostaglandin inhibitors seem of particular value, as they tend to quiet the excess uterine activity stimulated by the presence of the IUD. Preinsertion use of these agents is also helpful and should supplant local anesthesia for most cases.

TIMING OF INSERTION

A controversy has raged over the past 20 years as to when an IUD should be inserted [36, 56, 58, 73, 86, 90, 102]. After much discussion, most physicians agree that insertion during menses has many advantages. These are:

1. The cervix is already dilated and thus passage of the inserter is easier.
2. The continual menstrual flow seems to wash away bacterial contaminants and reduces immediate post-insertion infection.
3. One can be reasonably sure that the patient is not pregnant.
4. One does not have a second bleeding episode during the month.

IUD guidelines [36, 56, 73, 90, 102] have suggested that the IUD can be inserted any time during the cycle to ensure that some women would not be turned away because they presented at the wrong time or could not come in during menses. Random insertions are certainly easier to schedule. White et al. [125] found that the last half of the cycle (after day 11) is a better time to insert the TCu 200. It has been suggested that an IUD can be inserted postpartum [6, 18, 73, 90, 123, 126] or postabortally [48, 90, 127] (in the absence of a period). This is, indeed, technically true but probably not too prudent. The insertion of an IUD is almost invariably followed by some sort of bleeding episode. Furthermore, in the early postabortal period one can never be sure that the abortion was totally completed, so that any bleeding following the IUD insertion may be confusing. It is less confusing if the patient has experienced a normal period before the IUD is inserted. One should remember that an IUD insertion is intended to last for many years, and a little caution at the beginning may pay off over the long run.

SIDE EFFECTS AND COMPLICATIONS

Spotting, Bleeding, and Anemia

About a third of all patients who have IUDs inserted note a change in the character of their menstrual periods. The usual change is one of bleeding episodes becoming longer [73, 90], heavier, and frequently associated with increasing molimina (which may be a sign of ovulation in previous pill users). The occurrence of increased bleeding is not surprising, considering that the IUD increases the motility of the uterus. In fact, many of the problems with IUDs relate to the fact that the myometrium "resents" the foreign body being present and does its best to expel it.

Bleeding is also related to the size of the IUD and its relationship to the uterine walls. A tight-fitting IUD pressing against the walls seems to elicit more bleeding than one that is smaller and that does not exert lateral or vertical pressure [16, 55, 66, 118]. Bleeding is also increased by the presence of the tip of the IUD passing through the internal cervical os into the cervical canal. This may be a particular problem, for example, with the TCu 200, the Cu-7, and the Progestasert, all of which are 36 mm long and are rather easily pushed partially through the internal os in women with short cavities. It can also occur with the Lippes loop if the device has been inserted so as to leave the terminal piece protruding through the cervical os. This is why it is so important to *seat* the IUD after insertion to be sure that no part of it is protruding downward through the cervical os.

In some women a mild ascorbic acid deficiency is correlated with increasing menstrual flow. This can be checked with a petechiometer, and if more than four to six petechiae turn up in a square centimeter, the patient may show improvement with additional vitamin C and perhaps bioflavenoids to increase capillary strength. Vitamin C can be given conveniently in sustained-release capsules (which distribute the dose of ascorbic acid throughout the day); one 300 to 500 mg capsule b.i.d. should suffice. In the presence of capillary weakness, hesperidin, rutin, and citrus-bioflavenoids may be important adjuncts to the ascorbic acid.

If the menstrual flow is reported as being heavier for 3 or more months, the patient should be advised to use a hematinic to provide sufficient iron to compensate for the blood loss during the menses. The most effective hematinics use a chelated iron, such as ferrous fumerate, along with ascorbic acid, folic acid, and possibly B_{12} and desiccated liver. If the flow continues to be heavy and the hematocrit is falling despite the use of hematinics, it may be necessary to remove the IUD to prevent the development of a severe hypochromic anemia.

Some women benefit from the use of a vasoconstrictor during periods of heavy flow. Sudafed, 30 or 60 mg, or a combination of vasoconstrictor and antihistamine such as Actifed tablets or Ornade capsules have been advocated. These have proven to be beneficial to some women who have a very heavy flow. Prostaglandin inhibitors may also be of value as reported by Davies et al. [27].

Spotting, particularly around the time of ovulation, is also quite common with many women wearing IUDs. Sometimes the spotting occurs for several days premenstrually or postmenstrually. This may be particularly vexing in those cultures in which coitus is proscribed during episodes of bleeding.

Expulsion, Partial Expulsion, and Embedding

As mentioned in the preceding section, the uterus reacts frequently with strong contractions (which are similar in many ways to labor contractions) that can displace the IUD downward, pushing it through the cervical os. These contractions may partially expel the IUD, so that on visualization one can see the tip of the IUD protruding through the cervical os, or it may be felt by the partner during intercourse. Sometimes, particularly with the long-stemmed devices [22, 96], the displacement downward may be into the connective tissue of the cervix or through the lower uterine segment. When devices are deeply embedded, and they can, in fact, be partially perforated, they may be extremely difficult to remove. Pulling on the string may only break off the string without removing the IUD. It may be necessary to employ hysteroscopy [107] to back the IUD out of the false passage it is making and remove it under direct visualization.

Worse than that, the IUD may be completely expelled. Most expulsions occur in conjunction with menses, especially in the early months of use. If the patient notices the IUD on her napkin or tampon, then at least she will be aware that she has to use another form of contraception temporarily. Most IUD expulsions are accompanied by strong cramping, and patients should be instructed to look at their tampons and napkins before they discard them. However, in some women (particularly those of high parity who have a very lax internal os), the expulsion may be entirely silent, and the IUD can be lost in the toilet bowl. The unfortunate consequence of the unnoticed expulsion is often an unwanted pregnancy.

Perforation

It has been noted that perforation, when present, usually occurred at the time of insertion [20, 36, 80]. This is particularly true if the insertion takes place in the early puerperium or in the early postabortal period when the uterine walls are still soft. This tendency is especially marked in nursing women in whom the uterus by the sixth week is usually hyperinvoluted.

Perforations are rarely picked up at the time of insertion because the penetration through the uterine wall is generally quite symptomless. The first inkling might well be the missing of the period with evidence of an intrauterine pregnancy. However, serious problems such as bowel perforations [26, 36] have also been reported.

It was formerly thought that inert linear devices such as the Lippes loop could be left in situ if they perforated, but that closed devices such as the bow or the Antigon or Gräfenberg ring should be removed. It is now quite clear that all devices that perforate should be removed as soon as the perforation is detected. This can usually be done rather simply through a laparoscope. Zakin et al. [129–131] and Edelman et al. [36] have thoroughly reviewed data on embedding and perforation.

Pregnancy

Pregnancies occur, even with properly placed IUDs and while they are still in situ [3, 7, 36, 39, 69, 73, 90, 106]. It is true that should a partial expulsion or perforation take place, the possibility of pregnancy is increased. It is also true that if a silent expulsion or complete perforation takes place, pregnancy often will follow shortly after this event. However, pregnancies also occur while the IUD is entirely within the uterine cavity. This may relate to the size of the cavity: An IUD occupying less than 50 percent of the surface area is more likely to fail [16, 118]. It is also true that in a bicornuate uterus the presence of an IUD in one horn does not protect the woman against pregnancy occurring in the other horn.

Pregnancies, of course, pose problems [34]. A high percentage of women who become pregnant with IUDs will spontaneously abort [36]. Removing IUDs in early pregnancy has a tendency to increase the live birth rate [3] (as long as no intrauterine manipulation is required).

However, the experience in the 1970s of reports of midtrimester shock and death with the Dalkon shield [21, 24, 38, 42, 59, 63, 65] has led authorities to advise removal of the IUD should the tail be visible. Escherichia coli sepsis has been reported with a Cu-7 [92]. However, if the tail is not visible, one should not attempt to remove the IUD, unless permission to perform an abortion has been obtained. The patient should understand that trying to localize the IUD within the uterine cavity is quite likely to produce bleeding and possible abortion.

If the patient has decided to continue the pregnancy, no intrauterine manipulation should be carried out as the consequences are medicolegally quite disastrous. If the patient elects to carry on the pregnancy with an IUD in place, she should be advised to report immediately to the physician the occurrence of:

1. Any strange flulike symptoms in her pregnancy
2. The development of a purulent discharge
3. Abdominal pain or aching
4. Elevation of her temperature associated with backache or lower abdominal pain

At this time complete examination and the appropriate bacteriologic investigation should be made to try to avert development of serious intrauterine infection.

Ectopic Pregnancy

Another area of controversy has been the incidence of ectopic pregnancy [5, 54, 108, 110, 116] with respect to pregnancies occurring with the IUDs. The most recent review of this question by Sivin [108] was published in February of 1983. He concluded that there was no causal relationship between the use of nonmedicated or copper-bearing IUDs and ectopic pregnancy. While this may be true, it is equally true that a very high percentage of pregnancies occurring in women using IUDs are ectopic in location [17]. This is of particular importance to note, since many women have a bleeding episode after they have become pregnant with the IUD in place. An aberrant bleeding episode (a delay or diminishing of the flow) connected with any pregnancy symptoms should be followed by an investigation sufficient to rule in or out intrauterine pregnancy. Sivin did note an unusually high group of ectopics among users of the Progestasert, which might be the result of a tubal transport effect secondary to the release of intrauterine progesterone. Therefore, one should be especially alert to possible ectopic gestation in women using this device [110].

Lost IUD Strings and Difficult Removals

Because of movement of the IUD within the cavity, it is not unusual to have a string drawn up into the canal or perhaps entirely into the uterus so that neither the patient nor the clinician can detect it on pelvic examination. When this occurs, it is necessary to determine whether the IUD is still present [129–132]. This can usually be done rather simply with an ultrasound or x ray of the uterus performed with a sound in place. This will aid in delineating whether the IUD is in the uterus or the peritoneal cavity. Another method that may be used is hysterosalpingography with 0.5 ml of contrast media outlining the uterine cavity without obscuring the intrauterine device [17]. Hysteroscopy affords positive identification of IUD location and is especially helpful in cases of partial perforation.

Having determined that the IUD is in the cavity, one must then decide whether to bring down the tail or to leave it alone. If the woman is not having any symptoms, it may be prudent to leave the IUD where it is. If, on the other hand, she expresses concern, one may want to bring down the tail. This can be frequently done by passing a sterile cotton swab into the canal, twisting it, and bringing it down, or by using a helix-shaped instrument (designed for endometrial sampling) [46] by which one can bring down the tail with a twisting downward motion. If neither of these techniques works, it may be necessary to probe the uterine cavity with a plastic, flexible cannula such as a Karmen 3 mm cannula, a Novak curet, an IUD hook, or a MiMark (Helix) in an attempt to bring down the tail. If this is accomplished, and one notes that the IUD is present, then nothing further need be done. If, however, the tail does not come down, one may have to employ a paracervical block and use an IUD remover to bring the device down. Removal by hysteroscopy may be required [107].

IUDs and Pelvic Infection

Infection has been a major deterrent to the more widespread use of IUDs since their introduction in Germany in the first part of this century. Gräfenberg [49, 50] believed that a major contribution to the field of IUDs was the removal of the connection between the uterine cavity and the vagina. He felt that this continuity was the source of many of the infections seen in women using the Püst pessary and other tailed IUDs. Dickinson [33] was the most eloquent of the pioneers in the field of birth control who warned of infection with the use of IUDs. In his textbook *Control of Conception* he wrote:

All stems that reach from the vagina into the uterus, and more particularly those that have a disk in the vagina, furnish a ladder for infection to climb. They vitiate that remarkable provision of nature whereby the internal os is an effective barrier against the ascent of disease germs. The cervical canal in the non-pregnant woman may be actively infected, and yet there may be very little tendency to ascend, except during the period. Infection is sometimes carried in on the physician's uterine sound or by the curette, but most men have learned to render high respect for this defense, this portal of Curtis. Such natural protection the long stem disregards, and certain women pay a heavy penalty. The rings entirely within the uterus do not entail the same objection; but there is danger, in placing them, of carrying upward any infective material found inside the canal of the cervix.

The Population Council attempted to rule out the possibility of serious infection by publicizing a number of basic studies on the bacteriology and histology of the uterus after the introduction of IUDs. Data were presented at the Second International Conference on IUDs [103] held in New York City in October of 1964. Moyer and Mishell [78, 79] studied this problem for almost a decade, and in 1971 they concluded that almost all uteri became contaminated after the introduction of an IUD and that the bacteria thus introduced disappear within several months. This kind of study led to the introduction of sterile disposable introducers and sterilely packaged IUDs. Tietze and Lewit [121] concluded that there was no evidence showing a rise in infection owing to the presence of the IUD per se. There were, however, occasional reports of sepsis associated with IUDs, such as Agnew and Pritchard's paper [2]. Wright and Laemmle [128] noted an association between the use of IUDs and pelvic infection. Scott [100], in reviewing deaths for the first FDA report, noted a number of serious illnesses and deaths related to infection in association with the IUD. In 1972 at a Planned Parenthood Physicians' meeting, Burnhill [13] described a syndrome of progressive endometritis.

However, the profession's attention did not really become focused on the relationship between the IUD and pelvic infection until a number of deaths were associated with the Dalkon shield [65] and midtrimester pregnancy infections. At first the work consisted of a number of reports on the relationship between midtrimester infection and the presence of an IUD [21, 24, 34, 38, 42, 59, 63–65, 76, 92]. The general conclusions from these papers was that infections associated with intrauterine devices in the midtrimester of pregnancy are rare but could be very serious (and not infrequently lethal) because of the sudden change from a mild flulike syndrome to sudden overwhelming sepsis with vascular collapse. Most of the serious infections described were associated with the Dalkon shield. However, the current recommendation is to remove any IUD whose string is protruding through the cervical canal, should the woman become pregnant.

About the same time a number of authors began to record cases of pelvic abscesses associated with the use of the IUD. The striking thing about many of the case reports was that the abscesses were frequently unilateral, generally nongonococcal, and often in young women. Representative of these papers are the ones by Dawood and Birnbaum [32], Eschenbach et al. [40], Faulkner and Ory [41], Golde et al. [44], Golditch and Huston [47], Mead et al. [77], Niebyl et al. [81], Ory [83], Ostergard [85], Taylor et al. [117], Westrom et al. [124], Smith and Soderstrom [109], and Targum and Wright [113].

These studies showed an increased risk to users of IUDs of contracting serious pelvic inflammatory disease (PID) and led to warnings regarding the use of IUDs, particularly for young nulliparous women. The specter of sterility subsequent to the use of IUDs was not seriously considered until these reports were published. As most of this work had been triggered by Dalkon shield–related infections, investigators began to look for an etiologic factor that might have led to these infections.

Tatum et al. [115] noted that there seemed to be an association between the sheathed multifilament tail and ascending infection. The Dalkon Shield was the only device then on the market to be using a multifilament tail. Sparks et al. [111] at the University of Southhampton also noted a wicking effect of the tail, thus again focusing attention on the early prophetic words of Dickinson.

In the past 5 years a number of fine review studies have been completed. One of the most interesting group of studies are those published by Edelman and his group [35–37]. Their epidemiologic analysis of the PID papers indicates a general increase in the risk of infection among IUD users that is not related to the type of IUD used. They point out the importance of background PID rates and the age of the user population in attributing significance to the occurrence of PID in IUD users. Other recent articles include those by Kaufman et al. [67], Burkman [12], Lee et al. [68], Malhatra and Chaundhury [74], Ory [83], Osser et al. [84], Schmidt [99], the FDA itself [102], Tatum [115], the Population Report Studies [62, 63], and Senanayake [105].

These studies point to an increased risk of pelvic infection in IUD users. The Edelman group felt that, although the issue is quite complex owing to the rising and variable rates of pelvic inflammatory disease in this country, no difference could be shown between the different types of IUDs. However, as this chapter was being prepared, Lee et al. [68] published additional data from the Women's Health Study on IUDs, which indicated that the risk for pelvic inflammatory disease in Dalkon wearers was 8.3 times greater than that of the control group. This risk was 4 to 6 times greater than that associated with other IUDs, most of whose risk was in the first 4 months after insertion. The authors, along with almost all authorities, support the idea that *all* Dalkon shields should be removed. Immediate infection aside, there appears to be another syndrome in which a gradual contamination of the endometrial cavity takes place, which can result in a slow, progressive invasive disease, which may finally overwhelm the endometrial defenses and produce endometritis, myometritis, and parametritis. This process may take several months or longer. The syndrome was originally described by Burnhill [13] and its hallmark was the gradual onset of symptomatology, beginning with an increase in perimenstrual symptoms including bloating, spotting, low backache, and the development of an unpleasant or fishlike odor associated with the menses. This infection, if not treated, had a tendency to progress to a full-fledged inflammatory disease that was not caused by the usual sexually transmitted disease organisms.

When one begins to suspect the occurrence of pelvic inflammatory disease in an IUD wearer, then she should be warned of the possible sequelae. Appropriate bacteriologic tests should be performed, using both aerobic and anaerobic culture material. Gonococci, *Trichomonas*, and *H. gardnerella* should be ruled out as well. If the infection is identified and treated with appropriate antibiotics, the entire course of the disease may be reversed and the IUD wearer permitted to retain the device. If, however, the infection has been disseminated by the time the clinician has seen the patient and is already manifesting as tuboovarian abscesses with or without parametritis, then it is safer to remove the IUD (and culture it) to prevent any further seeding of the endometrial cavity through the passage of bacteria up the tail. The presence of uterine and adnexal tenderness has some ominous overtones and should not be lightly passed over in women wearing IUDs. A unilateral pelvic mass in an IUD wearer has been frequently described as due to a unilateral tuboovarian abscess. These can be treated with appropriate and sufficient antibacterial agents, provided the disease is recognized early. In this day and age, it is rarely necessary to perform emergency extirpative surgery unless the condition has been allowed to progress beyond the abilities of antimicrobial therapy.

Although this has not been described in the literature, it has been an observation of the author that this type of acquired, non-sexually-transmitted pelvic inflammatory disease (which has been largely described in U.S. women) is frequently associated with the use of tampons. Tampons have already been demonstrated in some rare cases to alter the microbiologic flora of the vagina, producing a toxic shock syndrome. It is therefore suggested that women who develop an inflammatory syndrome with IUDs be questioned as to their use of tampons and these be banned until the disease has been controlled.

Indeed, it is the suggestion of the author that all women using tampons while having an IUD in place should be cautioned to be prudent in their use of the tampons; that is, they should not use them when they are not flowing and not leave them intravaginally for prolonged periods of time.

Infections Produced by Actinomycosis

In 1967 Brenner and Gehring [11] reported a case of severe tubal actinomycosis with abscess formation in a 50-year-old woman who had been wearing a spring pessary for 25 years. In 1972 a tuboovarian abscess containing actinomycosis was removed by Henderson from a woman wearing a Majzlin spring [57]. Charnock and Chambers [23] reported five women with severe genital tract actinomycosis who had been using IUDs. Schiffer et al. [97, 98] also reported on IUD-associated actinomycosis. Seligman et al. [104] reported a serious case of PID related to actinomycosis. Not too much attention was paid to isolated case reports of these rare abscesses produced by actinomycosis until the organism was reported to be found frequently on Papanicolaou smears of women wearing IUDs. Spence et al. [112] noted that actinomycosis may have been missed in making the diagnosis of PID and recommended that the presence of actinomycosis be confirmed using immunofluorescent and microbiologic techniques. They further recommended removing the IUD until the Papanicolaou smear cleared.

Valicenti et al. [122] studied 69,925 cervical smears prospectively. Of this group 6,450 smears were from women using IUDs. Of these women 1.6 percent had actinomycosis proven by direct immunofluorescent techniques, 75 percent were asymptomatic, 20 percent had vaginal discharge, 10 percent had irregular bleeding, and 2 women had active pelvic inflammatory disease caused by actinomycosis. None of the non-IUD-wearing women had actinomycosis. They recommend removing the IUD and repeating the Papanicolaou smear after the next period in those cases where no symptoms of PID are present.

Symptomatic actinomycosis should be treated with penicillin, tetracycline, or, for severe cases not responding to these agents, clindamycin.

IUDs and Carcinogenicity

There is no evidence that the IUD is an etiologic agent in the genesis of cervical or uterine cancer. This subject was reviewed by Edelman et al. [36] and the Medical Device Advisory Committee of the Food and Drug Administration [102].

IUDs and Teratogenicity

There is no evidence that pregnancy occurring with an IUD in situ is more likely to produce a congenital abnormality than without the device [36, 102].

LENGTH OF TIME IUDS MAY BE LEFT IN SITU

Nonmedicated plastic IUDs may safely be left in place indefinitely if the woman remains asymptomatic [91]. Copper-carrying and progesterone-loaded IUDs should be replaced as indicated by the manufacturer's current instructions.

REMOVING IUDS

As indicated, there are a number of conditions in which IUD removal may be necessary, such as heavy bleeding, intolerable uterine cramping, partial expulsion, desire to switch to another form of contraception, or planning for pregnancy. In most cases, at least with the present IUDs, it is simply sufficient to grasp the thread of the IUD with a suitable Kelly clamp or uterine dressing forcep and use gentle downward traction to remove the IUD.

However, as indicated in the sections on embedding and difficult removals, the string may not be visible or the IUD may be partially embedded, so that either no strings are available or the IUD does not come down when one tugs on the string [94, 129–131]. If the IUD does not come down with modest traction, one should desist before the string is torn off or a uterine laceration is produced. Under those circumstances it is helpful to move to either hysterography [16, 118] or hysteroscopy [107] to determine whether the IUD is embedded. Hysteroscopy has the great virtue of determining absolutely whether the IUD is in the cavity, embedded, or partially perforated. It is also possible, if you have an operating hysteroscope, to guide a small alligator forceps into the cavity, grasp the IUD, and back it out of the perforation track or dislodge it from where it is embedded.

If the IUD thread is not available, a number of measures are available for determining where the IUD is. Intrauterine manipulations to remove an IUD are best carried out after a paracervical block (similar to the one used for inserting IUDs) is put in place. It is then usually possible (in the office) to dilate the cervix, using two or three small Pratt or Hegar dilators up to 6 or 7 mm. Then a universal IUD removal hook (Rocket of London) can be passed into the cavity and used to gently explore and locate the presence of the IUD. The IUD can be hooked and drawn downwards by the remover. One can also try to use a small alligator forcep (of the type used in laparoscopy or other endoscopic procedures) to grasp the IUD and bring it outward. This is frequently difficult to perform blindly and may have to be performed during hysteroscopy. If the IUD cannot be located and moved using the hook or al-

ligator forcep, then it is certain that hysterosalpingography, hysteroscopy, or ultrasound has to be used to further locate the presence and condition of the IUD.

INFORMED CONSENT AND PATIENT INSTRUCTIONS

Unfortunately, one reason for the decreased popularity of the IUDs these days relates to the number of malpractice actions that have been instituted against physicians having patients with IUD complications such as intrauterine pregnancy, ectopic pregnancy, and severe pelvic infections. Some of these problems have come about because of failure to properly inform the patient before insertion of the IUD about the side effects, complications, and limitations of this method.

It is mandatory that the patient be given some literature to read [56, 62, 102] that adequately describes the IUD and its problems. One of the best of these publications has been prepared by the American College of Obstetrics and Gynecology and is titled "The Intrauterine Device." Other publications are available from Planned Parenthood or from the U.S. Department of Health and Human Services. In addition to providing this literature, the physician should reinforce the main problems verbally to the patient. She should be shown the IUD and told

1. That it is made with plastic with or without metal (copper) or progesterone
2. That the IUD works primarily by preventing a fertilized egg from implanting
3. When you plan to insert the IUD and why you prefer to insert it during the menses (if that is your policy)
4. That about one in five women will have their IUDs removed within a year because of bleeding and cramping
5. That a small number of women become pregnant within several years of using the IUD; potential users should be very clear on the point that pregnancies can occur despite the presence of the IUD
6. That any drastic increase in menstrual flow or symptoms such as pelvic pain, backache, fishy odor, elevated temperature, etc. should be communicated to the clinician rapidly
7. That she may get some cramps during the insertion of the IUD and that you can probably prevent most of these by using a local anesthetic
8. That if she develops an elevated temperature within 3 days of the insertion of the IUD, a purulent discharge, or a soaking through more than two napkins an hour, she should call the physician
9. That the use of an additional barrier contraceptive

or spermicide during the first two periods after insertion of the IUD is recommended; it may lower the failure rate due to early expulsion

10. That she should be examined after one or two periods so that you can be sure that the IUD is not expelled
11. That she should not use tampons after IUD insertion
12. That if at any time her period is more than 7 to 10 days late, if she has a light period, or if she develops severe unilateral pain in the lower abdomen, she should call you and prepare to come in for almost immediate examination
13. That if she develops a yellow, creamy, puslike vaginal discharge or a fishy or ammoniacal vaginal odor she should come in for examination as soon as possible
14. That intrauterine contraceptive devices do not protect her from a sexually transmitted illness and if she is unsure of the state of her partner, it would be a good idea to use a barrier contraceptive as well (the condom is best suited to protect against the transmission of sexually transmitted disease)

An informed consent sheet should be used and signed by the patient in which she recognizes

1. That it is possible that she may become pregnant with an IUD in place
2. That her periods may change and become heavier
3. That she may have uterine cramping or bleeding disturbances
4. That it is possible to develop an infection while using the IUD
5. That she knows that she has no guarantee that this method will be free from side effects or problems

Using intrauterine devices requires cooperation and understanding. It requires the patient to provide feedback to the physician of any information that might indicate the development of either pregnancy, infection, or other IUD-related problems. The patient must understand that compliance with these principles is necessary for her continued safe use of a non-coitally-related effective method of contraception.

As was demonstrated by the failure of mass IUD programs in the 1960s, the IUD simply cannot be put in place and left without active cooperation of clinician and patient. An appropriately selected and counseled patient with a healthy reproductive tract of a size adequate to accommodate one of the current IUDs, who has a carefully and gently performed IUD insertion, can find the use of an IUD to be a very satisfactory and highly effective method of contraception. The overall risks are lower than those associated with the use of oral contraceptives [45].

REFERENCES

1. Acker, D., et al. Electrocardiogram changes with intrauterine device insertion. *Am. J. Obstet. Gynecol.* 115:458, 1973.
2. Agnew, H. N., and Pritchard, J. A. Abortion and bacterial shock induced with an intrauterine contraceptive device. *Obstet. Gynecol.* 28:332, 1966.
3. Alivor, G. T. Pregnancy outcome with removal of intrauterine device. *Obstet. Gynecol.* 41:894, 1973.
4. American College of Obstetricians and Gynecologists. The intrauterine device. *Tech. Bull.* 40, 1976, A. B. M. Anderson and J. H. Guillebaud.
5. Aznar, R., et al. Ectopic pregnancy rates in IUD users. *Br. Med. J.* 1:785, 1978.
6. Banharnsupawat, L., and Rosenfield, A. G. Immediate postpartum IUD insertion. *Obstet. Gynecol.* 38:276, 1971.
7. Bernard, R. P. IUD performance patterns: A 1970 world view. *Int. J. Gynaecol. Obstet.* 8:926, 1970.
8. Bernard, R. P. Factors governing IUD performance. *Am. J. Public Health* 61:559, 1971.
9. Birnberg, C. H., and Burnhill, M. S. A new intrauterine contraceptive device. *Am. J. Obstet. Gynecol.* 89:137, 1964.
10. Birnberg, C., and Burnhill, M. After office hours: Whither IUD? The present and future of intrauterine contraceptives. *Obstet. Gynecol.* 31:861, 1968.
11. Brenner, R. W., and Gehring, S. W. Pelvic actinomycosis in the presence of an endocervical contraceptive device. *Obstet. Gynecol.* 29:71, 1967.
12. Burkman, R. T. Intrauterine device use and the risk of pelvic inflammatory disease. *Am. J. Obstet. Gynecol.* 138:861, 1980.
13. Burnhill, M. S. The syndrome of progressive endometritis associated with intrauterine devices. *Adv. Plann. Parent.* (S. Lewit, ed.), 8, 1973.
14. Burnhill, M. S. Prescriptive Approaches to IUD Usage. In R. G. Wheeler, G. W. Duncan, and J. Speidel (eds.), *Intrauterine Devices: Development, Evaluation and Implementation.* New York: Academic, 1974. Pp. 78–89.
15. Burnhill, M. S. Teenage Pregnancy: Intrauterine Contraceptive Devices. In R. Russo (ed.), *Sexual Development and Disorders in Childhood and Adolescence.* New Hyde Park, N. Y.: Medical Examination, 1983. Pp. 192–196.
16. Burnhill, M. S., and Birnberg, C. H. Superimposition hysterography as a tool in the investigation of intrauterine contraceptive devices: Preliminary report. Proceedings of the 2nd International Conference on Intrauterine Contraception, New York, Oct. 1964. Pp. 127–134.
17. Burnhill, M. S., and Birnberg, C. The size and shape of the uterine cavity determined by hysterography with an intrauterine contraceptive device as a marker. *Int. J. Fer-*

til. 11:187, 1966.

18. Burnhill, M. S., and Birnberg, C. H. Contraception with an intrauterine bow inserted immediately postpartum. *Obstet. Gynecol.* 28:329, 1966.

19. Burnhill, M. S., and Birnberg, C. Uterine perforation with intrauterine contraceptive devices. *Am. J. Obstet. Gynecol.* 98:135, 1967.

20. Burnhill, M. S., and Birnberg, C. Improving the results obtained with current intrauterine contraceptive devices. *Fertil. Steril.,* 20:232, 1969.

21. Cates, W., et al. The intrauterine device and deaths from spontaneous abortion. *N. Engl. J. Med.* 295:1155, 1976.

22. Cederqvist, L. L., and Fuchs, F. Cervical perforation by the Copper-T intrauterine contraceptive device. *Am. J. Obstet. Gynecol.* 119:854, 1974.

23. Charnock, M., and Chambers, T. J. Pelvic actinomycosis and intrauterine contraceptive devices. *Lancet* 1:1239, 1979.

24. Christian, C. D. Maternal deaths associated with an IUD. *Am. J. Obstet. Gynecol.* 119:441, 1974.

25. Conrad, C. C., Ghazi, M., and Kitay, D. Z. Acute neurovascular sequelae of IUD insertion or removal. *J. Reprod. Med.* 11:211, 1973.

26. D'Amico, J., and Israel, R. Bowel obstruction and perforation with an intraperitoneal loop intrauterine contraceptive device. *Am. J. Obstet. Gynecol.* 129:461, 1977.

27. Davies, A. J., Anderson, A. B. M., and Turnbull, A. C. Reduction by naproxen of excessive menstrual bleeding in women using intrauterine devices. *Obstet. Gynecol.* 57:74, 1981.

28. Davis, H. J., and Lesinski, J. Mechanisms of action of IUDs in women. *Obstet. Gynecol.* 36:350, 1970.

29. Davis, H. J. The shield IUD: A superior modern contraceptive. *Am. J. Obstet. Gynecol.* 106:455, 1970.

30. Davis, H. J. *Intrauterine Devices for Contraception.* Baltimore: Williams & Wilkins, 1971. P. 8.

31. Davis, H., and Israel, R. Uterine Cavity Measurements in Relation to Design of Intrauterine Contraceptive Devices. In S. Segal, A. Southam, and K. Shafer (eds.), *Intrauterine Contraception* (International Congress Series, No. 86). Amsterdam: Excerpta Medica, 1965. Pp. 135–141.

32. Dawood, M. Y., and Birnbaum, S. J. Unilateral tuboovarian abscess and intrauterine contraceptive device. *Obstet. Gynecol.* 46:429, 1975.

33. Dickinson, R. L. *Control of Contraception.* Baltimore: Williams & Wilkins, 1938. Pp. 101–117.

34. Dreishpoon, I. H. Complications of pregnancy with an IUCD in situ. *Am. J. Obstet. Gynecol.* 121:412, 1975.

35. Edelman, D. A., et al. Pelvic inflammatory disease and the intrauterine device: A causal relationship? *Int. J. Gynaecol. Obstet.* 17:504, 1980.

36. Edelman, D. A., Berger, G. S., and Keith, L. *Intrauterine Devices and Their Complications.* Boston: Hall, 1979.

37. Edelman, D. A., Berger, G. S., and Keith, L. The use of

IUDs and their relationship to pelvic inflammatory disease: A review of epidemiologic and clinical studies. *Curr. Prob. Obstet. Gynecol.,* 6:5, 1982.

38. Eisenger, S. H. Second trimester spontaneous abortion, the IUD and infection. *Am. J. Obstet. Gynecol.* 124:393, 1976.

39. Erkkola, R., and Livukko, P. Intrauterine device and ectopic pregnancy. *Contraception* 16:569, 1977.

40. Eschenbach, D. A., Harnisch, J. P., and Holmes, K. K. Pathogenesis of acute pelvic inflammatory disease: Role of contraception and other risk factors. *Am. J. Obstet. Gynecol.* 8:838, 1977.

41. Faulkner, W. L., and Ory, H. W. Intrauterine devices and acute pelvic inflammatory disease. *J.A.M.A.* 235:1851, 1976.

42. Foreman, H., Stadel, B., and Schlesselman, S. Intrauterine device usage and fetal loss. *Obstet. Gynecol.* 58:669, 1981.

43. Gibor, Y., Deysach, L., and Lissen, C. H. Uterine length: Prognostic indicator for the successful use of the Cu-7 IUD. *J. Reprod. Med.* 11:205, 1973.

44. Golde, S. H., Israel, R., and Ledger, W. J. Unilateral tuboovarian abscess: A distinct entity. *Am. J. Obstet. Gynecol.* 127:807, 1977.

45. Guillebaud, J. The safety of intrauterine devices. *Stud. Fam. Plann.,* 10:174, 1979.

46. Guillebaud, J. Scheme for management of "lost" IUD threads. *IPPF Med. Bull.,* 14:1, 1980.

47. Golditch, I. M., and Huston, J. E. Serious pelvic infections associated with intrauterine contraceptive device. *Int. J. Fertil.* 18:156, 1973.

48. Goldsmith, A., et al. Immediate postabortal intrauterine contraceptive device insertion: A double blind study. *Am. J. Obstet. Gynecol.* 112:957, 1972.

49. Gräfenberg, E. An Intrauterine Contraceptive Method. In M. Sanger and H. J. Stone (eds.), *Practice of Contraception.* Baltimore: Williams & Wilkins, 1930.

50. Gräfenberg, E. The Intrauterine Method of Contraception. In *Sexual Reform Congress.* London: Kegan, Paul, Trench, Trubner Co. Ltd, 1930.

51. Hall, H., et al. The intrauterine ring for conception control. *Fertil. Steril.* 15:618, 1964.

52. Hall, H., Sedlis, A., and Chabon, I. Effect of intrauterine stainless steel ring on endometrial structure and function. *Am. J. Obstet. Gynecol.* 93:1031, 1965.

53. Hall, H., and Stone, M. Observations on the use of the intrauterine pessary with special reference to the Gräfenberg ring. *Am. J. Obstet. Gynecol.* 83:683, 1962.

54. Hallatt, J. G. Ectopic pregnancy associated with the intrauterine device: A study of seventy cases. *Am. J. Obstet. Gynecol.* 125:754, 1976.

55. Hasson, H. M., Berger, G. S., and Edelman, D. A. Factors affecting IUD performance: I. Endometrial cavity length. *Am. J. Obstet. Gynecol.* 126:973, 1976.

56. Hatcher, R. A., et al. *Contraceptive Technology, 1982–1983* (11th ed.). New York: Irvington, 1982. Pp. 72–97.

57. Henderson, S. R. Pelvic actinomycosis associated with an intrauterine device. *Obstet. Gynecol.* 41:726, 1973.

58. Huber, S. C., Piotrow, P. T., and Orlans, F. B. Intrauterine devices. *Popul. Rep.* [B] 2:48, 1975.

59. Hurt, W. G. Septic pregnancy associated with Dalkon shield device. *Obstet. Gynecol.* 44:491, 1974.

60. Ishihama, A. Clinical studies on intrauterine rings, especially the present state of contraception in Japan and the experiences in the use of intrauterine rings. *Yokohama Med. Bull.*, 10:89, 1959.

61. Ishihama, A. Clinical effects of Japanese IUDs: From our 15 years' clinical studies. *J. Iwate Med. Assoc.* 23:155, 1971.

62. Jennings, J. Report of safety and efficacy of the Dalkon shield and other IUDs. Prepared by the Ad Hoc Obstetric-Gynecologic Committee (to the United States Food and Drug Administration), Oct. 29–30, 1974.

63. Kahn, H. S., and Tyler, C. W. An association between the Dalkon shield and complicated pregnancies among women hospitalized for intrauterine contraceptive device-related disorders. *Am. J. Obstet. Gynecol.* 125:83, 1976.

64. Kahn, H. S., and Tyler, C. W., Jr. IUD related hospitalizations. *J.A.M.A.* 234:53, 1975.

65. Kahn, H. S., and Tyler, C. W., Jr. Mortality associated with use of IUDs. *J.A.M.A.* 234:57, 1975.

66. Kamal, I., et al. Dimensional and architectural disproportion between the intrauterine device and the uterine cavity: A cause of bleeding. *Fertil. Steril.* 22:514, 1971.

67. Kaufman, D. W., et al. Intrauterine contraceptive device use and pelvic inflammatory disease. *Am. J. Obstet. Gynecol.* 136:159, 1980.

68. Lee, N. C., et al. Type of intrauterine device and the risk of pelvic inflammatory disease. *Obstet. Gynecol.* 62:1, 1983.

69. Lewit, S. Outcome of pregnancy with intrauterine devices. *Contraception* 2:47, 1970.

70. Lippes, J. A Study of Intrauterine Contraception: Development of a Plastic Loop. In C. Tietze and S. Lewit (eds.), *Intra-Uterine Contraceptive Devices* (International Congress Series No. 54). Amsterdam: Excerpta Medica, 1962. Pp. 69–75.

71. Lippes, J. Contraception with intra-uterine plastic loops. *Am. J. Obstet. Gynecol.* 93:1024, 1965. (Also in A. J. Sobrero and S. Lewit (eds.), *Adv. Plann. Parent.* 2:148, 1967.)

72. Lippes, J. Observations after four years of experience with the intra-uterine plastic loop at the Buffalo Planned Parenthood Center. *J. Sex. Res.* 3:323, 1967.

73. Liskin, L., and Fox, G. (eds.). IUDs: An appropriate contraceptive for many women. *Popul. Rep.* [B]. 10:4, 1982.

74. Malhatra, N., and Chaundhury, R. R. Current status of intrauterine devices: II. Intrauterine devices and pelvic inflammatory diseases and ectopic pregnancy. *Obstet.*

75. Margulies, L. C. Permanent Reversible Contraception with an Intrauterine Plastic Spiral. In C. Tietze and S. Lewit (eds.), *Intrauterine Contraceptive Devices, Proceedings of the Conference* (International Congress Series No. 54). Amsterdam: Excerpta Medica, 1962.

76. Marshall, B. R., Hepler, J. K., and Kinguizi, M. S. Fatal *Streptococcus pyogenes* septicemia associated with an intrauterine device. *Obstet. Gynecol.* 41:83, 1973.

77. Mead, P. B., Beecham, J. B., and Malck, J. V. S. Incidence of infections associated with the intrauterine contraceptive device in an isolated community. *Am. J. Obstet. Gynecol.* 125:79, 1976.

78. Mishell, D. R., et al. The intrauterine device: A bacteriologic study of the endometrial cavity. *Am. J. Obstet. Gynecol.* 96:119, 1966.

79. Moyer, D. L., and Mishell, D. R., Jr. Reactions of human endometrium to the intrauterine foreign body: 2. Long-term effects on the endometrial histology and cytology. *Am. J. Obstet. Gynecol.* 111:66, 1971.

80. Nakamoto, M., and Buchman, M. Complications of intrauterine contraceptive devices. *Am. J. Obstet. Gynecol.* 94:1073, 1966.

81. Niebyl, J. R., et al. Unilateral ovarian abscess associated with the intrauterine device. *Obstet. Gynecol.* 52:165, 1978.

82. Oppenheimer, W. Prevention of pregnancy by the Grafenberg ring method: A re-evaluation after 28 years' experience. *Am. J. Obstet. Gynecol.* 78:446, 1959.

83. Ory, H. W. A review of the association between intrauterine devices and acute pelvic inflammatory disease. *J. Reprod. Med.* 20:200, 1978.

84. Osser, S., Liedholm, P., and Sjoberg, N. O. Risk of pelvic inflammatory disease among users of intrauterine devices, irrespective of previous pregnancy. *Am. J. Obstet. Gynecol.* 138:864, 1980.

85. Ostergard, D. R. The Dalkon shield intrauterine device: A review of current status. *J. Reprod. Med.* 14:64, 1975.

86. Ota, T. A study on the birth control with an intrauterine instrument. *Jpn. J. Obstet. Gynecol.* 17:210, 1934.

87. Paulson, J. D., and Kao, M. S. Cervical perforation by the Copper-7 intrauterine device. *Obstet. Gynecol.* 50:621, 1977.

88. Pharriss, B. B. Clinical experience with the intrauterine progesterone contraceptive system. *J. Reprod. Med.* 20:155, 1978.

89. Pharriss, B. B., et al. Progestasert: A uterine therapeutic system for long-term contraception: 1. Philosophy and clinical efficacy. *Fertil. Steril.* 25:915, 1974.

90. Piotrow, P., Rinehart, W., and Schmidt, J. (eds.). IUDs: Update on safety, effectiveness and research. *Popul. Rep.* [B]. 7:3, 1979.

91. Planned Parenthood Federation of America. IUD Use. *Medical Standards and Guidelines* (part 2, Sec. IV). New York, 1982.

Gynecol. Surv. 37:1, 1982.

92. Propper, N. S., and Moore, J. H. Association of *E. coli* sepsis in pregnancy with a CU-7 intrauterine device in place. *Obstet. Gynecol.* 48:765, 1976.

93. Püst, K. Ein brauchbarer frauenschutz. *Dtsch. Med. Wochenschr.* 49:952, 1923.

94. Rao, R. P. Lost intrauterine devices and their location. *J. Reprod. Med.* 20:195, 1978.

95. Richter, R. Ein mittel zur verhutung der konzeption. *Dtsch. Med. Wochenschr.* 35:1525, 1909.

96. Rienprayura, D., Phaosavasdi, S., and Somboonsuk, A. Cervical perforation by the CU-7 intrauterine device. *Contraception* 7:515, 1973.

97. Schiffer, M. A., et al. Actinomycosis infections associated with intrauterine contraception devices. *Obstet. Gynecol.* 45:67, 1975.

98. Schiffer, M. A., Elguezabal, A., and Allen, A. C. Actinomycosis infections associated with intrauterine contraceptive devices and a vaginal pessary. *Adv. Plann. Parent.* 7:183, 1978.

99. Schmidt, W. A. IUDs, inflammation and infection: Assessment after two decades of IUD use. *Hum. Pathol.* 13:878, 1982.

100. Scott, R. B. Critical illnesses and deaths associated with IUDs. *Obstet. Gynecol.* 31:322, 1968.

101. Scutchfield, R. D., and Long, W. N. Perforation of the uterus with the Lippes loop: Epidemiologic analysis. *J.A.M.A.* 208:2335, 1969.

102. *Second Report on Intrauterine Contraceptive Devices.* The Medical Device and Drug Advisory Committees on Obstetrics and Gynecology and the United States Department of Health, Education, and Welfare. Washington, D.C.: United States Government Printing Office, December 1978.

103. Segal, S. J., Southam, A. L., and Shafer, K. D. Intrauterine contraception. *Proceedings of the 2nd International Conference, Oct. 2–3, 1964, Belgium.* New York: Excerpta Medica, 1965.

104. Seligman, P. A., et al. Tuboovarian actinomycosis. *N. Y. State J. Med.* 76:278, 1976.

105. Senanayake, P. Contraception and the etiology of PID: New perspectives. International Symposium on Pelvic Inflammatory Disease, Apr. 1–3, 1980, United States Department of Health, Education, and Welfare, Atlanta, Ga. *Am. J. Obstet. Gynecol.* 38:852, 1980.

106. Shine, R. J., and Thompson, J. F. The in situ IUD and pregnancy outcome. *Am. J. Obstet. Gynecol.* 119:124, 1974.

107. Siegler, A. M., and Kemmann, E. Location and removal of misplaced or embedded intrauterine devices by hysteroscopy. *J. Reprod. Med.* 16:139, 1976.

108. Sivin, I. IUDs and ectopic pregnancy. *Stud. Fam. Plann.*, 14:57, 1983.

109. Smith, M. R., and Soderstrom, R. Salpingitis: A frequent response to intrauterine contraception. *J. Reprod. Med.* 16:159, 1976.

110. Snowden, R. The Progestasert and ectopic pregnancy. *Br. Med. J.* 1:1600, 1977.

111. Sparks, R. A., et al. The bacteriology of the cervix and uterus. *Br. J. Obstet. Gynaecol.* 84:701, 1977.

112. Spence, M. R., et al. Cytologic detection and clinical significance of *Actinomyces israelii* in women using intrauterine contraceptive devices. *Am. J. Obstet. Gynecol.* 131:295, 1978.

113. Targum, S. D., and Wright, N. H. Association of the IUD and pelvic inflammatory disease: Retrospective pilot study. *Am. J. Epidemiol* 100:262, 1974.

114. Tatum, H. J. Clinical aspects of intrauterine contraception: Circumspection 1976. *Fertil. Steril.* 28:3, 1977.

115. Tatum, H. J., et al. The Dalkon shield controversy: Structural and bacteriologic studies of IUD tails. *J.A.M.A.* 231:711, 1975.

116. Tatum, H. J., and Schmidt, F. H. Contraceptive and sterilization practices and extrauterine pregnancy: A realistic perspective. *Fertil. Steril.* 28:407, 1977.

117. Taylor, E. S., et al. The intrauterine device and tuboovarian abscess. *Am. J. Obstet. Gynecol.* 123:338, 1975.

118. Tejuja, S., and Malkani, P. K. Clinical significance of correlation between size of uterine cavity and IUCD: A study by planimeter-hysterogram technique. *Am. J. Obstet. Gynecol.* 105:620, 1969.

119. Tietze, C. Effectiveness and acceptability of intrauterine contraceptive devices. *Am. J. Public Health* 55:1874, 1965.

120. Tietze, C. Contraception with intrauterine devices, 1959–1966. *Am. J. Obstet. Gynecol.* 96:1043, 1966.

121. Tietze, C., and Lewit, S. Evaluation of IUDs: Ninth progress report of the Cooperative Statistical Program. *Stud. Fam. Plann.* 55:1, 1970.

122. Valicenti, J. F., et al. Detection and prevalence of IUD-associated *Actinomyces* colonization and related morbidity. *J.A.M.A.* 247:1149, 1982.

123. Weinberg, G., and Bailin, C. Postpartum insertion of the safety filament bow. *Obstet. Gynecol.* 41:925, 1973.

124. Westrom, L., Bengtsson, L. P., and Mardh, P. A. The risk of pelvic inflammatory disease in women using intrauterine devices as compared to non-users. *Lancet* 2:221, 1976.

125. White, M. K., et al. Intrauterine device termination rates and the menstrual cycle day of insertion. *Obstet. Gynecol.* 55:220, 1980.

126. World Health Organization Task Force on Intrauterine Devices for Fertility Regulation. IUD insertion following termination of pregnancy: A clinical trial of the TCU 220C, Lippes Loop D and Copper-7. 14:99, 1983.

127. World Health Organization Task Force on Intrauterine Devices for Fertility Regulation. IUD insertion following spontaneous abortion: A clinical trial of the TCU 220C, Lippes Loop D and Copper-7. 14:109, 1983.

128. Wright, N., and Laemmle, P. Acute pelvic inflammatory disease in an indigent population: An estimate of its inci-

dence and relationship to methods of contraception. *Am. J. Obstet. Gynecol.* 101:979, 1968.

129. Zakin, D., Stern, W, and Rosenblatt, R. Complete and partial uterine perforation and embedding following insertion of intrauterine devices: I. Classification, complications, mechanism, incidence and missing string. *Obstet. Gynecol. Surv.* 36:335, 1981.

130. Zakin, D., Stern, W., and Rosenblatt, R. Complete and partial uterine perforation and embedding following insertion of intrauterine devices: II. Diagnostic methods, prevention and management. *Obstet. Gynecol. Surv.* 36:401, 1981.

131. Zakin, D., Stern, W. Z., and Rosenblatt, R. Perforated and embedded intrauterine devices. *J.A.M.A.* 247:2144, 1982.

132. Zipper, J. A., et al. Metallic Cu as an adjunct to 'T' device. *Am. J. Obstet. Gynecol.* 105:1274, 1969.

VI. Other Methods of Contraception

24. Postcoital Contraception

A. Albert Yuzpe

The ability to control the timing of pregnancy has been a goal of individuals for centuries, and the desire to dissociate the act of coitus from pregnancy has resulted in the development of numerous contraceptive techniques, which span the range from primitive unphysiologic methods to highly sophisticated ones where single agents or combinations of drugs are administered at specific times during the menstrual cycle. With the current status of contraceptive technology, a woman may select one of many relatively safe and effective contraceptive methods. However, in cases where premeditated use of a method has not occurred yet unprotected exposure takes place, there may be a pressing need to provide the women with some form of contraception after the fact. Hence the need for postcoital contraceptive methods.

Two lines of direction have been pursued in postcoital contraceptive research. One has focused on its use as a single emergency treatment designed to prevent pregnancy following a single unprotected coital exposure. Such occasions may arise frequently following first coitus: It has been shown that 60 to 80 percent of such exposures are inadequately or completely unprotected [31, 33]. The value of this form of treatment has been demonstrated in cases of sexual assault or potential failure of a barrier method in situations such as condom rupture or displacement of a diaphragm, cervical cap, or contraceptive sponge. At the same visit that postcoital treatment is prescribed, the woman can also be counseled, and if the need for future contraception exists, a suitable ongoing method may be selected.

Another approach has involved the development of a postcoital agent that can be utilized as an ongoing method, whereby the drug is administered on each day that coitus occurs. The number of doses of any compound used with such a method varies greatly according to the number of exposure days. In such cases the regimen employed must be sufficient to prevent pregnancy following as few as a single exposure or as many as twenty or more exposure days per cycle. Hormonal agents (steroids) have been the drugs of choice.

Aside from pregnancy prevention, one of the major goals of the postcoital approach to contraception, regardless of the agent employed, is to limit drug exposure. By doing so, potential side effects might be reduced. Such a method could also be of value to those who elect to use steroidal contraception but whose frequency of exposure per cycle is sufficiently low as to fail to warrant daily administration of a standard combined oral contraceptive.

No drug has received marketing approval as a postcoital contraceptive medication from any drug regulatory agency in North America. However, steroids that are currently marketed for other indications are being used for this purpose. This chapter will include a discussion of the current postcoital methods employed for emergency as well as ongoing contraception. Nonsteroidal agents that may have some promise in this area will also be mentioned.

EMERGENCY HORMONAL POSTCOITAL CONTRACEPTION

To meet the needs of emergency postcoital contraception, steroidal and nonsteroidal estrogens alone or in combination with a progestin have been employed. Success with these steroids has varied from one clinical trial to another, with failure rates reported to range between 0 and 5 percent. Undesirable side effects such as nausea and vomiting are a problem. The potential risk of teratogenicity induced by such agents in the case of treatment failure, although minimal, may be a major stumbling block for the pharmaceutical industry in its efforts to market postcoital contraceptive agents. A medicolegal risk of the same nature exists for the prescribing physician.

In general, emergency postcoital contraception is provided for women who have experienced a single unprotected or inadequately protected act of intercourse. Administration should be confined to those exposed within the previous 72 hours; preferably treatment should be initiated as soon after exposure as possible. The dosage regimens vary greatly for the various drugs employed, as does the duration and number of doses per treatment.

Estrogens

Synthetic or conjugated natural estrogens have been employed individually as postcoital contraceptive agents since the original report in 1966 by Morris and van Wagenen [28]. Various dosage regimens of these steroids have been reported with varying success. Relatively high doses of these agents appear to be necessary in order to be effective with an apparent dose-response relationship demonstrable.

DIETHYLSTILBESTROL

Diethylstilbestrol (DES) and its diphosphate derivative were the first of the estrogens to be employed widely as postcoital agents. They have declined in popularity in recent years since DES use has been associated with vaginal adenosis and adenocarcinoma in female and genital abnormalities and dysfunction in male offspring of women who had taken this drug in the early stages of pregnancy (i.e., during the early stages of genital embryogenesis). No such problems have been reported when DES was used as a postcoital treatment nor are they likely to occur, since normally short-term exposure to the agent occurs before implantation (in the blastocyst stage). The adverse publicity received, however, has resulted in many women and their physicians avoiding its use.

Delay in the onset of menses after DES administration occurs in approximately 12 to 13 percent of cases, whereas 5.5 to 11 percent of women experienced a shortening of their cycle following treatment [11, 21]. Approximately one-half of women in one study noted no change in the amount of menstrual flow, whereas the remainder experienced either lighter or heavier menses [21].

Inconsistent results have been obtained with doses of DES less than 50 mg per day for 5 days. Some authors [20, 29] reported no failures with 25 mg per day, whereas Haspels [11, 12], on the other hand, did. It is impossible, however, to calculate the exact failure rate for the 25 and 30 mg per day regimens in Haspels' studies from the information reported. Doses of 10 mg per day for 5 days are definitely inadequate [26]. From the literature it appears that 50 mg per day for 5 days is the ideal dosage when DES is administered as a postcoital contraceptive agent [11]. Failure rates vary from 0 to 0.8 percent, with the failures occurring at doses of less than 50 mg per day for 5 days.

ETHINYL ESTRADIOL

Ethinyl estradiol (EE) has now become the most popular single estrogen employed for postcoital contraception as well as the major estrogenic constituent of the combined oral contraceptives. Its efficacy as a postcoital agent has been well established, with failure rates ranging from 0 to 0.6 percent [7, 22]. Menstrual patterns following EE treatment are similar to those following DES, with 13 percent experiencing a delay in menses and 11 percent a shortening (plus or minus 5 days) of their cycle [11].

The dosage shown to be most effective is 5 mg per day for 5 days. As with DES, the use of lower doses results in treatment failures.

CONJUGATED EQUINE ESTROGENS

Conjugated estrogens (CEE) are naturally occurring substances derived from equine urinary extracts. These agents have also been shown to be effective as emergency postcoital contraceptives, although Dixon et al. [7] suggest that at the dosages that they studied (5 mg EE and 30 mg CEE) EE appears to be more effective in preventing pregnancy. The intravenous route of administration was employed in 200 rape victims with no failures using 50 mg of CEE on each of 2 consecutive days [5]. Failure rates following oral administration range from 0 to 1.4 percent [6, 7].

As with EE and DES, CEE therapy results in menstrual delay in 13 percent and a shortening of menses in 19 percent (plus or minus 4 days). Seventy percent of women experienced no change in the character or bleeding pattern of their menses following treatment [34].

DEPOT ESTROGENS

Depot estradiol propionate injections administered to 12 women by Coutinho as a postcoital regimen resulted in two failures, both of which were ectopic pregnancies [5]. These results suggested to the investigator that the slower rate of achieving adequate blood levels with a depot estrogen may result in retardation of zygote transport. Schindler et al. [42] employed estradiol-benzoate 12.5 mg combined with 10 mg estradiol-phenylpropionate. The failure rate for 100 treated was 3 percent.

There does not appear to be any value in the use of intramuscular estrogen preparations for postcoital contraception at the present time, since the efficiency of this method does not approach that of the high-dose oral estrogen regimens.

SIDE EFFECTS OF POSTCOITAL ESTROGENS

As one would expect, high doses of estrogen may cause numerous side effects. These include nausea, vomiting, breast tenderness, headache, dizziness, menorrhagia, and abdominal pain. In addition, a case of pulmonary edema has been associated with high-dose estrogen administration [5]. The incidence of nausea and vomiting varies greatly from study to study and with the preparation employed. However, there is a suggestion that side effects associated with CEE may be milder and less frequent than those of DES or EE [34].

The incidence of ectopic pregnancy following postcoital estrogen administration has been reported to be 10 percent and has been compared to the ectopic rate with intrauterine device (IUD) use [30]. Whether this is a true statistic or merely suggestive of the fact that this treatment has no effect on tubal implantation and therefore provides no protection against ectopic pregnancy remains to be seen. The phenomenon of tubal locking seen in some animal species does not occur in humans and therefore cannot be responsible for the questionable predisposition to ectopic pregnancy in humans.

Estrogen-Progestin Combination

Two estrogen-progestin combinations have been employed for postcoital contraception. These include combinations of the nonsteroidal estrogen dienestrol with ethynodiol diacetate [45] and ethinyl estradiol with norgestrel [52]. Only one study [45] is available on the use of the dienestrol–ethynodiol diacetate combination; the failure rate was less than 1 percent.

Since the original pilot study employing the combination of ethinyl estradiol and norgestrel [52], numerous authors have reported on its use as an emergency postcoital contraceptive [10, 14, 37, 38, 41, 49, 53, 54]. The majority of these reports have been favorable, with success rates in the same range as those reported from estrogens alone. Tully [46], on the other hand, reported a failure rate of 5 percent for regularly cycling women exposed at midcycle. This is significantly greater than the failure rates reported by the other authors, which are in the range of 0 to 2 percent. The consensus of opinion among a number of the investigators is that the regimen consisting of 1 mg of norgestrel and 100 μg of ethinyl estradiol followed by the same dose 12 hours later is a safe and effective method of emergency postcoital contraception. As with the estrogens alone, treatment is confined to women reporting a single unprotected coital exposure within the previous 72 hours. In most studies treatment was administered regardless of the time in the cycle at which the exposure occurred. This is in contrast to other studies with estrogens alone, where the treatment was limited to those who were at midcycle or who showed evidence of sperm in the cervical mucus. The decision to treat all patients, regardless of the cycle day of exposure, has been predicated on the knowledge that pregnancy has been reported to occur on any day of the cycle, even though it is clear that the greatest risk occurs when exposure is at or just before midcycle.

The major side effects reported with the combined method are nausea and vomiting. Nausea has been reported to occur at rates ranging from 25 to 66 percent and vomiting in 5 to 24 percent of cases [14, 36, 37, 53, 54]. Concomitant antiemetic administration can significantly reduce the frequency and severity of these symptoms, whether associated with combined agents or estrogens alone.

Treatment success is indicated by the onset of menses. In the combined estrogen-progestin studies 98 percent of women treated began menses within 21 days following therapy [53, 54]. The remaining 2 percent or less were either pregnant or were experiencing a prolongation of their cycle. These women could be distinguished from one another by means of a sensitive pregnancy test by 21 days posttreatment. Delay in menses occurred in 7 percent of cases whereas shortening of the cycle was reported in 20 percent [53]. These results are in marked contrast to those with DES-, EE-, and CEE-treated subjects where more women experienced menstrual delay. The effect of treatment with the combined method is seen sooner and thus alleviates several days of anxiety associated with the anticipation of menses.

Since this regimen is not yet widely used and comparative data with estrogens alone are lacking, Van Santen and Haspels carried out a randomized, double-blind trial comparing this combined method with that of ethinyl estradiol alone [49]. A total of 187 women were treated, 96 in the ethinyl estradiol group and 91 in the combined therapy group. One pregnancy occurred during the entire study and that to one of the patients in the ethinyl-estradiol-only group. Further comparative trials are necessary to fully assess the combined therapy regimen.

Two advantages of the combination therapy are that it permits a significant reduction in both the total amount of steroid administered and in the total number of doses employed. The total dose of ethinyl estradiol administered as a single postcoital agent is 25 mg (2.5 mg b.i.d. for 5 days). This is equivalent to the administration for 2 years of a cyclic combined oral contraceptive drug that contains 50 µg of estrogen. In contrast, the combined therapy is equivalent to four tablets (days) of a similar standard preparation. In addition, by reducing the number of doses from 10 or 15 to 2, patient compliance can only be improved, especially in the face of side effects such as nausea and vomiting. Women are much more likely to comply with a two-dose schedule even if nausea or vomiting occurs, since these side effects are generally limited to a 12-hour period instead of 5 days as with estrogen therapy alone.

CONTINUING OR ONGOING POSTCOITAL CONTRACEPTION

Progestins such as quingestanol acetate [27, 40], d-norgestrel [18, 19, 44], and levonorgestrel [8] have been evaluated as ongoing forms of postcoital contraception. The last agent is currently employed in a marketed regimen in Hungary and is known as "Prostinor." With this preparation the maximum recommended dosage per cycle is four tablets of levonorgestrel, 0.750 mg per tablet. In any one cycle no more than 3 mg total dosage is recommended. Studies are currently being conducted by the World Health Organization to evaluate levonorgestrel as a postcoital contraceptive in the periovulatory period. Varying dosages of the other two progestins mentioned have been utilized with an apparent dose-response relationship demonstrated.

Cycle regularity is frequently disturbed when postcoital progestins are employed. In addition, other side

effects have been reported including nausea, vomiting, fatigue, breast tenderness, and headache. In many cultures irregularity of menstrual bleeding patterns is totally unacceptable, and thus postcoital progestin administration may have limited acceptability.

Assessment of Failures of Postcoital Hormonal Contraception

One of the most frequently posed questions when assessing the success or failure of a postcoital agent is "How many women would have become pregnant as a result of the particular exposure in question had no treatment been administered?" In addition, other confounding variables come into play including the fertility status of both the female and male partners and the possibility of other exposures having occurred during that cycle before or beyond the time when the particular treatment would exert its effects [51].

There is, of course, no answer to the first question. However, various investigators have produced probability tables based on mathematic models that suggest the chance of a specific act of intercourse leading to conception on any given day of the menstrual cycle. Using the first day of a significant rise in the basal body temperature (D) as a reference point, Barret and Marshall [2] found a maximum probability of conception on day D minus 2 days (D-2) of 0.30, whereas Schwartz et al. [43] calculated the probability on the same day to be 0.34. Royston [39] has recently confirmed these estimates.

A recently published prospective study by the World Health Organization [50] evaluated the probability of conception at specific times in the cycle. In this study the time of ovulation was assessed by evaluation of the vulvar and cervical mucus changes. The last day of "fertile-type mucus" (PD or peak day) has been shown by Billings et al. [4], Flynn and Linch [9], and Hilgers et al. [13] to closely correlate with the time of ovulation, with the fertile period calculated to be from the first day of recognizable mucus to 4 days after the PD. Coital exposure outside the fertile period resulted in a low probability of conception (0.004), whereas during the 3 days preceding the PD the probability rose to 0.55. On the PD the probability was 0.667, with the rate falling to 0.089 3 days later. Use of such probability tables partly overcomes the necessity of employing a control group in assessing the efficacy of a postcoital agent and avoids the ethical considerations of placebo administration.

Since the studies evaluating postcoital drugs used in emergency situations are of small numbers, failure rates are usually expressed as the percentage of women treated assuming that only one treatment is employed per cycle. This is in contrast to the failure rates for cyclic oral contraceptive therapy, which are expressed as pregnancies per 100 woman-years of use (Pearl formula) or as failures per 100 women initiating the method over the course of the following year (life-table analysis). Comparisons between the former (percentage) rates and the latter two methods are impossible. From the available literature it appears that for emergency postcoital contraception estrogens alone (EE, DES, or CEE) and EE combined with norgestrel are effective methods.

Mode of Action of Postcoital Hormonal Contraceptive Agents

Various modes of action can be postulated for postcoital hormonal contraceptive drugs, although it is unlikely that any one agent could affect all the physiologic mechanisms involved in conception. These actions include alteration or interference with sperm migration or capacitation, tubal transport, fertilization, luteal function, endometrial activity, implantation, embryonic viability, and even ovulation suppression.

It is highly unlikely that the drug, even if administered shortly after exposure, would exert its effects sufficiently rapidly to interfere with sperm migration or capacitation. Furthermore, antifertilization and cytotoxic effects of estrogen on the early embryo have not been shown in the human. Ovulation suppression would necessitate administration before the LH surge. Therefore, postcoital agents probably exert their effect upon the implantation process. Whether this is manifest through an alteration in endometrial enzymatic and/or metabolic activity or by other means remains to be established. It is known that estrogens reduce carbonic anhydrase activity in the endometrium as do intrauterine devices, although the role of such activity in implantation is still unclear.

An ideal animal model for assessing the effects of a postcoital agent in humans does not exist. Because of the mating habits of subhuman primates, testing must be limited to the periovulatory phase and not to other times. Toxicologic data are also difficult to obtain, since the frequency of administration and total dosage for continuing or ongoing postcoital methods are unpredictable.

ESTROGEN ONLY
High doses of estrogens have been shown to interfere with the process of implantation in the human [28]. This is the postulated mechanism of action when these steroids are employed for postcoital contraception and accounts for the selection of the term *pregnancy intercep-*

tion coined by Naqvi and Warren [32]. Several authors [5] have shown a reduction in plasma progesterone levels following the administration of DES and EE on the day of the basal body temperature rise or even 3 days later. Thus, a direct effect upon corpus luteum or luteinizing hormone (LH) function might be postulated. However, once implantation has occurred, human pregnancy is resistant to large doses of either exogenous EE or DES [1, 16, 17].

PROGESTINS ONLY
The progestins employed for continuing or ongoing regimens may act at several levels as may the estrogen-progestin combinations in the emergency regimen. Progestin administration results in the transformation of cervical mucus to the postovulatory type, which is thick and scant, lacks spinnbarkeit, and demonstrates poor sperm penetration qualities. However, this hostilelike effect would be too late to be of any value for postcoital contraception unless an overlapping phenomenon were to result from frequent administration. The endometrium may undergo variable response to progestins, but primarily it resembles that of inactivity. The effect upon ovulation is also highly variable. If anything, progestins retard tubal motility and might predispose to ectopic implantation (ectopic pregnancy). Therefore, one can safely say that the exact mechanism of action of postcoitally administered progestins requires further study.

ESTROGEN-PROGESTIN COMBINATIONS
Ling et al. [23, 24] has studied the endocrine and endometrial changes following the administration of 2 mg norgestrel combined with 200 μg of ethinyl estradiol. As has been seen with progestin-only administration, the effects are variable. With the combined therapy asynchronous development between glands and stroma in the endometrium is seen, with glandular development lagging. This has been confirmed by others [52]. Endocrine changes are variable but may be grouped into four categories: (1) no change in posttreatment levels of estradiol-17 beta and progesterone compared with those of pretreatment control cycles; (2) a reduction in both estradiol-17 beta and progesterone; (3) a reduction in estradiol only; and (4) a reduction in progesterone or a fluctuation of estradiol levels. Thus, varying types of luteal response may occur. In the majority of cases these responses are manifested by a shortened luteal phase and altered endometrium in the face of either reduced progesterone or estradiol levels (i.e., inadequate luteal phase). Where no reduction in the production of the steroids is seen, the effect may be postulated to occur at the cellular or subcellular level [24].

ADVANTAGES AND DISADVANTAGES OF POSTCOITAL HORMONAL CONTRACEPTION

Advantages

Emergency postcoital hormonal contraception, if used properly, can provide a means of avoiding unwanted pregnancy with its associated myriad of undesirable physical and psychosocial sequelae. The patient contacting a physician or family planning facility may be doing so for the first time. This not only allows the prescribing of an emergency postcoital treatment but also provides an opportunity for counseling and the institution of ongoing contraception.

Disadvantages

The major risk associated with postcoital contraception is failure and the dilemma that ensues concerning the subsequent management of the pregnancy. Since the majority of women for whom this method is selected are unmarried and frequently young, pregnancy termination is generally elected [3, 31, 33]. However, in some cases a woman may elect to continue the pregnancy. In this situation the question of teratogenicity must be considered. As previously mentioned, there is no reported case of a teratogenic effect occurring as a result of the postcoital administration of one of the estrogens when used alone or in the combined regimen. The blastocyst is relatively resistant to the effects of exposure to steroid hormones. The brief duration of therapy, especially with the combined medication, and the relatively short half-life of the steroids used make exposure of an implanted embryo (in cases of failure) highly unlikely. This may not be the case when progestins are employed on a continuing basis. In such instances continued exposure may occur in the face of an early unrecognized gestation. The embryo may be less resistant to steroid exposure with at least a potential risk of teratogenic effects resulting once implantation has occurred. This also can happen if an inaccurate history of sexual exposure and menstrual dates has been given.

Another disadvantage of postcoital contraceptives relates to their moral and ethical implications. A contraceptive method that exerts its effects after fertilization has occurred is, for some, unacceptable.

Finally, the potential for misuse of postcoital emergency treatment is always possible. Some women may begin to rely on repeated use of this form of treatment instead of employing an acceptable ongoing form of contraception. One may rationalize such repeated use since pregnancy rates are in the range of 2 percent. However, one must consider that these rates represent a risk of 2 percent per cycle, rather than 2 percent per year. Furthermore, the frequency of nausea, vomiting, and cycle disturbance associated with postcoital contraception would also rule out its use as a routine ongoing method.

OTHER AGENTS EMPLOYED FOR POSTCOITAL CONTRACEPTION

STS 557

The synthetic progestin STS 557 has been shown to have antiimplantation effects in baboons with a single dose of 0.4 mg administered within 3 to 6 hours of the onset of mating [35]. Phase I clinical trials are currently being conducted under the auspices of the World Health Organization. The safety of this compound must still be established, since it is a cyano derivative. Available toxicologic data do not, however, support this concern. Extensive clinical evaluation is still necessary before this agent can be considered as a postcoital contraceptive.

Centchromen

Centchromen has weak estrogenic and potent antiestrogenic properties. It also lacks progestational, androgenic, and antiandrogenic effects [15]. Although phase II clinical trials have been carried out with this drug, the side effects experienced, including marked ovarian enlargement, are significant enough that it may never reach further stages of development.

Chinese Home Visiting or Vacation Pills

As a result of the social structure in the People's Republic of China, some husbands and wives live apart and may spend only short periods of time together (1 or 2 weeks) during the course of a year (i.e., during their "vacations"). Vacation pills have been developed in order to prevent pregnancy during this short but concentrated period of coital exposure. These agents are not truly postcoital by definition, since their administration begins 1 or 2 days before the vacation and continues daily until the vacation ends. In some cases additional combined contraceptives are administered.

Nine such vacation pills have been developed including six different progestins, two progestin combinations, and one nonprogestin. A summary of the various agents employed as vacation pills are listed in Table 24-1. Well-controlled clinical trials are lacking with these regimens, despite the fact that large numbers of women have been treated.

Postcoital IUD Insertion

Lippes et al. [25] reported no pregnancies following the insertion of copper-T IUDs in 97 women after unpro-

Table 24-1. List of vacation pills used in People's Republic of China

Name	Dosage (mg)	Efficacy (% of cycles)	Mode of administration
Simple progestins			
Norethisterone	5	99.5	In case of vacation, one pill in the evening, then one pill each day for 10–14 days; change to pill No. 1 (norethisterone–ethinyl estradiol combination pill—various doses) or No. 2 (megestrol + ethinyl estradiol combination pill—various doses), if vacation longer than two weeks
Megestrol	2	99.6	One pill at midday before vacation and then in the evening; afterward one pill each day until the next day after vacation
Quingestanol	80	98.8	One pill for two weeks
Norgestrel	3	99.9	One pill 1–2 days before vacation, then one pill every day. Change to pill No. 1 or No. 2 if vacation longer than two weeks
R-2323	2.5	99.5	Similar to norgestrel
Norethisterone acetate-3-oxime	1	99.3	Similar to norgestrel
Progestin combinations			
Mequingestanol	Megestrol 0.55 Quingestanol 0.88	98.2	One pill at midday before vacation, then one pill postcoitally
Chlorquingestanol	Chlormadinone 0.25 Quingestanol 0.85	99.5	One pill at midday before vacation, then one pill every evening
Nonprogestin			
Anordrin	7.5	99.5	Was used as a postcoital agent. Results were equivocal

Woman-cycles, not woman-years.

tected coital exposure within the previous 5 days. Other studies have confirmed these results [47, 48].

The selection of such postcoital treatment may be ideal in some instances, such as situations where estrogens are contraindicated or where treatment is delayed beyond 72 hours or for the multiparous patient. It is less than ideal for the young nullipara, especially the one with multiple sexual partners. In the latter case IUD use may predispose to serious complications, such as the development of sexually transmitted disease and pelvic inflammatory disease (PID). The IUD may increase the risk of exacerbating a quiescent PID or predisposing to its development. However, when the ideal patient for such treatment is carefully selected, the method may serve not only as an effective postcoital contraceptive but also as a subsequent method of acceptable ongoing contraception. The Cu-7, the Cu-T 200, and the ML-Cu 250 have all been used for this purpose.

A major problem that might result from the use of the IUD in the event of its failure as a postcoital agent is the masking of an early gestation. This may occur since IUD insertion is often associated with varying degrees of irregular bleeding. When the steroidal method of postcoital contraception is employed, menstruation indicates the success of the treatment. However, an early gestation may still be present in the face of some irregular bleeding associated with the IUD. Thus, failures might not be detected until there is clinical evidence of uterine enlargement or a positive pregnancy test. The result could be a delay in further management of the pregnancy, whether it be by pregnancy termination or by removal of the IUD, if the patient wishes to continue the pregnancy.

SUMMARY

There is a pressing need for continued research in the development of postcoital contraceptive agents that are devoid of estrogenic activity, highly effective, and associated with a low incidence of risk and side effects. The prostaglandins, antiprogestins, LHRH agonists and antagonists, and hCG antagonists are all currently being evaluated as potential contraceptives. Their use may, at times, be postcoital in timing. Ideally, a single monthly treatment would induce menses regardless of the presence or absence of pregnancy. The World Health Organization Task Force on Postcoital, Once a Month and Menses Inducing Agents has been given the mandate of developing agents to meet these goals.

REFERENCES

1. Bacic, M., de Casparis, A. W., and Diczfalusy, E. Failure of large doses of ethinyl estradiol to interfere with early embryonic development in the human species. *Am. J. Obstet. Gynecol.* 107:531, 1970.

2. Barrett, J. C., and Marshall, J. The risk of conception on different days of the menstrual cycle. *Popul. Studies* 23:455, 1969.

3. Bauman, K. E. Selected aspects of the contraceptive practices of unmarried university students. *Am. J. Obstet. Gynecol.* 108:203, 1970.

4. Billings, E. L., et al. Symptoms and hormonal changes accompanying ovulation. *Lancet* 1:282, 1972.

5. Blye, R. P. The use of estrogens as postcoital contraceptive agents. *Am. J. Obstet. Gynecol.* 116:1044, 1973.

6. Crist, T., and Farrington, C. The use of estrogen as a postcoital contraceptive in North Carolina: Trick or treatment? *N.C. Med. J.* 34:792, 1973.

7. Dixon, G. W., et al. Ethinyl estradiol and conjugated estrogens as postcoital contraceptives. *J.A.M.A.* 244:1336, 1980.

8. Farkas, M. Post-coital contraception with Prostinor, a preparation containing 0.75 mg d-norgestrel. *Magyar Noorvosok Lapja* 41:474, 1978.

9. Flynn, A. M., and Lynch, S. S. Cervical mucus and identification of the fertile phase of the menstrual cycle. *Br. J. Obstet. Gynaecol.* 83:656, 1976.

10. Grillo, T. A., and Hatcher, R. The use of ethinyl estradiol and norgestrel pills as a morning after contraceptive. *Bull. Woodruff Med. Cent.* 11:183, 1980.

11. Haspels, A. A. Interception: Post-coital estrogens in 3016 women. *Contraception* 14:375, 1976.

12. Haspels, A. A., and Andriesse, R. The effects of large doses of estrogens post coitum in 2,000 women. *Eur. J. Obstet. Gynecol. Reprod. Biol.* 3:113, 1973.

13. Hilgers, T. W., Abraham, G. E., and Cavanagh, D. Natural family planning: I. The peak symptom and estimated time of ovulation. *Obstet. Gynecol.* 52:575, 1978.

14. Hutchinson, F. Post-coital birth control. Presented at the conference of the Pregnancy Advisory Service, London, Apr. 14, 1982.

15. Kamboj, V. P., et al. Biological profile of centchromen: A new post-coital contraceptive. *Indian J. Exp. Biol.* 15:1144, 1977.

16. Karnaky, K. J. Prolonged administration of diethylstilbestrol. *J. Clin. Endocrinol. Metab.* 5:279, 1945.

17. Karnaky, K. J. Estrogenic tolerance in pregnant women. *Am. J. Obstet. Gynecol.* 53:312, 1947.

18. Kesseru, E., Larranaga, A., and Parada, J. Post-coital contraception with d-norgestrel. *Contraception* 7:367, 1973.

19. Kovacs, L., and Seregely, G. D-norgestrel as post-coital anticoncipient in young women. Proceedings of the International Congress of Pediatric Gynecology (abstract). Tokyo, 1979.

20. Kuchera, L. K. Postcoital contraception with diethylstilbestrol. *J.A.M.A.* 218:562, 1971.

21. Kuchera, L. K. Postcoital contraception with diethylstilbestrol: Updated. *Contraception* 10:47, 1974.

22. Lehfeldt, H. Choice of ethinyl estradiol as a postcoital pill. *Am. J. Obstet. Gynecol.* 116:892, 1973.

23. Ling, W. Y., et al. Mode of action of dl-norgestrel and ethinyl estradiol combination in post-coital contraception. *Fertil. Steril.* 32:297, 1979.

24. Ling, W. Y., et al. Mode of action of dl-norgestrel and ethinyl estradiol combination in postcoital contraception: II. Effect of postovulatory administration on ovarian function and endometrium. *Fertil. Steril.* 39:292, 1983.

25. Lippes, J., Malik, T., and Tatum, H. J. The postcoital copper-T. *Adv. Plann. Parent.* 11:24, 1976.

26. Mears, E. In R. K. B. Hankinson et al. (eds.), *Proceedings of the Eighth International Conference of the International Planned Parenthood Federation.* London, 1967. P. 256.

27. Mischler, T. W., et al. Further experience with quingestanol acetate as a post-coital oral contraceptive. *Contraception* 9:221, 1974.

28. Morris, J. M., and van Wagenen, G. Compounds interfering with ovum implantation and development: III. Role of estrogen. *Am. J. Obstet. Gynecol.* 96:804, 1966.

29. Morris, J. M., and van Wagenen, G. Post-coital Oral Contraception. In A. J. Sobrero and S. Lewit (eds.), *Advances in Planned Parenthood.* Amsterdam: Excerpta Medica, 1969.

30. Morris, J. M., and van Wagenen, G. Interception: The use of postovulatory estrogens to prevent implantation. *Am. J. Obstet. Gynecol.* 115:101, 1973.

31. Munz, D., et al. Contraception knowledge and practice among undergraduates at a Canadian university. *Am. J. Obstet. Gynecol.* 124:499, 1976.

32. Naqvi, R. H., and Warren, J. C. Interception: Drugs interrupting pregnancy after implantation. *Steroids* 18:731, 1971.

33. Needle, R. H. The relationship between first sexual intercourse and ways of handling contraception among college students. *J. Am. Coll. Health Assoc.* 24:106, 1975.

34. Notelovitz, M., and Bard, D. S. Conjugated estrogen as a post-ovulatory interceptive. *Contraception* 17:443, 1978.

35. Oettel, M., et al. STS-557 as an interceptive in rodents and baboons. *Contraception* 21:537, 1980.

36. Parsons, A. D. The provision of a post-coital contraception

service. Presented to the conference of the Pregnancy Advisory Service. London, Apr. 14, 1982.

37. Percival-Smith, R. Post-coital contraception using dl-norgestrel/ethinyl estradiol combination. *Contraception* 17:247, 1978.

38. Percival-Smith, R., and Ross, A. Ethinyl estradiol dl-norgestrel combination as a morning-after pill: Preliminary report. *B.C. Med. J.* 18:240, 1976.

39. Royston, J. P. Basal body temperature, ovulation and the risk of conception, with special reference to the lifetimes of sperm and egg. *Biometrics* 38:397, 1982.

40. Rubio, B., et al. A new postcoital oral contraceptive. *Contraception* 1:303, 1970.

41. Schilling, L. H. An alternative to the use of high-dose estrogens for post-coital contraception. *J. Am. Coll. Health Assoc.* 27:247, 1979.

42. Schindler, A. E., et al. Postcoital contraception with an injectable estrogen preparation (Org 369-2). *Contraception* 22:165, 1980.

43. Schwartz, D., MacDonald, P. D. M., and Heuchel, V. Fecundability, and coital frequency and the viability of ova. *Popul. Studies* 34:397, 1980.

44. Spona, J., Matt, K., and Schneider, W. H. F. Study on the action of d-norgestrel as a postcoital contraceptive agent. *Contraception* 11:31, 1975.

45. Szontagh, F. E., and Kovacs, L. Post-coital contraception with dienestrol. *Med. Gynecol. Sociol.* 4:36, 1969.

46. Tully, B. Post coital contraception: A study. *Br. J. Fam. Plann.* 8:119, 1983.

47. Tyrer, L. The copper-7 and postcoital contraception. *Adv. Plann. Parent.* 15:111, 1980.

48. Van Santen, M. R., and Haspels, A. A. Interception by post-coital IUD insertion. *Contracept. Deliv. Syst.* 2:189, 1981.

49. Van Santen, M. R., and Haspels, A. A. Comparative randomized double-blind study of high dosage ethinyl estradiol versus ethinyl estradiol and norgestrel combination in postcoital contraception. *Acta Endocrinol.* (Suppl. 99):246, 1982.

50. World Health Organization Special Programme of Research in Human Reproduction, Task Force on Methods for the Determination of the Fertile Period. *Fertil. Steril.* In press, 1984.

51. Yuzpe, A. A. Postcoital hormonal contraception: Uses, risks and abuses. *Int. J. Gynaecol. Obstet.* 15:133, 1977.

52. Yuzpe, A. A., et al. Postcoital contraception: A pilot study. *J. Reprod. Med.* 13:53, 1974.

53. Yuzpe, A. A., and Lancee, W. J. Ethinyl estradiol and dl-norgestrel as a postcoital contraceptive. *Fertil. Steril.* 28:932, 1977.

54. Yuzpe, A. A., Percival-Smith, R., and Rademaker, A. W. A multi-centre clinical investigation employing ethinyl estradiol combined with dl-norgestrel as a postcoital contraceptive agent. *Fertil. Steril.* 37:508, 1982.

25. Coitus Interruptus

Malcolm Potts

Coitus interruptus, or male withdrawal, is certainly the oldest method of contraception. It is still widely used yet little analyzed and commonly misunderstood. It is the simplest method to comprehend, requires no professional advice or appliances, costs nothing—and cannot be forgotten when the couple go away for the weekend! It is explicitly mentioned in the Bible and the Koran, yet in the great explosion of scientific literature dealing with all aspects of family planning, only a handful of attempts have been made to accumulate objective data on this interesting and important contraceptive method [21, 23]. Many contemporary texts deal with the method in a pejorative way, copying unsubstantiated myths from one article to another.

Perhaps neglect of the method is related to the fact that it has no manufacturer to advertise its virtues and no clinicians to press its claims. Indeed, as it is a do-it-yourself method of contraception, those involved in the clinical practice of family planning almost by definition meet only those who, when they have used the method, have become dissatisfied with it for some reasons.

HISTORY

The Genesis passage concerning coitus interruptus is one of the oldest references to contraception in history and the only explicit one in the Bible: "Then Judah said to Onan, 'Go to your brother's wife, perform your duty as brother-in-law and raise up seed for your brother.' Onan knew that the descendants would not be his own, so whenever he had relations with his brother's wife, he let (the seed) be lost on the ground." The text has been subject to volumes of theological exegesis, but it remains uncertain whether Onan's sin was to practice coitus interruptus, to disobey his father, to want all property to go to his own heirs, or to show a lack of familial responsibility. The Talmud refers to coitus interruptus with the picturesque literary phrase "threshing inside and winnowing outside." The Babylonian Talmud says of the practice, "Whoever emits semen in vain deserves death." But this same condemnation is also used for those whose thoughts wander while reading scripture, and it seems unlikely that it was meant to be taken literally.

In Western theology the story of Onan has a pivotal position. Augustine, Aquinas, and the other early fathers of the Church refer to it [16]. St. Augustine, before his conversion to Christianity, was a Manichee and appears to have been faithful to the same woman for 11 years, during which time he had only one child. It is possible that he practiced the method that he was later to condemn. It should be noted that Augustine also condemned the use of periodic abstinence and, as Noonan [16] has pointed out, "In this history of the thought of theologians on contraception, it is, no doubt, piquant that the first pronouncement on contraception by the most influential theologian of teaching on such matters should be a vigorous attack on the one method to avoid procreation now accepted by twentieth-century Catholic theologians as morally lawful."

The prophet Mohammed was aware of the story of Onan and later Jewish commentary but adopted a more liberal interpretation. In the Traditions of the Prophet it is written, "Man said, 'O Prophet of God! I have a slave girl and I practice coitus interruptus with her, I dislike her becoming pregnant, yet I have the desires of men. The Jews believe that coitus interruptus constitutes killing a life in miniature form.' The Prophet replied, 'The Jews are liars. If God wishes to create it, you can never change it.'" When asked about what today would be called the possible psychologic side effects of the method, the prophet Mohammed replied, "Had this practice been injurious it would have harmed the Romans and Persians." The prophet, with an almost twentieth-century vision, prohibited the use of the method unless the woman consented [17]. The approval that the Koran extends to coitus interruptus has never been used as an integral part of family planning programs in any Islamic country, underscoring the unfortunate divorce that exists between traditional methods of fertility regulation and modern family planning programs.

While Islam gave a closely defined approval to *azl*, or coitus interruptus, the Christian church became increasingly obsessed with condemning the method. If the theologians and the writers of the medieval Penitentials are to be believed, coitus interruptus seems to have been well known and somewhat widespread throughout the Middle Ages [16]. In the eighth century St. Hubert condemned "spilling seed in coitus." The Bishop of Lyons (1270) wrote, "The sin against nature occurs when one contrives or consents that the seed be spilled in a place other than that allotted by nature" (although some theologians seem to have deliberately blurred the anatomic distinction between sodomy and coitus interruptus). Chaucer, in "The Parson's Tale," makes similar reference. Perhaps the earliest knowledge, attitude, and practice (KAP) study was that of St. Bernadine in the sixteenth century in Sienna who wrote, "Of one thousand marriages, I believe 999 are the devil's" (that is, employing the use of coitus interruptus). Unfortunately St. Bernadine does not record what methodology she used to conduct her prevalence survey.

DEMOGRAPHIC IMPACT

Historic demographers, largely using the records of baptisms, marriages, and deaths in European parishes

before the Industrial Revolution, have been able to measure some of the impact that coitus interruptus made on birth rates. Patient study of parish records enables the vital statistics of individual families to be reconstructed and birth intervals and birth rates to be established. Studies of this type were initiated in France and have been extensively carried out in England by Wrigley [29] and others and in Scandinavia by Utterstom [27].

In eighteenth-century rural France the average number of children per completed family was approximately eight if the woman married at 20, six if she married at 24, and four if she married at 30. There is little evidence in this group that there was any restraint on fertility other than that imposed by long intervals of breast-feeding. However, among the aristocracy a different story emerges. In Geneva the ruling classes appear to have begun to use birth control at the end of the seventeenth century, and Henry [9] has compared the fertility rates of the French aristocracy with those of the peasantry. The aristocracy have a lower fertility rate, suggesting that the decline of fertility was related to some form of voluntary limitation of fertility. Indeed, as there is some historic evidence that the aristocracy used wet nurses, on biologic grounds, one would expect their fertility to be higher, although this may have been offset to some extent by reduced coital frequency and access to alternative sexual partners, which aristocratic men probably enjoyed. The options available to lower fertility were induced abortion, possibly some herbal spermicides, and coitus interruptus, and there seems little doubt that the last was probably the largest contributor to the measured differentials in fertility. Henry concludes, "Birth control in marriage was certainly practiced in the French upper classes during the eighteenth century; the above mentioned study even leads us to suspect that it was already practiced at the end of the seventeenth."

Records of births and deaths for the aristocracy extend farther back into history than do those of the whole community. Peller [18] in a study of nearly 3,000 male members of European ruling families found that the average numbers of births per father in first marriages ranged from 6.1 in 1550 to 2.9 in 1921–1925. A slight decline begins in 1750. Hollingsworth [10] studied nearly 2,000 members of the British ducal families and worked out age-specific fertility rates for women of different cohort groups, demonstrating variations in the mean family size from 3.7 in 1330–1370 to 5.6 in 1730–1779. Again, it would seem that the use of coitus interruptus is the most likely explanation for the major part of the variations taking place. McKeown and Brown [14] suggest, "The only methods of limiting family size which would conceivably have been effective during the eighteenth century were abstinence, abortion and coitus interruptus." McKeown and Brown do not mention alternative forms of sexual congress, although they are possibilities that should not be overlooked.

While some degree of control of fertility, in which coitus interruptus probably played a major role, has been most extensively studied among the aristocracy of preindustrial Europe, evidence is now emerging that the peasantry also practiced an artificial restraint of fertility. Wrigley [29] has shown interesting variations in fertility in the Devonshire village of Colyton. Until about 1650 women were marrying at the mean age of 27 and, once married, had on average six or more children. In the seventeenth and early eighteenth centuries the mean age of marriage for women went up to the age of 30—in itself an example of remarkable restraint and concern over fertility. The later age of marriage was sufficient to reduce the expected family size from six to approximately five, but in practice the average fell to four, and within the group of women who married early, fertility fell off more sharply in the thirties and early forties than in the case of those women who married later in life. Once again, coitus interruptus was probably the most important factor operating.

Britain and France were not alone in Europe in the widespread practice of coitus interruptus. In nineteenth-century Spain fertility was 30 percent lower than in Prussia at the same time, and in Catalan it was lowest of all; again withdrawal is credited with much of the difference [13]. Wrigley [29] has pointed out that the demographic transition in the West "was achieved largely by 'pre-industrial' methods, by coitus interruptus and by procuring of abortions, both means which have been available to society centuries previously. The use of rubber sheaths, caps and spermicidal chemicals, which might be called 'post-industrial' methods of family limitation, played a comparatively minor role until well into the twentieth century."

Lewis-Faning [12] found evidence that in England in the 1940s only 16 percent of those women whose marriages had been contracted before 1910 had used an appliance method of contraception. The percentage rose slowly and for the 1920–1924 cohort the figure was 31 percent, rising to 57 percent for the 1940–1947 cohort. It would seem that the most rapid decline in birth rates in Western Europe occurred *before* the widespread adoption of condoms, spermicides, and other barrier methods. Wrigley [29] concludes, "The changes in marital fertility would have followed much the same pattern in all probability even if no new technique of contraception had been invented. In many ways much of the contemporary Third World is in the early stages of the demographic transition and is more similar socioculturally to, say, Britain in the interval from 1870 to 1900 than to the contemporary Western world. With this in mind, it is surprising that the role of coitus inter-ruptus in the contemporary developing world has not been looked at more carefully. It should also be expected that the contraceptive method that was most commonly used by our grandparents and great-grandparents would still find a role among individuals in the contemporary world."

EXTENT OF USE

It is easy to overlook the use of coitus interruptus. In response to the question "Do you use any form of contraception?" a respondent may easily answer "No," as coitus interruptus is not always categorized as a method of contraception, especially in the developing world where there is now a considerable awareness of such methods as oral contraceptives and intrauterine devices (IUDs). In Britain if a woman is asked, "Is your husband careful?" she may well answer "Yes," while she might have earlier replied that she did *not* use a contraceptive. In conducting surveys of contraceptive use it is important to know what euphemisms are common for coitus interruptus. Many countries have colloquial expressions that are of the type used in East Yorkshire, England, where coitus interruptus is described as "going to Beverley and getting off at Cottingham."

The difficulty of surveying the use of coitus interruptus is illustrated by the fact that when a representative sample of men and women are asked separately about their contraceptive practices, there is often considerable disagreement in the prevalence as reported by men and women. In England 39 percent of men but 46 percent of women claimed that they had used the method at some time or other [3]. Possibly the men were embarrassed to report the method or perhaps the women hoped it was being practiced when, indeed, it was not.

Less than 40 years ago in Britain the Royal Commission on Population found that 43 percent of all recently married couples used coitus interruptus as their only method of family planning, and among blue collar workers this proportion rose to 61 percent. The United States, unlike Western Europe from which it has drawn so many of its traditions, always reports a much lower prevalence of coitus interruptus; even in the 1950s only 5 percent of couples used it as a method of choice, and only 18 percent reported ever being users [8]. By 1976 the number of current users had dropped to 2 percent of currently married women aged 15 to 44. In other contemporary developed countries the use of coitus interruptus has also dropped (to use an appropriate verb) over recent decades (Table 25-1), although the method remains more widely used than periodic abstinence or the diaphragm in every country except the United States. In all developed countries coitus interruptus is relatively more prevalent among older couples than

Table 25-1. Percentage of women[a] using coitus interruptus in selected developed countries (World Fertility Survey 1976–1977)

	Coitus interruptus[b]	Pill	IUD	Sterilized[c]	All methods
Belgium	30	32	4	3	81
Spain	22	11	0.5	3	47
France	22	27	10	4	74
Hungary	17	36	10		73
Norway	6	16	28	7	71
United States	2	23	6	19	49

[a]Age varied 16–49 and 20–44 in some surveys.
[b]Includes use combined with periodic abstinence.
[c]Only voluntary sterilizations for contraceptive purposes included.

Table 25-2. Percentage of women using coitus interruptus in selected developing countries (World Fertility Survey data, 1970s)

	Coitus interruptus	Pills	All methods
Kenya	0.2	2.0	7
Indonesia	0.3	14.9	26
South Korea	2.6	8.4	35
Philippines	9.4	1.4	36
Turkey	16.7	6.1	38
Colombia	4.7	13.3	43
Haiti	4.7	3.3	19
Jamaica	1.4	11.9	39

Table 25-3. Percentage of respondents reporting ever use of selected methods—Turkey

Date	Ideal family size	Coitus interruptus	Condom	Pill
1963	3.2	14.5	9.8	1.1
1968	2.7	25.2	10.3	2.3

younger. For example, in Hungary 36 percent of couples where the wife is 35 to 39 use the method but only 15 percent of those 20 to 24. In the United States 7 percent of married women aged 35 to 44 reported that their husbands used coitus interruptus but only 2 percent of those from 20 to 24 [7]. Usage was remarkably constant across age, economic, and social groups.

World Fertility Survey (WFS) data from developing countries show a lower use of coitus interruptus than in developed communities, although compared with other methods it is still relatively important (Table 25-2), involving tens of millions of users [2, 11]. The WFS may underestimate use for reasons referred to above. For example, a few years earlier 60 percent of contraceptive users in Jamaica used the method [25] and 67 percent in Hungary [20]. The marked differences between Oriental (with the exception of the predominantly Christian Philippines) and Islamic nations, however, are almost certainly genuine. In Turkey use of the method grew rapidly, as ideal family size fell in the 1960s, the method spreading through the community much more rapidly than modern methods (Table 25-3). The method was used by 20 percent of a sample of doctors in Uttar Pradesh and 45 percent of upper caste Hindus in Calcutta [22].

Peterson [19] suggested that coitus interruptus is most likely to be used in a nuclear family where the responsibility for the children rests squarely on the father, rather than in the extended family where it is shared by a number of kinsfolk. Deys [5] was the first observer to attempt to categorize those adopting family planning by their marital roles. She observed that a group of couples in England where the husband uses condoms or coitus interruptus and then often goes on to seek a vasectomy and another group where the woman uses pills, IUDs, or diaphragms and then goes

on to ask for tubal ligation can be distinguished by certain aspects of their marital lives. She learned that the men in the first group were often role dominant in their marriages and had strongly masculine occupations, commonly employed at jobs which women rarely or never do; they were policemen, firemen, long distance lorry drivers, coal miners. (Deys once vasectomized all the men who wanted no more children on one of Her Majesty's submarines!) Such role-dominant men were usually wage earners rather than salaried and gave their wives "housekeeping money." They were reluctant to share domestic chores, such as doing the washing after a meal or changing the baby's diapers, unless the wife was sick and physically incapable of doing these tasks. By contrast, female methods of contraception commonly were associated with marriages where the two partners shared many decisions, sometimes the wife had a professional job, and the partners pooled their incomes. Household tasks were undertaken by whoever was available.

Health professionals who counsel men in vasectomy services may find themselves dealing with an individual who has used coitus interruptus for many years. Sometimes the man will seek vasectomy not because the method has failed but simply because he is getting older and feels that he has the family he wants. The man has probably discussed the operation with his wife but quite likely would not expect her to be interviewed by clinic staff before his operation. Sometimes men will have used coitus interruptus for so many years that it has become virtually a reflex, and they may need to be reminded that they will have to relearn their coital technique if they are to take full benefit from the vasectomy.

CLINICAL

A great deal of nonsense has been written about the side effects of contraception, and coitus interruptus still carries more than its fair share of myths. Sjovall [23] speculates that a man using the method may be involved in a "vicious circle" of impotence, although she does agree that the dangers of frigidity and unresponsiveness in the woman have been exaggerated. As recently as 1963 Calderone [1] reported that "urologists. . . were unanimous in condemning the practice for men by attributing various prostatic difficulties to it." Such myths are interesting more as illustrations of the biases of physicians than as a commentary on coitus interruptus. They are the historic descendants of such lurid treatises as that by the Dutch Pastor Osterwald (1700) *Traite des sources de la corruption qui regne aujord'hui parmi les Chretiens* and of *The Crime of Onan, or the Heinous Vice of Self-Defilement,** published in England in 1717 [15].

In 1878 Dr. Rugh, addressing the Obstetric Section of the British Medical Association, declared that "the moral and physical evils likely to follow [coitus interruptus] affect the whole population." He claimed that "conjugal onanism" caused metritis, leucorrhoea, "ovarian dropsy," sterility, nymphomania, nervous prostration, mental decay, galloping cancer, and suicide. Even pioneers of family planning, such as Marie Stopes, condemned coitus interruptus as "harmful to the nerves as well as unsafe."

In reality, coitus interruptus is obviously acceptable to many users if not to those who provide family planning services. A study of 750 women from the Birmingham FPA Clinic in 1956 [6] who gave up the recommended clinic method found that 58 percent *chose* coitus interruptus as an alternative; the investigator

*The *Crime of Onan* puts its most severe warnings into verse for each memory.
At Judgement Day:

"The great Account Book then shall lie,
Open to every Offender's Eye
To try his Self-Defilements by.

Then sits the Judge upon his Throne
And makes all Self-Defilements known
When each Onanian knows HIS OWN" [23].

commented: "Dependence on coitus interruptus is so widespread that many women think of it not as a contraceptive but rather as a normal part of sexual intercourse. In a number of instances, the husband had become so accustomed to withdrawal that he was unable to give up the practice when the wife wore a cap."

In a survey of nearly 2,000 British women questioned in 1967–1968 by Cartwright [3], among 311 who had discontinued the use of the method 60 percent did so because they thought it was unreliable, only 31 percent because they found it unpleasant to use, and a mere 4 percent because they believed it harmful to health. By contrast, among 381 former condom users 54 percent abandoned the method because they found it unpleasant to use. Ten years later Chamberlain [4] showed that only 6 percent of mothers from a socially disadvantaged group in Leeds, England, were in favor of the method. How much this disapproval was spontaneous and how much the result of medical condemnation is difficult to unravel. If a couple love one another, there seems every reason to assume that they can have a sexually satisfying life and use coitus interruptus if this is what they choose.

The side effects ascribed to coitus interruptus, as with many other contraceptive methods, go back to a moral condemnation of the method, and sometimes what is really being condemned is contraception itself.

EFFECTIVENESS

As long ago as 1949 the Royal Commission on Population in Britain reported that "no difference has been found between users of appliances and users of non-appliance methods as regards the average number of children." Among those relying on nonappliance methods of all kinds (of which withdrawal was, of course, the most popular) the pregnancy rate was 8 per 100 years of exposure. In the Princeton study the overall pregnancy rate for those couples practicing withdrawal was 17 per 100 women-years compared with 14 for the condom and diaphragm and 38 for the "safe period" [28]. The Indianapolis study revealed a failure rate of only 10, compared with an average rate of 12 for all other methods, and among high-income couples the rate was precisely the same as for the diaphragm. In Calcutta an extensive survey revealed that pregnancy rates were lower at each occupational level for those employing withdrawal than for those using other traditional methods.

It is commonly suggested that withdrawal is unreliable because preejaculatory loss of fluid from the penis may contain sperm. The origin of this hypothesis goes back to Abraham Stone [24] in 1931 who was puzzled as to why coitus interruptus ever failed at all. He asked several of his friends who had microscopes to examine preorgasmic secretion for sperm. He finally collected 24 slides from 18 individuals. Two showed many spermatozoa, two contained a few, and one occasional sperm. Stone rightly reported that the figures were "insignificant for a definite conclusion." Today, when the physiology of fertilization is more clearly understood, many biologists would consider the risk of fertilization to be minimal unless a high concentration of sperm is present in the tubes. To obtain this concentration, many millions must be deposited in the vagina. In addition, the sperm in the preejaculatory fluid will have been stored at body temperature since the last ejaculation and are therefore unlikely to have retained their fertilizing ability. Nevertheless, the myth that such sperm make coitus interruptus unreliable is copied uncritically from one textbook to another.

MORTALITY

The only recorded mortality from the use of coitus interruptus is that of Onan for, whatever his sin, it "did displease Yahweh, who killed him."

CONCLUSION

Anyone who wishes to attempt to understand the overall pattern of fertility control within a community must pay attention to the prevalence, acceptability, and failure rate of coitus interruptus, which still ranks as a widespread method of family planning in the world. Certainly more couples use this method and more births are averted by this method than by vaginal barrier methods, prostaglandins, or hormone injectables and implants, yet these contraceptive techniques have accumulated a body of research and literature that is, literally, a thousand times greater than that concerned with coitus interruptus. While those who counsel individuals and couples about family planning are unlikely to find themselves teaching the method, their professional wisdom will be greater and their usefulness to the couple increased if they have a general understanding of coitus interruptus and some of the characteristics of those who use the method.

In broad terms, it seems established that coitus interruptus played a predominant role in the fertility decline that accompanied industrialization in the West. The method remained the single most important contraceptive choice through the years of low birth rates associated with economic depression in Europe in the 1930s. It continued to be the most common method after World War II in Eastern Europe among those societies that first achieved zero population growth.

Many doctors and nurses belong to marriage partnerships that involve joint decision making (the opposite of a role-dominant marriage), so they are often ill equipped to understand and set up family planning services that appeal primarily to a group with a different lifestyle. It may be this fact that accounts for some of the history of vasectomy services themselves. Characteristically, family planning programs and many "expert" advisers often discount the possibility that vasectomy could be acceptable, for example, in Latin America with its macho traditions. However, they may be proved wrong when one or more adventurous individuals actually sets up such services. It is interesting that de Castro in Sao Paulo, Brazil, like Deys in London and Simcock in Australia, found that it is predominantly blue collar workers, many of whom have used condoms or coitus interruptus, who apply for vasectomy services. While it is useful to add vasectomy to the category of choices available in routine family planning clinics, this step, of itself, may not lead to very large numbers of men coming forward for the operation. In order to appeal to a socially different group, a vasectomy service is often required to have its own identity, patterns of communication, and style of service. It is not just that vasectomy involves men but that it involves men from a group of marriages with a different social setting, different pattern of thinking, and commonly different patterns of contraceptive use than those partnerships that employ female methods of contraception.

Coitus interruptus is like a bicycle or buffalo cart; no doubt there are better methods of transport or better methods of contraception, but for a great many people it represents a practical solution to an everyday problem. Instead of criticizing the method, one should capitalize on it. When those who use it feel the need, they will move to more modern methods. To change the metaphor, health professionals who denigrate coitus interruptus can be likened to a university chancellor who condemns primary education because children who leave school cannot do calculus. There should be nothing contradictory about promoting coitus interruptus and at the same time hoping that it will be replaced by something better.

REFERENCES

1. Calderone, M. *Manual of Family Planning and Contraceptive Practice*. Baltimore: Williams & Wilkins, 1970. P. 437.
2. Carrasco, E. The prevalence of natural family planning through results of WFS surveys. Presented at the United Nations Fund for Population Activity/World Health Organization meeting on Natural Family Planning. Quoted

in R. L. Kleinman, *Periodic Abstinence for Family Planning*. London: International Planned Parenthood Federation, 1983.

3. Cartwright, A. *Parents and Family Planning Services*. London: Routledge and Kegan Paul, 1970.

4. Chamberlain, A. Gin and hot baths. *New Society*, July 15th, 1976.

5. Deys, C. M. Cultural aspects of male sterilization. Clinical Proceedings of International Planned Parenthood Federation, Southeast Asia and Oceanic Regional Medical and Scientific Congress, Sydney, 1972. *Aust. N.Z. J. Obstet. Gynaecol.* p. 187.

6. Florence, L. S. *Progress Report on Birth Control*. London: FPA, 1956.

7. Ford, K. Contraceptive use in the United States 1973–1976. *Fam. Plann. Perspect.* 10:264, 1978.

8. Freedman, R., Whelpton, P. K., and Campbell, A. *Family Planning, Sterility and Population Growth*. New York: McGraw-Hill, 1959.

9. Henry, L. *Anciennes Familles Genevoise*. Paris, 1950.

10. Hollingsworth, T. M. A demographic study of the British ducal families. *Popul. Stud.* 11:4, 1957.

11. Leriden, H. Les facteurs de la fecondite dans les pays developpés. *Proceedings of the World Fertility Survey Conference*, London, 1980. Vol. 1, p. 411.

12. Lewis-Faning, E. *Family Limitation and its Influence on Human Fertility during the Past Fifty Years*. London: HMSO, 1969.

13. Livi-Bacci, M. Fertility and population growth in Spain in the eighteenth and nineteenth centuries. *Daedalus* 97:523, 1968.

14. McKeown, T., and Brown, R. G. Medical evidence related to English population changes in the eighteenth century. *Popul. Stud.* 9:119, 1955.

15. McLaren, A. *Birth Control in Nineteenth Century England*. London: Croom Helm, 1978.

16. Noonan, J. T. *Contraception: A History of Its Treatment by the Catholic Theologians and Canonists*. Cambridge, Mass.: Harvard University Press, 1965.

17. Omran, A. R. A Resume of Islam's Position on Family Planning and Abortion. In I. R. Nazer (ed.), *Induced Abortion: a Hazard to Public Health?* Beirut: IPPF, 1972.

18. Peller, S. Births and Deaths Among Europe's Ruling Families Since 1500. In E. V. Glass and D. E. C. Eversley (eds.), *Population in History*. London: E. Arnold & Co., 1965. P. 87.

19. Peterson, W. *Population*. London: Macmillan, 1969.

20. Potts, M. Abortion in Eastern Europe. *Eugenics Rev.* 60, 1967.

21. Potts, D. M. Coitus Interruptus: Clinical Proceedings of International Planned Parenthood Federation. Southeast Asia and Oceanic Regional Medical and Scientific Congress, Sydney, 1971. *Aust. N.Z. J. Obstet. Gynaecol.* 241, 1972.

22. Sinha, J. N. *All India Conference on Family Planning*. Bombay: Lucknow, Family Planning Association, 1955.

23. Sjovall, E. Coitus Interruptus. In M. S. Calderone (ed.), *Manual of Family Planning and Contraceptive Practice*. Baltimore: Williams & Wilkins, 1970. P. 433.

24. Stone, A., and Himes, N. E. *Practical Birth Control Methods*. New York: Viking, 1938.

25. Stycos, J. M., and Back, W. K. *The Family and Population Control*. Chapel Hill, N.C.: University of North Carolina, 1955.

26. United States Department of Health and Human Services. *Contraceptive Efficacy Among Married Women Aged 15–44 Years: United States*. Bethesda, Md.: National Center for Health Sciences, 1980.

27. Utterstrom, G. In D. V. Glass and E. D. C. Eversley (eds.), *Population and History*. London: E. Amdd & Co., 1965.

28. Westoff, C. F., Herrera, L. F., and Whelpton, P. K. Social and psychological factors affecting fertility. *Milbank Mem. Fund Q.* 31:291, 1953.

29. Wrigley, E. A. *Population and History*. London: Weidenfeld and Nicolson, 1969.

26. Contraception by Periodic Abstinence or Lactational Anovulation

Elizabeth B. Connell

For centuries people have attempted to control their fertility using any and every means at their disposal. In some instances individuals have desired to do this without the use of drugs or devices, either for personal or religious reasons. A number of techniques have been devised to try to attain this goal. The earliest name for this approach was *rhythm* or *the safe period*. This term was then replaced by *natural family planning*. Currently many people use the phrases *ovulation detection, fertility awareness,* or *periodic abstinence* to describe these techniques. Regardless of the name, the basic concept and goal are the same—to attempt to predict impending ovulation, using one or more techniques, and to avoid sexual intercourse during the fertile interval. This approach to contraception became feasible only when modern science began to study the reproductive process in both men and women. In 1650 Leeuwenhoek first saw sperm through his microscope and identified them as the probable source of male fertility; however, the clear elucidation of the events of the menstrual cycle and the actual visualization of ovulation and fertilization are comparatively recent events [3, 18, 19, 54].

As research in human fertility gradually received higher priority, the cyclic hormonal patterns and their biologic effects on the female reproductive tract were progressively better documented. It was ultimately determined that an ovum is capable of being fertilized for 12 to 24 hours following ovulation [17, 19]. Sperm, however, were found to be viable for 48 hours or, in some cases, up to 5 or more days, being stored in cervical crypts and subsequently released into the endometrial cavity [1, 13, 23, 36–38, 49]. It was also discovered that ovulation usually occurs approximately 14 days before the onset of the menstrual flow [30, 40].

Cyclic changes in cervical mucus play a major role in the female reproductive process. These alterations form the basis for the cervical mucus method. The mucus is secreted from the crypts lining the endocervical canal and is composed of mucin, a glycoprotein with a chain-link pattern, in which inorganic salts and numerous organic compounds are dispersed. Before ovulation, cervical mucus is thick, sparse, and impenetrable by sperm. Under the influence of estrogen, periovulatory mucus becomes elastic, thin, and watery. Parallel chains (micelles) form, permitting the passage of sperm. During the luteal phase, the mucus again becomes thick and unfavorable for sperm migration. Based on these discoveries, several methods of contraception utilizing periodic abstinence were developed.

When assessing the effectiveness of any contraceptive technique, it is important to recognize that two different types of rates are reported. The first of these is method effectiveness, the rate obtained when a method is used perfectly; it is classically found in the early evaluation of a new technique when subjects are carefully selected, meticulously trained, and intensively followed. Failures, as would be expected, are lowest in this group. The second rate is use-effectiveness. This is the value obtained with wider, less controlled usage, including both correct and incorrect application, and is, therefore, lower. The lowest values are those known as extended use-effectiveness rates; in this situation, the method is in widespread use by many individuals receiving varying levels of care.

Statistically valid data on the various methods of natural family planning have, until fairly recently, been quite limited. The best currently available rates will be included for each technique. Effectiveness rates vary considerably from one study to another, as training and motivation play important roles. In general, the calendar method has the lowest use-effectiveness rates, cervical mucus the next, and symptothermal the best. Use of more than one technique improves the results [45].

When effectiveness rates are determined for different centers, even in the same study, considerable variation is often encountered. For example, in a World Health Organization (WHO) study [58], pregnancy rates varied from 128 (Manila) to 27.9 (Auckland). In Mauritius, the natural family planning program has been quite successful, but the time spent in training and follow-up is extensive, visits being as often as 1 to 2 times a week for the first three cycles and weekly to 3 to 4 times a year thereafter [45].

A considerable amount of time must be spent in teaching natural family planning methods. Often individual success or failure can be traced to the quality of the woman's training. While instruction has often been carried out by members of the health care profession, in many programs this is successfully done by peers who are often themselves users [57].

CALENDAR METHOD

In the 1930s Ogino [40] in Japan and Knaus [30] in Austria devised formulas for the calculation of the fertile and infertile portions of a woman's menstrual cycle. Their methods were based on the observation that ovulation preceded menstruation by a fixed number of days, regardless of the total length of the cycle. Ogino postulated an 8-day fertile period and Knaus, 5 days. A critical review in 1962 [19] favored the longer time period. The fertile period is determined in three steps:

1. Identification of the shortest and longest cycle from the 12 previous cycles
2. Calculation of the first day of the probable fertile period, using the shortest cycle minus 18 days

3. Calculation of the last day of the probable fertile period, using the longest cycle minus 11 days

With this method a woman whose previous cycles had varied from 26 to 32 days would calculate her fertile period as follows:

1. First day of the fertile period: $26 - 18 = 8$
2. Last day of the fertile period: $32 - 11 = 21$

Therefore her fertile period would be estimated to be from the eighth to the twenty-first day. Calendar rhythm is widely practiced, but failure rates are generally high. Reported pregnancy rates range from 14.4 to 47.0 per 100 woman-years of use [19, 45].

Since many women have mildly to moderately irregular menstrual cycles, their potentially fertile periods are quite lengthy [51]. Close adherence to their schedules, therefore, demands a considerable number of days of abstinence each month. This may put a great strain on couples attempting to use this technique. Thus, it is not surprising to find that continuation rates are rather low and pregnancy rates are rather high with the calendar method.

TEMPERATURE METHOD

When basic research on the menstrual cycle was carried out, it was observed that as progesterone levels increased just after ovulation, the basal body temperature (BBT) also rose 0.3 to 0.5°C [42]. This observation made possible a second type of contraception by periodic abstinence: the temperature method. Couples attempting to use this technique must abstain from coitus from the time menses cease until 3 days after the rise in the BBT. This method has been found to have the highest effectiveness rates when all the rules are carefully followed. Several studies have shown the pregnancy rates to range from 0.3 to 6.6 per 100 woman-years of use [33, 45, 48]. The temperature method has several disadvantages. First, a woman must take and record her temperature daily before arising. Second, other factors such as an intercurrent infection or use of drugs may also produce an increase in body temperature. Finally, and most important, this method demands long periods of abstinence and thus is unacceptable to many couples.

COMBINED CALENDAR AND TEMPERATURE METHOD

With the combined calendar and temperature method the presumed start of the fertile period is determined using the Ogino calendar method. The end of the fertile period is assumed to be 3 days after the temperature elevation has taken place. The advantage of this approach is that the required period of abstinence is shorter than is the case with the temperature method.

OVULATION DETECTION METHOD (CERVICAL MUCUS METHOD)

Another observation made during the evaluation of the changes occurring throughout the menstrual cycle was that the cervical mucus underwent characteristic and predictable cyclic alterations. The technique described by the Drs. Billings [4–6] of Australia is based upon the fact that the cervical mucus mirrors closely the levels of estrogen. Following the end of menstruation, little to no cervical mucus is produced. Then, for a variable number of days rather thick, sticky, gray, opaque mucus is noted. Shortly before ovulation occurs, the mucus becomes more profuse, watery, slippery, stretchy, and transparent, resembling raw egg white. The day when these changes are most pronounced is known as the "peak day" and has been found to coincide very closely with the time of ovulation [21]. Following this, the mucus returns to its previous sticky state or may actually disappear.

Women using this method are required to check the mucus at the introitus daily. They may have intercourse during the dry days following the menses. Once mucus is noted, abstinence must be practiced until the fourth postpeak day.

This particular technique has several advantages over the previously described methods. First, it does not require the daily taking and recording of the BBT. Second, for women with irregular cycles it is easier to follow and demands fewer days of abstinence. However, mistakes can be made when the mucus findings are complicated by vaginal discharge, secretions caused by sexual stimulation, or the use of vaginal lubricants and medications.

The ovulation detection method has use-effectiveness rates that are better than those of calendar rhythm but not as good as those of the symptothermal technique. Pregnancy rates range from 5.3 to 32.1 per 100 woman-years [45].

SYMPTOTHERMAL METHOD

It has also been found possible to combine the temperature method with the identification of the physical changes associated with ovulation, including cervical mucus detection. As ovulation approaches, many

women experience some of the following symptoms: breast tenderness and enlargement, pelvic or abdominal cramping, pelvic pain (mittelschmerz), abdominal bloating, low backache, vulvar swelling, and/or mild vaginal bleeding or spotting [20]. In addition, repeated palpation of the cervix will frequently disclose a softening at about the same time [27].

When using this method, women may have intercourse until they notice vaginal wetness. Then they must practice abstinence until the third day after the temperature rise or the fourth day after the peak of mucus production [28].

In general, the more indicators a woman uses, the more apt she is to be successful in preventing unwanted pregnancies. However, the problems noted separately for the temperature and ovulation methods also apply to their combined use.

The symptothermal method has the best use-effectiveness rates; reported pregnancy rates range from 4.9 to 34.4 per 100 woman-years, most studies averaging around 15. In a recent WHO study of the ovulation method the pregnancy rates varied from 17.7 per 100 woman-years in Dublin to 31.0 in Auckland.

WORLD HEALTH ORGANIZATION STUDIES

Multiple studies [29, 55] on the ovulation method have been carried out. In an attempt to evaluate the ovulation method as a means of contraception, the World Health Organization Task Force on Methods for the Determination of the Fertile Period set up a prospective multicenter trial in five countries (El Salvador, India, Ireland, New Zealand, and the Philippines). This study was completed in June 1979. The first report [57] dealt primarily with the teaching phase; it was found that despite wide variations in sociocultural and educational backgrounds 94 percent of the women in the study were able to recognize the record changes in cervical mucus. The second report [58] addressed the issue of effectiveness. The overall cumulative net probability of discontinuation after 13 cycles was found to be 35.6 percent, with 19.6 percent due to pregnancy. When the pregnancy rates per 100 woman-years were calculated, it was found that 15.4 percent were attributable to conscious departures from the rules, 3.5 percent to inaccurate application of instructions, 2.8 percent to method failure, and 0.4 percent to inadequate teaching; 0.5 percent were of uncertain etiology.

CONGENITAL ANOMALIES

In recent years concern has been expressed about the possible increase in congenital abnormalities in babies born as the result of failure of the use of one of these methods [50]. In addition, a number of papers in the medical literature show that the fertilization of post mature ova in a variety of animals will result in chromosomal anomalies, fetal demise, and the birth of congenitally malformed offspring [7–9, 11, 59].

With regard to the possibility of similar problems in the human, two papers published in 1968 [14, 56] pointed out the increased incidence of pregnancy wastage and birth defects in women using periodic abstinence. A report that appeared in 1970 [22] suggested that pregnancies conceived at the end of the fertile period were more likely to end in an early spontaneous abortion or an abnormal infant.

Another author [24] reported a higher incidence of retarded children born to parents using calendar rhythm. A number of additional studies [2, 16, 26] have been carried out, attempting to determine whether or not there are health hazards to fetuses conceived from "aged gametes." In a small study reported in 1968 [32] no correlation was found between the time of fertilization and spontaneous abortion. A prospective study done in 1976 [39] also showed no relationship. However, a study [25] comparing the incidence of central nervous system defects and Down's syndrome in various parts of the world concluded that the risks were higher in those areas where periodic abstinence was the major form of contraception.

A 1976 prospective study [39] showed no statistically significant difference in the rate of serious birth defects in infants of women using periodic abstinence as compared with women in the total group. A 1977 retrospective study of children with neural tube defects [31] showed no relationship to the use of periodic abstinence as compared with normal siblings.

There is still considerable debate as to whether there is a real risk involved with the use of these methods and, if so, what the order of magnitude might be. It is anticipated that continued study will help to clarify this issue.

Another approach to this problem that has been suggested is the use of barrier contraception during the fertile period by those couples to whom this is acceptable. This would serve two purposes: It would increase the overall effectiveness of these techniques, and it would reduce the potential for abnormal pregnancies.

ADVANTAGES AND DISADVANTAGES

Use of these methods by many couples in recent years has permitted the following conclusions to be drawn.

The primary advantages are

1. Safety—no medications or devices with potential side effects are required

2. Effectiveness—given strict adherence to the method
3. Little or no cost
4. Acceptable to certain religious groups
5. Increases communication and strengthens marital bonds for some couples

The primary disadvantages are

1. Interference with sexual spontaneity.
2. High level of motivation required.
3. Cooperation of male partner(s) sometimes difficult to achieve.
4. Psychosexual stresses produced by periods of abstinence.
5. Considerable training time needed.
6. Accurate record keeping required.
7. Minor user deviation results in high failure rate.
8. Potential for abnormalities in pregnancy.

LACTATION

For centuries lactation has been a major form of contraception. It has played a key role in birth spacing and continues to do so in many parts of the world [46]. In certain cultures its effectiveness is augmented by the fact that intercourse is not practiced during lactation. While the majority of women in developed countries do not breast-feed and use medical methods of contraception, the time between births is similar to that found in developing countries where women traditionally nurse their infants until they become pregnant again [10, 12, 34, 53].

The length of time before ovulation is resumed varies considerably and depends upon a number of factors. Primary among these are the frequency and intensity of suckling and the use of supplementary feeding. The first two tend to increase and maintain the flow of milk through a neurohormonal mechanism [52]. The addition of infant formulas and foods, however, tends to decrease lactation and leads to the earlier return of ovulation.

In some areas of the world lactational amenorrhea may last for as long as 2 to 3 years and is associated with suppressed ovarian activity [35]. The levels of prolactin are directly related to the number and duration of suckling episodes, the introduction of supplementary food producing a decrease in both, with a gradual resumption of ovarian function [35]. In nonlactating women, on the other hand, cyclic ovarian activity is usually resumed by 9 weeks postpartum [35].

Thus, any woman who is not fully breast-feeding is at risk of pregnancy. Those who do not wish to become pregnant must use some form of contraception. Oral contraceptive pills have been used, although some suppression of lactation has been noted, particularly with higher dose medications, leading some doctors to recommend the use of the minipill [41]. It is known that hormones will be transmitted to breast milk, although no adverse effects have been noted with the current low-dose preparations [47]. Intrauterine devices are effective when inserted either immediately postdelivery or later.

When periodic abstinence is the method of choice during lactation, variability in cervical mucus patterns may cause problems and mandate long periods of abstinence. Reports have shown low pregnancy rates in lactating women (e.g., 9.1 per 100 woman-years when the majority were totally breast-feeding) [15, 43, 44]. Traditional abstinence with prolonged breast-feeding, practiced for cultural reasons and as a child-spacing technique, has had a major impact on fertility in the past in many societies, but its use is rapidly disappearing [45].

REFERENCES

1. Belonoschkin, B. Determination of the fertilizing ability of sperm. *Int. J. Fertil.* 4(1):1, 1959.
2. Berger, C. J. Medical risks associated with "natural" family planning. *Adv. Plann. Parent.* 15(1):1, 1980.
3. Bergman, P. Sexual cycle, time of ovulation and time of optimum fertility in women. *Acta Obstet. Gynecol. Scand. (Suppl. 24)*:1, 1950.
4. Billings, E. L., and Billings, J. J. The idea of the ovulation method. *Aust. Fam. Physician* 2:81, 1973.
5. Billings, E. L., Billings, J. J., and Catarinich, M. *Atlas of the Ovulation Method* (3rd ed.). Melbourne Advocate Press, 1977.
6. Billings, E. L., et al. Symptoms and hormonal changes accompanying ovulation. *Lancet* 1:282, 1972.
7. Blandau, R. J. The female factor in fertility: 1. Effects of delayed fertilization on the development of the pronuclei in rat ova. *Fertil. Steril.* 3:349, 1952.
8. Blandau, R. J., and Jordan, E. S. The effect of delayed fertilization on the development of the rat ovum. *Am. J. Anat.* 66:275, 1941.
9. Blandau, R. J., and Young, W. C. The effect of delayed fertilization on the development of the guinea pig ovum. *Am. J. Anat.* 64:303, 1939.
10. Bonte, M., and van Balen, H. Prolonged lactation and family spacing in Rwanda. *J. Biosoc. Sci.* 1:97, 1969.
11. Chang, M. C. Effects of delayed fertilization on segmenting ova, blastocysts and fetuses in rabbits. *Fed. Proc.* 11:14, 1952.
12. Chen, L. C., et al. A prospective study of birth interval dynamics in rural Bangladesh. *Popul. Studies* 28:277, 1974.
13. Collins, W. P. The physiological basis for natural family planning. *International Seminar on Natural Methods of Family Planning*, Department of Health, Dublin, Ireland, Oct. 8–9, 1979. In collaboration with the World Health Organization, Dublin, Ireland. Pp. 24–41.
14. Cross, G. Anencephalus and spina bifida. *Br. Med. J.* 2:253, 1968.
15. Gross, B. A. The hormonal and ecological correlates of lactation infertility. Presented to the First General Assembly of the International Federation for Family Life Promotion, Cali, Colombia, June 22–29, 1977.
16. Guerrero, R., and Rojas, O. I. Spontaneous abortion and aging of human ova and spermatozoa. *N. Engl. J. Med.* 293:573, 1975.
17. Guerrero, R., Rojas, O., and Cifuentes, A. Natural Family Planning Methods. In E.S.E. Hafez (ed.), *Human Ovulation, Mechanisms, Prediction, Detection and Induction.* New York: North-Holland, 1979.
18. Hartman, C. G. *Time of Ovulation in Women: A Study on the Fertile Period in the Menstrual Cycle.* Baltimore: Williams & Wilkins, 1936.
19. Hartman, C. G. *Science and the Safe Period: A Compendium of Human Reproduction.* Baltimore: Williams & Wilkins, 1962.
20. Hilgers, T. W. Natural family planning: III. Intermenstrual symptoms and estimated time of ovulation. *Obstet. Gynecol.* 58:152, 1981.
21. Hilgers, T. W., Bailey, A. J., and Prebil, A. M. Natural family planning: IV. The identification of postovulatory infertility. *Obstet. Gynecol.* 58:345, 1981.
22. Iffy, L., and Weingate, M. B. Risks of rhythm method of birth control. *J. Reprod. Med.* 5:11, 1970.
23. Insler, V., et al. Sperm storage in the human cervix: A quantitative study. *Fertil. Steril.* 33:288, 1980.
24. Jongbloet, P. H. The intriguing phenomenon of gametopathy and its disastrous effects on human progeny. *Maandschrift voor Kindergeneesk.* 37:261, 1970.
25. Jongbloet, P. H., and Van Erkelens-Zwets, J. H. J. Rhythm methods: Are there risks to the progeny? In J. Sciarra (ed.), *Risks, Benefits and Controversies in Fertility Control*: Hagerstown, Md.: Harper & Row, 1977.
26. Jongbloet, P. H., and Zwets, H. J. Preovulatory over-ripeness of the egg in the human subject. *Int. J. Gynaecol. Obstet.* 14:111, 1976.
27. Keefe, E. F. Self-observation of the cervix to distinguish days of possible fertility. *Bull. Sloane Hospital for Women.* 8:129, 1962.
28. Kippley, J., and Kippley, S. *The Art of Natural Family Planning.* Cincinnati: Couple to Couple League International, 1975.
29. Klaus, H., et al. Use-effectiveness and client satisfaction in six centers teaching the Billings ovulation method. *Contraception* 19:613, 1979.
30. Knaus, H. *Die Periodische Frucht- und Unfruchtbarkeit des Weibes Zentralblatt fuer Gynaekologie.* 57:1393, 1933.
31. Kuhr, M. D. Neural-tube defects and mid-cycle abstinence: A test of the "over-ripeness" hypothesis in man. *Dev. Med. Child Neurol.* 19:589, 1977.

32. Marshall, J. Congenital defects and the age of spermatozoa. *Int. J. Fertil.* 13:110, 1968.

33. Marshall, J. A field trial of the basal-body-temperature method of regulating births. *Lancet* 2:8, 1968.

34. Martin, W. J., Morley, D. C., and Woodland, M. Interval between births in a Nigerian village. *J. Trop. Pediatr.* 10:82, 1964.

35. McNeilly, A. S., Howie, P. W., and Houston, M. J. Relationship of Feeding Pattern, Prolactin, and Resumption of Ovulation Postpartum. In G. I. Zatuchni, M. H. Labbok, and J. I. Sciarra (eds.), *Research Frontiers in Fertility Regulation*. Hagerstown, Md.: Harper & Row, 1980.

36. Moghissi, K. S. Sperm Migration in the Female Genital Tract. In G. I. Zatuchni et al. (eds.), *Vaginal Contraception: New Developments*. Hagerstown, Md.: Harper & Row, 1979.

37. Moghissi, K. S. Prediction and detection of ovulation. *Fertil. Steril.* 34:89, 1980.

38. Odell, W. D., and Moyer, D. I. Sperm and Ovum Transport. In W. D. Odell and D. L. Moyer (eds.), *Physiology of Reproduction*. St. Louis: Mosby, 1971.

39. Oechsli, F. W. *Studies of the Consequences of Contraceptive Failure: Final Report*. Berkeley, Calif.: University of California, 1976.

40. Ogino, K. Ovulationstermin und konzeptionstermin. *Zentrabl. Gynakol.* 54:464, 1930.

41. Oral Contraceptives in the 1980's. *Popul. Rep.* [A]. No. 6, May–June, 1982.

42. Palmer, A. The diagnostic use of basal body temperature in gynecology and obstetrics. *Obstet. Gynecol. Surv.* 4:1, 1949.

43. Perez, A. Lactational Amenorrhea and Natural Family Planning. In E. S. E. Hafez (ed.), *Human Ovulation: Mechanisms, Predictions, Detection and Induction*. Amsterdam: North-Holland, 1979.

44. Perez, A. Post partum return of fertility: Ovulation method initiated after childbirth: Preliminary report. Presented to the International Federation for Family Life Promotion, Second International Congress. Navan, Ireland, Sept. 24–Oct. 1, 1980.

45. Period Abstinence—How Well Do New Approaches Work? *Popul. Rep.* [1] No. 3, Sept., 1981.

46. Potter, R. G. Birth intervals: Structure and change. *Pop. Studies* 17:155, 1963.

47. Potts, M., and Whitehorne, E. Contraception and the Lactating Woman. In G. L. Zatuchni, M. H. Labbok, and J. J. Sciarra (eds.), *Research Frontiers in Fertility Regulation*. Hagerstown, Md.: Harper & Row, 1980.

48. Rice, F. J., Lanctot, C. A., and Garcia-Devasa, C. Biological effectiveness of the sympto-thermal rhythm method: An international study: A preliminary report. *Acta Med. Rom.* 16:349, 1978.

49. Silverman, E. M., and Silverman, A. G. Persistence of spermatozoa in the lower genital tracts of women. *J.A.M.A.* 240:1875, 1978.

50. Simpson, J. L. Genetic Consequences of Aging Sperm or Aging Ova: Animal Studies and Relevance to Humans. In J. Sciarra (ed.), *Risks, Benefits and Controversies in Fertility Control*. Hagerstown, Md.: Harper & Row, 1977.

51. Treloar, A. E., et al. Variation of the human menstrual cycle through reproductive life. *Int. J. Fertil.* 12:77, 1967.

52. Tyson, J. E., et al. Significance of the Secretion of Human Prolactin and Gonadotropin for Puerperal Lactational Infertility. In K. Elliott and D. W. Fitzsimms (eds.), *Breast-Feeding and the Mother*. Amsterdam: Exerpta Medica, 1976.

53. Vis, H. L., et al. The health of mother and child in rural Central Africa. *Stud. Fam. Plann.* 6:437, 1975.

54. Vollman, R. F. *The Menstrual Cycle*. Philadelphia: Saunders, 1977.

55. Wade, M. E., et al. A randomized prospective study of the use-effectiveness of two methods of natural family planning: An interim report. *Am. J. Obstet. Gynecol.* 134:628,1979.

56. Witschi, E. Natural control of fertility. *Fertil. Steril.* 19:1, 1968.

57. World Health Organization Task Force on Methods for the Determination of the Fertile Period, Special Programme of Research, Development, and Research Training in Human Reproduction: A prospective multicentre trial of the ovulation method of natural family planning. 1. The teaching phase. *Fertil. Steril.* 36:152, 1981.

58. World Health Organization Task Force on Methods for the Determination of the Fertile Period, Special Programme of Research, Development and Research Training in Human Reproduction: A prospective multicentre trial of the ovulation method of natural family planning. II. The effectiveness phase. *Fertil. Steril.* 36:591, 1981.

59. Zimmerman, L., and Rugh, R. Effect of age on development of the egg of the leopard frog, *Rana pipiens*. *J. Morphol.* 68:329, 1941.

27. Immunologic Approaches to Fertility Regulation

Nancy J. Alexander
Deborah J. Anderson

Immunization, the technique introduced by Louis Pasteur in 1830, is still one of the most powerful medical techniques known to man. It has been unequaled in its effect on the control of human disease. The global acceptance and enormous impact of vaccines have stemmed from their ease of application, low cost, long-term effects, and minimal adverse reactions.

Population pressures in certain regions of the world are demanding new approaches to fertility regulation, and vaccines offer a potentially effective answer to the problem. The developing embryo and reproductive systems of both men and women contain unique molecules; these could provide suitable antigens for contraceptive vaccines. Documented cases of infertility attributable to natural autoimmunity to reproductive and embryonic antigens further indicate that immunization can provide a safe and effective method of fertility regulation in human beings. In this chapter we review the immunoanatomy of the male and female reproductive systems, discuss the most promising candidates for contraceptive vaccines, and summarize recent biochemical and technologic advances.

BACKGROUND ON VACCINES AND IMMUNIZATION

Vaccines are classically comprised of inactivated organisms (bacteria, virions) or antigen extracts that stimulate the immune system to respond to and eliminate organisms bearing these antigenic determinants. The unique characteristics of the immune system that permit the success of this approach are (1) precise specificity of the response, (2) amplification of specific immune-cell populations after immunization, and (3) long-term memory. Most vaccines are administered by injection with or without adjuvants (discussed in detail later) to induce a systemic humoral immune response. However, oral administration of live attenuated organisms (i.e., polio vaccine) can also result in both systemic and local secretory immune responses. Vaccines are most commonly administered to children and are given in an initial series of one to three injections, with booster injections every few years when continued protection is required. Vaccination of adults produces more varied responses, which are affected by age, sex, immune status, and prior exposure to the immunizing antigen. Few, if any, of the current vaccines achieve a 100 percent immunity rate, but the spread of infectious organisms can be effectively controlled if a large percentage of the population is protected [83].

The work described in this chapter, Publication No. 1247 of the Oregon Regional Primate Research Center, was supported by National Institutes of Health Grants RR-00163 and CA 32132.

Passive immunization (administration of preformed antibodies to nonimmune persons) is also widely used in the control of certain infectious diseases and to manage other pathologic phenomena such as Rh sensitization after pregnancy. Antibodies are obtained from animals or human beings that have been vaccinated or that have a natural immunity to the infectious agent. This technique provides immediate but relatively short-term (a few weeks) protection because the antibodies are gradually cleared from the system. Frequent administration of specific antibodies for long-term protection in humans has not been possible because animal antisera induce sensitization and serum sickness, and human antisera are expensive and potentially hazardous because of transfer of pathologic viruses. The recent development of human monoclonal antibodies, a breakthrough in this area, will soon provide an economical source of well-defined human antibodies for this procedure.

PREREQUISITES OF A CONTRACEPTIVE VACCINE FOR USE IN HUMANS

The first step in the development of a human contraceptive vaccine is the identification of an appropriate antigenic determinant that is unique to the target (is not found on any other tissues or molecules). The target antigen must have a physiologic function relevant to fertility that can be blocked by antibody or be located on a cell that can be lysed by complement. The reproductive hormones and several antigens isolated from the zona pellucida, sperm, embryonic, and fetal tissue appear to qualify.

Second, the antigen must be immunogenic and available in large quantities at a reasonable cost. This requirement originally was a major obstacle to the development of human contraceptive vaccines because human reproductive antigens are weaker immunogens than the pathogens commonly used in vaccines and are not available in large quantities. However, several of the reproductive antigens appear to have been evolutionarily conserved (i.e., found in many species) and can be extracted from a more accessible species for subsequent use in humans. The most exciting advance in this area is the recent development of genetic engineering technology, which offers a means to produce large quantities of specific proteins at low cost. Once appropriate antigens are identified, large-scale production of human proteins for use in vaccines could begin.

The third characteristic of the ideal contraceptive is reversibility. There is a need for permanent sterilization techniques, but a method that is highly effective and reversible would gain much wider acceptance. Unfortunately, it is difficult to reverse immunologic sensitization, especially in a system that is frequently boosted by natural appearance of antigen (this booster effect occurs to varying degrees with all the antigens proposed for use in reproductive systems). Some predict that it may be particularly difficult to reverse immunity to sperm antigens in persons for whom coitus provides frequent immunologic stimulation. Induction of immunologic tolerance or immunosuppression is an effective way to achieve a decreased active immune response. Immunosuppressive drugs have been used successfully by several clinical investigators to treat immunologic infertility in both men and women [4, 49], but such approaches are not without risk.

IMMUNE STATUS OF THE REPRODUCTIVE ORGANS AND NATURAL IMMUNITY TO REPRODUCTIVE ANTIGENS

Male Reproductive Tract

Mature spermatozoa are first produced in the male testes at puberty, long after immunologic self-tolerance has been established. These cells express unique autoantigens but they are isolated from the immune system. Tight junctions between Sertoli cells form a blood-testis barrier that isolates sperm within the seminiferous tubules from blood components such as lymphocytes and immunoglobulins. The impermeability of the blood-testis barrier prevents sensitization of the host to sperm-specific antigens. Throughout the remainder of the sperm duct system, sperm are isolated by tight junctions between epithelial cells. The rete testis is a weak barrier (the cuboidal epithelium has discontinuous junctions) and is a likely initial site of immune-mediated damage following immunization to sperm, as is the efferent duct region (where the arrangement of junctional ridges is not as parallel as that between Sertoli cells). Under normal circumstances, sperm are sufficiently isolated to prevent immune sensitization [31, 46, 75]. These barriers and possibly other mechanisms such as immunosuppressive factors produced by germ cells [50] and several of the reproductive organs [7] maintain a balance between the immune system and the autoantigenic haploid cells of the testes; autoimmune responses to spermatozoa are rarely detected in young men with no history of testicular trauma. However, the numerous documented cases of antisperm immunity and associated infertility indicated that this balance can be overturned [2, 60, 77]. Spermatogenesis can be disrupted in the testes by cellular and humoral autoimmune responses directed against germ cell antigens. There is no evidence that a local secretory immune system exists in male reproductive tissues, but humoral antisperm antibodies can transude

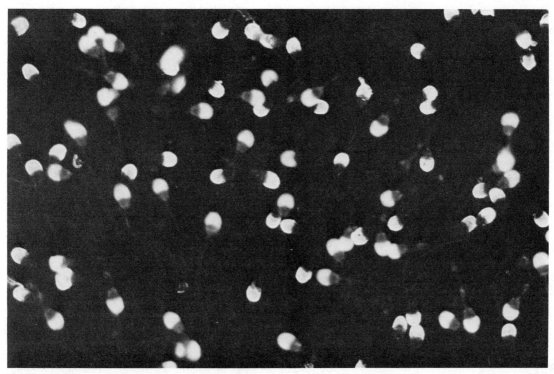

Fig. 27-1. Animals and human beings that have been immunized with sperm or vasectomized develop antisperm antibodies. This micrograph shows antibodies to the acrosomal region of spermatozoa found in human vasectomy serum.

from the serum into the accessory organs [76] and cause infertility by agglutinating or immobilizing sperm upon ejaculation. Few cases of systemic pathologic side effects have been reported in men with high titers of antisperm antibodies and chronic immunologic infertility, but immunization of experimental animals with germ-cell antigens can result in autoimmune orchitis [107] (Figs. 27-1 and 27-2). Furthermore, studies of vasectomized mice with sperm autoimmunity have shown a significant increase in spontaneous tumor development [6], and research in vasectomized monkeys has demonstrated more severe atherosclerosis [3, 22]. Before sperm immunity can seriously be considered as a contraceptive approach in men, a safe procedure with well-defined sperm antigens must be assured.

Female Reproductive Tract

The female reproductive tract is not an immunologically privileged site; antibodies produced by a systemic immune response do enter the uterus and vagina and could exert an immunocontraceptive effect. Serum antibody transudates are found in the human vagina [109] and uterus [65]. Evidence from animal studies indicates that transudation of serum proteins into the uterus is under hormonal control and is positively affected by estrogens [116].

The human cervix has its own secretory immune defense system, and cervical secretions contain relatively high levels of IgA antibodies at certain stages of the menstrual cycle. Based on this discovery, reproductive immunologists have proposed eliciting a local secretory immune response to sperm membrane antigens to achieve infertility in women; the antibodies would bind to sperm as they swam through the cervix, a strategic "Straits of Gibraltar," and would impede their motility and fertilizing capacity. However, there are conceptual problems with this approach.

First, the IgA levels in cervical mucus fluctuate widely and are lowest at midcycle, just when antibodies would be needed for contraception [84] (Figs. 27-3 and 27-4). Homing of IgA plasma cells to the cervix appears to be under hormonal control. The number of IgA-producing plasma cells increases during the late secretory phase of the menstrual cycle but decreases in the early secretory phase of the cycle and in pregnancy; it is proposed that progesterone induces homing to the

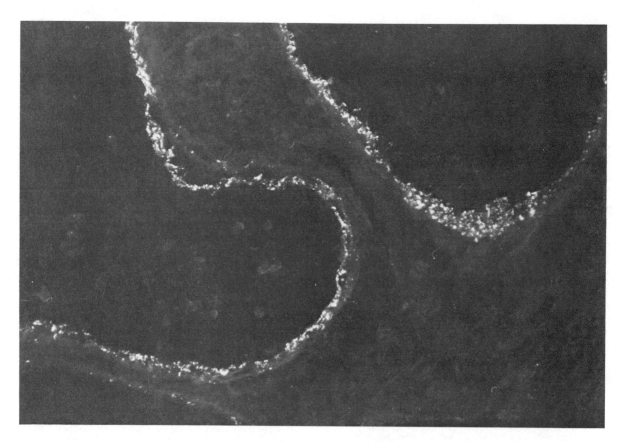

Fig. 27-2. When circulating sperm antibodies are present, immune complexes can become deposited in the testis. In this section of vasectomized rabbit testis, such immune complex deposition is evidenced by the bright dots (due to fluorescent tagged anti-IgG) around each seminiferous tubule.

cervix, but that human chorionic gonadotropin (hCG) and luteinizing hormone (LH) block this effect [68]. Furthermore, the number of cervical epithelial cells containing secretory component (a small peptide chain that stabilizes IgA in secretions) is small at midcycle and increases in the late secretory phase of the menstrual cycle and in pregnancy (Fig. 27-5).

Second, IgA antibodies do not fix complement by the classic pathway and therefore cannot cause a cytotoxic effect when they bind to sperm. The antifertility effect would have to be produced by blockage of sperm receptors or interference with motility.

Third, local secretory immune responses are stimulated in the gastrointestinal tract. Uncommitted B cells are apparently instructed to respond to specific antigens in Peyer's patches in the gut, and the IgA antibodies produced by plasma cells that subsequently home to various mucosal tissues are generally directed against enteric organisms [112]. Gut activation of an immune response gives rise to the possibility of orally administering sperm antigens to achieve local secretory antisperm antibody production in the cervix. In one

recent study female mice administered spermatozoa through the gastrointestinal tract had reduced fertility [23]. The approach of the oral administration of vaccines is attractive because of the convenience and the elicitation of a local rather than systemic response (with possible side effects). Research has revealed that the oral administration of antigens can (1) elicit a secretory immune response, (2) elicit humoral immune responses, including allergic responses, and (3) induce suppressor cells that inhibit any immune responses to the antigen [97].

That reproductive processes in women are vulnerable to immunologic intervention has been best documented by the numerous reports of natural infertility in women with antisperm antibodies [51, 52] and anti–

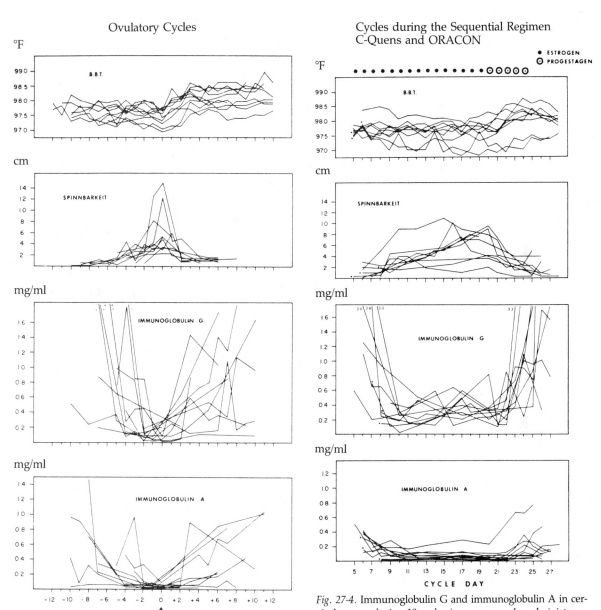

Fig. 27-3. Immunoglobulin G and immunoglobulin A, obtained by microradial immunodiffusion techniques, in cervical mucus during 10 ovulatory cycles. The last day of low basal body temperature was designated as day zero and the curves were arranged accordingly. Both IgG and IgA are lowest at midcycle. (From G. F. B. Schumacher. Soluble Proteins of Human Cervical Mucus. In M. Elstein, K. S. Moghissi, and R. Borth [eds.], *Cervical Mucus in Human Reproduction.* Copenhagen: Scriptor, 1973.)

Fig. 27-4. Immunoglobulin G and immunoglobulin A in cervical mucus during 10 cycles in women under administration of sequential contraceptives (C-Quens, E. Lilly & Co.; ORACON, Mead Johnson & Co.). Because of the exogenous steroids, it is easier to evaluate immunoglobulin cyclic response. IgA levels seem lower than in Figure 27-3. Both IgA and IgG levels are low at midcycle, the time when high levels would be important for an antisperm vaccine to be effective. (From G. F. B. Schumacher. Soluble Proteins of Human Cervical Mucus. In M. Elstein, K. S. Moghissi, and R. Borth [eds.], *Cervical Mucus in Human Reproduction.* Copenhagen: Scriptor, 1973.)

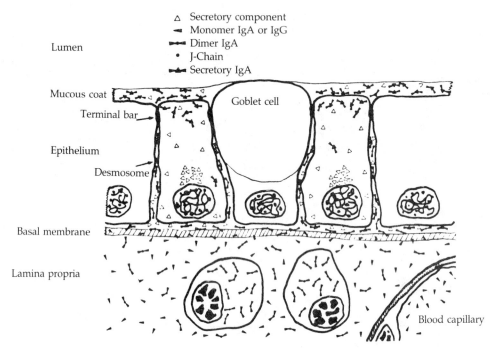

Fig. 27-5. Plasma cells secrete IgA, which becomes stabilized by a secretory component secreted by the cervical epithelial cells. Dimeric secretory IgA is then released in the mucus. The number of epithelial cells containing the secretory component is hormonally dependent and lowest at midcycle. (From J.-P. Vaerman and J. Férin. Local immunological response in the vagina, cervix and endometrium. *Acta Endocrinol.* [Suppl.] [Copenh.] 78:281, 1975.)

zona pellucida antibodies [87]. Furthermore, it is suspected that some frequent aborters are autoimmune to embryonic or placental antigens [13, 96]. However, we must also mention that female reproductive processes are associated with various safeguards which protect against immune responses that could affect fertilization and pregnancy. Although spermatozoa are antigenic and can elicit immune responses in women, they rarely do so because seminal plasma contains potent immunosuppressive factors that directly suppress lymphocyte function, inhibit complement-mediated lysis, and alter the expression of antigens on the sperm surface [7, 61, 95]. Uterine secretions have been ascribed immunosuppressive properties and may protect the early preimplantation embryo from immunologic rejection [13, 67]. A host of immunoprotective mechanisms seem to be operative during the later stages of normal pregnancy:

The placenta provides an immunologic barrier to protect the fetus [114].

Maternal suppressor T cells are activated [21].

Humoral "blocking" antibodies coat antigenic sites on the placenta and protect the fetus from cellular immune responses [62].

Numerous cellular immunosuppressive factors are produced by the placenta [12].

It appears that both humoral and cellular immune responses to fetal antigens develop during the course of normal pregnancy [47, 72] and that pregnancy is usually not affected. Such natural protective mechanisms may also block some of the immunocontraceptive approaches directed at pregnancy termination.

ADMINISTRATION OF CONTRACEPTIVE VACCINES

Since most reproductive antigens are weak immunogens, contraceptive vaccines will probably be administered with adjuvants, agents that act nonspecifically to achieve effective systemic immune responses. The mechanisms underlying the immunopotentiating effects of adjuvants are (1) slowing of antigen release; (2) denaturation of antigens and a consequent increase in immunogenicity; (3) recruitment of reactive cells; and

(4) stimulation of proliferation and differentiation in immunocompetent cells. The macrophage appears to be the cell directly affected by many of the adjuvants: Adjuvants may facilitate macrophage–B-cell interaction and thus bypass the need for helper T lymphocytes in B-cell differentiation and antibody production, and they may increase the efficiency of macrophage stimulation of helper T cells. However, one well-known adjuvant, bacterial endotoxin lipopolysaccharide (LPS), is a B-cell mitogen, and its adjuvant effect is due to direct stimulation of B lymphocytes. When cultured with endotoxin, B cells produce antibodies to T-dependent antigens without the assistance of helper T cells. The various adjuvants produce significantly different overall immune effects and can be classified according to whether humoral or cell-mediated immune responses are favored and which antibody class predominates [5].

Freund's adjuvant is one of the most powerful immunopotentiators known. Incomplete Freund's adjuvant primarily stimulates antibody formation, and complete Freund's adjuvant (CFA) (containing mycobacteria) elicits both cell-mediated and humoral immune responses. Unfortunately, Freund's adjuvants cannot be used in humans because the mineral oil is not degraded; it persists at the injection site and elicits the formation of granulomas. Furthermore, the complete adjuvant also sensitizes the recipient to mycobacterial antigens. Such a powerful adjuvant can induce autoimmune reactions, especially if the immunizing antigen is related to other molecules found in host tissues.

Two adjuvants show promise for use with human contraceptive vaccines: (1) liposomes, biodegradable nonimmunogenic concentric spheres of phospholipids separated by aqueous compartments, which target antigens to macrophages and greatly enhance the immunogenicity of an antigen preparation; and (2) N-acetylmuramyl-L-alanyl-D-isoglutamine (muramyl dipeptide or MDP), a synthetic glycopeptide structurally similar to a structure of the mycobacterium cell wall that can substitute for mycobacterium in CFA. A recent report [20] showed that immunologic castration of male mice can be achieved through the administration of luteinizing hormone releasing hormone (LHRH) conjugated to MDP in an aqueous medium. Also, animal data indicate that MDP can be used orally to stimulate immune responses, and it may be a candidate for the oral vaccine approach to stimulating secretory immune responses.

The nature of the immune response is affected by the type of antigen, the type of adjuvant, the route and timing of immunization, and host factors. Considerable experimentation with various antigen/adjuvant combinations and immunization protocols may be required to achieve effective immunocontraception in people.

POTENTIAL CONTRACEPTIVE VACCINE ANTIGENS

Antigens of the Oocyte

The initial stages of oogenesis occur very early in life, but oocytes undergo final maturation in women immediately before ovulation. Several unique antigenic substances are associated with oocyte development and may provide suitable targets for immunologic contraception in women.

Zona Pellucida

Because of the small number of mature follicles present at any time, the oocyte is a logical candidate for immunocontraception. There are two possible approaches: (1) permanent sterilization by annihilation of all oocytes, or (2) blockage of fertilization of mature oocytes.

Recent studies strongly suggest that the zona pellucida, a noncellular, gelatinlike layer surrounding the mature oocyte, may be an excellent target for immunologic inactivation [26, 79]. It surrounds the egg, and its integrity is important for both fertilization and early embryonic development (Fig. 27-6). It remains intact after fertilization and persists until just before implantation, when either pulsations of the blastocyst or uterine proteolytic activity break the zona and allow hatching of the blastocyst. Antigens of the zona pellucida, which are unique to the reproductive tract, are immunogenic.

During oocyte development fibrils deposit, enlarge, and coalesce to form the zona pellucida, which is comprised of nonhomogeneous regions [70] (Figs. 27-7 and 27-8). Bleil and Wassarman [14] have recently provided evidence that the three major mouse zona pellucida glycoproteins are secreted by the growing oocyte.

Sperm binding to the zona is the first stage of fertilization. In vivo such attachment involves the plasma membrane in the cap region of the sperm head and the zona pellucida. When capacitated sperm penetrate the zona and touch the egg surface, cortical granules break down and a trypsinlike protease is released into the perivitelline region [98]; this enzyme subsequently hydrolyzes part of the zona proteins and alters the sperm receptor sites so that they can no longer bind sperm [113]. The zona reaction, this sequence that results in an increased resistance to sperm penetration and a decrease in sperm binding, is thought to prevent polyspermia [11, 43, 117]. Hybrid fertilization of zona pellucida–intact eggs is very rare, an indication that the zona sperm receptor is species-specific. The mouse zona sperm receptor has been biochemically characterized and is a glycoprotein of approximately 83,000 molecular weight [14].

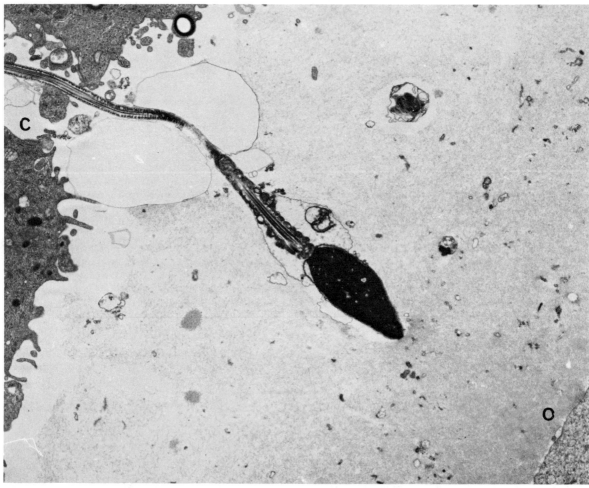

Fig. 27-6. Partially reacted human spermatozoon, which has penetrated about halfway through the zona of a two-cell embryo (its tail is still between two corona cells). Note that the inner half of the zona is denser and more compact than its outer half. C = corona radiata; O = ovum (48 hours after insemination) ($\times$9100). (From A. H. Sathananthan et al. Ultrastructural observations on the penetration of human sperm into the zona pellucida of the human egg in vitro. *J. Androl.* 3:356, 1982.)

The zona pellucida protects and physically isolates the newly forming embryo [42]. This isolation is particularly important in the period of compaction during morula formation when the dividing cells become much more adhesive. The zona pellucida also provides an osmotic environment that encourages a normal cell cleavage pattern [63] and prevents early egg adherence in the oviduct [64].

Antibodies to zonae pellucidae have been found in some fertile women [80, 87] and more commonly in infertile, pregnant, and menopausal women [25]. Whether those fertile women with antibodies simply have a titer that is insufficient to cause infertility is not clear. Nonetheless, the presence of such naturally occurring antibodies to the zona pellucida, without ill effects, indicates that the use of these antibodies as contraceptive agents may be feasible.

Many studies on zona pellucida antigens involved hamster, rabbit, mouse, and rat zonae, but current efforts have focused on bovine and porcine zonae because of the availability of greater amounts of tissue. Screening procedures, which include washing minced ovarian tissue through a series of decreasing meshes or use of collagenase, allow the collection of thousands of oocytes in a few hours [30, 45].

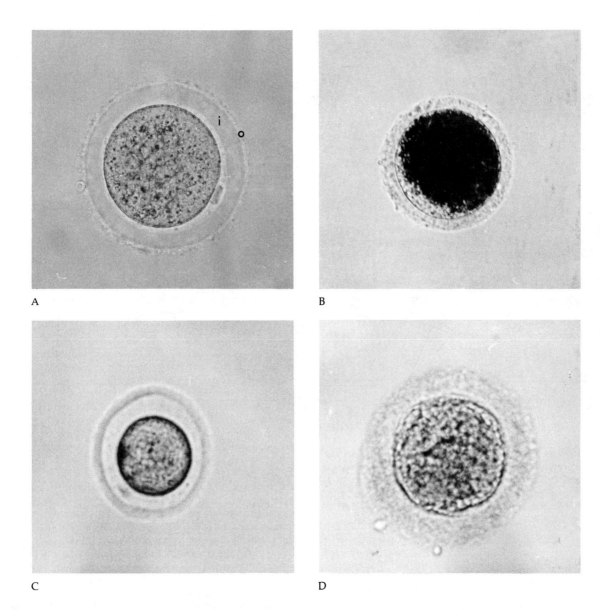

A

B

C

D

Fig. 27-7. Zonae pellucidae surrounding oocytes obtained from various species. (A) Rabbit zona. Note the two distinct layers comprising the zona—an inner homogeneous layer (*i*) and an outer, more coarsely granular layer (*o*) (×605). (B) Pig zona (×385). (C) Mouse zona (×625). (D) Human zona (×455). (From A. G. Sacco. Immunocontraception: Consideration of the zona pellucida as a target antigen. *Obstet. Gynecol. Annu.* 10:1, 1981.)

Antibodies directed against the zona pellucida can be detected in several ways. When antibodies to the zonae are mixed with antigen, a precipitation layer forms around the outside of the zonae which results in modification of the light-scattering properties (Fig. 27-9). Adding a specific fluorescence-tagged second antibody is another way to detect the presence of antibodies to the zona (Fig. 27-9). Since antibody-treated zonae dissolve considerably more slowly than untreated ones, a third approach is to evaluate the inhibi-

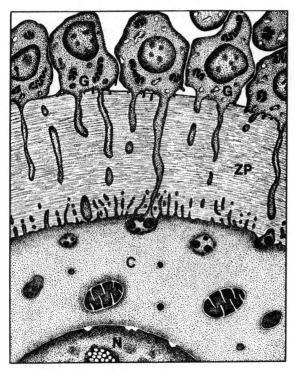

Fig. 27-8. Structure of fully formed zona pellucida (*ZP*) around an oocyte in graafian follicle. Microvilli arising from oocyte interdigitate with processes from granulosa cells (*G*). These processes penetrate into the cytoplasm of oocyte (*C*). It is obvious that the zona pellucida is composed of several constituents. *N* = oocyte nucleus. (From T. G. Baker. Oogenesis and Ovulation. In C. R. Austin and R. V. Short [eds.] *Reproduction in Mammals, Book 1, Germ Cells and Fertilization* [2nd ed.]. Cambridge: Cambridge University Press, 1982.)

tion of zona lysis. When oocytes surrounded by their zonae are exposed to antibody and subsequently to sperm, the sperm do not become attached. The amount of sperm binding is inversely related to the concentration of antibody that was added to the zona. The most sensitive assays for evaluating antizona antibodies involve the use of radiolabeled or enzyme-linked zona antigens.

At least one and as many as four antigens [29] specific for zonae pellucidae have been described. Data obtained by two-dimensional gel electrophoresis indicate that porcine, rabbit, and mouse zonae are comprised of three major glycoprotein antigens [15, 28] (Fig. 27-10). At least two of the zona pellucida antigens do not appear to be species specific, and use of antibodies produced in response to these antigens may be relevant to human contraception. The third antigen,

termed ZP3, is the sperm receptor and is species specific [14, 113].

In vitro studies have revealed that when eggs are exposed to antizona antibodies, fertilization is prevented [105]; presumably this occurs because the antibody interferes with the sperm receptor sites on the surface of the zona. Passive immunization (injecting the antibody fraction of serum from one animal into another animal) has also clearly indicated an inhibition of fertility. In these studies the females were immunized with the antiserum before or shortly after mating. Later their reproductive tracts were excised and cleaved eggs, embryos, and implantation sites were counted [78, 104]. With passive immunization the period of infertility is short (10 to 33 days) but longer than a single cycle [73, 78, 103, 119]. The length of this infertile period suggests that the antibodies bind to maturing oocytes in addition to ovulated oocytes. Ova recovered from passively immunized animals have an immune precipitate on the outer regions of the zona and exhibit an increased resistance to lytic agents [73, 102, 103]. Passive immunization may, in addition to preventing fertilization, prevent hatching of the blastocyst before implantation. Such an approach, which has potential as a "morning-after" method, would be attractive to persons desiring a reversible contraceptive.

For longer immunity, active immunization with zona antigen is a possibility [44]. Active immunization of rats with zona antigens has demonstrated that long-term suppression of fertility is possible [1]. Immunization of rabbits with porcine zona pellucida glycoproteins resulted in infertility and appears also to have affected immature eggs and/or normal ovarian function [27, 118]. We still are far from having a marketable vaccine; studies must be conducted on the correlation of antibody titer and infertility, the effectiveness of booster injections, and possible side effects. Purification of the various zona antigens and subsequent immunization will result in a greater monospecific response.

In summary, studies on immunization with zona pellucida antigens for contraception suggest some distinct advantages: (1) The method blocks fertilization, (2) a limited number of zonae would be exposed at any time so low amounts of antibody might be sufficient, and (3) because zona antigens of several animal species are immunologically cross reactive, sources of material are readily available [26].

Sperm Antigens

Human sperm express several autoantigens that could provide suitable material for contraceptive vaccines if it could be shown that antibodies directed against them block sperm function. However, few of these antigens have been adequately characterized. Studies using

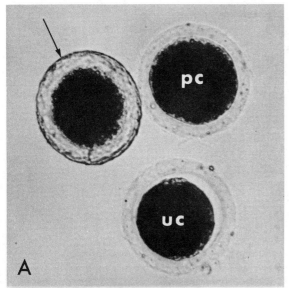

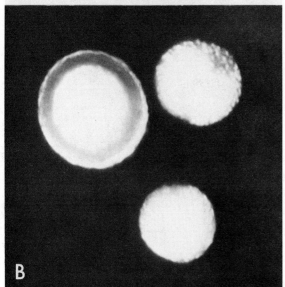

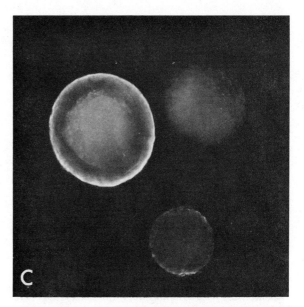

Fig. 27-9. Porcine zonae treated with rabbit antiporcine zona pellucida gamma globulin. Control zonae are either untreated (*uc*) or have been treated with rabbit preimmune gamma globulin (*pc*). The same oocytes are shown in all three photographs. (A) Appearance of the precipitation layer (*arrow*) on the outer surface of the zona as observed by bright field microscopy. Note absence of precipitation layer on control zonae (×330). (B) Appearance of precipitation layer as observed using dark-field optics (×330). (C) Appearance of antibody-treated zona using the indirect fluorescent antibody technique. Bright fluorescence is present on outer surface of antibody-treated zona. Fluorescein-conjugated antirabbit gamma globulin used as the second antibody (×330). (From A. G. Sacco. Immunocontraception: Consideration of the zona pellucida as a target antigen. *Obstet. Gynecol. Annu.* 10:1, 1981.)

monoclonal antibodies to identify purity and determine the function of sperm antigens will soon provide the information for the development of a sperm vaccine.

The best characterized sperm antigen with the greatest contraceptive potential is lactate dehydrogenase-C_4 (LDH-C_4). This enzyme is completely absent from the female and is found only on male germ cells. This C_4 isoenzyme of lactate dehydrogenase, the most abundant LDH of spermatozoa, has been purified to crystalline homogeneity [33].

Initial studies [34, 35] demonstrated that active immunization of female rabbits and mice with this sperm-specific isoenzyme results in a significant reduction in pregnancies of female mice and rabbits. Subsequent studies [37] showed that immunization of female baboons results in circulating antibody titers and a substantial reduction in fertility. The effect appears to occur in the oviduct most likely by causing agglutination of sperm or complement-mediated cell lysis, thus preventing fertilization [57, 58]. Since oviductal fluid is a transudate of serum, high circulating antibody levels probably result in sufficient quantities of antibody in the oviduct. Ovulatory cycles are not altered by the immunization procedure. Success of the vaccine is as-

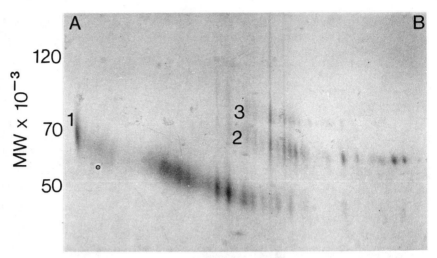

Fig. 27-10. High-resolution two-dimensional polyacrylamide gel electrophoresis of porcine zonae pellucidae. This pattern illustrates the three major glycoprotein families detected by Coomassie Blue staining. (Electrophoresis was carried out as described by B. S. Dunbar, C. Liu, and D. W. Sammons. Biol. Reprod. 24:1111, 1981.)

sociated with high antibody titers to LDH-C₄. When the antibody titers fall, normal pregnancies ensue. The conceptions that do occur result in normal fetuses.

The use of such a natural product as LDH-C₄ is limited to the amount available. Recent studies have been directed toward the development of a synthetic peptide that would elicit an immune response to the native protein [115]. Residues 152 to 159 of mouse LDH-C₄ contain a unique antigenic determinant [39] (Table 27-1). This peptide is an eight-residue loop, lying mostly on the surface of LDH-C₄.

The data on immunized baboons suggest that immunization to LDH-C₄ is effective, does not impair embryonic development, does not damage the reproductive system, and is reversible [37].

In more recent work two additional peptide fragments that bind antibody to LDH-C₄ were identified. These consist of residues 5 to 16, the intersubunit arm, and residues 211 to 220. These peptides were conjugated to bovine serum albumin (BSA) or diphtheria toxoid (DT) and injected into rabbits. Each peptide-carrier combination provoked antibodies that reacted with native LDH-C₄. These results lend strong support to the goal of constructing a synthetic vaccine [36].

Other interesting work from this laboratory involves the development of monoclonal antibodies to LDH-C₄ [38]. Four hybridomas produce monoclonal antibodies that differed in their affinities among species of LDH-C₄. These findings suggest only partial conservation of the antigenic determinants of LDH-C₄. One of the monoclonal antibodies has been mapped to residues 101 to 114, the coenzyme binding loop. The difference of a serine in rat LDH-C₄ from a threonine in mouse LDH-C₄ at residue 108 reduces the binding affinity of

Table 27-1. Sequences of various LDH isozymes at segment 152–159

Isozyme	Amino acid sequences
Mouse C	Ile-Ser-Gly-Phe-Pro-Val-Gly-Arg
Dogfish A	Leu-Ser-Gly-Leu-Pro-Met-His-Arg
Chicken A	Ile-Ser-Gly-Phe-Pro-Lys-His-Arg
Pig A	Ile-Ser-Gly-Phe-Pro-Lys-Asp-Arg
Chicken B	Leu-Ser-Gly-Leu-Pro-Lys-His-Arg
Pig B	Leu-Ser-Gly-Leu-Pro-Lys-His-Arg

Source: From V. Gonzales-Prevatt, T. E. Wheat, and E. Goldberg. Identification of an antigenic determinant of mouse lactate dehydrogenase C₄. Mol. Immunol. In press, 1984.

the monoclonal antibody by half. These results illustrate the exquisite sensitivity of hybridoma technology in assessing epitope diversity in homologous proteins of several species.

Embryonic Antigens

Embryonic and fetal tissues express differentiation antigens that are immunologically foreign to the adult immune system. Immunization of syngeneic adult inbred mice with embryonic tissue has produced antisera that detect a system of embryonic antigens present on sper-

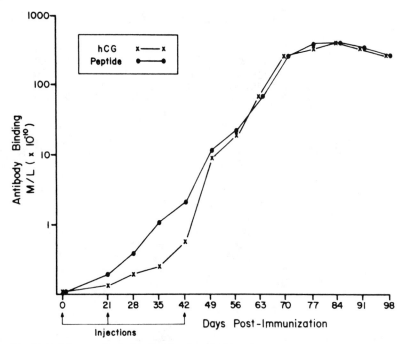

Fig. 27-11. Mean antibody binding levels of hCG and peptide 109-145 from five rabbits immunized with a beta-hCG peptide 109-145–tetanus toxoid conjugate. (From J. E. Powell et al. Characteristics of antibodies raised to carboxy-terminal peptides of hCG beta subunit. *J. Reprod. Immunol.* 2:1, 1980.)

matozoa and the embryo at various stages of development [8]. Antibodies to oncofetal antigens have been found in vitro to affect compaction and embryo development (anti-F9 antibodies on mouse embryos) but not to react with other somatic cells [56]. Furthermore, many of these embryonic antigens appear to have been evolutionarily conserved: Antiembryonic antibodies produced by syngeneic immunization of mice react with sperm from every species tested, including man, as well as several human teratocarcinoma cell lines [19, 53]. Many of the embryonic antigenic determinants appear to be glycosylation products and cannot be studied by conventional protein biochemistry techniques. Two monoclonal antibodies produced to stage-specific embryonic antigens in mice cross-react with human teratocarcinoma cell lines and appear to react with ABO-blood-group–related carbohydrate antigens [40].

Studies are under way to identify human embryonic antigens through analysis of antibodies in human pregnancy and infertility sera. Such naturally occurring antibodies might indicate which embryonic determinants are immunogenic and are not associated with immunologic-mediated pathologic changes.

Human Chorionic Gonadotropin

As early as 1903 Dobrowski passively immunized animals with antiplacental serum and disrupted pregnancies [59], but it was not until the 1970s that large-scale practical experiments were begun. The hormone hCG, which is synthesized by the placenta, is the focus of this work. Human chorionic gonadotropin is produced by the trophoblastic layer shortly after fertilization and perhaps before implantation occurs. This hormone prevents degeneration of the corpus luteum and subsequent decline in progesterone, which results in menstruation. In women hCG is detectable by the sixth to eighth day postfertilization [82]. The levels rise rapidly and peak at about 47 IU per milliliter in serum at the eighth to tenth week of pregnancy [18]. Antibodies to hCG have been demonstrated to terminate pregnancy in baboons [100], marmosets [48], rats [10], and mice [101].

Although the alpha subunit of this pregnancy hormone is similar to other pituitary hormones, its beta subunit has a unique amino acid sequence. Either the whole molecule or the beta subunit can be used for immunization (Fig. 27-11), but use of only the beta subunit can minimize the likelihood of cross-reactions with other hormones.

The whole molecule, which is biologically the most effective for neutralizing hCG action, has been coupled to the diazonium salt of sulfanilic acid in order to increase its antigenicity. This vaccine, however, generates antibodies that neutralize LH as well as hCG [90, 94]. Large areas of amino acid sequence homology of beta hCG with beta hLH allow the development of cross-reacting antibodies [24, 69, 86, 99]. A comparison of the first 110 amino acid residues of hCG and hLH beta subunits reveals 94/110 (85%) identity [66]. The beta hCG is 30 residues longer than the beta hLH (145 versus 115). This observation of a cross-reaction of hCG with LH after injections into both human beings and monkeys [89] has led to concern that immunizations might cause autoimmune damage to the pituitary or ovarian cells that have receptors for LH or might cause glomerulonephritis owing to the accumulation of LH-antibody complexes in the kidney. Immunized women, however, have not shown any signs of altered pituitary, ovarian, or kidney function [24].

Since the beta subunit itself is not sufficiently antigenic, Nash and associates [69] have linked it to tetanus toxoid. Diphtheria and tetanus toxoids have consistently been effective carriers for enhancing antibody responses to peptides [92].

Because of the concern about cross reactivity, peptides from the carboxy-terminal region of beta hCG are being considered as potential antigens for vaccine development. The region used for immunization must be sufficiently large to cause the production of antisera that react with more than one site on the hCG molecule, so that resulting antigen-antibody complexes will be large enough to be removed rapidly from the circulation. A length of at least 35 amino acid residues is considered appropriate [74, 89]. Peptides with amino acid spacers elicit higher antibody responses than peptides without spacers [93]. However, since yields of peptides from the digestion of beta hCG are small, synthetic peptides are being considered.

A second problem associated with active immunization to hCG is that the immune response varies greatly among individuals. In order to be assured of a response, one needs conjugates or adjuvants that cause a heightened immune response. Studies so far [85] have found a wide variation in the development of peak titers among batches of the vaccine and among individuals treated with the same batch. In many cases maximum titers of circulating antibodies to hCG do not seem to occur until 4 to 5 months, and then titers quickly decline. Even booster injections provide no sustaining effect. Although Shahani's study was not designed to test contraceptive efficacy, one cannot overlook the fact that 10 pregnancies occurred in eight women. Most pregnancies occurred when the antibody titer was probably low, an indication that pregnancy does not act as a booster for a secondary immune response. Fortunately, the antibodies have had no adverse effect on fetal development.

Recent studies have attempted to determine which adjuvants are the most effective in significantly enhancing antibody responses to hCG-peptide conjugates. Mice and rabbits have been used to evaluate adjuvants as well as to determine the best delivery system for both antigen and adjuvant. Two hydrophilic adjuvants, NAc-nor-Mur-L.ala-D.isoGln,CGP 11,637 and NGlycol-nor-Mur-L.α-abu-D.isoGln,DT-l, are particularly effective in stimulating antibody production to both hCG peptides. Antibody levels with these adjuvants are higher than those obtained when CFA was used. An emulsion containing squalene-water stabilized with arlacel A proved to be a superior vehicle. Combinations of adjuvants may be the most effective approach to vaccine formulation [92]; phase I clinical trials are planned for 1984 [91].

Genetic engineering may provide a source of material. Recent studies have mapped hCG genes and shown that the beta subunit is encoded by at least eight genes arranged both in tandem and as inverted pairs [16].

Investigators have suggested another use of hCG vaccines, namely, for cancer therapy. This hormone is produced ectopically by gastrointestinal tract carcinomas [17] as well as by trophoblast tumors and testicular tumors [110]. Immunization against beta hCG allows destruction of these tumors by removing the immunosuppressive effect of hCG so that the tumor antigens can be recognized by the host immune system.

In summary, although no overt symptoms of dysfunction have resulted from immunization to hCG, the initial enthusiasm for this approach has somewhat waned because of (1) possible cross-reactions with LH and the chance that cytotoxic cellular immune responses to pituitary cells could result, and (2) the problem of maintaining high antibody levels for sustained contraceptive effects. Perhaps such cross-reactions will prove to be of more theoretical than practical interest since no pituitary or immune complex damage has been found in animals that have been immunized with hCG. Nonetheless, the development of synthetic molecules that have enough homology to hCG to cause a polyvalent immune response but no cross reaction with LH is encouraging and, coupled with the use of immunologic adjuvants that promote a more effective response, should go a long way toward providing a consistent immune response [92, 93, 108].

An exciting possibility is the use of human monoclonal anti-hCG antibodies. Recently, numerous clones of antibodies that neutralize the effect of hCG have been developed [41]. Generation of highly specific monoclonal antibodies obviates the problem of cross-reactions with other pituitary hormones, and such antibodies should be safe and well tolerated. They could be administered as a single injection for morning-after contraception or as a depot for protection of longer duration. Use of a depot approach would provide a strong immunologic tool for fertility regulation. The major drawback would be the logistics of repeated injections of large populations [54].

Other Hormones

The hCG beta subunit vaccine has the advantage of producing antibodies to a hormone that is present infrequently; thus, there is little risk of immune complex disease and tissue damage. Other female reproductive hormones, both steroids and peptides, have been tested as immunogens for contraception with less successful results.

Because steroids are poor immunogens, they have not been extensively studied as vaccines. In one study [55] female rats immunized against estrogen conceived and had normal pregnancies, but the LH surge was suppressed; although some of the rats immunized against progesterone conceived, none delivered healthy offspring. Progesterone levels remained high in these animals despite circulating antibodies against progesterone.

Every vaccine that has been described in this chapter has been intended for use in women. Antibodies to follicle-stimulating hormone (FSH) have been suggested for use in men, but it is not clear whether suppression of FSH can result in termination of spermatogenesis. In one simian study spermatogenesis was initially suppressed but returned to normal levels even with active immunization during the third year [71]. Before any conclusions can be drawn from preliminary studies of this nature, further information is needed on the precise role of FSH in the maintenance of human spermatogenesis and on whether suppression of FSH by antibodies would have detrimental immunologically mediated effects.

A vaccine comprised of LHRH, a decapeptide that is not species specific, has been considered as a possible agent for fertility control [32]. LHRH has a low molecular weight (1,183); its structure is known, it can be easily synthesized, and it is readily available in purified form. Because of its low molecular weight, it is not immunogenic upon injection unless attached to a carrier molecule. In females immunized against LHRH ovulation ceases and estrogen levels are considerably lowered. In the male, antibodies to LHRH result in a marked decrease in testicular size, cessation of spermatogenesis, and a severe reduction in testosterone levels [20]. Immunologic castration may prove an important veterinary tool to increase meat production, but its use in the human appears remote. Use of agonists and antagonists to LHRH may have more contraceptive

value than immunologic approaches [111] because this approach is reversible and can be more precisely controlled.

PASSIVE IMMUNIZATION AS AN APPROACH TO FERTILITY REGULATION

The availability of human monoclonal antibodies with any desired antigenic specificity will revolutionize the role of passive immunization in the prevention and cure of human disease. Human hybridoma antibodies have already been produced by several laboratories [54, 88], but better myeloma cell lines and in vitro B-cell sensitization techniques are needed before the potentialities of this field can be fully realized. The advantages of using human hybridoma antibodies for passive immune transfer are (1) they are an inexpensive source of unlimited quantities of well-defined and very specific serologic reagents; (2) their effects are short term and fully reversible; (3) the degree of immunity is directly proportional to the amount of administered antibody and is not subject to individual variation in immune responsiveness; and (4) since they are human proteins, severe sensitization to the antibodies themselves does not develop, and they can be administered several times (however, it is theoretically possible that with repeated injections, antibodies to allotypic regions or to the antigenic combining site [idiotypic region] would develop and impair the function of subsequently administered antibodies) [54].

Human monoclonal antibodies have several foreseeable applications in human fertility regulation: (1) early pregnancy termination induced by systemic or intrauterine administration of antibodies with activity directed against embryonic or placental antigens or other factors necessary for the maintenance of pregnancy; (2) short-term contraception by injection of antibodies with specificity for antigenic determinants on reproductive hormones or gametes; (3) longer-term contraception through passive administration in a long-acting depot form; and (4) local barrier immunologic protection by incorporation of antisperm antibodies into vaginal foams or jellies.

The major disadvantage to the passive immunization approach is its short duration and the necessity of frequent administration for a continuous effect. However, passive immunization provides a good backup or adjunct for long-term contraceptive vaccines.

A CAUTIONARY NOTE

With vaccines against infectious organisms the level of immunity achieved can be affected by a variety of factors including age, sex, immunogenetic factors, prior exposure to the antigen, illness, and immunosuppressive agents. It has not been necessary to work out the conditions for a 100 percent immunization rate with vaccines in the past; however, in the case of contraceptive vaccines it will be essential to achieve and sustain immunity in all vaccinated individuals. New techniques to accomplish absolutely effective immunization must be explored, and follow-up serologic studies should be conducted in the initial clinical trials to ensure that persistent immunity has been obtained.

Reproductive tissues, gametes, and early embryos all express foreign antigens, but natural protective mechanisms have evolved to prevent sensitization to these antigens and to suppress immune responses should sensitization occur. Such natural protective mechanisms are not fully understood and will probably interfere with the antifertility effects of certain of the contraceptive vaccines.

It will be absolutely essential to test for short-term and long-term pathologic side effects of contraceptive vaccines. It will be necessary to establish conclusively that the immune response generated to a reproductive antigen does not cross-react with antigens on any other tissue.

With a vaccine directed against plentiful reproductive antigens, there will be a risk of immune complex disease, which can produce extensive or subtle arterial and glomerular damage. With vaccines against embryonic or other pregnancy-associated antigens, there obviously also exists the risk of teratogenesis. A less obvious potential risk is the possibility of enhanced tumor growth. Malignant cells often express embryonic antigens, which serve as targets for immunosurveillance. Tumors often grow better in animals that have been immunized with embryonic tissue than in nonimmunized animals, because the embryonic antigens are masked by blocking non-complement-fixing antibodies or because natural antitumor immune responses are inhibited by specific suppressor cells that were generated by the immunization procedure [106]. The possibility that these very serious pathologic side effects could develop in healthy people as a result of a contraceptive vaccination program absolutely demands that a cautious solid scientific approach be taken. Vaccine candidates must be well characterized and well tested in animal models before use in clinical trials.

SUMMARY

Immunologic approaches to human fertility regulation are now feasible owing to recent biochemical advances and the new technologies of human monoclonal antibody production and genetic engineering. It remains to be decided which reproductive antigens will elicit the best immunologic protection with the least risk of side effects. Since most reproductive antigens are weak immunogens, suitable adjuvants must also be developed and tested with each antigen system. Unlike vaccination against infectious diseases, contraceptive vaccines must achieve a near 100 percent efficacy level to be acceptable.

Women are better candidates than men for contraceptive immunization because of reproductive periodicity and accessibility of their reproductive target tissues. A mixture of immunizing antigens would achieve the most effective immunization of a large heterogeneous population. An effective mixed vaccine might comprise gamete antigens, which would serve as primary targets, and pregnancy-associated antigens, which would be backup targets in case of contraceptive failure. Immunization against the alpha subunit or regions of the beta subunit of hCG would also provide a dual-target antigen system. The primary effects of this immunization would be inhibition of LH, which shares considerable structural homology with hCG, and prevention of ovulation; however, in case of failure, a secondary effect would be interference with the function of hCG, which plays an important role in the maintenance of early pregnancy. Appropriate vaccines must be selected on a cultural as well as on a physiologic basis. The vaccines comprised of embryonic or other pregnancy-associated antigens must be rigorously tested for possible teratogenic or tumor-promoting side effects.

Reversibility may prove to be a major problem, especially with sperm vaccines, since intercourse would provide frequent antigen boosts of the immune response. Passive immunization with human monoclonal antibodies promises to be an effective and safe method for short-term (reversible) contraception and early pregnancy termination.

REFERENCES

1. Aitken, R. J., and Richardson, D. W. Immunization Against Zona Pellucida Antigens. In J. P. Hearn (ed.), *Immunological Aspects of Reproduction and Fertility Control.* Baltimore: University Park Press, 1980. Pp. 173–201.

2. Alexander, N. J. Sperm Antibodies and Infertility. In A. T. K. Cockett and R. L. Urry (eds.), *Male Infertility: Workup, Treatment, and Research.* New York: Grune & Stratton, 1977. Pp. 123–143.

3. Alexander, N. J., and Clarkson, T. B. Vasectomy increases the severity of diet-induced atherosclerosis in *Macaca fascicularis. Science* 201:538, 1978.

4. Alexander, N. J., Sampson, J. H., and Fulgham, D. L.

Pregnancy rates in patients treated for antisperm anti-bodies with prednisone. *Int. J. Fertil.* 28:63, 1983.

5. Allison, A. C. Mode of action of immunological adjuvants. *J. Reticuloendothel. Soc.* (Suppl. 26):619, 1979.

6. Anderson, D. J., et al. Spontaneous tumors in long-term-vasectomized mice: Increased incidence and association with antisperm immunity. *Am. J. Pathol.* 111:129, 1983.

7. Anderson, D. J., and Tarter, T. H. Immunosuppressive effects of mouse seminal plasma components in vivo and in vitro. *J. Immunol.* 128:535, 1982.

8. Artzt, K., et al. Surface antigens common to mouse cleavage embryos and primitive teratocarcinoma cells in culture. *Proc. Natl. Acad. Sci. U.S.A.* 70:2988, 1973.

9. Baker, T. G. Oogenesis and Ovulation. In C. R. Austin and R. V. Short (eds.), *Reproduction in Mammals, Book 1, Germ Cells and Fertilization* (2nd ed.). Cambridge: Cambridge University Press, 1982. Pp. 17–45.

10. Bambra, C. S., and Gombe, S. The role of placental gonadotropins (PMSG and hCG) in pregnancy in the rat. *J. Reprod. Fertil.* 53:109, 1978.

11. Barros, C., and Yanagimachi, R. Polyspermy-preventing mechanisms in the golden hamster egg. *J. Exp. Zool.* 180:251, 1972.

12. Beer, A. E., and Billingham, R. E. *The Immunobiology of Mammalian Reproduction.* Englewood Cliffs, N.J.: Prentice-Hall, 1976.

13. Beer, A. E., and Billingham, R. E. Immunoregulatory aspects of pregnancy. *Fed. Proc.* 37:2374, 1978.

14. Bleil, J. D., and Wassarman, P. M. Mammalian sperm-egg interaction: Identification of a glycoprotein in mouse egg zonae pellucidae possessing receptor activity for sperm. *Cell* 20:873, 1980.

15. Bleil, J. D., and Wassarman, P. M. Structure and function of the zona pellucida: Identification and characterization of the proteins of the mouse oocyte's zona pellucida. *Dev. Biol.* 76:185, 1980.

16. Boorstein, W. R., Vamvakopoulos, N. C., and Fiddes, J. C. Human chorionic gonadotropin β-subunit is encoded by at least eight genes arranged in tandem and inverted pairs. *Nature* 300:419, 1982.

17. Braunstein, G. D., et al. Ectopic production of human chorionic gonadotropin by neoplasms. *Ann. Intern. Med.* 78:39, 1973.

18. Braunstein, G. D., et al. Serum human chorionic gonadotropin levels throughout normal pregnancy. *Am. J. Obstet. Gynecol.* 126:678, 1976.

19. Buc-Caron, M.-H., et al. Presence of a mouse embryonic antigen on human spermatozoa. *Proc. Natl. Acad. Sci. U.S.A.* 71:1730, 1974.

20. Carelli, C., et al. Immunological castration of male mice by a totally synthetic vaccine administered in saline. *Proc. Natl. Acad. Sci. U.S.A.* 79:5392, 1982.

21. Clark, D. A., McDermott, M. R., and Szewczuk, M. R. Impairment of host-versus-graft reaction in pregnant mice: II. Selective suppression of cytotoxic T-cell generation correlates with soluble suppressor activity and with successful allogeneic pregnancy. *Cell. Immunol.* 52:106, 1980.

22. Clarkson, T. B., and Alexander, N. J. Long-term vasectomy: Effects on the occurrence and extent of atherosclerosis in rhesus monkeys. *J. Clin. Invest.* 65:15, 1980.

23. Curtis, G. L., and Ryan, W. L. Infertility in mice following gastrointestinal immunization with spermatozoa. *IRCS Medical Science: Biochemistry* 10:202, 1982.

24. Das, C., et al. Discriminatory effect of anti-Pr-β-hCG TT antibodies on the neutralization of the biological activity of placental and pituitary gonadotropins. *Contraception* 18:35, 1978.

25. Dietl, J., Knop, G., and Mettler, L. The frequency of serological anti–zona pellucida activity in males, females and children. *J. Reprod. Immunol.* 4:123, 1982.

26. Dunbar, B. S. Morphological, Biochemical and Immunochemical Characterization of the Mammalian Zona Pellucida. In J. Hartmann (ed.), *Mechanism and Control of Fertilization.* New York: Academic, 1984.

27. Dunbar, B. S. Personal communication.

28. Dunbar, B. S., Liu, C., and Sammons, D. W. Identification of the three major proteins of porcine and rabbit zonae pellucidae by high resolution two-dimensional gel electrophoresis: Comparison with serum, follicular fluid, and ovarian cell proteins. *Biol. Reprod.* 24:1111, 1981.

29. Dunbar, B. S., and Raynor, B. D. Isolation and characterization of porcine zona pellucida antigens. *Fed. Proc.* 38:466, 1979.

30. Dunbar, B. S., Wardrip, N. J., and Hedrick, J. L. Isolation, physiochemical properties, and the macromolecular composition of the zona pellucida from porcine oocytes. *Biochemistry* 19:356, 1980.

31. Dym, M. The fine structure of the monkey (*Macaca*) Sertoli cell and its role in maintaining the blood-testis barrier. *Anat. Rec.* 175:639, 1973.

32. Fraser, H. M. Inhibition of Reproductive Function by Antibodies to Luteinizing Hormone Releasing Hormone. In J. P. Hearn (ed.), *Immunological Aspects of Reproduction and Fertility Control.* Baltimore: University Park, 1980. Pp. 143–171.

33. Goldberg, E. Amino acid composition and properties of crystalline lactate dehydrogenase-X from mouse testes. *J. Biol. Chem.* 247:2044, 1972.

34. Goldberg, E. Infertility in female rabbits immunized with lactate dehydrogenase X. *Science* 181:458, 1973.

35. Goldberg, E. Effects of immunization with LDH-X on fertility. *Acta Endocrinol.* [Suppl.] (Copenh.) 78(194):202, 1975.

36. Goldberg, E. Personal communication.

37. Goldberg, E., et al. Reduction of fertility in female baboons immunized with lactate dehydrogenase C_4. *Fertil. Steril.* 35:214, 1981.

38. Goldman-Leikin, R. E., and Goldberg, E. Characterization of monoclonal antibodies to the sperm-specific lac-

tate dehydrogenase isozyme. *Proc. Natl. Acad. Sci. U.S.A.* 80:3774, 1983.

39. Gonzales-Prevatt, V., Wheat, T. E., and Goldberg, E. Identification of an antigenic determinant of mouse lactate dehydrogenase C_4. *Mol. Immunol.* 19:1579, 1982.

40. Gooi, H. C., et al. Stage-specific embryonic antigen involves $\alpha 1 \rightarrow 3$ fucosylated type 2 blood group chains. *Nature* 292:156, 1981.

41. Gupta, S. K., Ramakrishnan, S., and Talwar, G. P. Properties and characteristics of an anti-human chorionic gonadotropin monoclonal antibody. *J. Biosci.* 4:105, 1982.

42. Gwatkin, R. B. L. Studies on the zona pellucida of the mouse egg. *J. Reprod. Fertil.* 6:325, 1963.

43. Gwatkin, R. B. L., et al. The zona reaction of hamster and mouse eggs: Production in vitro by a trypsin-like protease from cortical granules. *J. Reprod. Fertil.* 32:259, 1973.

44. Gwatkin, R. B. L., Williams, D. T., and Carlo, D. J. Immunization of mice with heat-solubilized hamster zonae: Production of anti-zona antibody and inhibition of fertility. *Fertil. Steril.* 28:871, 1977.

45. Gwatkin, R. B. L., Williams, D. T., and Meyenhofer, M. Isolation of bovine zonae pellucidae from ovaries with collagenase: Antigenic and sperm receptor properties. *Gamete Res.* 2:187, 1979.

46. Hamilton, D. W. Structure and Function of the Epithelium Lining the Ductuli Efferentes, Ductus Epididymidis, and Ductus Deferens in the rat. S. R. Geiger (executive ed.), *Handbook of Physiology, Section 7, Endocrinology, Vol. V, Male Reproductive System*. Washington, D.C.: American Physiological Society, 1975. Pp. 259–301.

47. Hamilton, M. S., and Anderson, D. J. Antibodies to antigens on teratocarcinoma cells are associated with parity in mice. *Biol. Reprod.* 27:104, 1982.

48. Hearn, J. P. Long Term Suppression of Fertility by Immunization with hCG-β Subunit and its Reversibility in Female Marmoset Monkeys. In G. P. Talwar (ed.), *Recent Advances in Reproduction and Regulation of Fertility*. Amsterdam: Elsevier, 1979.

49. Hendry, W. F., et al. Steroid treatment of male subfertility caused by antisperm antibodies. *Lancet* 2:498, 1979.

50. Hurtenbach, U., Morgenstern, F., and Bennett, D. Induction of tolerance in vitro by autologous murine testicular cells. *J. Exp. Med.* 151:827, 1980.

51. Ingerslev, H. J. Antibodies against spermatozoal surface-membrane antigens in female infertility. *Acta Obstet. Gynecol. Scand.* (Suppl. 100):1, 1981.

52. Isojima, S., Li, T. S., and Ashitaka, Y. Immunologic analysis of sperm-immobilizing factor found in sera of women with unexplained sterility. *Am. J. Obstet. Gynecol.* 101:677, 1968.

53. Jacob, F. Mouse teratocarcinoma and embryonic antigens. *Immunol. Rev.* 33:3, 1977.

54. Kaplan, H. S., Olsson, L., and Raubitschek, A. Monoclonal Human Antibodies: A Recent Development with Wide-Ranging Clinical Potential. In A. J. McMichael and

J. W. Fabre (eds.), *Monoclonal Antibodies in Clinical Medicine*. New York: Academic, 1982. Pp. 17–35.

55. Kaushansky, A., et al. Endocrine and reproductive repercussions of immunization against progesterone and oestradiol in female rats. *Acta Endocrinol.* 84:795, 1977.

56. Kemler, R., et al. Surface antigen in early differentiation. *Proc. Natl. Acad. Sci. U.S.A.* 74:4449, 1977.

57. Kille, J. W., and Goldberg, E. Female reproductive tract immunoglobulin responses to a purified sperm specific antigen [LDH-C_4]. *Biol. Reprod.* 20:863, 1979.

58. Kille, J. W., and Goldberg, E. Inhibition of oviducal sperm transport in rabbits immunized against sperm-specific lactate dehydrogenase (LDH-C_4). *J. Reprod. Immunol.* 2:15, 1980.

59. Laffont, A. S., and Théron, G. Trois cas de stérilisation biologique temporaire. *Bull. Soc. Obstet. Gynecol.* (Paris) 23:207, 1934.

60. Linnet, L., Hjort, T., and Fogh-Andersen, P. Association between failure to impregnate after vasovasostomy and sperm agglutinins in semen. *Lancet* 1:117, 1981.

61. Lord, E. M., Sensabaugh, G. F., and Stites, D. P. Immunosuppressive activity of human seminal plasma: I. Inhibition of in vitro lymphocyte activation. *J. Immunol.* 118:1704, 1977.

62. McCormick, J. N., et al. Immunohistological and elution studies of the human placenta. *J. Exp. Med.* 133:1, 1971.

63. Mintz, B. Experimental study of the developing mammalian egg. *Science* 138:594, 1962.

64. Modlinski, J. A. The role of zona pellucida in the development of mouse eggs in vivo. *J. Embryol. Exp. Morphol.* 23:539, 1970.

65. Moghissi, K. S. Human fallopian tube fluid: I. Protein composition. *Fertil. Steril.* 21:821, 1970.

66. Morgan, F. J., Birken, S., and Canfield, R. E. Human chorionic gonadotropin: A proposal for the amino acid sequence. *Mol. Cell. Biochem.* 2:97, 1973.

67. Mukherjee, A. B., Ulane, R. E., and Agrawal, A. K. Role of uteroglobin and transglutaminase in masking the antigenicity of implanting rabbit embryos. *Am. J. Reprod. Immunol.* 2:135, 1982.

68. Murdoch, A. J. M., Buckley, C. H., and Fox, H. Hormonal control of the secretory immune system of the human uterine cervix. *J. Reprod. Immunol.* 4:23, 1982.

69. Nash, H., et al. Observations on the antigenicity and clinical effects of a candidate antipregnancy vaccine: β-Subunit of human chorionic gonadotropin linked to tetanus toxoid. *Fertil. Steril.* 34:328, 1980.

70. Newport, A., and Carroll, J. Structure and composition of the zona pellucida of the mouse oocyte. *Biochem. Soc. Trans.* 4:896, 1976.

71. Nieschlag, E., and Wickings, E. J. Immunological neutralization of FSH as an approach to male fertility control. *Int. J. Androl.* 5:18, 1982.

72. Nymand, G., et al. Occurrence of cytotoxic antibodies during pregnancy. *Vox Sang.* 21:21, 1971.

73. Oikawa, T., and Yanagimachi, R. Block of hamster fertilization by anti-ovary antibody. *J. Reprod. Fertil.* 45:487, 1975.

74. Powell, J. E., et al. Characteristics of antibodies raised to carboxy-terminal peptides of hCG beta subunit. *J. Reprod. Immunol.* 2:1, 1980.

75. Ross, M. H. The Sertoli cell and the blood-testicular barrier: An electronmicroscopic study. *Adv. Androl.* 1:83, 1970.

76. Rümke, P. The origin of immunoglobulins in semen. *Clin. Exp. Immunol.* 17:287, 1974.

77. Rümke, P., et al. Prognosis of fertility of men with sperm agglutinins in the serum. *Fertil. Steril.* 25:393, 1974.

78. Sacco, A. G. Inhibition of fertility in mice by passive immunization with antibodies to isolated zonae pellucidae. *J. Reprod. Fertil.* 56:533, 1979.

79. Sacco, A. G. Immunocontraception: Consideration of the zona pellucida as a target antigen. *Obstet. Gynecol. Annu.* 10:1, 1981.

80. Sacco, A. G., and Moghissi, K. S. Antizona pellucida activity in human sera. *Fertil. Steril.* 31:503, 1978.

81. Sathananthan, A. H., et al. Ultrastructural observations on the penetration of human sperm into the zona pellucida of the human egg in vitro. *J. Androl.* 3:356, 1982.

82. Saxena, B. B., et al. Radioreceptor assay of human chorionic gonadotropin: Detection of early pregnancy. *Science* 184:793, 1974.

83. Schiff, G. M. Active immunizations for adults. *Annu. Rev. Med.* 31:441, 1980.

84. Schumacher, G. F. B. Soluble Proteins of Human Cervical Mucus. In M. Elstein, K. S. Moghissi, and R. Borth (eds.), *Cervical Mucus in Human Reproduction*. Copenhagen: Scriptor, 1973. Pp. 93–113.

85. Shahani, S. M., et al. Clinical and immunological responses with Pr-β-hCG-TT vaccine. *Contraception* 25:421, 1982.

86. Shastri, N., et al. Differential affinity of anti-Pr-β-hCG-TT antibodies for hCG and hLH. *Contraception* 18:23, 1978.

87. Shivers, C. A., and Dunbar, B. S. Autoantibodies to zona pellucida: A possible cause for infertility in women. *Science* 197:1082, 1977.

88. Shoenfeld, Y., et al. Production of autoantibodies by human-human hybridomas. *J. Clin. Invest.* 70:205, 1982.

89. Stevens, V. C. The Current Status of Anti-Pregnancy Vaccines Based on Synthetic Fractions of hCG. In J. P. Hearn (ed.), *Immunological Aspects of Reproduction and Fertility Control*. Baltimore: University Park Press, 1980. Pp. 203–216.

90. Stevens, V. C. Vaccines Against Pregnancy. In C. C. Fen, D. Griffin, and A. Woolman (eds.), *Recent Advances in Fertility Regulation*. Geneva: Atar S. A., 1981. Pp. 211–227.

91. Stevens, V. C. Personal communication.

92. Stevens, V. C., et al. Preparation and formulation of a human chorionic gonadotropin antifertility vaccine: Selection of adjuvant and vehicle. *Am. J. Reprod. Immunol.* 1:315, 1981.

93. Stevens, V. C., et al. Preparation and formulation of a human chorionic gonadotropin antifertility vaccine: Selection of a peptide immunogen. *Am. J. Reprod. Immunol.* 1:307, 1981.

94. Stevens, V. C., and Crystle, C. D. Effects of immunization with hapten-coupled hCG on the human menstrual cycle. *Obstet. Gynecol.* 42:485, 1973.

95. Stites, D. P., and Erickson, R. P. Suppressive effect of seminal plasma on lymphocyte activation. *Nature* 253:727, 1975.

96. Stolp, W., et al. Occurrence of HL-A-antibodies in sera of sterile women. *Int. J. Fertil.* 18:141, 1973.

97. Strober, W., Richman, L. K., and Elson, C. O. The regulation of gastrointestinal immune responses. *Immunol. Today* 2:156, 1981.

98. Szollosi, D. Development of cortical granules and the cortical reaction in rat and hamster eggs. *Anat. Rec.* 159:431, 1967.

99. Talwar, G. P. Anti-hCG immunization. *Contraception* 18:19, 1978.

100. Talwar, G. P., et al. Immunization Against hCG: Efficacy and Teratological Studies in Baboons. In T. C. Anand Kumar (ed.), *Non-Human Primate Models for Study of Human Reproduction*. Basel: Karger, 1980. Pp. 190–201.

101. Talwar, G. P., Gupta, S. K., and Tandon, A. K. Immunologic Interruption of Pregnancy. In N. Gleicher (ed.), *Reproductive Immunology*. New York: Alan R. Liss, 1981. Pp. 451–459.

102. Tsunoda, Y., and Chang, M. C. Effect of anti–rat ovary antiserum on the fertilization of rat, mouse and hamster eggs in vivo and in vitro. *Biol. Reprod.* 14:354, 1976.

103. Tsunoda, Y., and Chang, M. C. The effect of passive immunization with hetero and isoimmune anti-ovary antiserum on the fertilization of mouse, rat and hamster eggs. *Biol. Reprod.* 15:361, 1976.

104. Tsunoda, Y., Soma, T., and Sugie, T. Inhibition of fertilization in cattle by passive immunization with anti–zona pellucida serum. *Gamete Res.* 4:133, 1981.

105. Tsunoda, Y., and Sugie, T. Effect of antibody to detergent solubilized zonae pellucidae on in vivo and in vitro fertilization in the mouse. *Gamete Res.* 6:73, 1982.

106. Tung, K. S. K. Antifertility vaccines: Considerations of their potential immunopathologic complications. *Int. J. Fertil.* 21:197, 1976.

107. Tung, K. S. K., and Alexander, N. J. Autoimmune Reactions in the Testis. In A. D. Johnson and W. R. Gomes (eds.), *The Testis*. New York: Academic, 1977. Vol. 4., pp. 491–516.

108. Twining, S. S., and Atassi, M. Z. Antibody-combining sites can be mimicked synthetically. Surface-simulation synthesis of the immunoglobulin new combining site to the gamma-hydroxyl derivative of vitamin K_1. *J. Biol. Chem.* 253:5259, 1978.

109. Vaerman, J.-P., and Férin, J. Local immunological response in the vagina, cervix and endometrium. *Acta Endocrinol.* [Suppl.] (Copenh.) 78(194):281, 1975.

110. Vaitukaitis, J. L. Immunologic and physical characterization of human chorionic gonadotropin (hCG) secreted by tumours. *J. Clin. Endocrinol. Metabol.* 37:505, 1973.

111. Vickery, B. H., McRae, G. I., and Stevens, V. C. Suppression of luteal and placental function in pregnant baboons with agonist analogs of luteinizing hormone–releasing hormones. *Fertil. Steril.* 36:664, 1981.

112. Walker, W. A., and Isselbacher, K. J. Intestinal antibodies. *N. Engl. J. Med.* 297:767, 1977.

113. Wassarman, P. M., Florman, H. M., and Greve, J. M. Receptor Mediated Sperm-Egg Interactions in Mammals. In C. B. Metz and A. Monroy (eds.), *Biology of Fertilization.* New York: Academic. In press, 1984.

114. Wegmann, T. G., et al. The ability of the murine placenta to absorb monoclonal anti–fetal H-2K antibody from the maternal circulation. *J. Immunol.* 123:1020, 1979.

115. Wheat, T. E., and Goldberg, E. Immunologically Active Peptide Fragments of the Sperm-Specific Lactate Dehydrogenase C$_4$ Isozyme. In D. H. Rich and E. Gross (eds.), *Peptides: Synthesis—Structure—Function.* Pierce Chemical Company, 1981. Pp. 557–560.

116. Wira, C. R., and Sandoe, C. P. Hormonal regulation of immunoglobulins: Influence of estradiol on immunoglobulins A and G in the rat uterus. *Endocrinology* 106:1020, 1980.

117. Wolf, D. P., and Hamada, M. Induction of zonal and egg plasma membrane blocks to sperm penetration in mouse eggs with cortical granule exudate. *Biol. Reprod.* 17:350, 1977.

118. Wood, D. M., Liu, C., and Dunbar, B. S. Effect of alloimmunization and heteroimmunization with zonae pellucidae on fertility in rabbits. *Biol. Reprod.* 25:439, 1981.

119. Yanagimachi, R., Winkelhake, J., and Nicolson, G. L. Immunological block to mammalian fertilization: Survival and organ distribution of immunoglobulin which inhibits fertilization in vivo. *Proc. Natl. Acad. Sci. U.S.A.* 73:2405, 1976.

Index

Index